CT Virtual Hysterosalpingography

Patricia Carrascosa • Carlos Capuñay
Carlos E. Sueldo • Juan Mariano Baronio

CT Virtual Hysterosalpingography

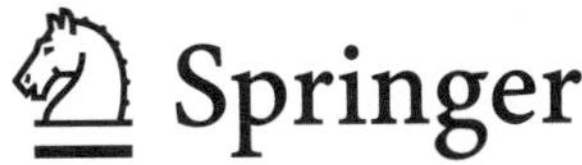 Springer

Patricia Carrascosa, MD, PhD
Diagnóstico Maipú
Buenos Aires
Argentina

Carlos Capuñay, MD
Diagnóstico Maipú
Buenos Aires
Argentina

Carlos E. Sueldo, MD
University of California
San Francisco, CA
USA

Juan Mariano Baronio, MD
CEGYR
Buenos Aires
Argentina

ISBN 978-3-319-35541-2   ISBN 978-3-319-07560-0   (eBook)
DOI 10.1007/978-3-319-07560-0
Springer Cham Heidelberg New York Dordrecht London

Prologue

It is with great pleasure that I introduce this book on virtual hysterosalpingography. Virtual hysterosalpingography (VHSG) is a new non-invasive diagnostic technique that allows the evaluation of the entire gynecologic tract in a single study, by combining the benefits of hysterosapingography with multidetector computer tomography (CT). The advantages of this imaging modality are that the addition of the CT allows an amazing 3-D visualization of the uterine cavity, fallopian tubes, and extrauterine structures, very helpful in the diagnosis of polyps, myomas, uterine anomalies, and tubal pathology with a high degree of accuracy. The images represent what a surgeon would see in the OR and are an invaluable preoperative test. The procedure is simple, quick, and fairly painless and provides maximum imaging of the reproductive organs of the patient.

This book is laid out in a very logical sequence, starting with general information about virtual hysterosalpingography, followed by a description of the technique in detecting pathology of the cervix, uterine cavity, congenital uterine abnormalities, and tubal pathology. The third section covers limitations and diagnostic errors. This book is very practical and filled with beautiful images.

The book is written and edited by the leaders in the field. The editors have vast experience with this new technology, and have performed the largest volume of cases. We congratulate the editors on this excellent contribution to the field of reproductive imaging with this comprehensive review of this new technology. This will be an essential addition to radiologists, reproductive endocrinologists, and gynecologists who would want to learn about or gain experience with this new imaging technique.

Laurel Stadtmauer, MD, PhD
Jones Institute for Reproductive Medicine at Eastern Virginia Medical School,
Norfolk, VA, USA

Acknowledgement

The authors kindly thank Dr. Graciela Fernández Alonso for her dedicated reading of the manuscript, Nicolás Page for the translation assistance and Daniel Cirigliano for the illustration work. And Diagnóstico Maipú that made the realization of this production a possibility.

Contents

Contributors

Graciela Fernández Alonso, MD, PhD Department of Pathology and High Complexity Laboratory, Diagnóstico Maipú, Buenos Aires, Argentina

Juan Mariano Baronio, MD Department of Fertility, CEGYR, Buenos Aires, Argentina

Carlos Capuñay, MD Departments of Computed Tomography and Magnetic Resonance, Diagnóstico Maipú, Buenos Aires, Argentina

Patricia Carrascosa, MD, PhD Department of Computed Tomography and Magnetic Resonance, Diagnóstico Maipú, Buenos Aires, Argentina

Carlos E. Sueldo, MD Department of Obstetrics and Gynecology, University of California, San Francisco, CA, USA

Javier Vallejos, MD Departments of Computed Tomography and Magnetic Resonance, Diagnóstico Maipú, Buenos Aires, Argentina

Ana Vasconcelos, MD Departments of Computed Tomography and Magnetic Resonance, Diagnóstico Maipú, Buenos Aires, Argentina

Part I

Generalities of Virtual Hysterosalpingography

Technical Aspects of Multislice Computed Tomography

Computed tomography (CT) is the imaging diagnosis method of high complexity most used in clinical practice. It was born in the 70s by the hand of English engineer Sir Godfrey N. Hounsfield [1–3] and has been subject to, over the past four decades, numerous technological changes, transforming into, today, the pillar of all imaging methods utilized in the study of patients with tumors located outside of the central nervous system. The development of the helical (spiral) or volume CT in the early 90s, and the incorporation of the multislice technology at the end of this decade, generated a great impact on the diagnostic capability of the technique [4–10]. The medical community disposes of a variety of non-invasive CT studies that over time have modified the traditional prevention and treatment algorithms. Among them, the angiographies in diverse vascular territories, including the coronary arteries and the pulmonary venous mapping in patients with refractory atrial fibrillation who are candidates for a radiofrequency ablation, or the CT brain perfusion on patients with acute cerebral ischemia. A separate group of studies is one that includes those that utilize virtual imaging reprocessing, highlighting the virtual colonoscopy, a diagnosis procedure that, for the past 15 years, has managed to earn a place in screening for colorectal cancer, as well as the recently developed virtual hysterosalpingography technique.

It is important to make emphasis on the fact that the excellent performance and current role of CT in the decision-making of a diversity of different clinical entities is due to the arrival of the new multidetector row units, which supply an excellent space-time resolution, and in this way, optimize the use of intravenous contrast substances and, with the incorporation of innovative techniques in the processing of raw data, achieve a significant reduction in the radiation dose to which patients are exposed to on a daily basis [11–17].

Before delving into the concepts of this new generation of CT scanners, a brief description of its technique and evolution from its origins will take place.

Basic Concepts

The CT equipment is used to obtain axial (transversal) images on the axis of the human body, basing its operation on the measurement of attenuation that the X-rays beam undergoes in each voxel when crossing the different anatomical structures of the region subject to study. This absorption of the ionizing radiation is established by the lineal coefficient particular to each matter or substance that is pierced by the X-rays beam. The final product is a matrix of numbers, to each of which is assigned a shade of gray to produce the typical CT image. The Hounsfield units are universally used in the scale, in which water is assigned the value 0, and air −1,000.

Components of a CT Scanner

Gantry

Based on the introduction of slip ring technology, continuous rotation of the X-ray tube and the detector became possible. Larger volume coverage in shorter scan times and improved longitudinal resolution became feasible after the introduction of multislice CT systems in 1998. The gantry constitutes the frame on which the following are assembled (Fig. 1.1): the X-ray tube, the crown of detectors, the high voltage generator and the data measurement system. In these third-generation CT scanners, the X-ray tube and detector are built onto a rotation system that rotates around the patient, covering a scan field of view of 50 cm. The main challenge is the stability of both focal spot and detector position during rotation, in particular with regard to the high rotational speeds (0.20 s) and gravitational forces of latest CT systems. Also in the gantry are assembled the cooling system, the position and speed censors, the hydraulic apparatus for the inclination of the gantry, the system used for the ascent, descent, and braking of the CT table, and finally the microphones and loudspeakers used for intercommunication with the patient.

P. Carrascosa et al., *CT Virtual Hysterosalpingography*,
DOI 10.1007/978-3-319-07560-0_1, © Springer International Publishing Switzerland 2014

X-Rays Generating System

Collimator and X-Rays Tube

The tube is the vacuum device that generates the X-rays beam. A state-of-the-art X-ray tube provides a peak power of 70 kW at various voltages (80 kV, 100 kV, 120 kV, 140 kV). It is formed, on one end, by the cathode (tungsten filament), which when circulating an electrical current, and turned incandescent, generates a flow of electrons towards the anode where they impact. When the electrons, which posses a great kinetic energy, hit the anode, they transfer all their energy, which converts mostly into heat (99 %), and 1 % into X-rays. The size of the anode plate determines the heat storage capacity and the performance level of the tube/generator unit. In the present, fast anode cooling (e.g. the rotating envelope tube design) and high power scans in rapid succession can be performed.

The surface on which said impact takes place is called the focal spot, and its characteristics will depend on the generated X-rays beam's quality. An image with great detail is obtained with a small focal spot. The X-rays tube is encapsulated in a metal or glass structure, surrounded by a shield (dome) which offers protection against secondary radiation (Fig. 1.2).

Generator

The high-tension generator is the power circuit that supplies the X-rays tube with the correct voltage for its operation. In other words, it provides the necessary current to heat the cathode filament, as well as to accelerate the electrons. The sharpness and contrast of the CT image taken is highly influenced by the generator's characteristics. They can be of high or low frequency, continuous or pulsating. Currently, the system most used is the continuous emission one that transforms the web tension into a continuous tension, and then transmits it to a converter that transforms it into a squared pulse beam with a frequency of 15 kHz, with a pulse width that will depend on the kilovoltage, on the miliamperage and on the exposure time chosen.

Detection System

Detectors

In general, CT systems use solid state detectors. Each detector element consists of a radiation-sensitive solid-state material, which converts the absorbed X-rays into visible light. This

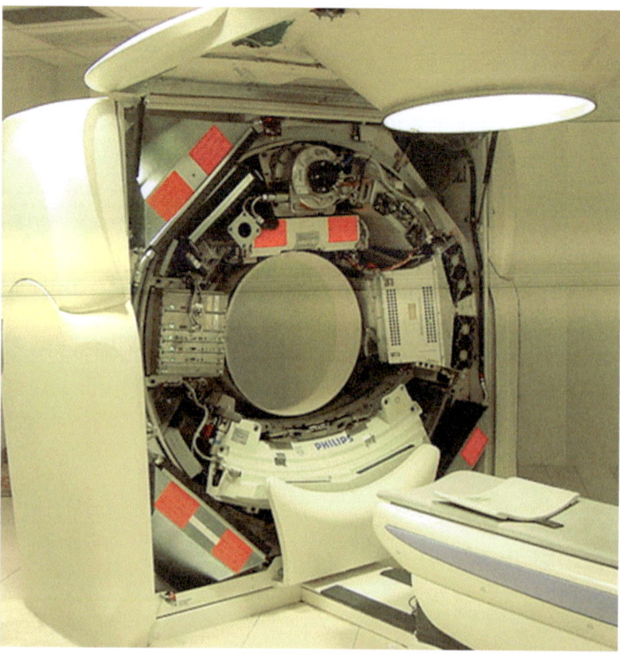

Fig. 1.1 Photo of gantry of a third generation MSCT scanner

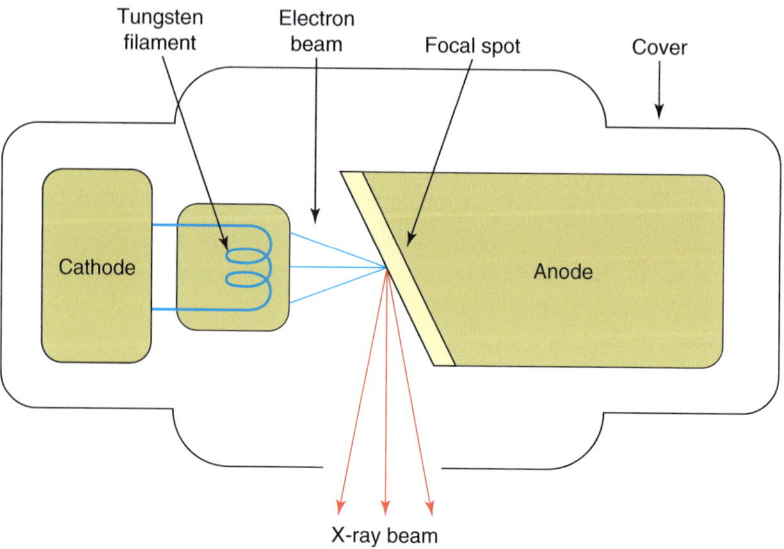

Fig. 1.2 Layout of an X-ray tube

light is detected by a photodiode and the electrical current is amplified and converted into a digital signal, which then will be used in the imaging reconstruction process. These devices measure the quantity of photons that pass through the section of study, the signal received being proportional to the density of the elements that constitute the object of study. The structure of the detectors is alternating. Their composure, size and design shift constantly so as to find a fast response speed to the variations in radiation. They must be stable, with an ample dynamic range, little dependence on temperature, and low decay times. There are three classes of detectors: (i) with photomultipliers; (ii) with semiconducting photodiodes; (iii) and with pressurized Xenon gas chambers (Fig. 1.3).

Data Measurement Unit

It constitutes the link between the detectors and the processing and storage of data system. This unit integrates the electrical signals received from the detectors, amplifies, and sends them in the form of numbers, using a binary code, to the computer. It generates a digital and analogical conversion. The stream of data generated by the current CT systems is a challenge for data transmission off the gantry and for real-time data processing in the subsequent image reconstruction systems.

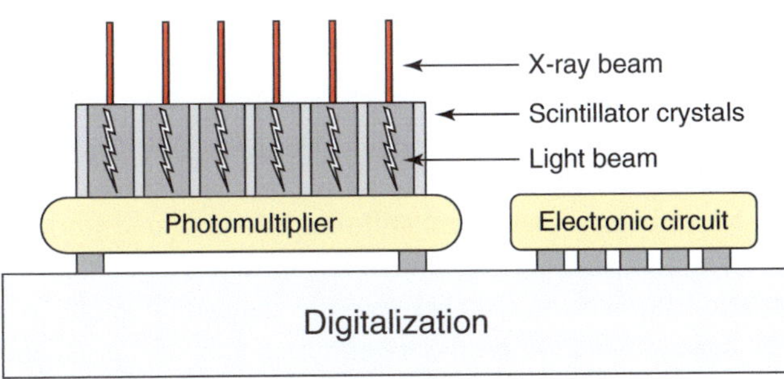

Fig. 1.3 Diagram of a CT detector

Data Management Console

Imaging Processing and Reconstruction

The traditional CT image formation process belongs to the first generation of imaging reconstruction methods and is called filtered back-projection. This algorithm is characterized for its speed in deteriorating the high noise in the image, which is accomplished with the use of filters (Kernels) and an exposure to a higher radiation dose. A diversity of image reconstruction algorithms have been created to obtain, today, images with a diagnostic quality that upholds three premises: prevention of artifact; preservation of natural appearance; improvement in the image quality. The result today is the fourth generation of imaging reconstruction methods, denominated advanced iterative reconstruction (Fig. 1.4). Taking into account these premises, this new technique in reconstruction prevents the generation of lineal artifacts before the creation of the image, maintaining an adequate texture. The artificial appearance the image used to have is overcome by utilizing the previous generations of iterative reconstruction. With this algorithm, it is possible to enhance the image's quality and/or reduce the radiation dose levels beyond those used in conventional reconstructions of filtered back-projection by 80 %, maintaining an image with diagnostic quality [18].

Types of Computed Tomography

Conventional CT

In the early 70s, Electrical and Musical Industries Ltd. (EMI), a company based in London, built the first conventional CT scanner, designed to obtain images of the head. Its prototype was installed in the Atkinson Morley's Hospital,

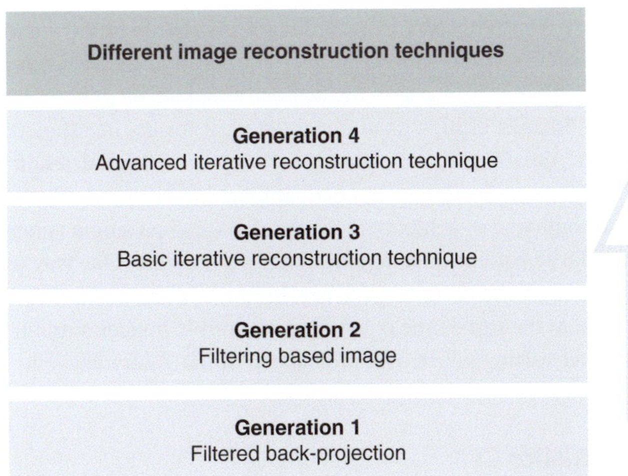

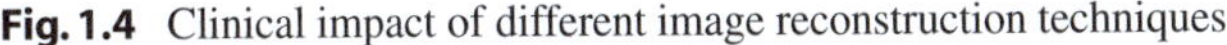

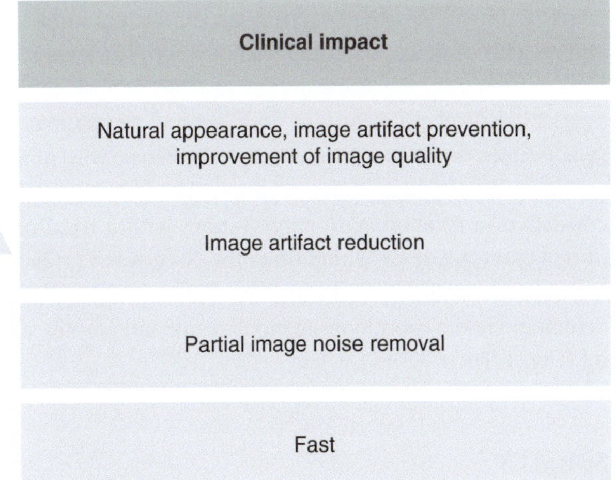

Fig. 1.4 Clinical impact of different image reconstruction techniques

also in London, where on October 1st 1971 the first tomographic image with clinical ends was taken on a patient with suspicions of a frontal tumor [1, 2]. The EMI Mk1 took between 4.5 and 20 min to take each image, with a matrix of 80×80 pixels and a 3 mm $\times$ 3 mm $\times$ 13 mm voxel size. The processing of the images obtained during the day was carried out in the same factory during the night. This stage took approximately 20 min per image, which were returned to the center in the morning. Modifications in the image's reconstruction algorithms and a rise in the number of detectors per slice permitted its successor, the CT1010, achieve images with a matrix of 160×160 or 320×320 pixels, on a field of vision of 210 mm and with an acquisition time of 1 min. The first images of the abdomen obtained on a prototype machine dedicated to body tomography, the CT5000, were achieved only in December of 1974, and Hounsfield himself joined the research team. This CT scanner generated an image with a matrix of 320×320 pixels in barely 20 s, and a field of vision of 240, 320, and 400 mm [3].

CT scanners from the first and second generations utilized a translation/rotation technology. In the first generation, a thick, collimated pencil X-ray beam faced a detector. Both were then moved covering the object of study, rotated 1°, and moved again and so on until covering a rotation of 180°. During the translation, X-rays are emitted and the data is collected. The resolution of the resulting image is low and the acquisition time very prolonged. In the second generation, the principle to achieve the image is similar; the difference lies in a wider X-rays beam, with a coverage angle of 5°, and a variable number of detectors. This modification permits the acquisition time of data to diminish to a couple of minutes. Another inconvenience with these devices was the instability of the detector, a sodium iodide crystal, and the need to calibrate at the end of each translation, which limited the scanning speed. The CT scanners of third and fourth generation appeared in 1976. The third generation systems are based on a rotation/rotation system, an X-rays beam with a wide coverage width of 30–60°, covering the entire region of study and an arch of detectors composed of multiple elements [3]. In these devices, the X-rays tube and the line of detectors assembled on the gantry turn 360° around the patient. The sweep times are reduced to less than 5 s, along with a better, and less wasteful, use of the radiation. The fourth generation consists of a rotation/stationary system, with a fixed crown of detectors inside of which turns the X-rays tube, reaching high speeds, and thus reducing the scanning time. Plus, the detectors yield a more homogenous result and greater stability (Fig. 1.5).

early 90s. This innovative system of volumetric image acquisition without a doubt constituted the fundamental base for future developments, and put the spotlight on a completely unknown spectrum of new diagnostic applications that generated a rebirth of the method, overshadowed slightly by the growth that magnetic resonance imaging began having around those years [19–24].

Taking into account the better temporal resolution, the image acquisition time lower than 1 s and the possibility of obtaining volumetric information of a certain region, allowed the spiral CT the chance of achieving, for the first time, a volume data without the danger of miss- or double-registration of anatomical details. These third generation CT scanners utilize a slip-ring technology to transmit electrical power for its functioning, disposing of the need for cables in the assembly of the gantry, and are able to achieve a volumetric acquisition of continuous images due to the constant spin of the X-rays tube and the detector system, mounted onto a rotating gantry. The temporal resolution is increased, with acquisition times below 1 s [25–27].

In parallel to the described technological development, an informatics advance of similar magnitude happened, with the appearance of workstations: specially created computers with programmes that offer diverse imaging post-processing techniques to visualize and analyze CT images, such as the multiplanar reformations, the maximum and minimum intensity projections, the three-dimensional surface shaded displays, the volume rendering techniques, and the virtual endoscopy images [28–30].

Nevertheless, there were still things to continue working on. The fundamental problem of the spiral CT is the inverse relationship which exists between the acquisition length and the space resolution on the longitudinal axis of the patient. The smallest unit that constitutes the CT image is the voxel. Isotropic images are those which are constituted by voxels, whose x, y and z axis are equal; this is a cubical or isotropic voxel [10]. In the spiral CT, images are constituted by voxels whose length in the x axis are longer in relation to the x and y axis (Fig. 1.6). Although this configuration yields a very good space resolution on the acquisition plane by generating axial images of high anatomical detail, it results insufficient in the creation of multiplanar or three-dimensional reconstructions with a high diagnostic impact. In the spiral CT era, the challenge of achieving isotropic images in a single apnea and large volume coverage were not yet possible. One way to increment the longitudinal resolution and obtain a cubic voxel at the same time is to acquire multiple images simultaneously, using a faster rotation speed of the gantry as well.

Spiral CT

One of the most transcendent and important feats in CT history was the introduction of the spiral (helical) CT in the

Multislice CT

Based on this premise, a new line of CT scanners with a tray of 4 rows of detectors burst into the radiologic world in

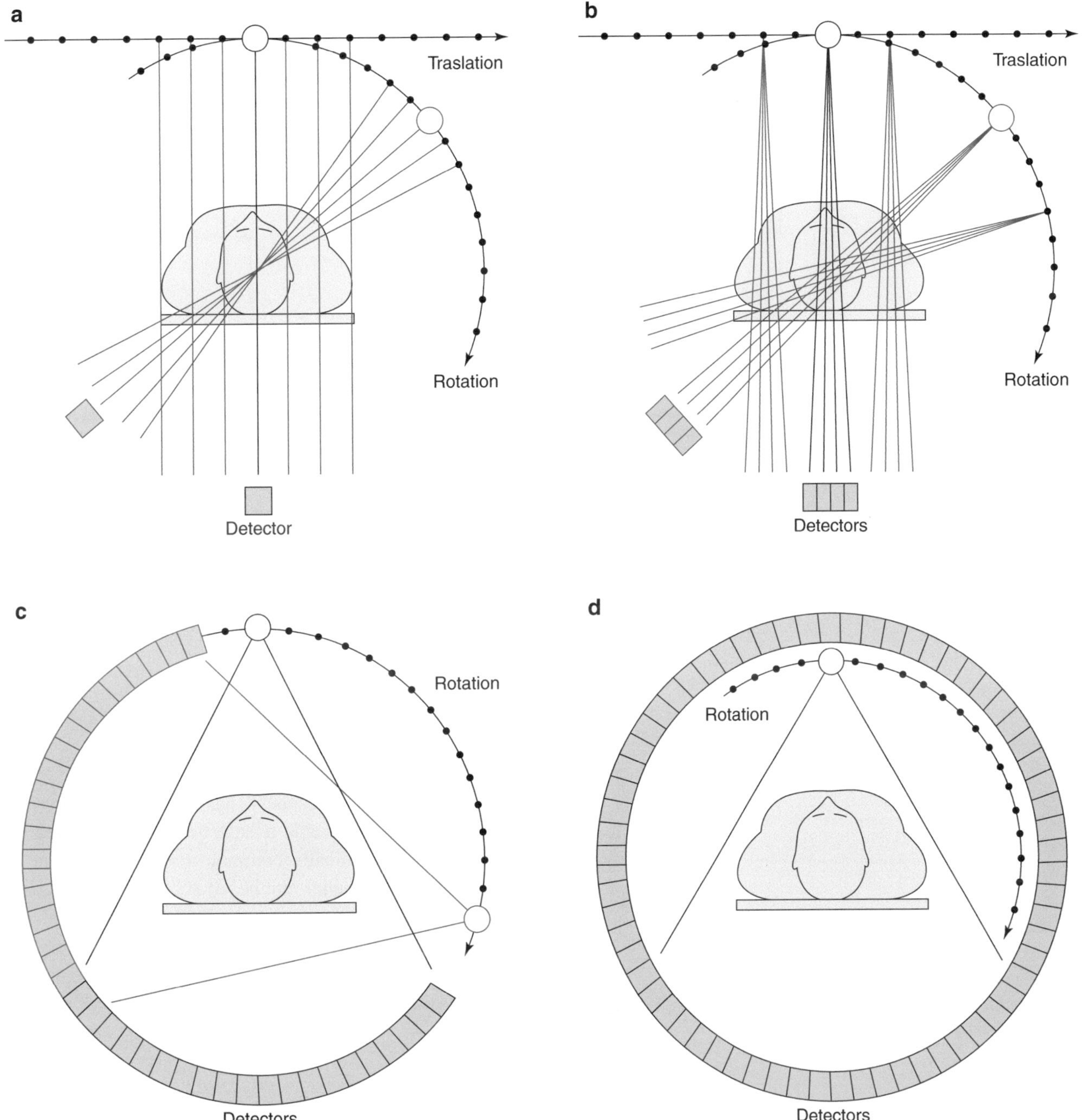

Fig. 1.5 CT systems. (**a**) First generation. (**b**) Second generation. (**c**) Third generation. (**d**) Fourth generation

1998. To count with more than one row of detectors in the direction of the scan allows the obtaining of, for each turn the X-rays tube and the detectors give around the patient, as many images as there are rows of detectors. The era of the multislice CT (MSCT), also called multidetector CT [5, 6, 31–34], is born. Depending on the configuration of the tray of detectors, the number of rows of detectors can vary between 4 and 320, the latter ones reaching only one rotation up to a length of 16 cm on the z axis [35–37]. The gantry rotation speed occupies the same important status, variable

between different machines from 200 to 500 ms. The conjunction between a high space and time resolution allows the achievement of a volumetric acquisition of continuous submillimetric (0.3–0.6 mm) images constituted of isotropic voxels, covering an extended area of the z axis in a matter of seconds [31–33].

The MSCT offers a wide range of acquisition protocols due to a great amount of parameters to take into account when programming a study (type of scan; type of collimation; pitch; gantry rotation speed; amongst the most important)

Fig. 1.6 CT voxel configuration

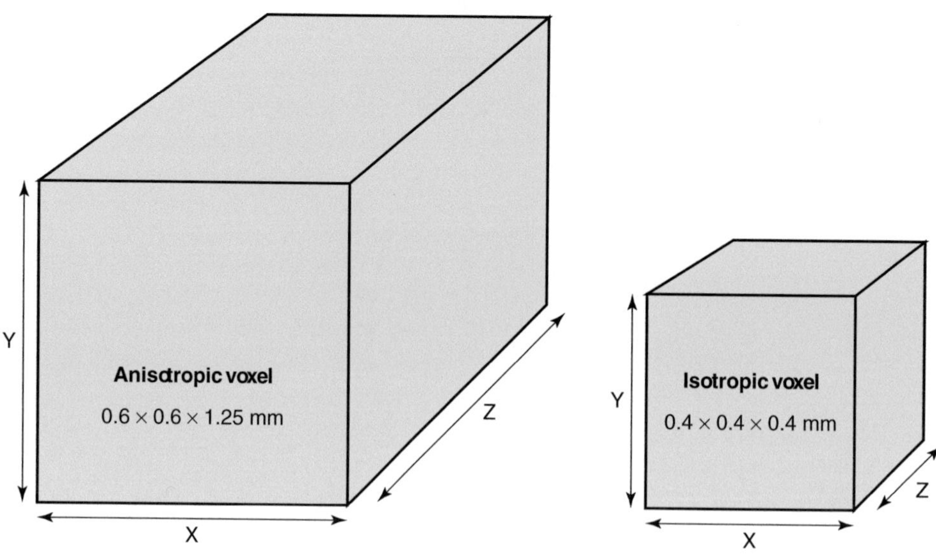

Table 1.1 MSCT acquisition parameters

Type of CT acquisition
Helical
Axial
Length of CT scan
CT scan direction
Cephalic
Caudal
Table speed
Pitch
Gantry rotation time
X-ray collimation
X-ray voltage (kV)
X-ray current (mA)
Z-axis automatic modulation
Real time modulation
Raw data reconstruction algorithm
Filtered back projection
Advanced iterative reconstruction
Adaptive filter (Kernel)
Image resolution
Image matrix

(Table 1.1). Once the raw data from the images is collected, there exists a series of variables to consider before deciding how the information will be reconstructed and presented for its analysis (slice thickness; reconstruction intervals; image filter). In MSCT a fundamental difference exists between how the images are acquired and how they are visualized at the time of making the diagnosis [36]. Unlike the spiral CT, the MSCT technology allows to reconstruct images with a thickness different to the one chosen at the time of scanning (e.g. 1.25; 2.5; 3.75; 5 and 10 mm). This depends on the original collimation used and is feasible due to the possibility of combining the signals obtained from contiguous detectors. It is of vital importance to consider the purpose of the study when choosing a certain type of image acquisition and reconstruction protocol [37–39].

Design of Detectors

CT detectors design should provide alternative slice thicknesses to adjust the best scan speed, longitudinal resolution and image noise for each different clinical application. Each manufacturer of CT scanners has introduced alterative detector designs. To be able to select different slice widths, the scanners electronically combine a variable number of detector rows to a smaller number of slices according to the selected beam collimation and the desired slice thickness. Regarding the detector design, three detector types have been commonly used (Fig. 1.7).

A. The fixed array detector design: formed by parallel rows of detector elements of equal sizes in the longitudinal direction.

B. The adaptive array detector design: the rows comprise detectors with different sizes in the longitudinal direction, which increases from the central region towards the peripheral areas of the detector tray.

C. The hybrid array detector design: the central rows comprise detectors with the less width (0.; 0.625; 0.75 mm, on the outer zones, detectors with double the thickness (1 mm; 1.25 mm; 1.5 mm respectively) are located.

Depending then on the configuration of the tray, the number rows of detectors can be less, equal or greater than the number of images reconstructed per rotation of the gantry. For most of the multislice CT scanners, the lowest thickness of cut is equal to the thickness of each individual row of detectors. For example, in a CT scanner with a detector configuration of 64×0.5, the lowest slice thickness is 0.5 mm.

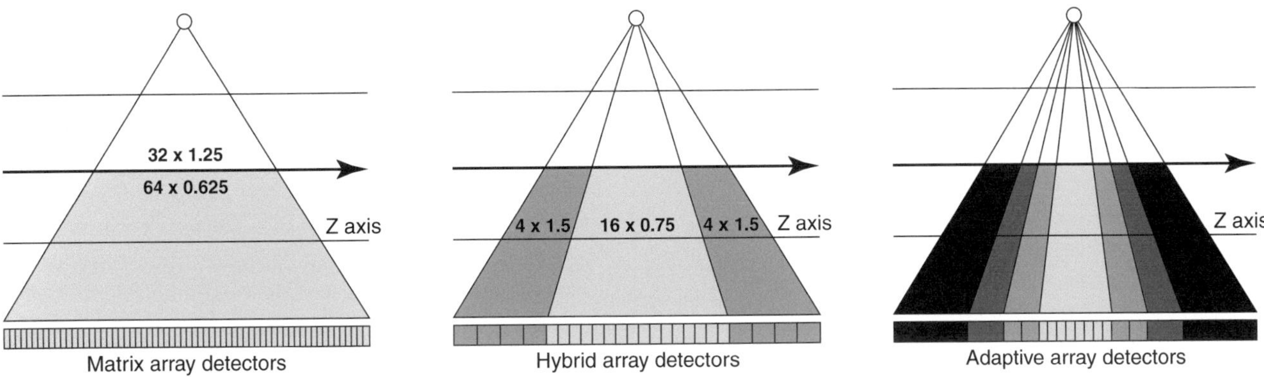

Fig. 1.7 Type of MSCT detectors

In the spiral CT, the X-ray beam that generates an image must run in a perpendicular plane to the transversal axis of the patient (z axis). In the MSCT this premise is not fulfilled entirely, due to the fact that the projection of the X-rays beam is tilted by the so-called cone angle in relation to the center plane. This angle is null for the detectors in the centre, while larger for the ones located at the edges, and becomes higher as the number of rows of detectors is increased. It is for this reason that the peripheral detectors are less efficient than the ones in the centre. In the new MSCT systems, different reconstruction algorithms have been implemented to reduce this problem, like the adaptive reconstruction on multiple planes [32–34].

Inter-detector Interval

This concept is unique to the multislice technology, and makes reference to the space that exists between two adjacent detectors on the patient's longitudinal axis. The radiation which falls in these spaces is of a lower intensity and does not take part in the formation of the image, being discarded. At a higher number of detectors, more is the number of inter-detector intervals, and less efficient is the radiation dose.

Pitch

In the spiral CT, the meaning of the term pitch is simple and implies the relationship between the advance of the CT table (in mm) across the gantry during the 360° rotation, and the width of the X-rays beam (in mm).

$$\boxed{\text{Pitch} = \text{CT table advance} / \text{Width of X-rays beam}}$$

In MSCT, the position of the detectors on the z-axis and the collimations vary from one device to another, generating confusion over the concept of pitch. Therefore, it is necessary to distinguish between two definitions of pitch:

The detector pitch, the least used, is defined as the advance of the CT table (in mm) across the gantry during a 360° rotation, in relation to the width of the chosen detector (in mm).

$$\boxed{\text{Detector pitch} = \text{CT table feed per rotation} / \text{Width of the detector}}$$

The beam pitch, the most used, consists in the relation between the movement of the CT table (in mm) across the gantry during a 360° rotation and the width of the X-rays beam, which is determined by multiplying the number of detectors used by the width of the chosen detector (in mm).

$$\boxed{\begin{aligned}\text{Beam pitch} &= \text{CT table feed per rotation} / \text{Width of the detector} \\ &\quad \times \text{Number of active detectors}\end{aligned}}$$

For example, a 64-row CT scanner with a collimation of 0.625 mm, a CT table movement of 19 mm/s and a rotation time of 0.4 s, has a pitch equal to: $(19/2.5)/(64 \times 0.625) = 0.19$.

This last concept in beam pitch, applicable to the spiral CT as well as to the MSCT, is the one recommended to use when comparing the exposure to radiation between both technologies [40].

Rotation Time

The rotation time indicates the time it takes the X-ray tube to turn 360° around the CT table. The improvements achieved in the rotation time have been fundamental for achieving a temporary resolution that allows reducing the scan time, diminishing the moving artifacts and of obtaining a better view of the contrast bolus in vascular studies.

In the spiral CT, the rotation time was approximately one second in every device, whereas in the MSCT it has been reduced considerably, reaching in last generation of CT scanners 0.20 s, being 0.5 s the rotation time used daily in most studies. The concept of acquisition speed is the number of slices acquired per second, reflecting the multislice equipment's potential strength, due to the number of detector rows and the rotation speed used. For example, in a 64-row CT

Table 1.2 Advantages of MSCT

Shorter scan time
Movement artifacts reduction
Pediatric patients
Politrauma patients
Dyspneic patients
Optimization of intravascular contrast usage
Volume contrast reduction
Homogenous opacification
Well define arterial and venous phases
Greater z-axis scan coverage
Isotropic image acquisitions
High quality multiplanar and 3D images
Lower radiation exposure
Post CT scan slice thickness modification

scanner, choosing a rotation time of 0.5 s, it would be possible to acquire 128 images per second.

It must also be taken into account that the rotation speed influences the quality of the image. Fast rotation speeds jointly reduce the radiation doses as well as the image's quality [41].

Advantages of Multislice CT

The most important advantages of MSCT are the image acquisition speed, the isotropic space resolution, the reduction in the volume of vascular contrast utilized and the less quantity of effective radiation doses to which the patient is subject to (Table 1.2). The possibility to study obese patients is also mentioned, with weights reaching 400 lb (300 kg), as well as the incorporation of new image reconstruction algorithms (advanced iterative reconstruction) which prevent the technical artifacts created by low exposure, increase the space resolution and permit an additional reduction of the radiation dose by up to 80 %.

Conclusion

The introduction of multislice CT technology accompanied by great advances in hardware and software generated, in this new millennium, a resurgence of the CT. The last generations of CT scanners of 64 and 256-rows allow to obtain a volume of sub-millimetric and isotropic images of vast areas of the body in a matter of seconds, to create bidimensional and tridimensional reconstructions in any plane of space, and to apply more sophisticated processing and acquisition algorithms like the virtual endoscopy or the electrocardiographic synchronization of cardiac images.

As a result, this new technology puts the CT in a place of privilege, despite of having to face the obstacle which the use of ionizing radiation presents. The knowledge of the basic physics principles of the MSCT along with a correct choice of the acquisition parameters according to the study, and region of body under study, are important to optimize, individually according to each patient, the best study protocol. The incorporation of the advanced iterative reconstruction of images, along with the use of filters, new detector designs, collimators and systems of automatic selection of the X-rays tube's current, that adapts it according to the physical contexture of the patient, allow to fully adjust the minimum radiation dose necessary to generate a CT image with diagnostic quality, in accordance with the ALARA (As Low As Reasonable Achievable) principle which makes reference to the phrase "as low as reasonably achievable" that recommends the establishment of adequate cut points and the modification of the acquisition parameters to fully optimize the radiation dose, while maintaining an image quality acceptable in all CT studies. This subject is explained in detail in the chapter on radiation (see Chap. 14).

References

1. Hounsfield GN. Computerised transverse axial scanning (tomography): part 1. Description of system. Br J Radiol. 1973;46:1016–22.
2. Ambrose J. Computerised transverse axial scanning (tomography): part 2. Clinical application. Br J Radiol. 1973;46:1023–47.
3. Beckmann EC. CT scanning the early days. Br J Radiol. 1976;79:5–8.
4. Kelly DM, Hasegawa I, Borders R, et al. High-resolution CT using MDCT: comparison of degree of motion artifact between volumetric and axial methods. AJR Am J Roentgenol. 2004;182:757–9.
5. McCollough CH, Zink FE. Performance evaluation of a multi-slice CT system. Med Phys. 1999;26:2223–30.
6. Rydberg J, Buckwalter KA, Caldemeyer KS, et al. Multisection CT: scanning techniques and clinical applications. Radiographics. 2000;20:1787–806.
7. Mansfield SD, Scott J, Oppong K, et al. Comparison of multislice computed tomography and endoscopic ultrasonography with operative and histological findings in suspected pancreatic and periampullary malignancy. Br J Surg. 2008;95:1512–20.
8. Holzapfel K, Rummeny EJ, Hannig C, et al. MSCT for staging and response evaluation of esophageal cancer. Radiology. 2007;47:101–9.
9. Imbriaco M, Smeraldo D, Liuzzi R, et al. Multislice CT with single-phase technique in patients with suspected pancreatic cancer. Radiol Med. 2006;111:159–66.
10. Kobayashi S, Nagano H, Marubashi S, et al. Multidetector computed tomography for preoperative prediction of postsurgical prognosis of patients with extrahepatic biliary cancer. J Surg Oncol. 2010;101:376–83.
11. Ji H, Rolnick JA, Haker S, et al. Multislice CT colonography: current status and limitations. Eur J Radiol. 2003;47:123–34.
12. Cohnen M, Vogt C, Beck A, et al. Feasibility of MDCT colonography in ultra-low-dose technique in the detection of colorectal lesions: comparison with high resolution video colonoscopy. AJR Am J Roentgenol. 2004;183:1355–9.
13. Iannaccone R, Laghi A, Catalano C, et al. Detection of colorectal lesions: lower-dose multidetector row helical CT colonography compared with conventional colonoscopy. Radiology. 2003;229:775–81.
14. Hara AK, Johnson CD, MacCarty RL, et al. CT colonography: single- versus multi-detector row imaging. Radiology. 2001; 219:461–5.

15. Pickhardt PJ, Choi JR, Hwang I, et al. Computed tomographic virtual colonoscopy to screen for colorectal neoplasia in asymptomatic adults. N Engl J Med. 2003;349:2191–200.

16. Carrascosa P, Capuñay C, Castiglioni R, et al. Virtual colonoscopy: single vs. multislice CT. Eur Radiol. 2001;Suppl 1:364. Abstract.

17. Castiglioni R, Carrascosa P, Capuñay C. Actualización en colonoscopía virtual: experiencia con tomógrafo Multislice. Rev Argent Coloproctol. 2001;12:72–5.

18. Renker M, Ramachandra A, Schoepf UJ, et al. Iterative image reconstruction techniques: applications for cardiac CT. J Cardiovasc Comput Tomogr. 2011;5:225–30.

19. Baile EM, King GG, Muller NL, et al. Spiral computed tomography is comparable to angiography for the diagnosis of pulmonary embolism. Am J Respir Crit Care Med. 2000;161:1010–5.

20. Rubin GD, Dake MD, Napel SA, et al. Three dimensional spiral CT angiography of the abdomen: initial clinical experience. Radiology. 1993;186:147–52.

21. Vining DJ, Gelfand DW, Bechtold RE, et al. Technical feasibility of colon imaging with helical CT and virtual reality. Am J Roentgenol. 1994;62(Suppl):104.

22. Remy-Jardin M, Remy J, Wattinne L, et al. Central pulmonary thromboembolism: diagnosis with spiral volumetric CT with the single-breath-hold technique comparison with pulmonary angiography. Radiology. 1992;185:381–7.

23. Baron RL, Oliver Jr JH, Dodd Jr GD, et al. Hepatocellular carcinoma: evaluation with biphasic, contrast-enhanced, helical CT. Radiology. 1996;199:505–11.

24. Polverosi R, Vigo M, Baron S, et al. Evaluation of tracheobronchial lesions with spiral CT: comparison between virtual endoscopy and bronchoscopy. Radiol Med (Torino). 2001;102:313–9.

25. Kalender WA. Computed tomography. Munich: Publicis MCD Verlag; 2000. p. 35–55.

26. Hsieh J. Computed tomography. Bellingham: SPIE; 2003. p. 1–12.

27. Lee JKT, Sagel SS, Stanley R, et al. Computed body tomography with MRI correlation. 4th ed. Philadelphia: Lippincott Williams & Wilkins; 2006. p. 1–28.

28. Caoili EM, Paulson EK. CT of small-bowel obstruction: another perspective using multiplanar reformations. AJR Am J Roentgenol. 2000;174:993–8.

29. Bhalla M, Naidich DP, McGuinness G, et al. Diffuse lung disease: assessment with helical CT – preliminary observations of the role of maximum and minimum intensity projection images. Radiology. 1996;200:341–7.

30. Johnson CD, Dachman AH. CT colonography: the next colon screening examination? Radiology. 2000;216:331–41.

31. Hu H, He HD, Foley WD, et al. Four multidetector row helical CT: image quality and volume coverage speed. Radiology. 2000;215:55–62.

32. Prokop M. General principles of MDCT. Eur J Radiol. 2003;45 Suppl 1:S4–10.

33. Rydberg J, Liang Y, Teague SD. Fundamentals of multichannel CT. Radiol Clin North Am. 2003;41:465–74.

34. Mahesh M. Search for isotropic resolution in CT from conventional through multiple-row detector. Radiographics. 2002;22:949–62.

35. Mori S, Endo M, Obata T, et al. Properties of the prototype 256-row (cone beam) CT scanner. Eur Radiol. 2006;16:2100–8.

36. Hoe H, Toh KH. First experience with 320-row multidetector CT coronary angiography scanning with prospective electrocardiogram gating to reduce radiation dose. J Cardiovasc Comput Tomogr. 2009;3:257–61.

37. Napoli A, Fleischmann D, Chan FP, et al. Computed tomography angiography: state-of-the-art imaging using multidetector-row technology. J Comput Assist Tomogr. 2004;28:S32–45.

38. Cademartiri F, Luccichenti G, van Der Lugt A, et al. Sixteen-row multislice computed tomography: basic concepts, protocols, and enhanced clinical applications. Semin Ultrasound CT MR. 2004;25:2–16.

39. Cody DD, Moxley DM, Krugh KT, et al. Strategies for formulating appropriate MDCT techniques when imaging the chest, abdomen, and pelvis in pediatric patients. AJR Am J Roentgenol. 2004;182:849–59.

40. Wang G, Vannier MW. The effect of pitch in multislice spiral/helical CT. Med Phys. 1999;26:2648–53.

41. Mahesh M, Scatarige JC, Cooper J, et al. Dose and pitch relationship for a particular multislice CT scanner. AJR Am J Roentgenol. 2001;177:1273–5.

The Birth of a New Diagnostic Technique

Twelve years ago, in an imaging diagnosis center in Vicente López, a northern area of Greater Buenos Aires, the idea of investigating the uterine cavity and fallopian tubes using a computed tomography (CT) based technique similar to the one of the traditional X-ray hysterosalpingography (HSG) arose: it was the early days of the virtual hysterosalpingography (VHSG).

In this chapter, the first steps of the technique and its changes and growth over the years and hand of technological advances will be described, as well as the beginning of its clinical application, until becoming the everyday method known today.

For this purpose, this chapter is divided into five stages:

Stage I: VHSG's birth with spiral CT equipment.

Stage II: Improvement of the new technique with the incorporation of 4-slice CT technology.

Stage III: Advances of the VHSG due to the introduction of 16-slice CT units.

Stage IV: Technique's optimization with 64-slice CT scanners. The beginning of VHSG clinical applications.

Stage V: Introduction of 256-slice CT scanners a new reaches of the VHSG. Real-time CT image acquisitions with ultra-low radiation doses.

Stage I

VHSG appears in early 1998. In those times, all virtual CT studies were, fundamentally, exams utilized for the evaluation of the colon. Virtual colonoscopy, also called CT Colonography, was born by the hand of Dr. Vining [1] in 1994 and soon other clinical applications were explored like virtual bronchoscopy, virtual gastroscopy, virtual ureteroscopy and cystoscopy, among other studies [2–5]. Nevertheless, applications for the evaluation of the gynecologic apparatus hadn't yet been developed. It is for this reason that the study of the cervix, uterus and tubes through CT generated a new expectation.

The CT units used in those times were spiral CT scanners which allowed volumetric image acquisitions. Nevertheless, due to the fact that these CT units were not fast (tube rotation times of 1 s), the image acquisition was long and still had thick cuts (4 mm), which did not permit detecting small lesions. Also, the acquisition of isotropic images without loss of resolution in the different planes of space was not feasible. In spite of these limitations, the Diagnóstico Maipú research team carried out an investigational protocol to verify how far the acquisition of information of the feminine genital apparatus utilizing the available CT equipment and virtual CT algorithms was possible. The results obtained through conventional X-ray HSG, radiologic study of preference to evaluate the gynecologic apparatus, were compared with the first attempts at HSG via CT, which was denominated VHSG (virtual hysterosalpingography). The CT unit used was a single-slice CT scanner (Picker, model PQ5000). The technique employed in the initial stage of the VHSG was similar to that used in X-ray HSG studies. With the patient on the CT table in gynecologic position, with prior asepsis cleansing of the perineum, a speculum is placed to distend the vaginal cavity. After that, asepsis of the cervical canal is carried out and the cervical neck is clamped, placing then a metallic cannula into the external cervical canal through which pure iodine contrast media is instilled to distend the uterine cavity (Fig. 2.1). Following this description, the procedure is practically the same as the X-ray HSG examination; hence the patient discomfort is the equal. The only advantage of the CT virtual study in this first stage is that the patient was not required to move during the image acquisition, as was necessary in the traditional radiologic exam. Moreover, the total time of the new procedure was significantly shorter (15 min versus 30 min). The CT image acquisition lasted approximately 45 s, with a slice thickness of 4 mm. The prolonged scanning length and the thick 4 mm slices did not allow evaluation of the Fallopian tubes; nevertheless a visualization of the endometrial cavity was possible. This achievement generated great enthusiasm among researchers due to the

P. Carrascosa et al., *CT Virtual Hysterosalpingography*,
DOI 10.1007/978-3-319-07560-0_2, © Springer International Publishing Switzerland 2014

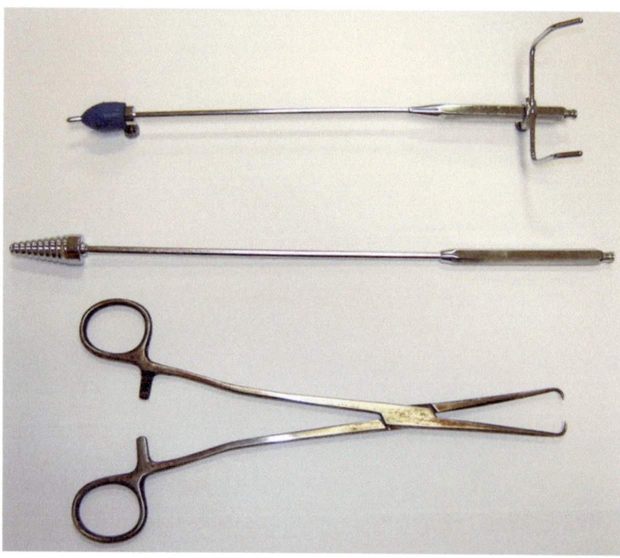

Fig. 2.1 Instruments utilized in the conventional HSG exam. Metallic cannula with rubber end; metallic cannula with metallic end; tenaculum

fact that this new modality made possible the evaluation of the uterine pathology from different angles using 2D or 3D images and virtual endoscopic views (Fig. 2.2). In this way, the VHSG had, although few, some more advantages for the patient in terms of the execution of the study; it permitted a complete evaluation of the uterine cavity providing precise information and facilitated a more accurate diagnostic result. Nevertheless, the primary limitation was the impossibility of evaluating the Fallopian tubes. For this reason, the VHSG was not yet able to compete with the traditional X-ray exam that granted a complete view of the gynecologic apparatus. The first results of the VHSG experience were shown in the 21st International Radiology Congress which took place in Argentina in September 2000.

Stage II

As of November 1999 it was possible with the incorporation of a 4-slice CT scanner (the first in the country), to make certain changes in the CT acquisition parameters and have new and better reprocessing tools, which had great impact on the VHSG procedure's final result. This new CT scanner (Picker-Marconi; Mx8000), was much faster than the CT units used until that moment. This new CT scanner had a rotation time of 0.5 s (double the speed of the spiral CT scanner) and offered 8 images per second. This improvement in the CT acquisition time allowed the VHSG to be performed in a shorter scan time of 25 s (average). At the same time, the slice thickness was reduced to 2 mm, hence the space resolution was enhanced and endocavitary lesions of scarce millimeters began to be detected. The images obtained were

isotropic, which means they were constituted by cubic voxels, which avoids the loss of resolution when changing position in multiplanar reformats, tridimensional images or endoscopic views. The uterine cavity could be visualized better, but the Fallopian tubes still could not be opacified and visualized correctly in most studies (Figs. 2.3 and 2.4). For this reason the changes and improvements failed to achieve a breakthrough in the performance of the procedure [6].

Stage III

Only in the year 2004, with the incorporation of a 16-slice CT scanner, significant improvements in VHSG studies could be achieved. These CT scanners had a rotation time similar to the 4-slice CT units (0.4 s), but thanks to a greater number of detector rows, they offered up to 40 images per second. Hence the studies could be acquired in only 12 s. In addition, improvements in space resolution with 1 mm slice thickness generated the possibility of a better evaluation of the Fallopian tubes, very limited until then. During this stage, research studies were carried out comparing the VHSG and the X-ray HSG in the evaluation of the uterine pathology and the Fallopian tubes. It was concluded from these studies that the VHSG correctly evaluated the cervical canal and uterine cavity pathology in the totality of the patients. However, only in 50 % of the cases, the visualization and evaluation of the Fallopian tubes were feasible. Despite the substantial improvements achieved by the VHSG technique, it wasn't enough to compete with the X-ray HSG because in a large percentage of patients, Fallopian tube assessment could not be achieved [7, 8].

Simultaneously, another improvement was developed, the use of iodine-containing, nonionic, hypo-osmolar contrast media. Given its viscosity, these contrast media generated less discomfort in patients when distending the uterine cavity, and even more so in its passage to the peritoneal cavity. Afterwards, this type of iodine contrast agents began to be used diluted in saline solution, due to the fact that the density of the pure iodine contrast instilled in the cervix, uterus and tubes was high and, in certain cases, produced image artifacts which made impossible a precise view and diagnosis of endoluminal pathology. These contrast media dilutions allowed clear improvements in the image quality. During this stage, the physicians and technologist who performed the procedure remained in the CT room during the image acquisition to instill the contrast media into the uterine cavity, which was done manually.

With the purpose of transforming this new imaging diagnostic modality in a non invasive study, a series of changes in the way the study was performed were carried out: (i) traction of the uterine neck at the moment of the image acquisition was canceled; (ii) the use of tenaculum to clamp and

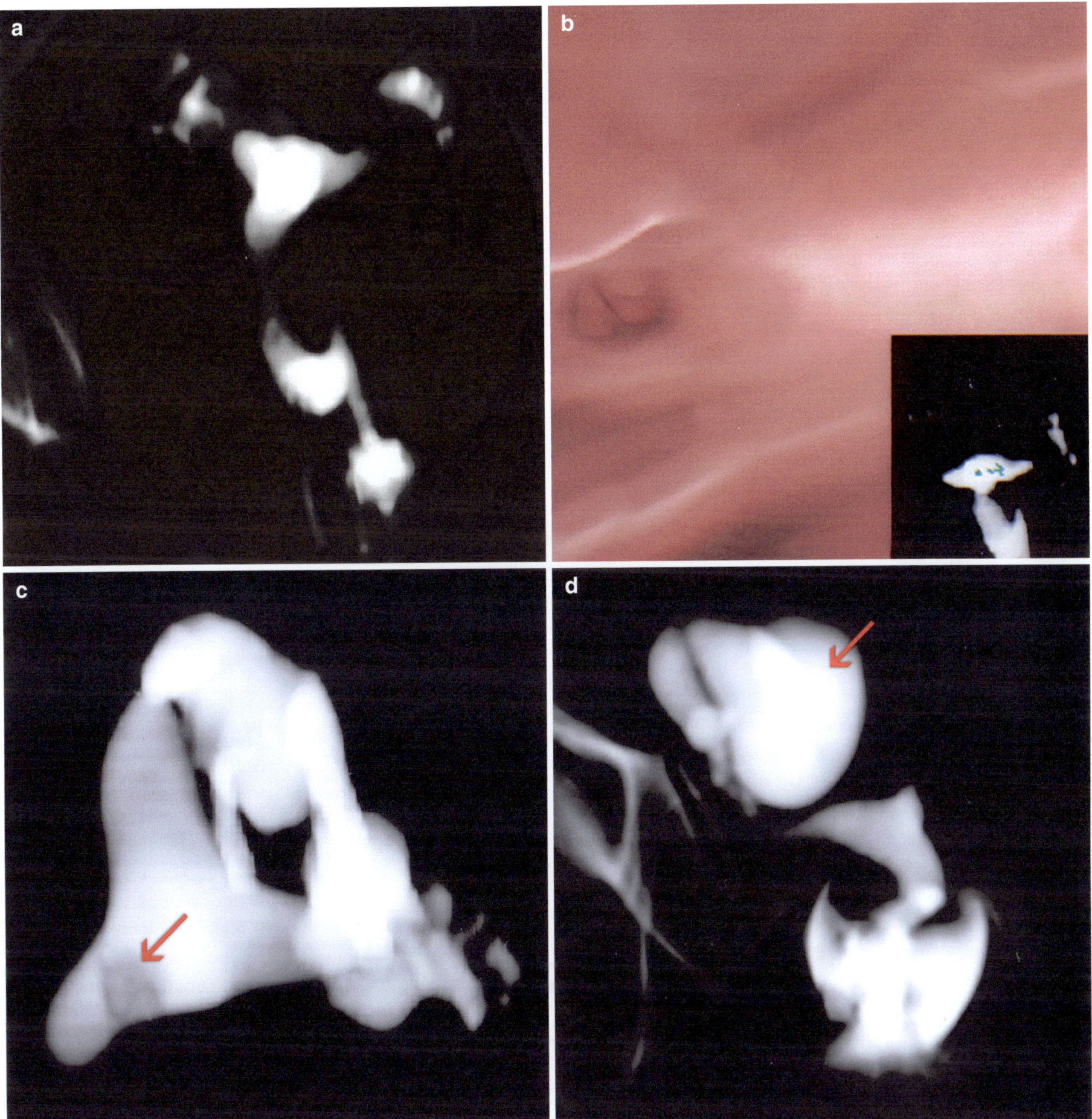

Fig. 2.2 VHSG images obtained with a helical CT scanner. (**a**) Coronal multiplanar reconstruction which shows a normal uterine silhouette. (**b**) Virtual endoscopy image of the uterine cavity. (**c**) Axial multiplanar reconstruction which shows a filling defect over the right uterine horn compatible with an endometrial polyp (*arrow*). (**d**) Coronal multiplanar reconstruction which shows a large right hydrosalpinx (*arrow*)

tract the neck was annulled; (iii) a plastic cannula with a rubber olive on its end which is simply positioned in the external cervical orifice was implemented (Fig. 2.5).

The MSCT obtains volumetric information which then? Can be reproduced in any plane of space and allows a spread, throughout the different types of reconstructions, of the anatomical structures that might overlap each other resulting in a great advantage over the older traditional radiologic procedure. The X-ray HSG requires an obligatory traction of the uterus to manage a spread, not overlapped, image of the gynecologic organs and provide diagnostic information. The transformation of the VHSG in a non invasive study generated great acceptance among the patients, who had a great fear of invasiveness, pain and soreness related to the traditional X-ray HSG exam. On the other hand this change in the exam procedure reduces the number of probable

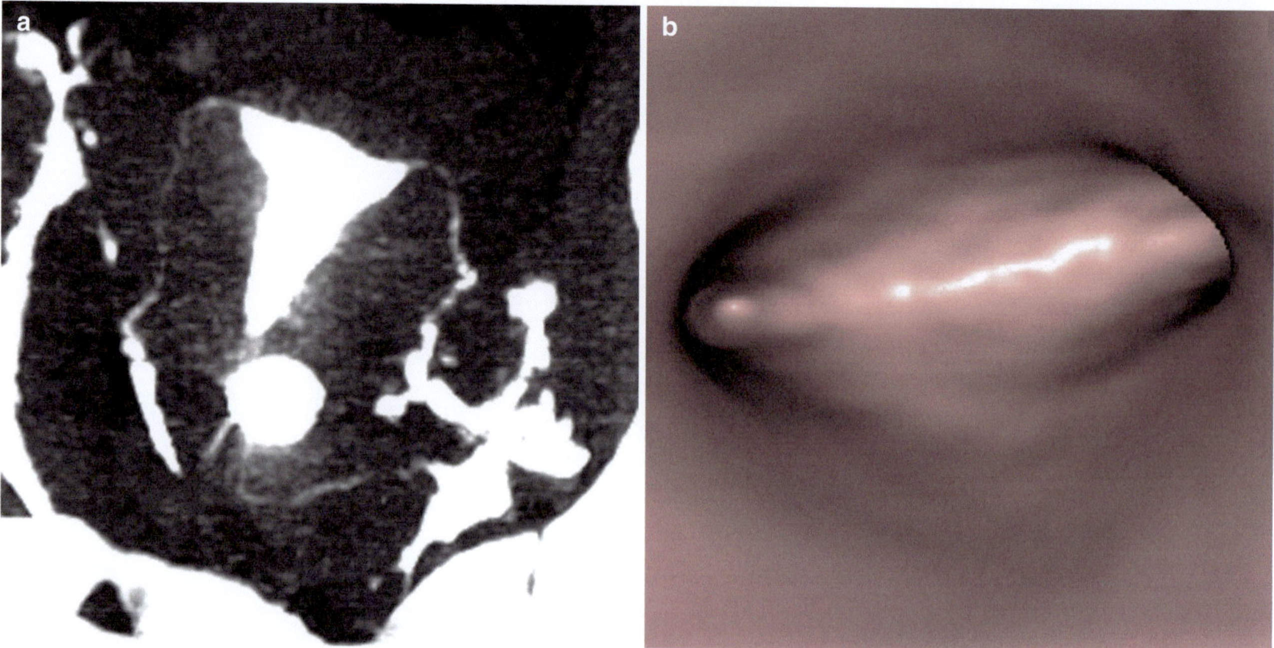

Fig. 2.3 VHSG images obtained with a 4-slice CT scanner. Normal study. (**a**) Coronal maximum intensity projection image. (**b**) Virtual endoscopy image

complications due to the fact that the possibility of bleeding, tearing or infection was dramatically dropped with the absence of cervical clamping.

In this stage, the obtained CT image quality allows a diagnosis of cervical and endometrial cavity lesions of very small size, which in the X-ray HSG study was not visible. As previously mentioned, the evaluation of the Fallopian tubes was still sub-optimal (Figs. 2.6, 2.7 and 2.8). The results obtained in the research works were presented in diverse congresses and published in national and international medical journals.

Stage IV

During October 2006, Diagnóstico Maipú incorporated a new 64-slice CT scanner (Brilliance 64; Philips Medical Systems). This CT unit offers 120 images per second, and at the same time, because of having very thin detectors, allows acquiring the studies with 0.9 mm slice thickness. These technological advances enabled the VHSG to be performed with a higher image resolution and in only 4.5 s. This was the most important and revolutionary change because the VHSG could now evaluate the Fallopian tubes in 100 % of patients (Figs. 2.9, 2.10, and 2.11). In addition, the adjustment of the CT image acquisition parameters of kilovoltage and tube current to the physical body of each patient allowed the reduction of the effective dose of radiation in VHSG studies to an average of 0.9 mSv. During this stage new comparative studies were carried out with the X-ray HSG and also with the diagnostic hysteroscopy to determine the sensitivity, specificity, positive and negative predictive values of the VHSG in comparison with the traditional techniques. These obtained excellent results, validating the diagnostic capacity of the VHSG allowed beginning its implementation in a clinical setting. The results obtained were presented in congresses and published in diverse radiological and gynecological journals, which permitted the spread of the method throughout the medical community and to place the procedure in the diagnostic algorithm of the infertile patient [8–12].

An innovative change of incredible value was introduced at this stage. The studies began to be performed without the need of the physician staying in the CT room during the scan. Because of this, the research team at Diagnóstico Maipú designed a device that allowed connecting the cannula to the injector pump in order to make the instillation of the contrast dilution fully automatic (Fig. 2.12). This accomplishment fulfilled two objectives: (i) that the contrast could be applied at a slow and constant flow rate, reducing the discomfort experienced by the patient during the distention of the uterine cavity; (ii) that the physician who carried out the procedure did not expose himself to radiation during the exam.

However, new uncertainties arose. One of them was the impossibility of carrying out the VHSG studies on patients allergic to iodine. Based on our experience of doing CT vascular studies with gadolinium, a non-iodine contrast used usually in magnetic resonance imaging examinations, on patients allergic to iodine contrasts [13, 14], the

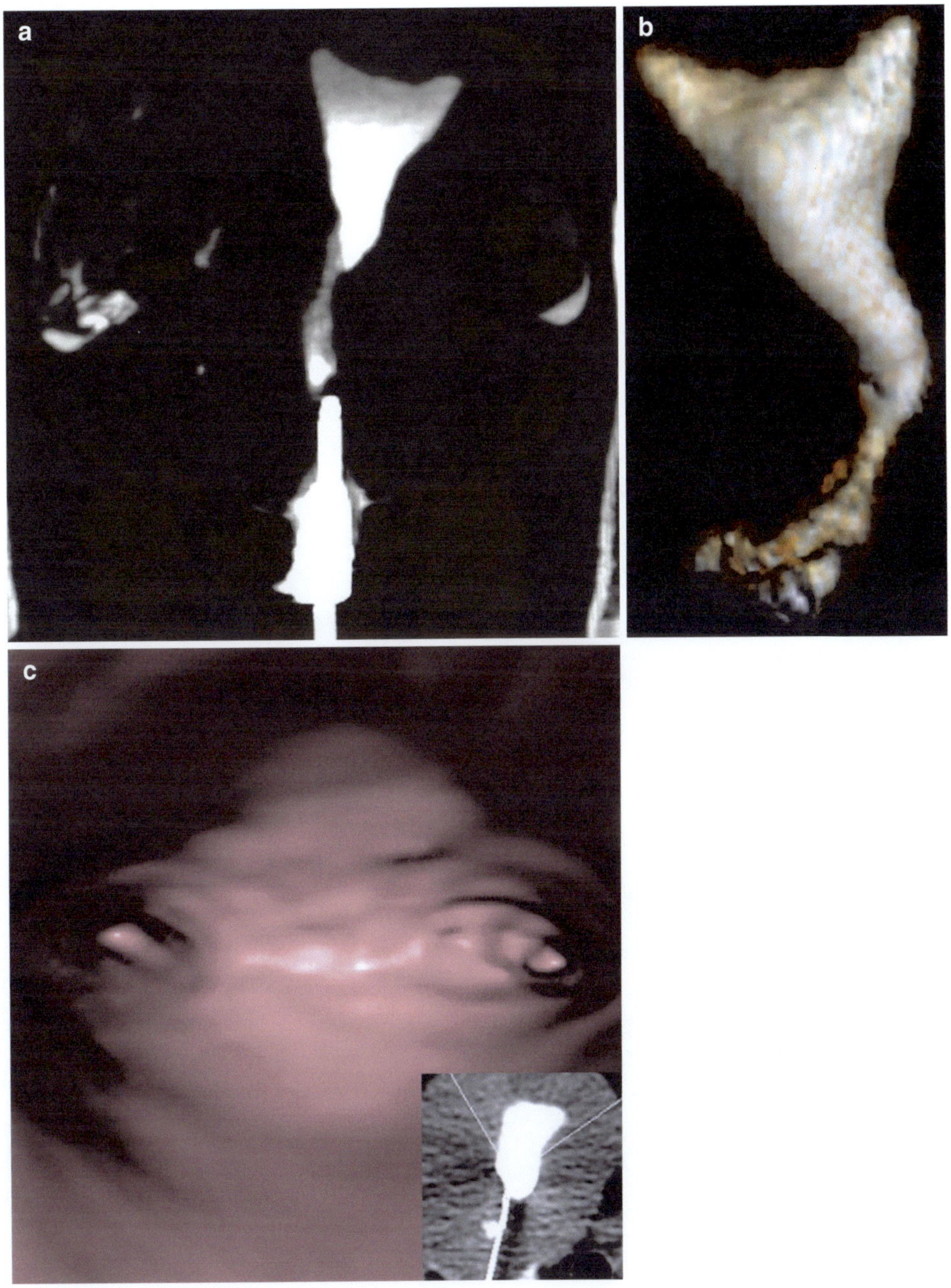

Fig. 2.4 VHSG images obtained with a 4-slice CT scanner. Poor visualization of the Fallopian tubes. (**a**) Coronal maximum intensity projection image. (**b**) Oblique coronal 3D volume rendering image. (**c**) Virtual endoscopy image

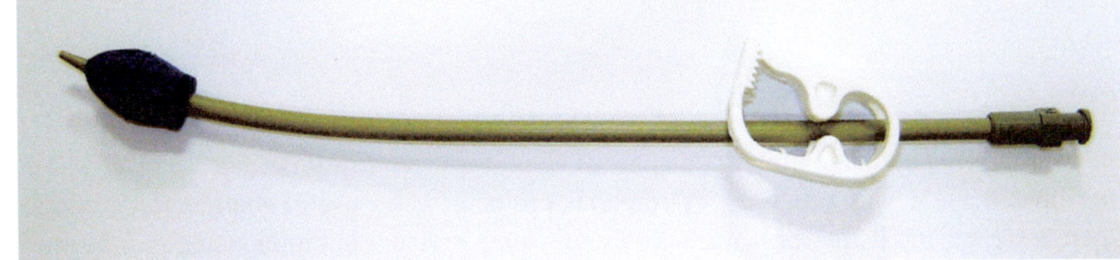

Fig. 2.5 Instrument utilized in the VHSG study. Plastic cannula with rubber end

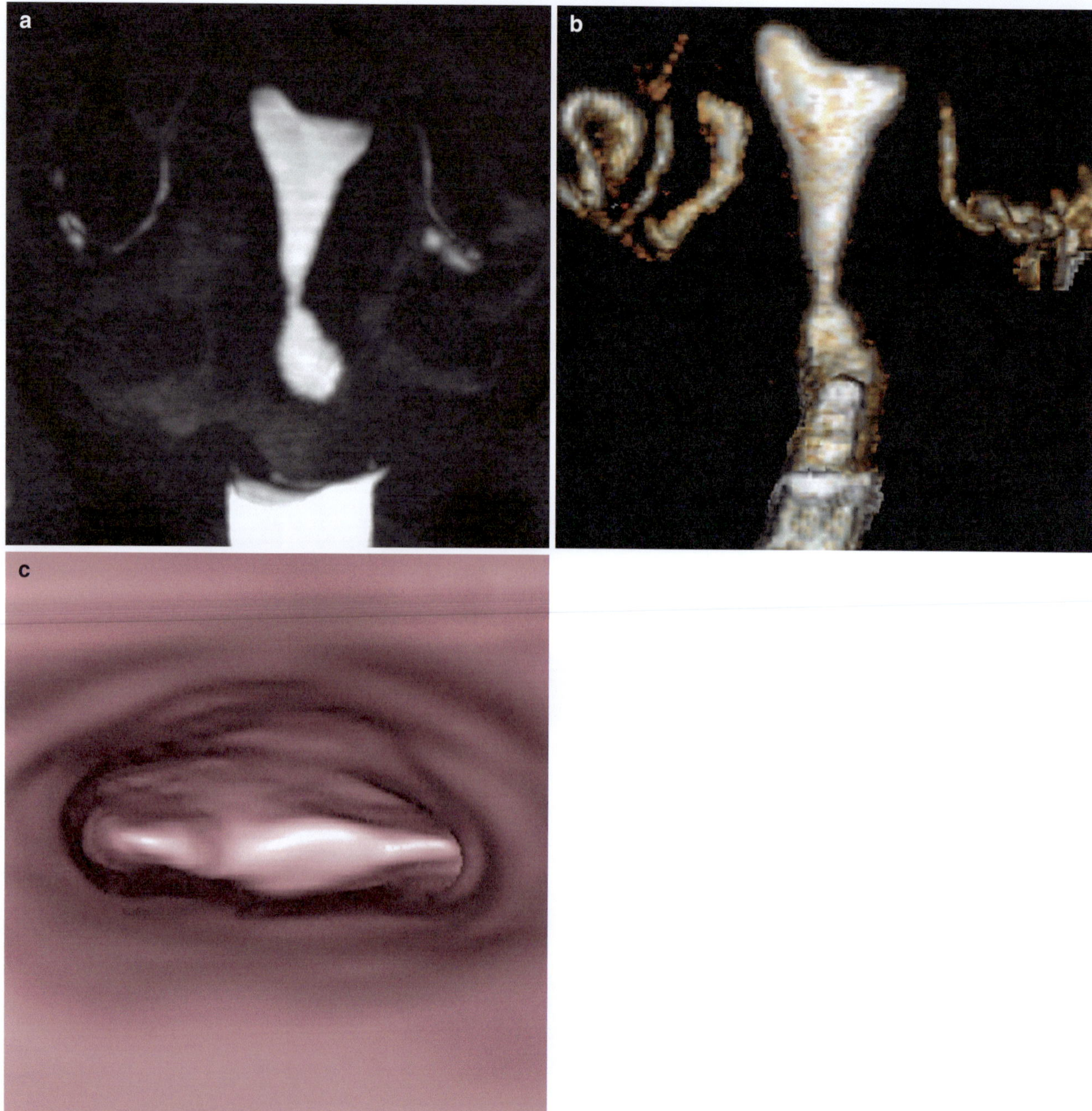

Fig. 2.6 VHSG images obtained with a 16-slice CT scanner. Incomplete visualization of the Fallopian tubes. (**a**) Coronal maximum intensity projection image. (**b**) Oblique coronal 3D volume rendering image. (**c**) Virtual endoscopy image

possibility of using gadolinium as a contrast agent for uterine opacification was proposed. A research protocol was then designed and its performance was tested. Comparative studies were done to evaluate the best dilution to use, the opacification obtained, the image quality and the diagnostic results (Fig. 2.13). It was concluded that gadolinium was a useful contrast to be utilized in this group of patients without influencing the diagnostic accuracy of the method [15]. Its only limitation is its cost, three times greater than the iodine contrast media.

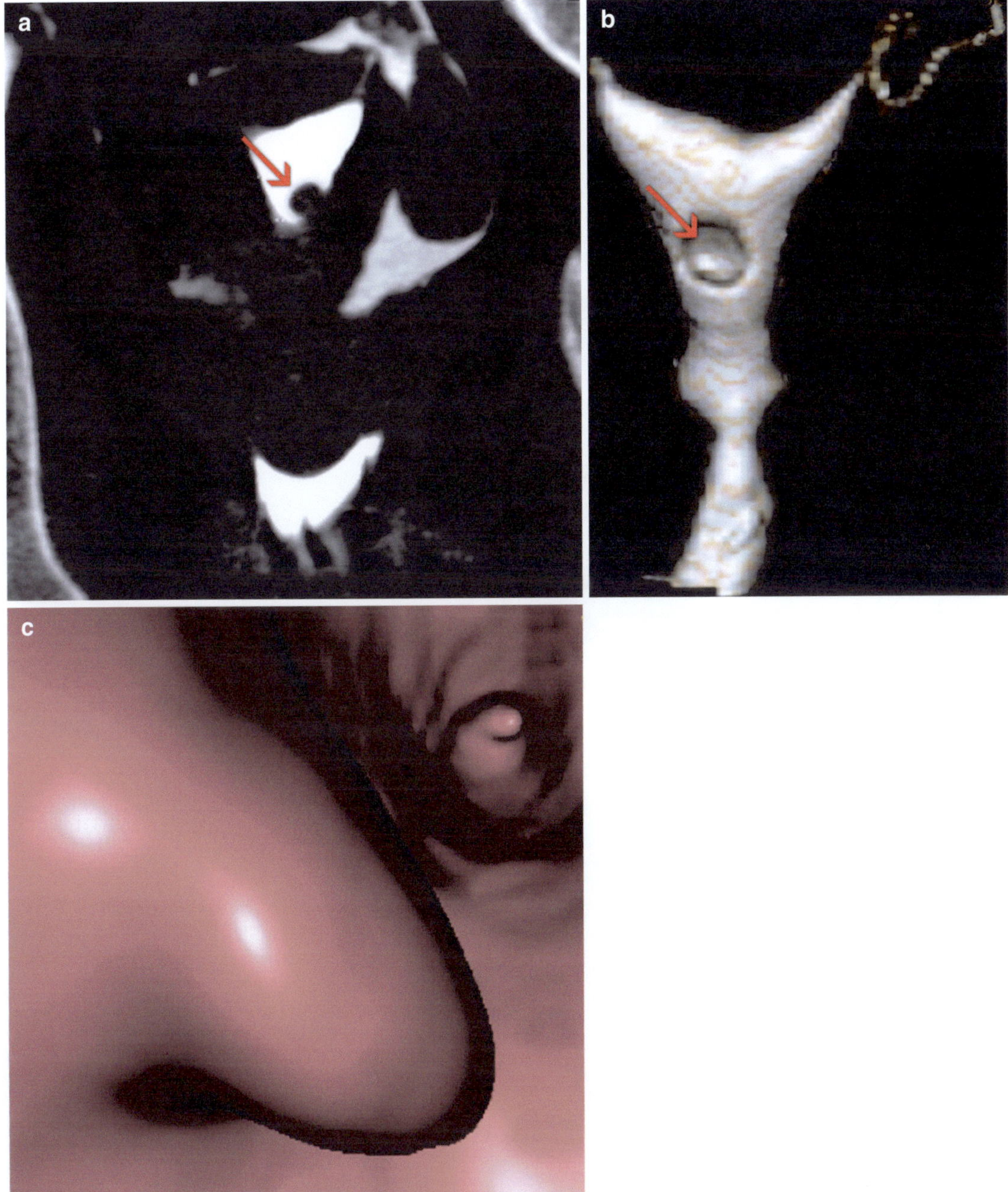

Fig. 2.7 VHSG images obtained with a 16-slice CT scanner. Endometrial polyp (*arrow*). (**a**) Coronal multiplanar reconstruction. (**b**) Coronal 3D volume rendering image. (**c**) Virtual endoscopy image

Stage V

On December 2010, VHSG studies began to be performed with a 256-slice CT scanner (Brilliance CT; Philips Medical Systems). This CT unit possessed a rotation time of 0.27 s and allowed acquiring the study in only 1.5 s, making the procedure a real-time exam. The adjustment of technical parameters according to the physical characteristics of the patient, and the usage of a iterative reconstruction, permitted utilizing only 80 kVp and 100 mAs, substantially reducing the effective radiation dose in these studies to only 0.3 mSv (Figs. 2.14, 2.15 and 2.16) [5–16].

Fig. 2.8 VHSG images obtained with a 16-slice CT scanner. Bilateral hydrosalpinx. (**a**) Coronal maximum intensity projection image. (**b**) Oblique coronal 3D volume rendering image. (**c**) Virtual endoscopy image of the right uterine tube

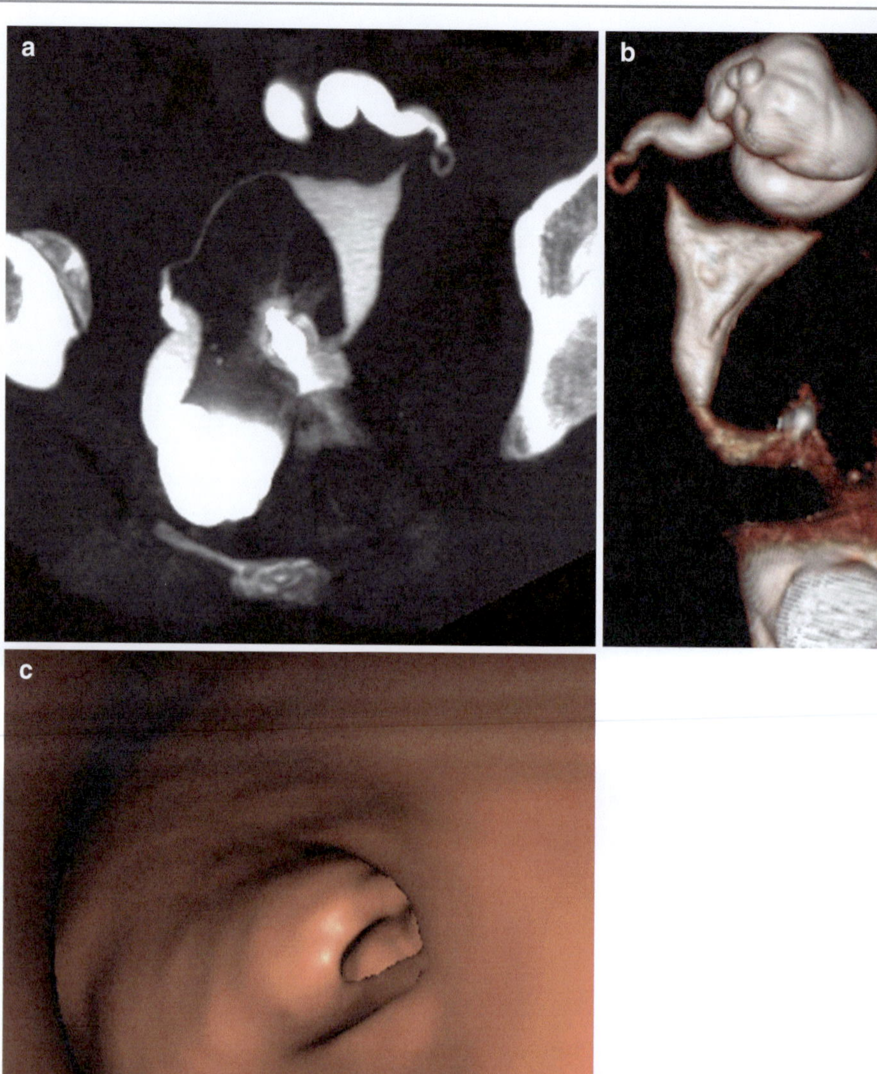

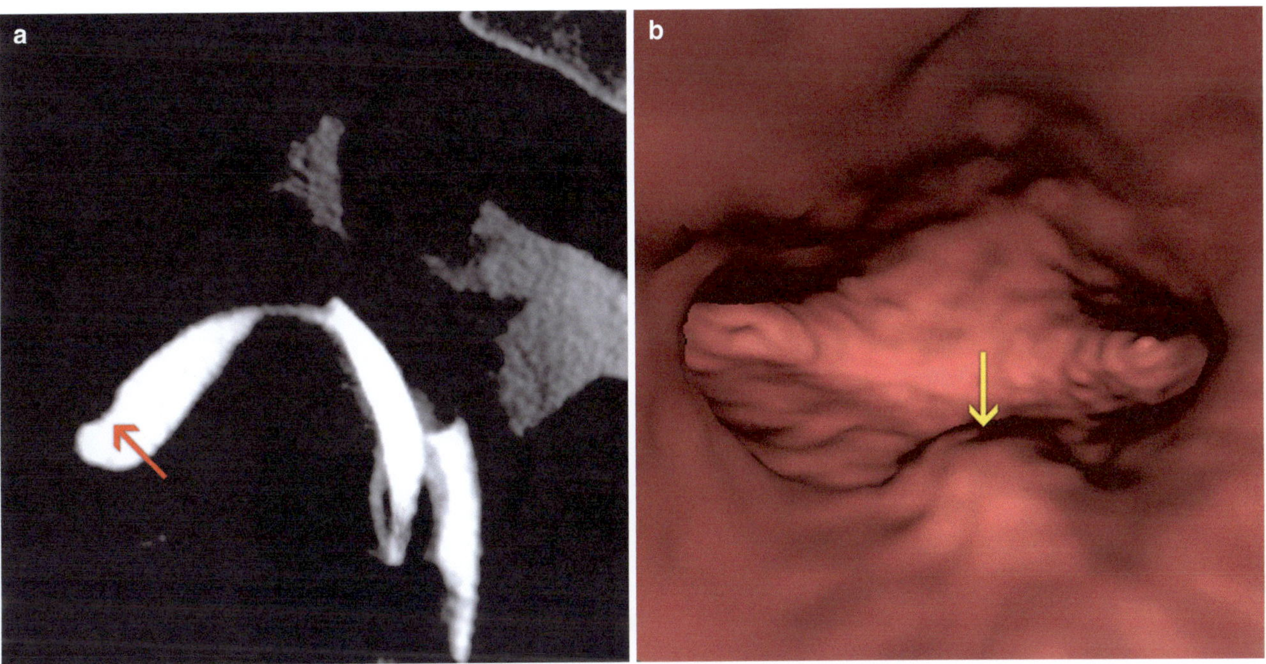

Fig. 2.9 VHSG obtained with a 64-slice CT scanner. Submucosal myoma (*arrows*). (**a**) Sagittal maximum intensity projection image. (**b**) Virtual endoscopy image

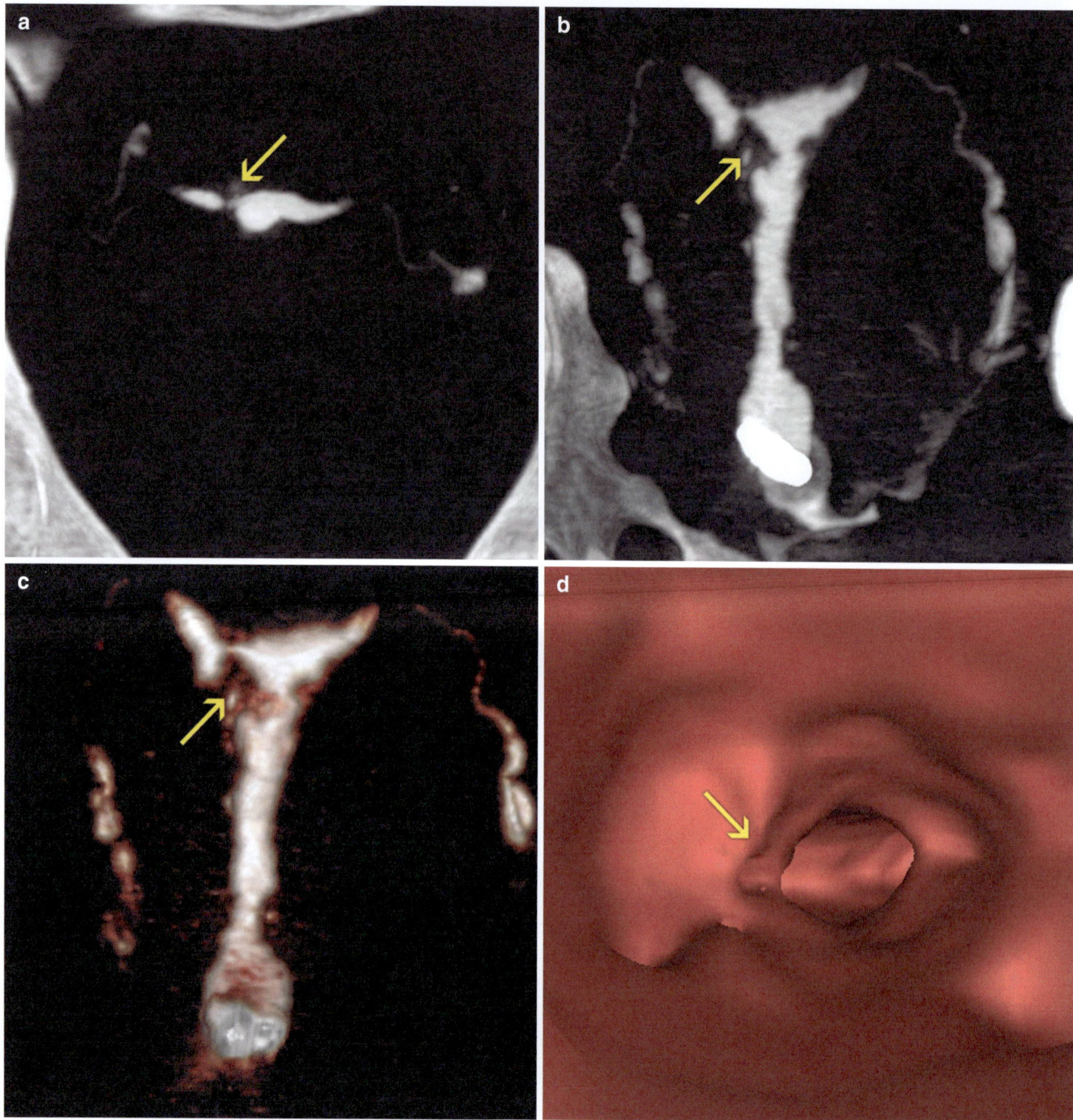

Fig. 2.10 VHSG images obtained with a 64-slice CT scanner. Uterine synechiae (*arrows*). (**a**) Axial maximum intensity projection (MIP) image. (**b**) Coronal MIP image. (**c**) Coronal 3D volume rendering image. (**d**) Virtual endoscopy image

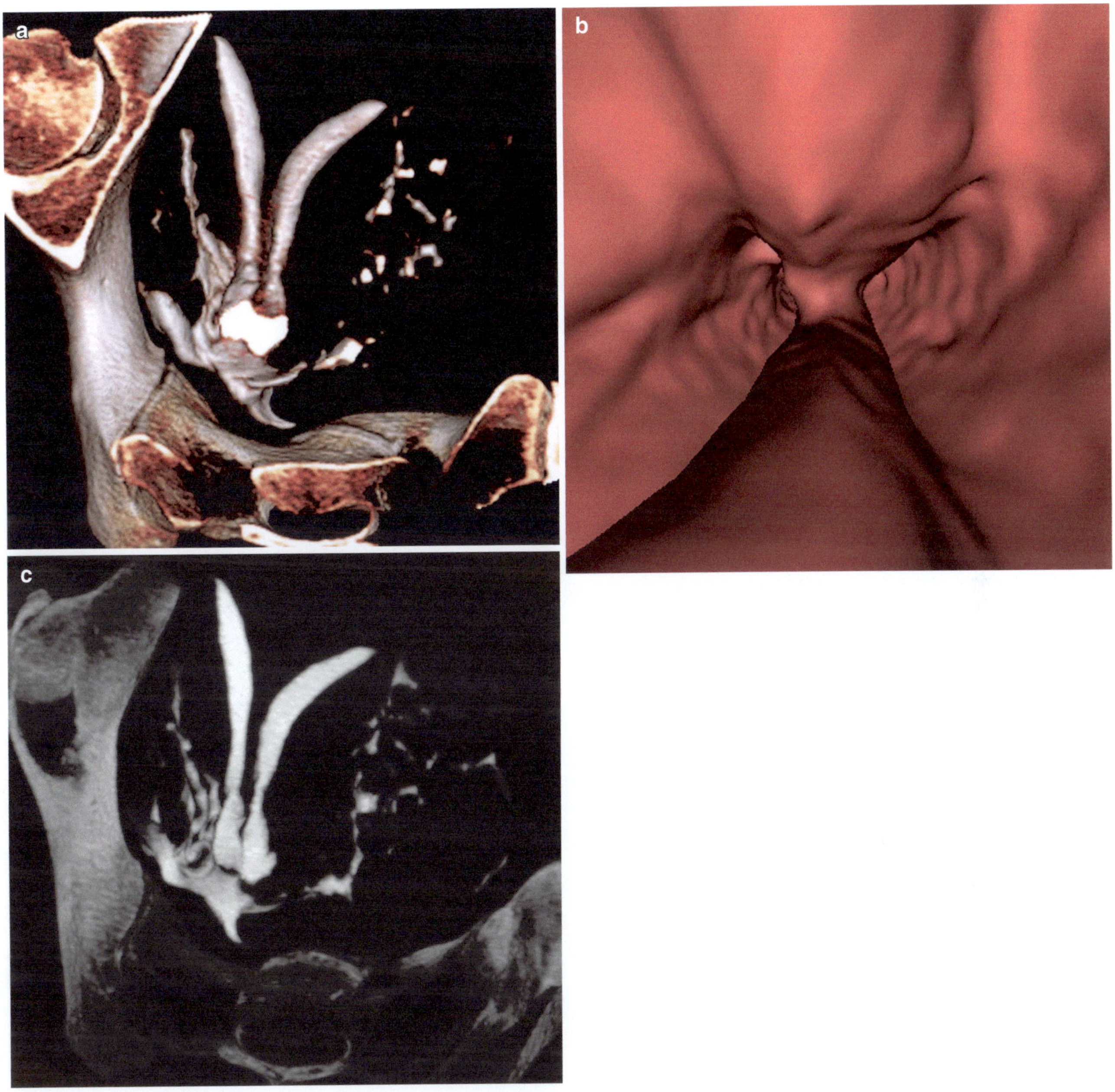

Fig. 2.11 VHSG images obtained with a 64-slice CT scanner. Complete septate uterus. (**a**) Coronal maximum intensity projection image. (**b**) Coronal 3D volume rendering image. (**c**) Virtual endoscopy image

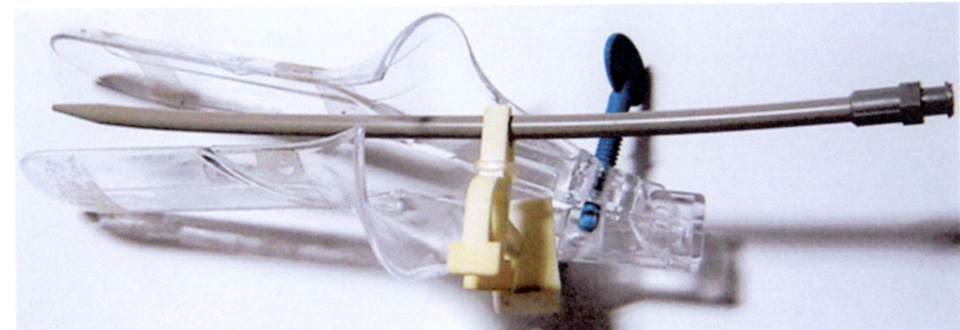

Fig. 2.12 Device designed to carry out the VHSG procedure

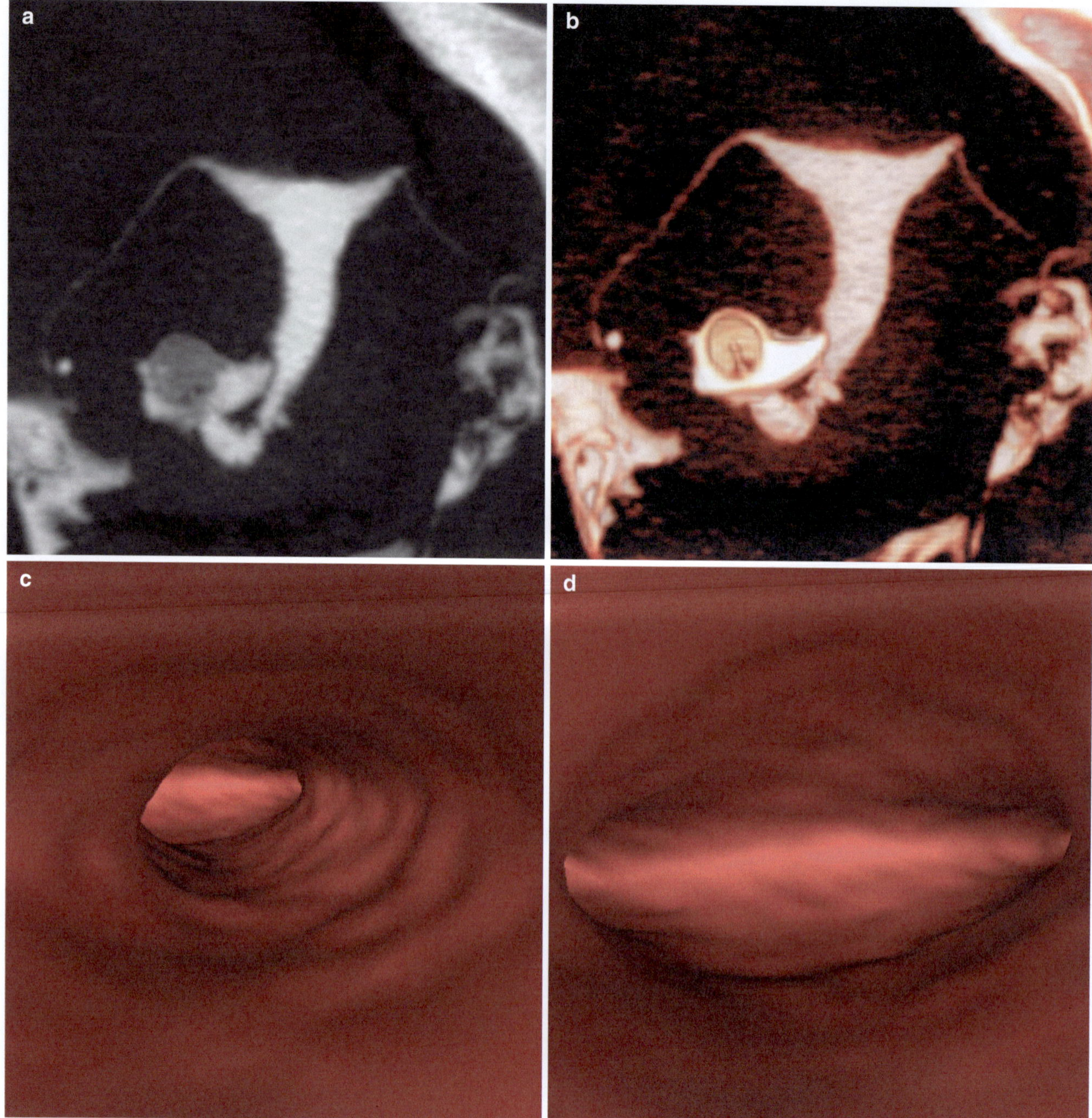

Fig. 2.13 VHSG images obtained with a 64-slice CT scanner with the use of gadolinium. (**a**) Coronal maximum intensity projection image. (**b**) Coronal 3D volume rendering image. (**c**, **d**) Virtual endoscopy images

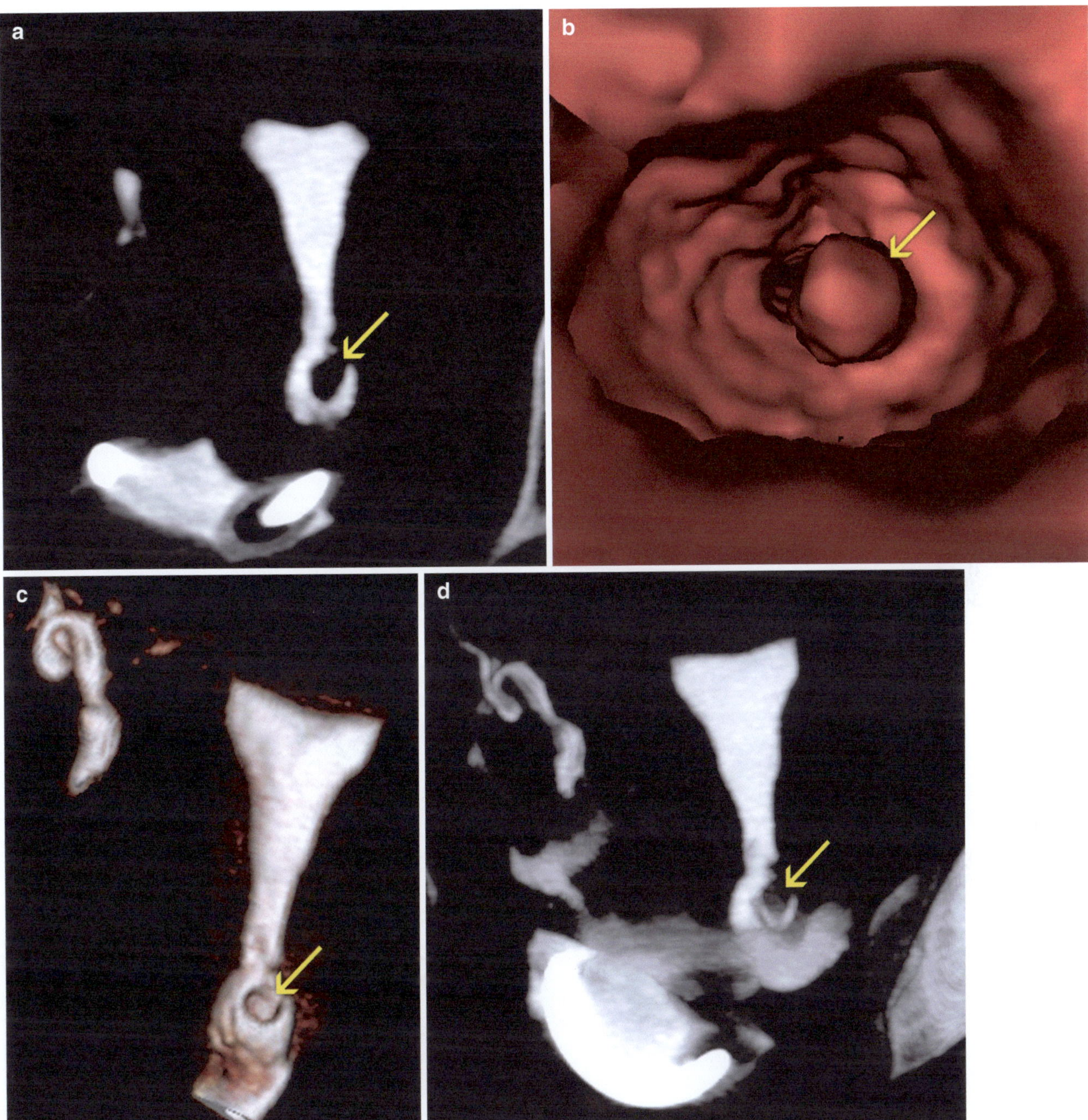

Fig. 2.14 VHSG images obtained with a 256-slice CT scanner. Cervical polyp (*arrows*). Left tubal blockage is also appreciated. (**a**) Coronal multiplanar reconstruction. (**b**) Coronal maximum intensity projection image. (**c**) Coronal 3D volume rendering image. (**d**) Virtual endoscopy image

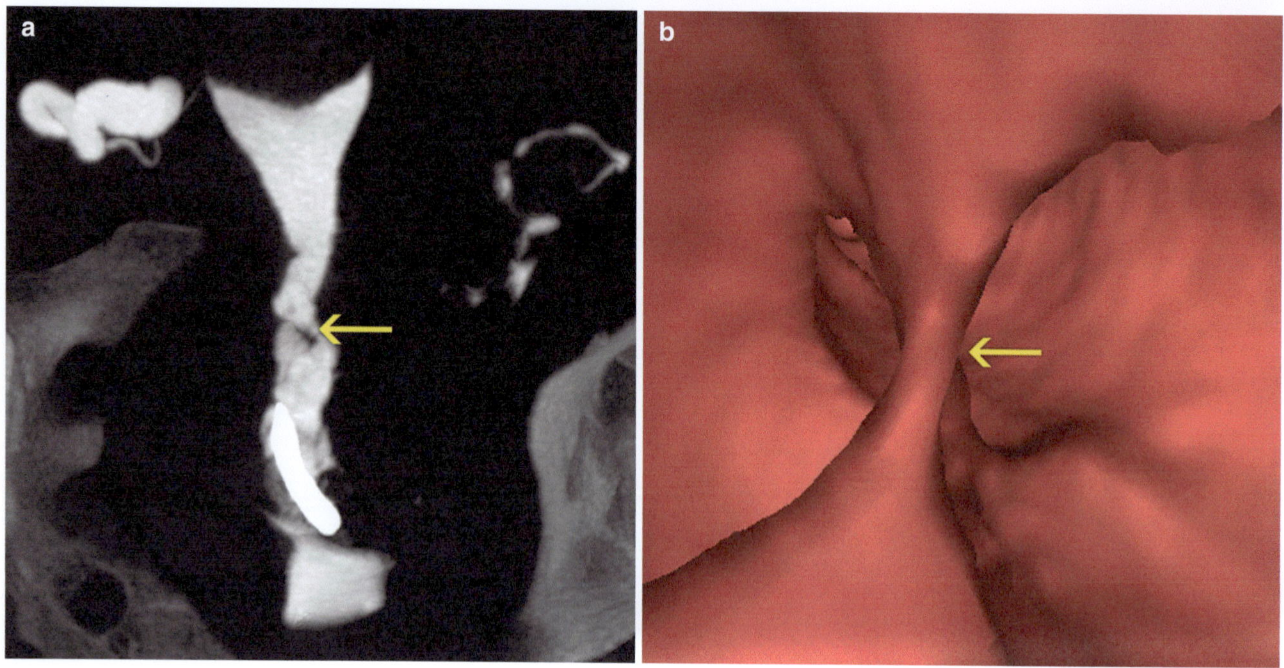

Fig. 2.15 VHSG images obtained with a 256-slice CT scanner. Cervical synechiae (*arrows*). Mild right distal tubal dilatation is also appreciated. (**a**) Coronal maximum intensity projection image. (**b**) Virtual endoscopy image

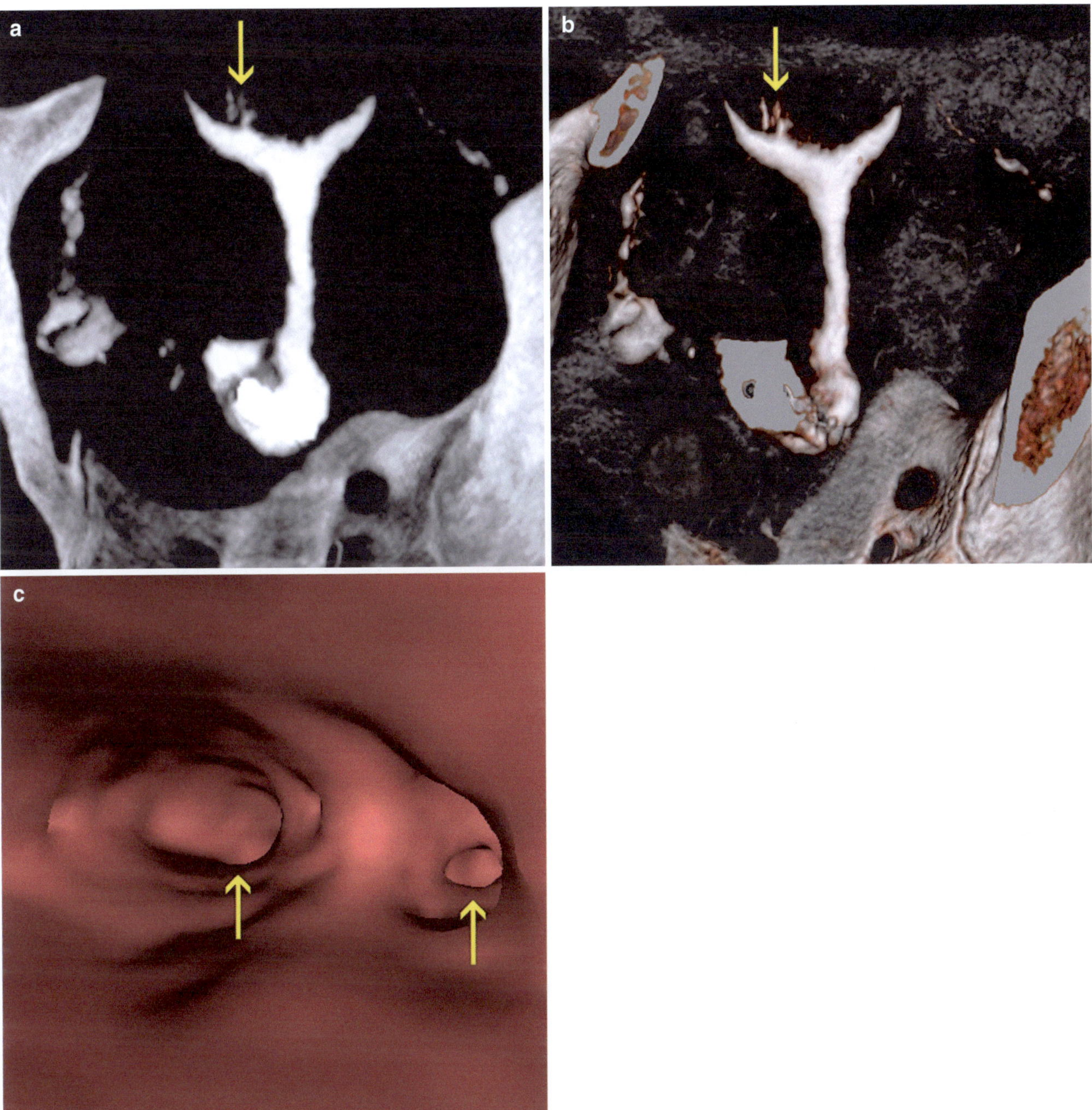

Fig. 2.16 VHSG images obtained with a 256-slice CT scanner. Uterine adenomyosis at the uterine fundus (*arrows*). (**a**) Coronal maximum intensity projection image. (**b**) Coronal 3D volume rendering image. (**c**) Virtual endoscopy image

Conclusion

The technological advances and developments of the procedure have permitted the VHSG to constitute a diagnostic study that offers integral information of the cervix, uterus, Fallopian tubes and extra-gynecologic structures in real time, with scarce discomfort and a minimum radiation dose.

This exam allows the physician to obtain complete and accurate diagnostic information on the female reproductive apparatus in just one step, reserving other complementary studies for more complex diagnostic situations.

References

1. Vining DJ, Gelfand DW, Bechtold RE, et al. Technical feasibility of colon imaging with helical CT and virtual reality. Am J Roentgenol. 1994;62(Suppl):104.
2. Carrascosa P, Capunay C, Ulla M, et al. Elevated gastric lesions: virtual gastroscopy. Abdom Imaging. 2006;31:261–7.
3. Higgins W, Ramaswamy K, Swift R, et al. Virtual bronchoscopy for three-dimensional pulmonary image assessment: state of the art and future needs. Radiographics. 1998;18:761–8.
4. Fenlon H, Bell T, Ahari H, et al. Virtual cystoscopy: early clinical experience. Radiology. 1997;205:272–5.
5. Capuñay C, Carrascosa P, Martín López E, et al. Multidetector CT angiography and virtual angioscopy of the abdomen. Abdom Imaging. 2009;34:81–93.
6. Carrascosa P, Baronio JM, Borghi M, et al. Histerosalpingoscopía virtual. Una técnica novedosa y no invasiva para diagnosticar patología intrauterina. Reproduccion. 2006;21:19–26.
7. Carrascosa P, Capuñay C, Mariano B, et al. Virtual hysteroscopy by multidetector computed tomography. Abdom Imaging. 2008;33: 381–7.
8. Carrascosa P, Baronio M, Capuñay C, et al. Multidetector computed tomography virtual hysterosalpingography in the investigation of the uterus and fallopian tubes. Eur J Radiol. 2008; 67:531–5.
9. Carrascosa P, Baronio M, Capuñay C, et al. Clinical use of 64-row multislice computed tomography hysterosalpingography in the evaluation of female factor infertility. Fertil Steril. 2008;90(5): 1953–8. Rg.
10. Carrascosa P, Capuñay C, Baronio M, et al. 64- Row multidetector CT virtual hysterosalpingography. Abdom Imaging. 2009;34: 121–33.
11. Baronio M, Carrascosa P, Capuñay C, et al. Diagnostic performance of CT virtual hysteroscopy in 69 consecutive patients. Fertil Steril. 2010;94(Supplement):S77.
12. Carrascosa P, Capuñay C, Vallejos J, et al. Virtual Hysterosalpingography: a new multidetector CT technique for evaluating the female reproductive system. Radiographics. 2010;30:643–61.
13. Carrascosa P, Merletti PG, Capuñay C, et al. New approach to noninvasive coronary angiography by multidetector computed tomography: initial experience using gadolinium. J Comput Assist Tomogr. 2007;31:441–3.
14. Carrascosa P, Capuñay C, Bettinotti M, et al. Feasibility of gadolinium-diethylene triamine pentaacetic acid enhanced multidetector computed tomography for the evaluation of coronary artery disease. J Cardiovasc Comput Tomogr. 2007;1:86–94.
15. Carrascosa P, Capuñay C, Vallejos J, et al. Gadolinium vs iodine virtual hysterosalpingography: an alternative for allergic patients? Fertil Steril. 2008;90(Supplement S157):S1–528.
16. Vardhanabhuti V, Loader R, Roobottom CA. Assessment of image quality on effects of varying tube voltage and automatic tube current modulation with hybrid and pure iterative reconstruction techniques in abdominal/pelvic CT: a phantom study. Invest Radiol. 2013;48:167–74.

The VHSG is a novel non invasive diagnostic modality which allows a complete evaluation of the gynecologic system (cervix, uterus and Fallopian tubes) in a single study [1–5]. It is performed with multislice computed tomography (MSCT) that obtains volumetric acquisitions in few seconds. Images can then be post-processed on diverse planes without loss of definition [6–8]. The MSCT achieves the concept of isotropy where, despite the acquisition of the image on the axial plane, it can evaluate the anatomy or the pathology in any other plane with similar image quality [9, 10] (Fig. 3.1).

VHSG needs multislice CT of 64 or more rows to acquire the images in less than 5 s. The objective of the study is to analyze all of the gynecologic system: cervix, uterus and Fallopian tubes. The structures most difficult to assess are the Fallopian tubes due to the fact that they are philliform and require optimum contrast distention during scanning to be evaluated. They opacify and empty very quickly, so it is essential that the scanning last the shortest time possible.

The VHSG study, provides useful information of the gynecologic apparatus and, simultaneously, evaluates intrapelvic structures (Fig. 3.2).

The way the study is performed is detailed in the present chapter. It consists in:

- Preparation of the patient before the study.
- Preparation of the patient during the study.
- Technical parameters
- Ways of reprocessing and analyzing the information.
- Final report on findings and presentation of the study to the referring physician.
- Complications.
- Patient's acceptance and discomfort to the VHSG study.

Preparation of the Patient Before the Study

A similar preparation to the conventional hysterosalpingography (HSG) procedure is required. A fact that stands out is that, being the VHSG a non invasive technique that does not require clamping the uterine cervix, a prophylactic treatment with antibiotics is not necessary.

The indications against carrying out the VHSG include pregnancy and active pelvic infection.

The study is performed between the 6th and 11th day of the menstrual cycle to avoid the interruption of any possible pregnancy. From the interruption of the menstrual bleeding until 48 h after the study, the patient must abstain from sexual intercourse.

Preparation of the Patient During the Study

The patient lies down on the CT table in the gynecologic position (Fig. 3.3).

The perineum is cleansed with Povidone-Iodine solution and sterilized gauze. Later, a speculum is placed at the vaginal level so as to have access the external cervical orifice which is also sanitized with sterilized gauze and Povidone-Iodine solution [4].

A digital explorer radiography is carried out (Scout View) previous to the study acquisition (Fig. 3.4). A plastic cannula of 10 F is placed in the external cervical orifice (Fig. 3.5) and approximately 15 ml of a mix of contrast and physiological solution of 70 % is instilled. The solution is applied with an injector pump at a speed of 0.3 ml/s (Fig. 3.6). The aim of doing it automatically is achieving a constant and smooth speed and pressure which reduces the discomfort during the procedure and assures an optimal uterine distention.

The acquisition initiates 30 s after beginning the contrast instillation.

As mentioned before, CT scanners of 64 or more rows that acquire images in less than 5 s are necessary to carry out the VHSG studies. CT scanners with lower number of detectors rows acquire studies in more prolonged times, of 10–12 s approximately, making the correct evaluation of the Fallopian tubes almost impossible in many cases.

The MSCT units of 256 or 320 detectors rows perform this technique in only 1.5 s, transforming this modality into

P. Carrascosa et al., *CT Virtual Hysterosalpingography*,
DOI 10.1007/978-3-319-07560-0_3, © Springer International Publishing Switzerland 2014

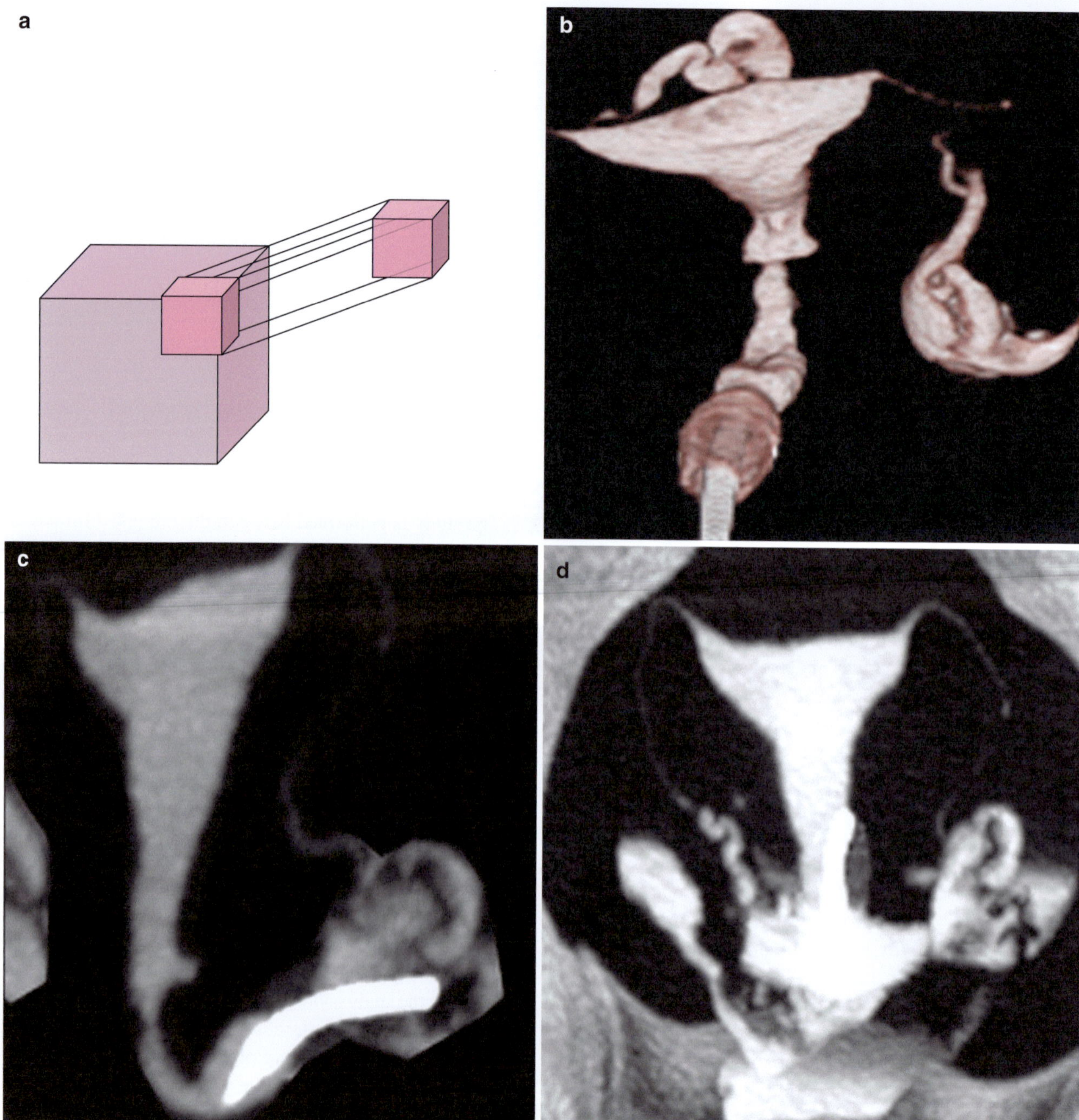

Fig. 3.1 MSCT isotropic reconstruction. (**a**) The cube represents the acquired volume of the CT scan. The axial CT acquisition obtained with a thin slice thickness and 50 % image overlapping enables to reconstruct the CT data in any plane without loss of resolution. This is known as isotropy. (**b**) 3D volume rendering image. It exhibits the neck, uterine silhouette and Fallopian tubes. (**c**, **d**) Maximum intensity projection (MIP) images that show the gynecologic apparatus in its totality with this three-dimensional format. The MIP images identify very well the uterine tubes. (**e**, **f**) Virtual endoscopy images display endoluminal views of the isthmic and cervical region and the uterine fundus

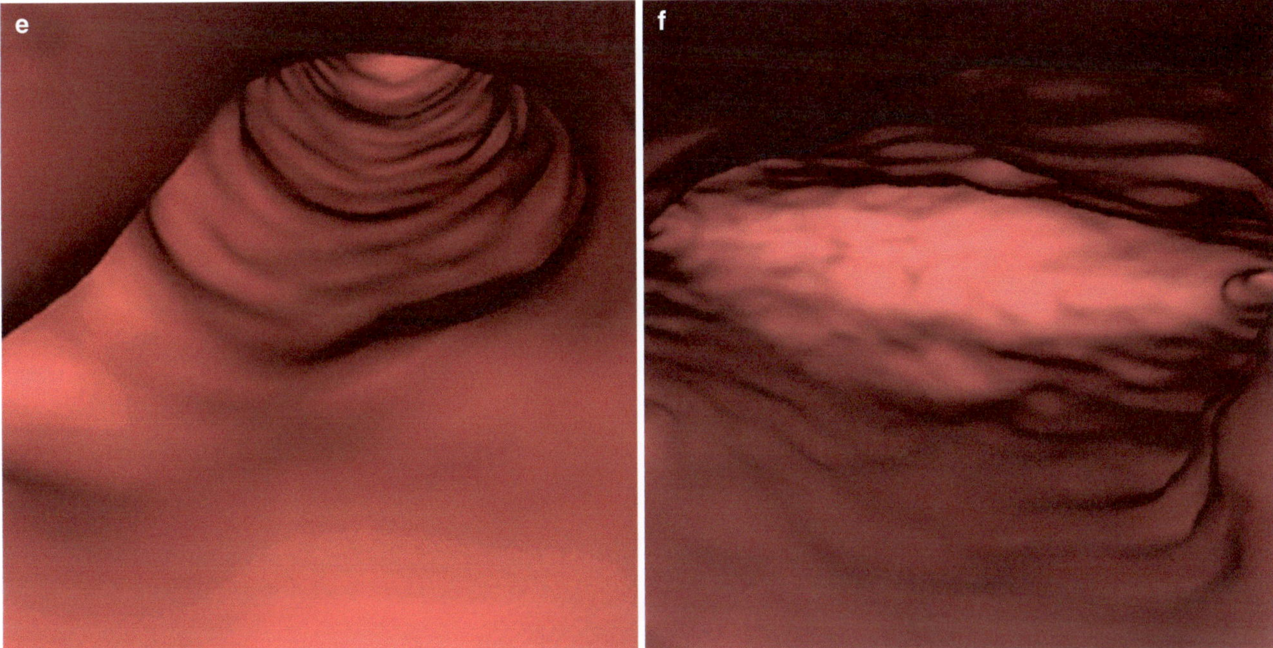

Fig. 3.1 (continued)

a real time study because it can show the contrast passing from the ampullary region to the perineum [11–13] (Fig. 3.7), transforming this modality into a real time study.

Technical Parameters to Use on the Units

The technical parameters used depend on the CT scanner used (Table 3.1).

An automatic tube current modulation which reduces the radiation dose is used during the study. Furthermore, new scanners allow the so called iterative reconstruction that helps further diminish the radiation dose, without losing the image quality [14].

Once acquired, the images are transferred to a workstation where diverse types of reconstructions are carried out.

Ways of Reprocessing and Analyzing the Information

Various post-processing algorithms that consist of multi-plane reconstructions, maximum intensity projection (MIP) reconstructions, volume rendering reconstructions and endo-scopic views (EV) are used [15, 16].

Multiplanar Reconstructions

Coronary, sagittal and oblique reconstructions with soft tissue windows allow the evaluation of the cervix, uterus, Fallopian tubes and extra- uterine structures (Figs. 3.8 and 3.9).

The curve multiplanar reconstructions are able to display, in only one plane, all of the gynecological apparatus, avoid-ing the superposition of anatomical structures and allowing a detailed evaluation of them in a single plane (Fig. 3.10).

Measurements of the polyps, myomas, etc. are carried out on bidimensional images, since they provide the most preci-sion [17–19].

Maximum Intensity Projection Images

This post-processing method is used to obtain images of the cervix, uterus and the Fallopian tubes in shades of gray, in a tridimensional format. It provides excellent anatomical detail, especially of the Fallopian tubes.

Normal tubes are slim and difficult to evaluate in axial or bidimensional images (Fig. 3.11). This reprocessing method easily identifies the diverse ampullar pathologies (Fig. 3.12), hydrosalpinx (Fig. 3.13), unilateral tubal occlusion (Fig. 3.14) or bilateral tubal occlusion (Fig. 3.15).

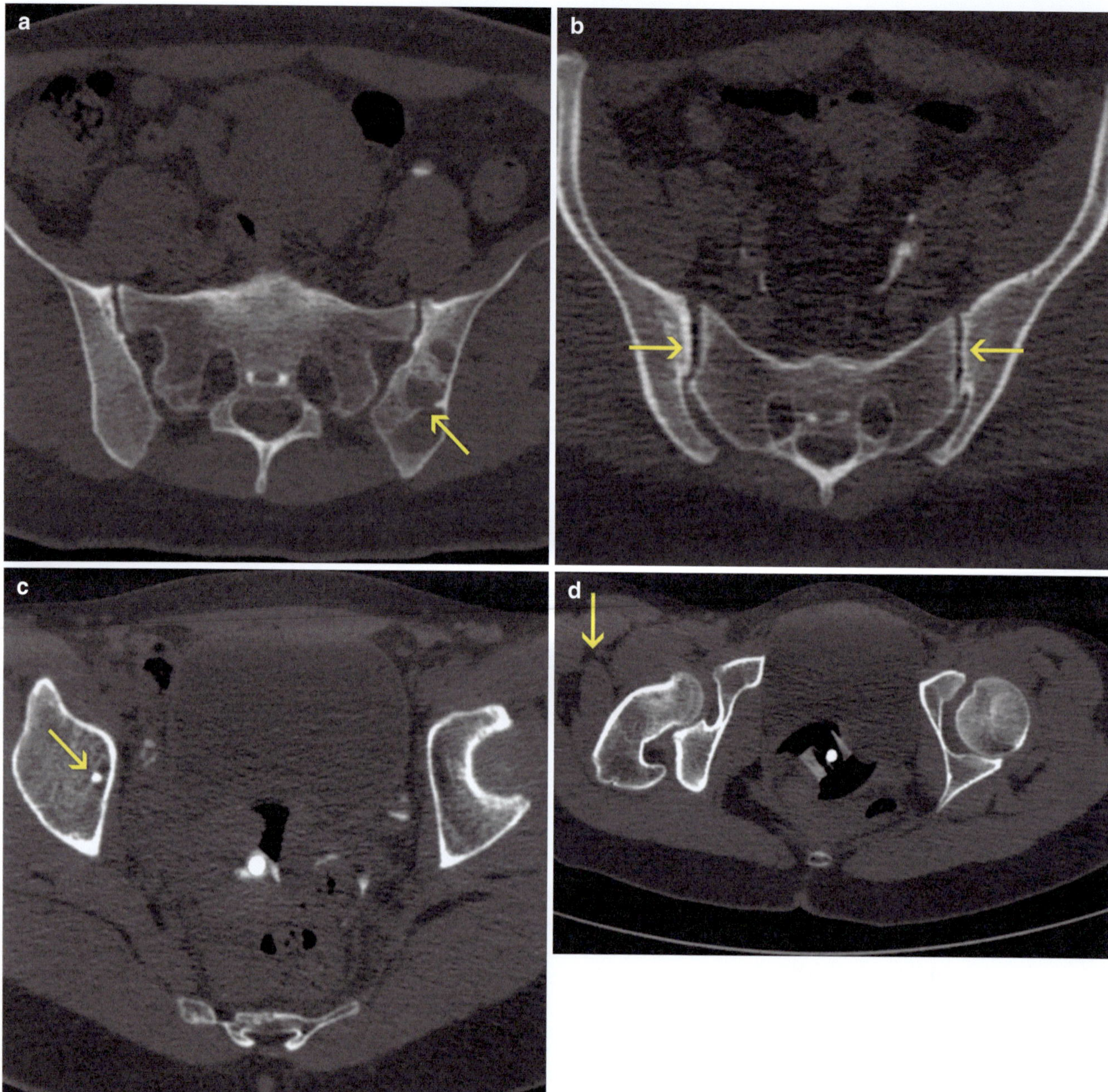

Fig. 3.2 Associated findings. The VHSG study permits the evaluation of the intra-pelvic extra-gynecologic structures, offering complementary information. The findings can be of diverse etiology. (**a**) Osteolytic lesion in the left iliac bone (*arrow*). (**b**) Bilateral sacroiliac arthrosis (*arrow*). (**c**) Bone island on right acetabular roof (*arrow*). (**d**) Muscular atrophy in right pelvic region (*arrow*)

Fig. 3.3 Patient's position on the CT table to perform the VHSG study

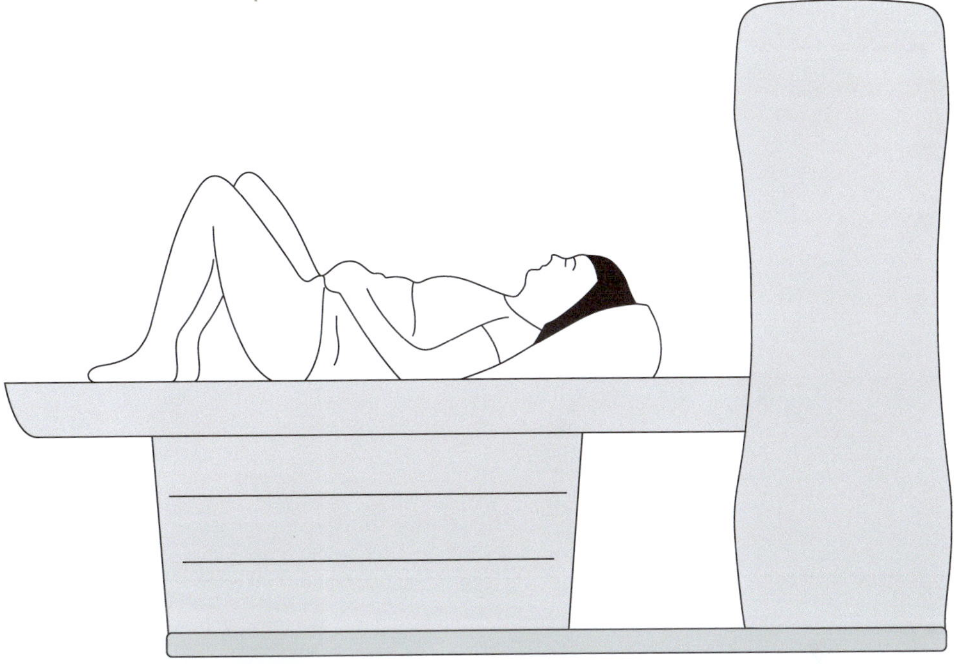

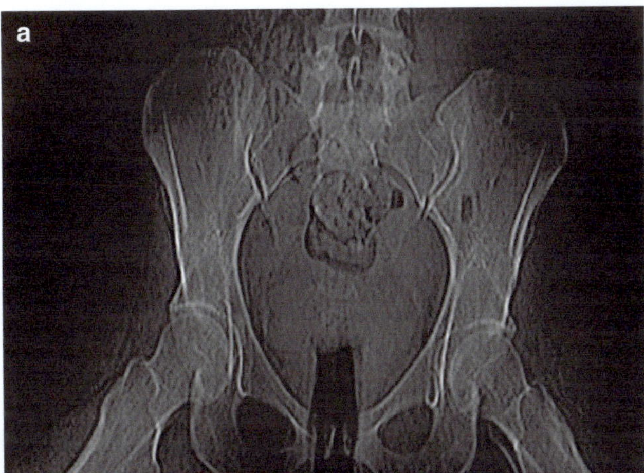

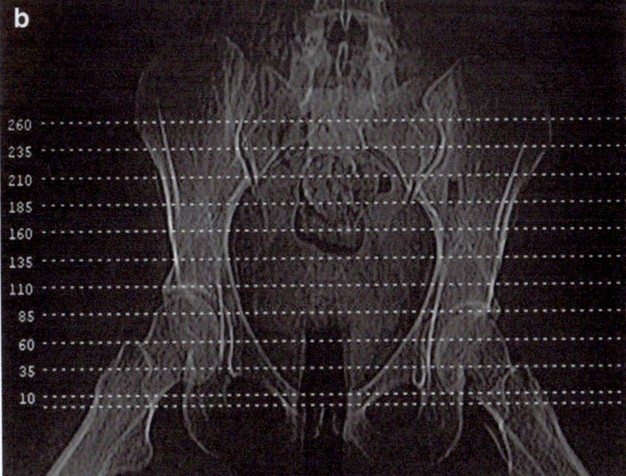

Fig. 3.4 (**a**) Scout view of the pelvis. (**b**) Scout view with the subsequent CT examination planned

Fig. 3.5 10F cannula utilized in the VHSG study

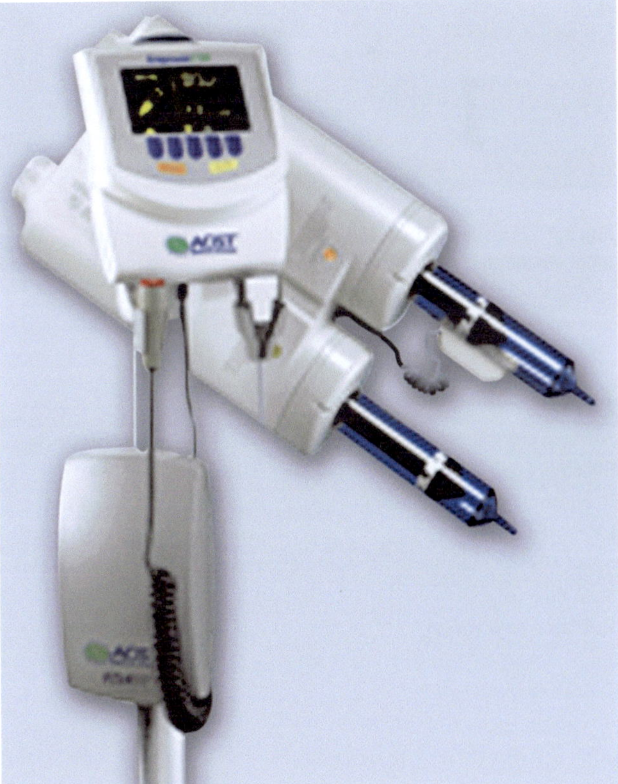

Fig. 3.6 Injector pump for automatic contrast administration

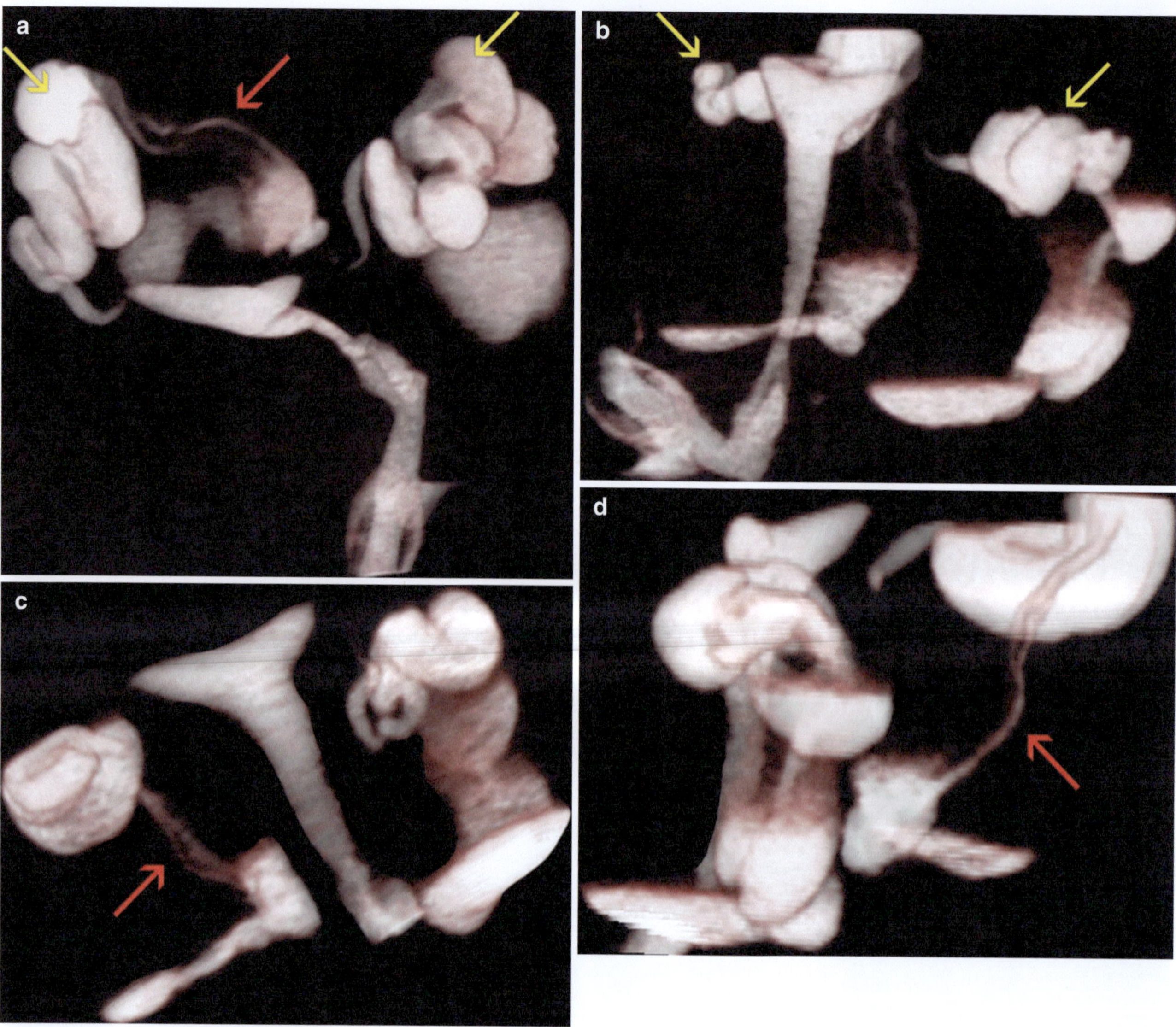

Fig. 3.7 256-slice VHSG study in real time. (**a–d**) Volume rendering images in different views that show a uterus of normal morphology. Bilateral tubal dilatation (*yellow arrows*) with contrast spillage into the peritoneal cavity (*red arrows*)

Table 3.1 Technical parameters of VHSG according to CT scanner

Scanner	64-slice	256-slice
Slice thickness (mm)	0.9	0.625
Reconstruction interval (mm)	0.45	0.3
kV	80–100	80–100
mAs	100–150	100–150
Scan time (s)	3.2	1.5
Radiation dose (mSv)	0.6	0.3

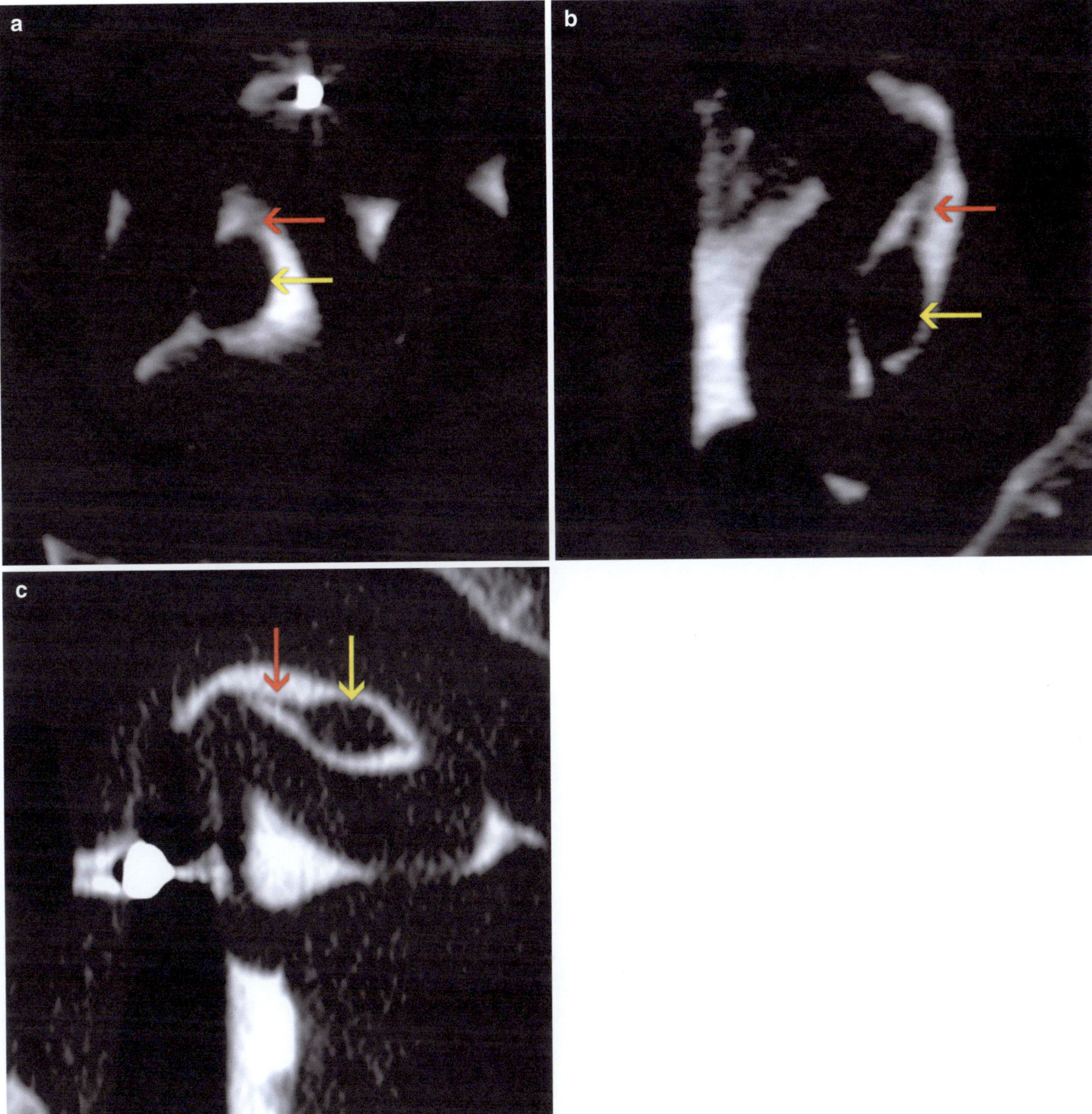

Fig. 3.8 Multiplanar reconstruction (MPR) images. Endometrial stalked polyp. (**a**) Magnified axial image of retroverted uterus which shows a stalked polyp. The head (*yellow arrow*) and the stalk (*red arrow*) of the polyp that extends to the cervix can be clearly observed. (**b**) Oblique MPR image. (**c**) Sagittal MPR image

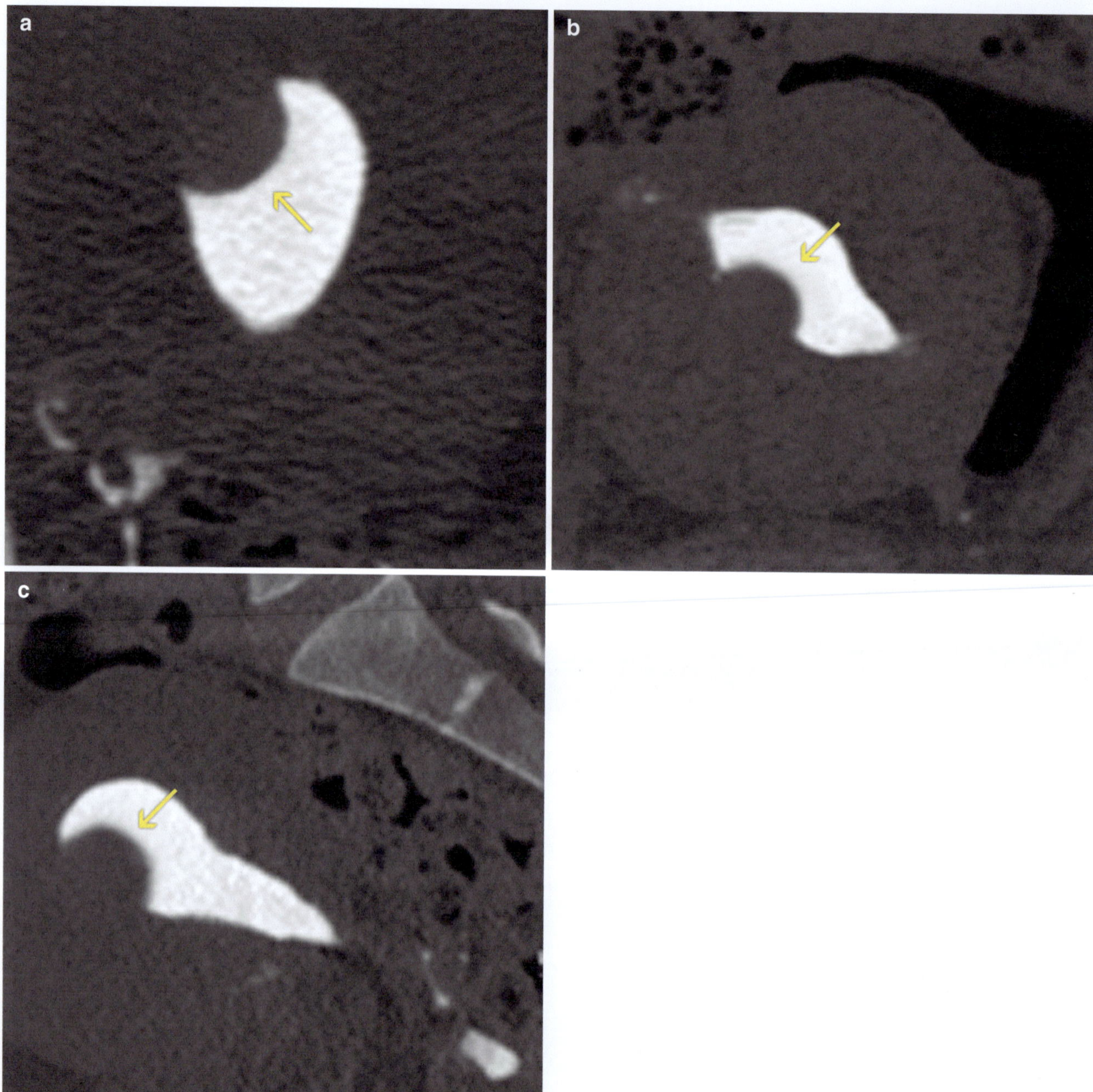

Fig. 3.9 Multiplanar reconstruction (MPR) images of submucosal myoma with endocavitary projection (*arrows*). (**a**) Axial image that exhibits an elevated lesion which projects from the right lateral wall towards the uterine cavity compatible with submucosal myoma. (**b**) Coronal MPR image. (**c**) Sagittal MPR image

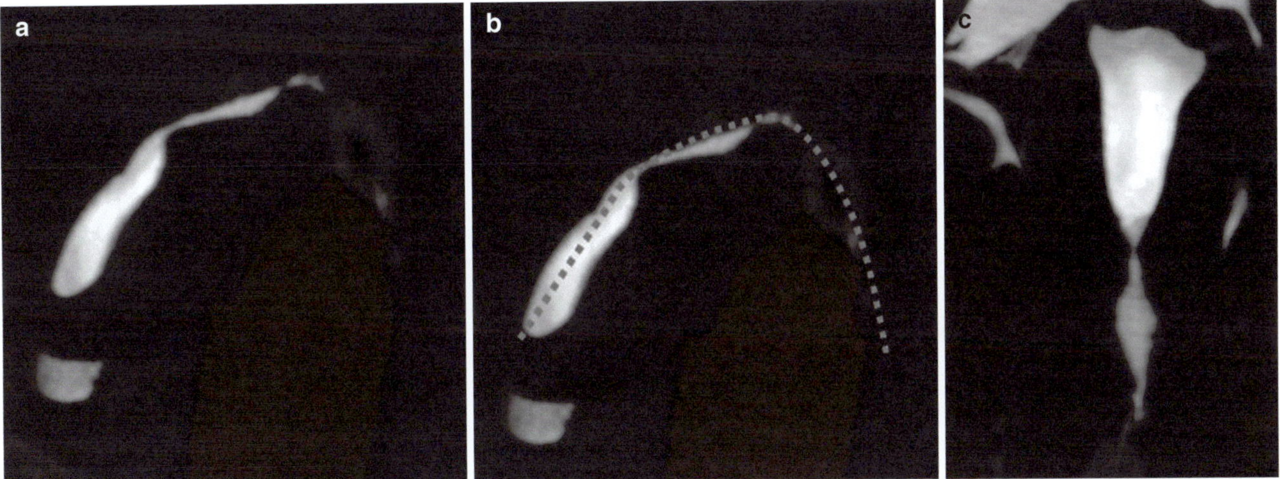

Fig. 3.10 Curved multiplanar reconstruction (cMPR) image of the cervix, uterus and tubes. (**a**) A sagittal multiplanar reconstruction image shows an anteverted uterus. (**b**) A line is traced through the central axis of the cervix and uterus to display the gynecologic apparatus in a single plane with no superposition of the anatomical structures. (**c**) cMPR image which shows the gynecological apparatus displayed bidimensionally

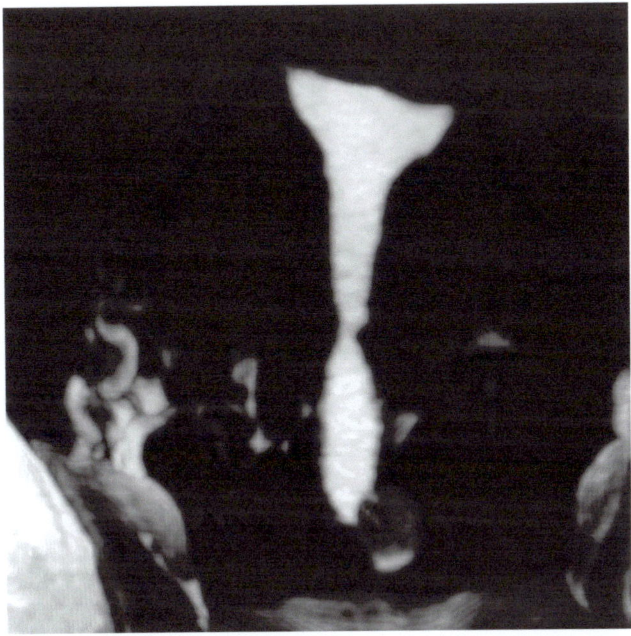

Fig. 3.11 Maximum intensity projection image of normal uterine tubes. Tubes are easily visualized despite their thin caliber

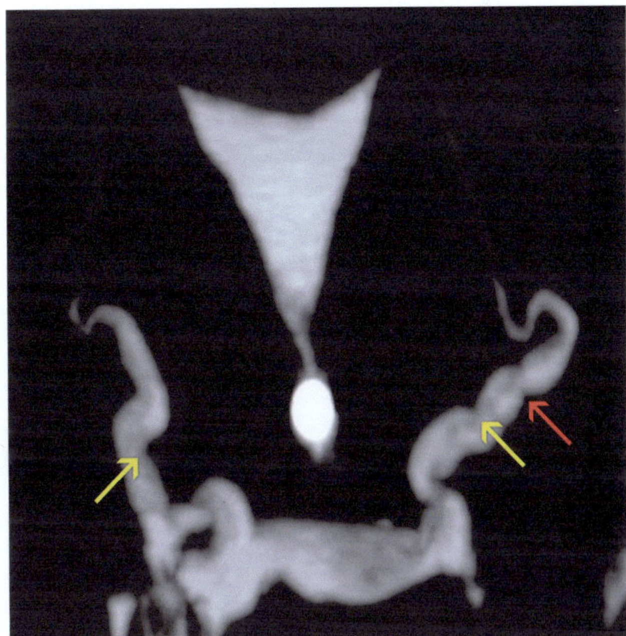

Fig. 3.12 Maximum intensity projection image of uterine tubes. Bilateral ampulla dilatation is observed (*yellow arrows*) with thick folds in their lumen (*red arrow*)

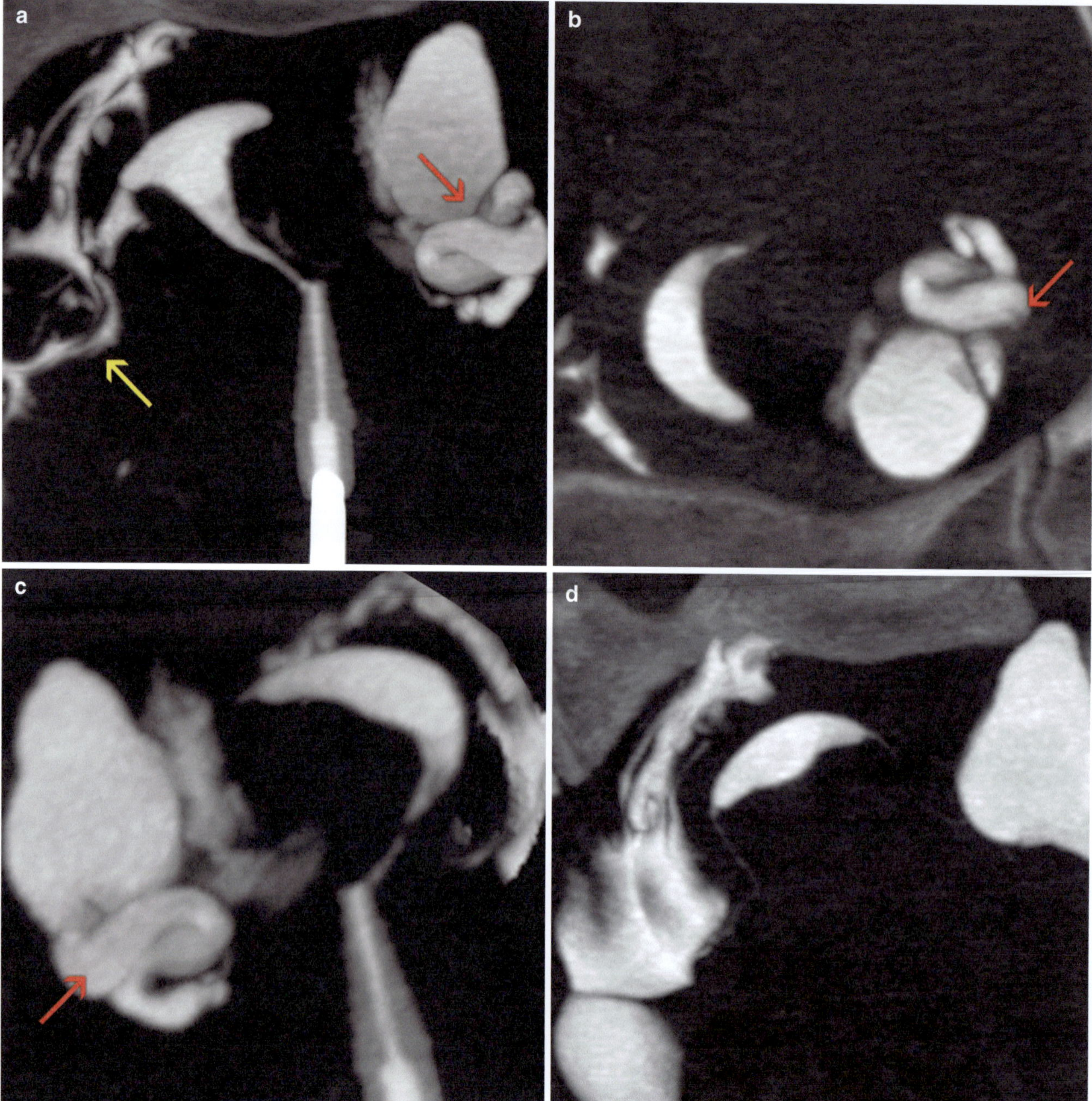

Fig. 3.13 Left hydrosalpinx. (**a–d**) Maximum intensity projection images in different views that show a normal right Fallopian tube (*yellow arrow*) and a dilated left tube (*red arrow*)

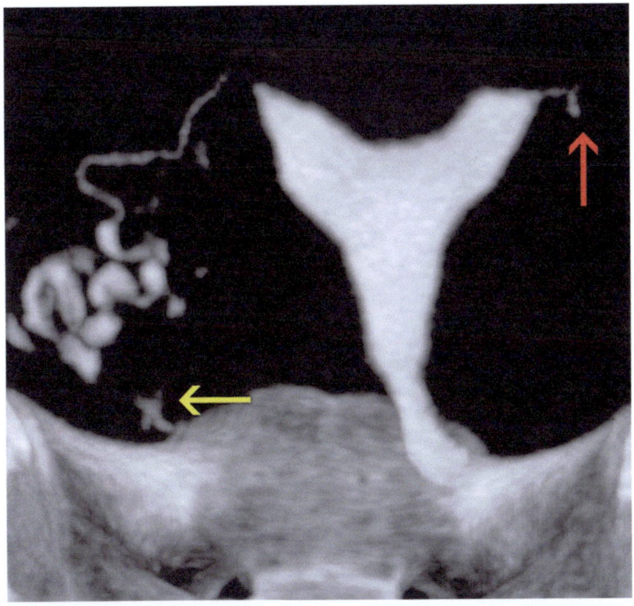

Fig. 3.14 Unilateral tubal occlusion. Maximum intensity projection image of arcuate uterus. Normal right uterine tube with spillage of contrast into the peritoneal cavity (*yellow arrow*). The left uterine tube is occluded (*red arrow*)

Nevertheless, this post-processing technique is not useful in the detection of intrauterine lesions, which require other reprocessing methods (Fig. 3.16).

3D Volume Rendering Reconstructions

This reconstruction provides tridimensional views of the gynecologic system with a window which recognizes the endoluminal contrast. It detects a wide range of pathologies, such as stenosis, parietal irregularities, polyps and hydrosalpinx. It also permits the confirmation of suspicious lesions in other forms of evaluation (Figs. 3.17, 3.18, 3.19 and 3.20).

Virtual Endoscopy

This reprocessing algorithm complements the previous ones, allows the confirmation of findings in the previously mentioned post processing modalities, and also provides intra-luminal information similar to a conventional hysteroscopy study [20].

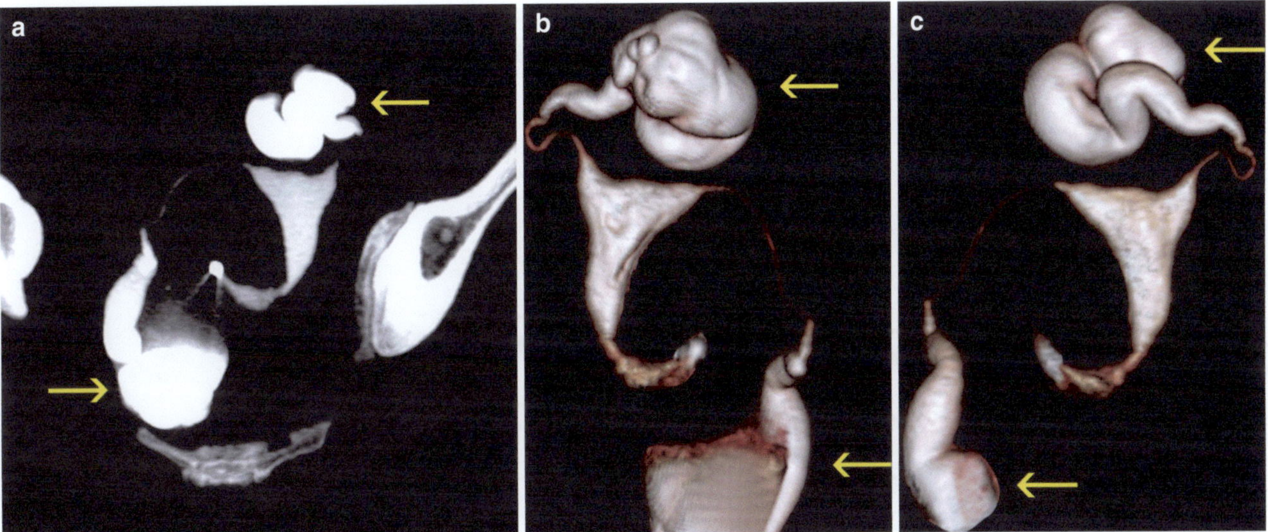

Fig. 3.15 (**a**) Left hydrosalpinx. Maximum intensity projection image which shows bilateral hydrosalpinx with absence of spillage of contrast into the peritoneal cavity – negative Cotte test (*arrows*). (**b**, **c**) Volume rendering images in different views which show similar findings (*arrows*)

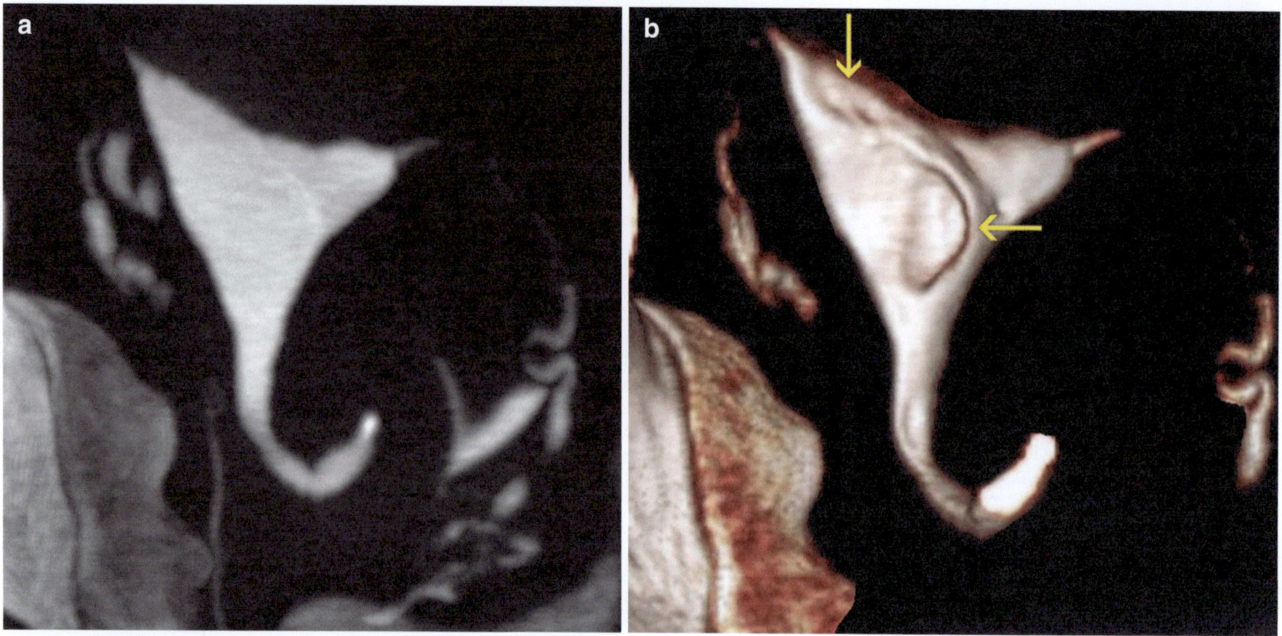

Fig. 3.16 Submucosal myoma: maximum intensity projection (MIP) versus volume rendering (VR) evaluation. (**a**) MIP image of the uterus without evidence of pathology. (**b**) VR image displays two images of filling defect in the uterine cavity (*arrows*) not identifiable in the MIP image

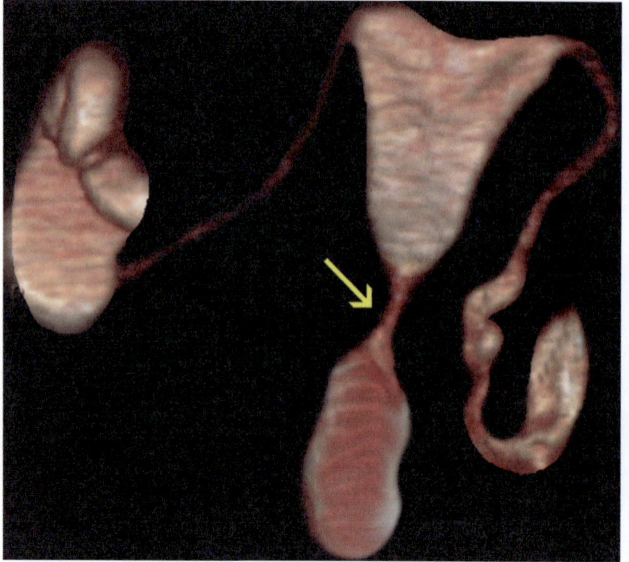

Fig. 3.17 Volume rendering image of cervical stenosis. A diffuse narrowing of the endocervical canal is observed (*arrow*)

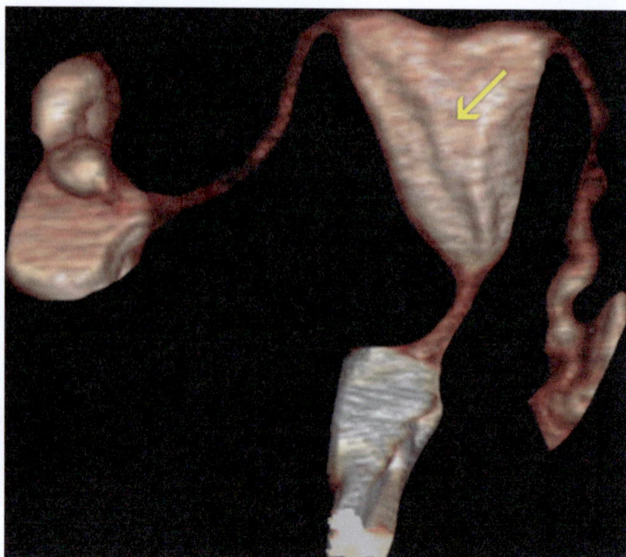

Fig. 3.18 Volume rendering image of uterine wall irregularities. Irregular uterine margins secondary to thick myometrial folds (*arrow*)

The images can have different orientations. They can be viewed from the cervix towards the uterine fundus or vice versa (Figs. 3.21). It is central to always check the orientation indicator which is shown on the bottom left margin which indicates the image's position and orientation.

Final Report on Findings and Presentation of the Study to the Referring Physician

The images are saved fixed and in movie format, which allows one to view the navigation in movement. Hence, a CD and printed images are sent.

Complications

The number of complications in a VHSG study is low due to the fact it is a non invasive technique which does not require cervical clamping or uterine traction, and therefore the chance of bleeding is null.

The risk of infection is also considerably reduced. Since 2006, a total of 11,500 cases have been studied and we have had not a single case of bleeding or infection.

Minor complications like extravasations of the contrast to venous plexus are more common but, usually when this finding is observed, it is not associated with symptomatology in the patient. The extravasations can be small, moderate or extensive (Figs. 3.22 and 3.23). In only a low percentage of cases may it be related to an allergic reaction. We have had a 5 % of patients with extravasations of the contrast and in only one case did we observe a mild allergic reaction that was reversed with corticoid agents. To reduce the risk of allergy, it is useful to use a hypo-osmolar contrast, and in

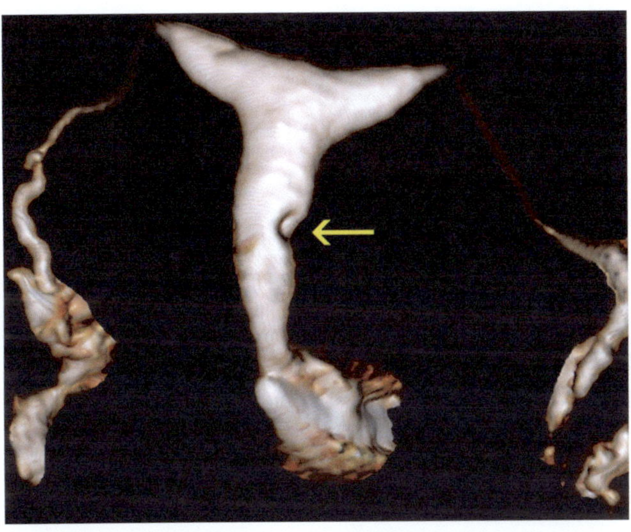

Fig. 3.19 Volume rendering image of an endometrial polyp. An elevated lesion is observed on the left lateral uterine wall (*arrow*)

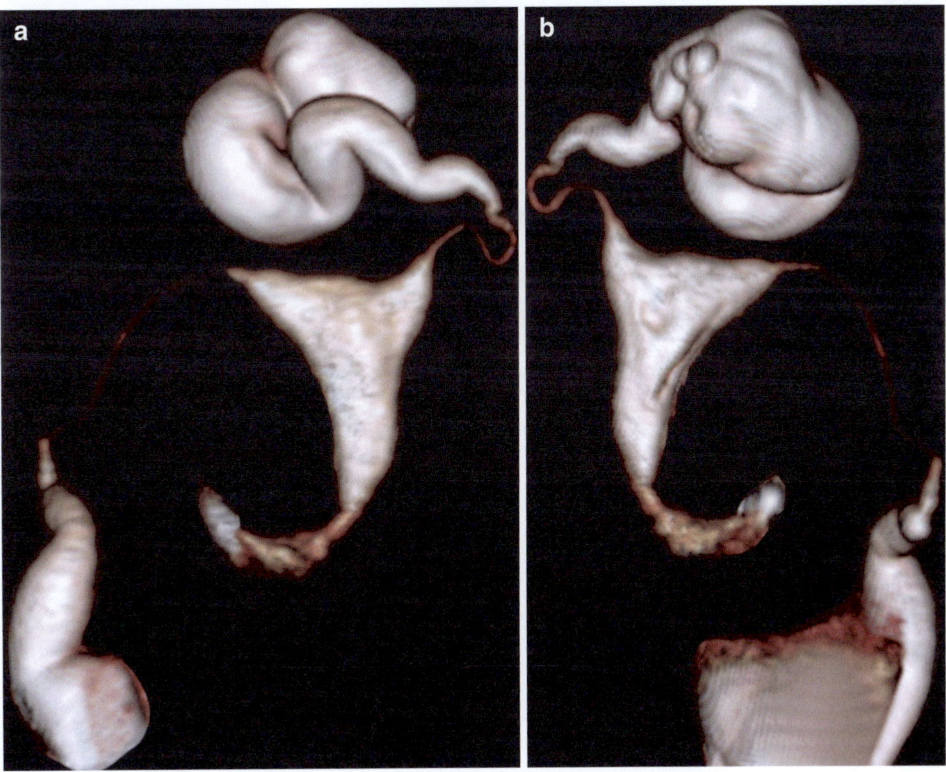

Fig. 3.20 (**a**, **b**) Volume rendering images of bilateral hydrosalpinx

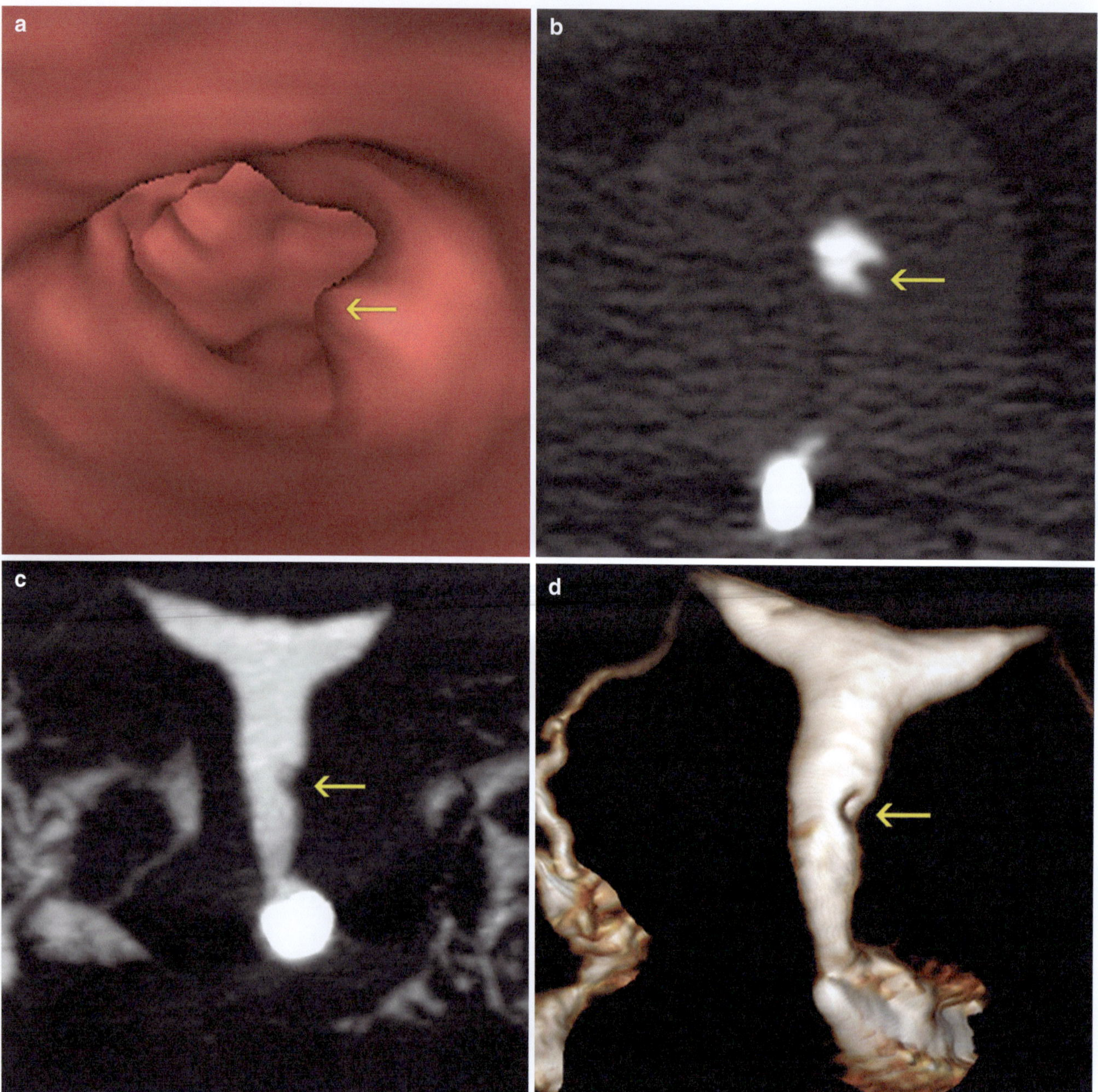

Fig. 3.21 Endometrial polyp (*arrows*). (**a**) Virtual endoscopy image that shows an elevated lesion compatible with an endometrial polyp. This finding is corroborated with other reprocessing formats. (**b**) Axial CT image. (**c**) Maximum intensity projection image. (**d**) Volume rendering image

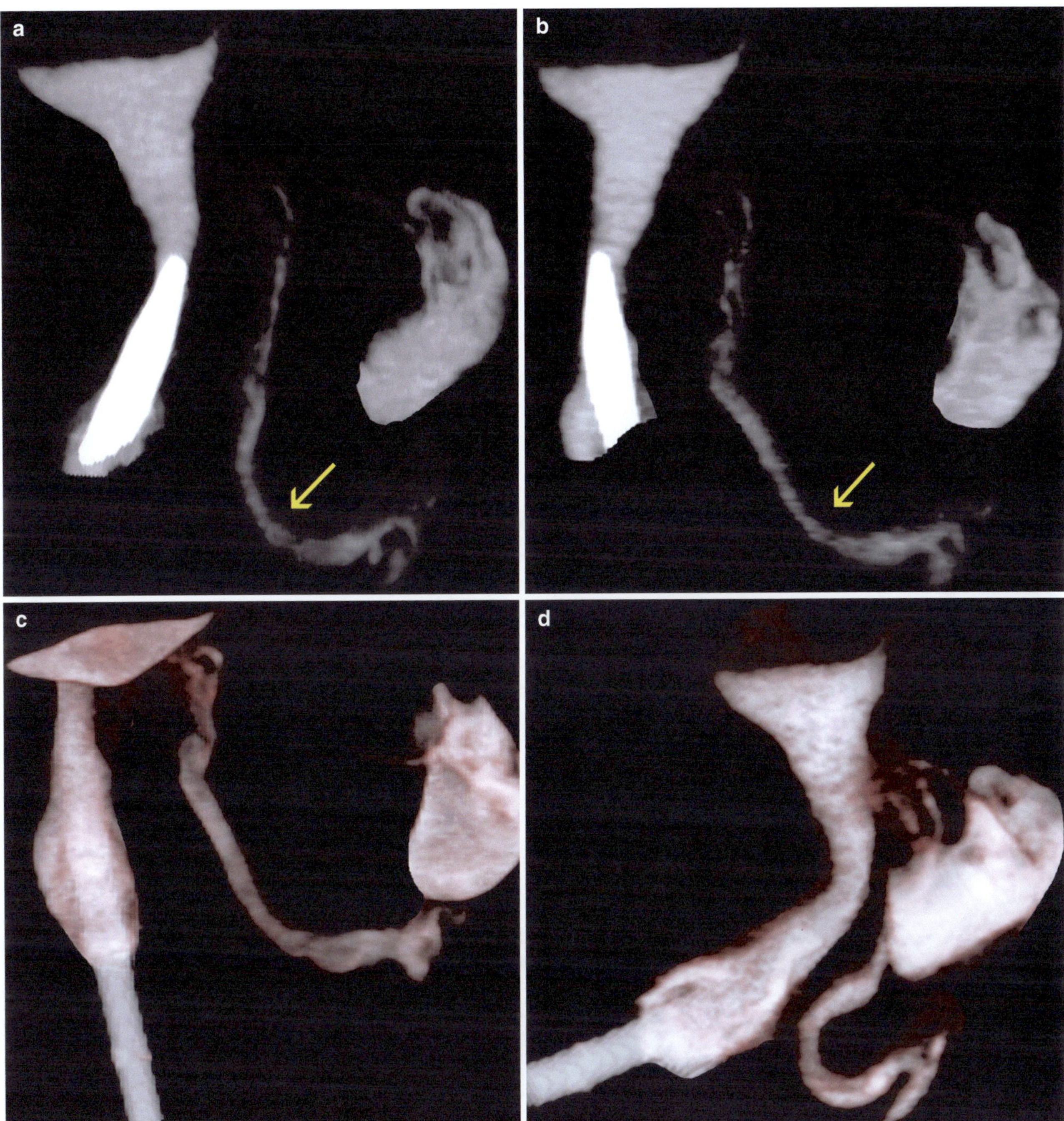

Fig. 3.22 Moderate contrast venous intravasation during a VHSG procedure (*arrow*). (**a**, **b**) Maximum intensity projection images. (**c**, **d**) Volume rendering images

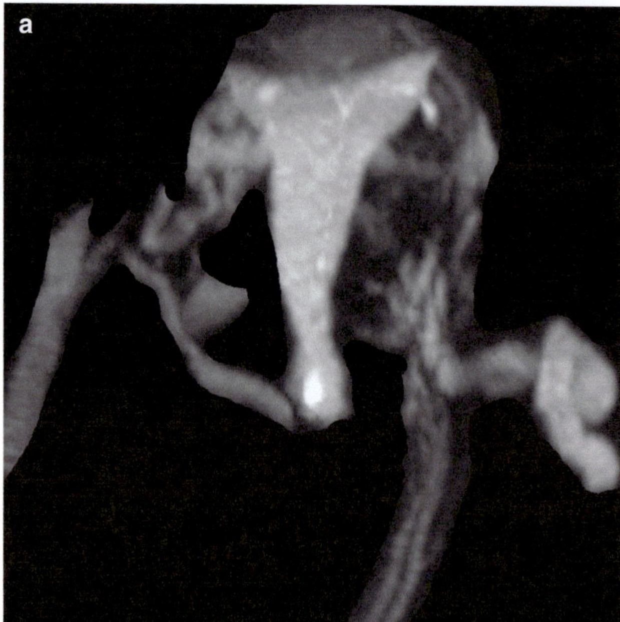

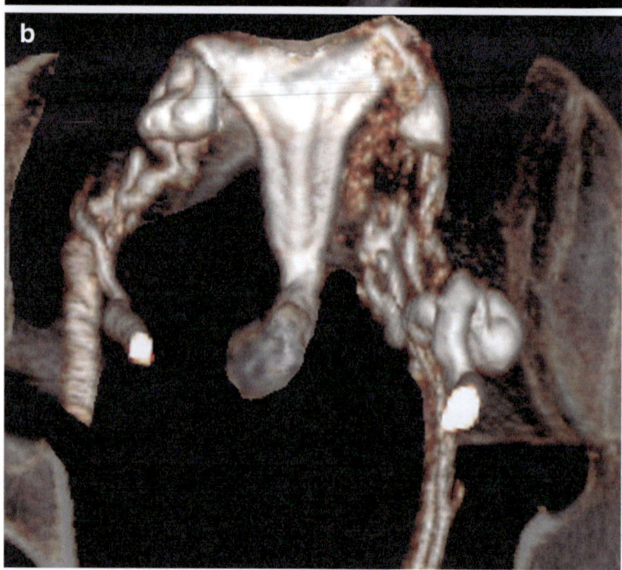

Fig. 3.23 Severe contrast venous intravasation during a VHSG procedure. (**a**) Maximum intensity projection image. (**b**) Volume rendering image

known cases of allergy to iodine, gadolinium (paramagnetic contrast which does not produce allergy). See Chap. 13. Gadolinium is not routinely utilized because of its higher costs compared with the iodine contrast.

Patients' Acceptance and Discomfort to the VHSG Study

The patients have accepted this new diagnostic technique due to the fact that it is pretty well tolerated and in the majority of cases, produces a slight or directly no discomfort, in comparison with other diagnostic techniques which are more bothersome like the HSG [21, 22] and the sonohysterography [23].

In the case of the HSG, it is required that the uterine neck be clamped and pulled with the aim of spreading the overlapped anatomical structures. When carrying out the clamp and pull, pain is generated, and at the same time, complications like bleeding or infection are plausible.

In the sonohysterography, a catheter ball is introduced in the uterine neck and is insufflated to occlude the uterine cavity so as to allow its study. Said catheter generates pains in the patient and makes difficult the evaluation because the ball is located in the area of study.

Since October of 2006, we have performed a total of 11,500 VHSG studies. The patients were questioned and they completed a form to inform us on the level of discomfort experienced by them during the VHSG study.

The discomfort was classified in levels:

- Level 0: no discomfort.
- Level I: slight discomfort
- Level II: moderate discomfort.
- Level III: severe discomfort.
- Level IV: intolerable discomfort.

Most of the patients (81 %) did not inform any type of pain; 11 % said they experienced slight discomfort; 4.5 % moderate; 2.5 % severe and 1 % intolerable.

It is worth stating that the patients who had been subject to previous conventional HSG studies had a better acceptance for the virtual study than those who were experiencing the diagnostic method for the first time. The reason for this could be higher expectations for the new method and the impossibility of comparison with the conventional technique.

Conclusion

The VHSG is a diagnostic modality which permits the evaluation of the totality of the female gynecologic apparatus in only one study. A correct preparation, respecting the adequate days to perform the study, an adequate acquisition technique utilizing multislice scanners of 64 or more detectors rows and an interpretation by trained physicians in the analysis of these images, make this technique an integrated procedure of extreme value in the study of the infertile woman.

The combined and systemized analysis of the axial images, the multiplanar reconstructions, the tridimensional images in maximum projection intensity (volume rendering), along with the virtual endoscopy, allow the achievement of the best diagnostic outcome, facilitating the recognition of normal anatomy and pathological processes, diminishing the number of errors.

References

1. Carrascosa P, Baronio M, Capuñay C, et al. Multidetector computed tomography virtual hysterosalpingography in the investigation of the uterus and fallopian tubes. Clinical Imaging. 2009;33:165.
2. Carrascosa P, Capuñay C, Mariano B, et al. Virtual hysteroscopy by multidetector computed tomography. Abdom Imaging. 2008;33(4):381–7.
3. Carrascosa P, Capuñay C, Baronio M, et al. 64- Row multidetector CT virtual hysterosalpingography. Abdom Imaging. 2009;34: 121–33.
4. Carrascosa P, Capuñay C, Vallejos J, et al. Virtual hysterosalpingography: a new multidetector CT technique for evaluating the female reproductive system. Radiographics. 2010;30:643–61.
5. Carrascosa P, Capuñay C, Vallejos J, et al. Virtual hysterosalpingography: experience with over 1000 consecutive patients. Abdom Imaging. 2011;36(1):1–14.
6. Hsieh J. Computed tomography. Bellingham: SPIE; 2003. p. 1–12.
7. Hu H, He HD, Foley WD, et al. Four multidetector row helical CT: image quality and volume coverage speed. Radiology. 2000;215:55–62.
8. Mahesh M, Scatarige JC, Cooper J, et al. Dose and pitch relationship for isotropic resolution in CT from conventional through multiple-row detector. Radiographics. 2002;22:949–62.
9. Kulama E. Scanning protocols for multislice CT scanners. Br J Radiol. 2004;77:S2–9.
10. Mc Collough CH, Zink FE. Performance evaluation of a multi-slice CT system. Med Phys. 1999;26:2223–30.
11. Mori S, Endo M, Tsunoo T, et al. Physical performance evaluation of a 256-slice CT-scanner for four-dimensional imaging. Med Phys. 2004;31(6):1348–56.
12. Endo M, Mori S, Kandatsu S, et al. Development and performance evaluation of the second model 256-detector row CT. Radiol Phys Technol. 2008;1(1):20–6.
13. Ritschl L, Sawall S, Knaup M, et al. Iterative 4D cardiac micro-CT image reconstruction using an adaptive spatio-temporal sparsity prior. Phys Med Biol. 2012;57(6):1517–25.
14. Beister M, Kolditz D, Kalender WA. Iterative reconstruction methods in X-ray CT. Phys Med. 2012;28(2):94–108.
15. Sebastian S, Kalra MK, Mittal P, et al. Can independent coronal multiplanar reformatted images obtained using state-of-the-art MDCT scanners be used for primary interpretation of MDCT of the abdomen and pelvis? A feasibility study. Eur J Radiol. 2007;64(3):439–46.
16. Kirchgeorg MA, Prokop M. Increasing spiral CT benefits with post-processing applications. Eur J Radiol. 1998;28(1):39–54. Review.
17. Baronio M, Carrascosa P, Capuñay C, et al. Diagnostic performance of CT virtual hysteroscopy in 69 consecutive patients. Fertil Steril. 2010;94(Suppl):S77.
18. Capuñay C, Baronio M, Carrascosa P, et al. CT virtual hysterosalpingography in the evaluation of uterine myomas. Fertil Steril. 2010;94(Suppl):S211.
19. Carrascosa P, Baronio JM, Borghi M, et al. Histerosalpingoscopía virtual. Una técnica novedosa y no invasiva para diagnosticar patología intrauterina. Reproduccion. 2006;21:19–26.
20. Chalazonitis A, Tzovara I, Laspas F, et al. Hysterosalpingography: technique and applications. Curr Probl Diagn Radiol. 2009;38(5):199–205.
21. Lee A, Ying YK, Novy MJ. Hysteroscopy, hysterosalpingography and tubal ostial polyps in infertility patients. J Reprod Med. 1997;42(6):337–41.
22. Radić V, Canić T, Valetić J, et al. Advantages and disadvantages of hysterosonosalpingography in the assessment of the reproductive status of uterine cavity and fallopian tubes. Eur J Radiol. 2005;53(2):268–73.
23. Hamed HO, Shahin AY, Elsamman AM. Hysterosalpingo-contrast sonography versus radiographic hysterosalpingography in the evaluation of tubal patency. Int J Gynaecol Obstet. 2009;105(3):215–7.

In the 6th week of the embryo development the morphological sexual characteristics of both sexes start to establish themselves. In every embryo, on both sides of the middle line, the following structures are present: (i) a genital septum; (ii) a Wolf mesenteric duct, beside the genital septum; (iii) a paramesonephric Müllerian duct that consists of three segments: (a) a vertical cranial sector beside the Wolf duct; (b) a middle horizontal sector that passes in front of the Wolf duct; and (c) an inferior or caudal sector. According to the established sex at the moment of fertilization, the absence of the Y chromosome clears the way for the differentiation in the female sense, establishing the retraction of the Wolf ducts, the development of the structures derived of the Müller paramesonephric ducts and the formation of the ovaries [1–3].

The uterovaginal primordial is formed from the fusion of the Müllerian ducts. They have a Y shape, with a medial and caudal direction reaching the urogenital middle. The cranial and middle sectors are the origins of the Fallopian tubes, while the caudal portion forms the uterus and 4/5 of the vagina. The fusion begins in the inferior section with a caudal-cephalic direction, completing itself in 11th or 13th week of the mentioned period. Once finalized and the uterine silhouette formed, the reabsorption of the septum which divides both conduits to constitute the endometrial cavity, the cervical canal and part of the vagina begins (Fig. 4.1). This phase concludes after the 3rd month of the fertilization [2, 4–6].

In this chapter, the normal feminine reproductive apparatus and its radiological manifestation in virtual hysterosalpingography (VHSG) studies is described.

Uterus

The uterus is a muscular organ, of triangular shape located in the lower pelvis behind the bladder and in front of the rectum, with the cranial base and the neck on its inferior side, extending to the vagina. It possesses a virtual cavity, and its size varies depending on the age of the patient and her gestational history. In the nulliparous women it measures approximately $9 \times 6 \times 3$ cm. It is formed of three layers: (i) the serose one, referring to the visceral leaf of the peritoneum that covers it; (ii) the myometrium, which conforms the middle layer and is characterized by the presence of intertwined smooth muscular fibers; (iii) the endometrium, which constitutes the inner glandular mucosa layer. The uterus divides into: cervix, body or corpus, and the isthmus as barrier between the first two segments.

Position of the Uterus

The position of the uterus is determined by the orientation of the neck in relation to the vagina (version) and the body in relation to the neck (flexion) [7]. The most common, anteversio-anteflexio, occurs when the neck is flexed forward over the vagina, and in the same way, the uterine body over the neck. The uterus can adopt different positions considered as normal variants. These are shown in Fig. 4.2

Cervix and Isthmus

The uterine cervix is the lowest fibromuscular region of the uterus, thin and round with an average length of 4 cm and a diameter of 2.5 cm. Its lower part denominated vaginal portion or tenca snout, penetrates in the vagina while the upper portion remains on top and joins the muscular body of the uterus at the level of the internal cervical orifice in the isthmic region. The shape and size of the uterine neck suffers variations according to the age, moment of menstrual cycle and number of pregnancies of the patient. In a nulliparous women, the neck is fusiform and the external os is

P. Carrascosa et al., *CT Virtual Hysterosalpingography*,
DOI 10.1007/978-3-319-07560-0_4, © Springer International Publishing Switzerland 2014

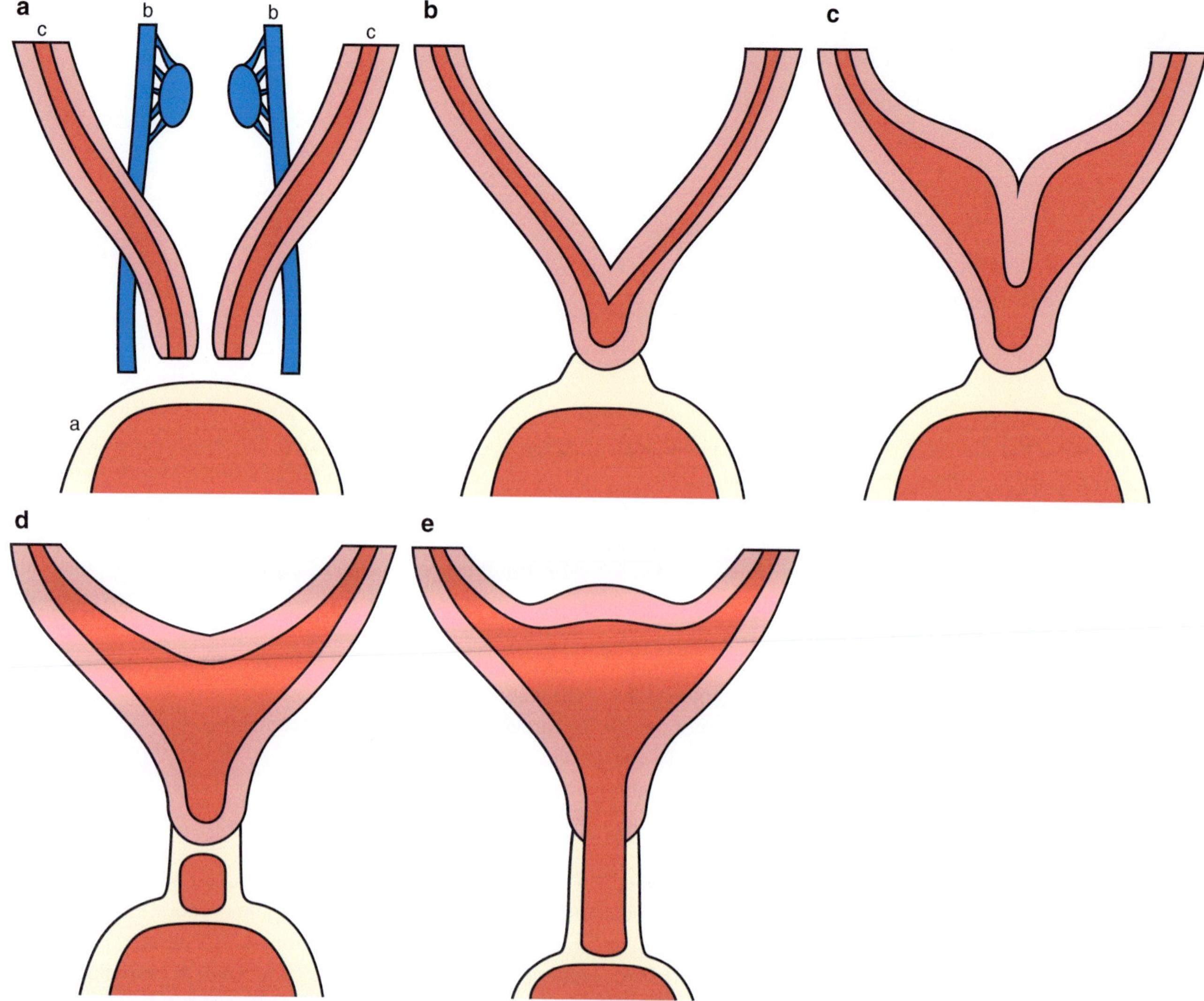

Fig. 4.1 Embryologic development. (**a–e**) Process of female sexual differentiation (**a** urogenital septum; **b** Wolf mesonferic duct; **c** paramesonephric Müllerian duct)

small, round and located in the center; on the other hand, in a woman who has already had a child, it is of great volume and the external os presents the aspect of a wide elongated clift.

The cervical canal passes through the endocervix. It communicates the vagina with the uterine cavity through the internal and external cervical os. Its length and diameter present a great variation according to the age and the moment of the patient's hormonal cycle (Fig. 4.3). The cervical canal is covered by the cylindrical epithelium, also known as the glandular epithelium. This epithelium is not a smooth and flat surface in the canal, it is made of multiplane longitudinal folds that project towards the lumen of the canal and give place to papillary projections. At the same time, it produces in the cervical estroma invaginations that constitute crypts, also known as endocervical glands (Fig. 4.4). In the VHSG studies, these glands are seen as sacular structures of small size projected on the walls of the cervical canal. On occasions, when dilated, they can be prominent, and observed as pseudodiverticular outgrowths (Fig. 4.5).

The isthmus is the shortest portion of the uterus, located between the upper part of the neck and the lower part of the uterine body (Fig. 4.6).

Body and Fundus

The uterine fundus conforms the upper dome-like portion of the uterus. It is constituted by a thick layer of muscular fibers, and is located on top of the insertion zone of the Fallopian tubes. The external configuration of the uterus is of utmost importance in the classification of uterine malformations. The final result of the complete fusion of the müllerian ducts during the embrionary period determines the external convex configuration. The uterine body corresponds to the principal portion of the uterus, containing a unique endometrial cavity, of triangular shape and covered by the endometrium (Fig. 4.7). The alterations in the process of fusion of the paramesonferic ducts that determine the appearance of the external uterine fundus, plus the alterations that occur during the process of

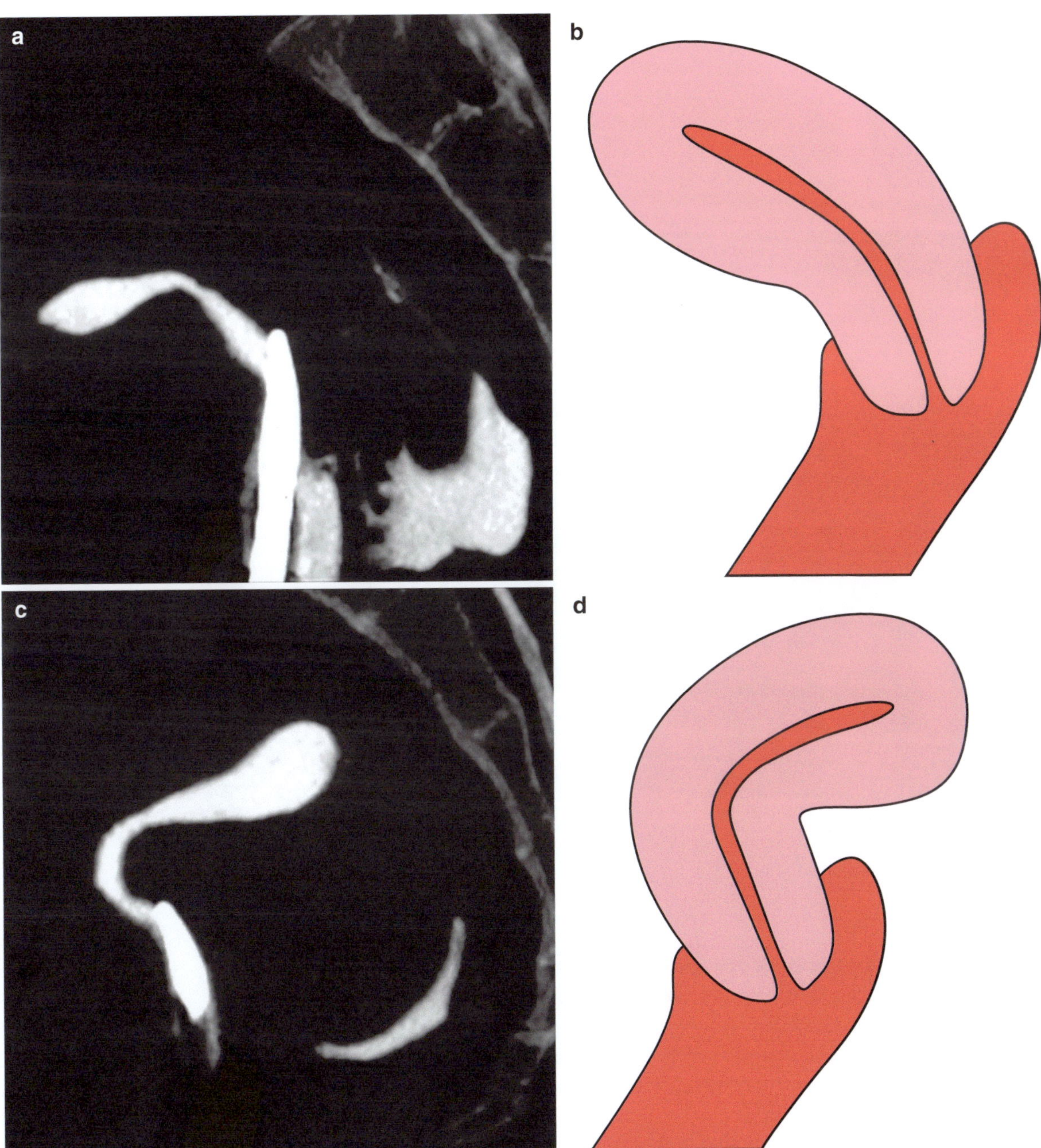

Fig. 4.2 Position of uterus in the lower pelvis. Maximum intensity projection VHSG images which show the different positions, determined by the orientation of the cervical neck in relation to the vagina and of the body in relation to the cervical neck. (**a**, **b**) Anteversio-anteflexio uterus. (**c**, **d**) Anteversio-retroflexio uterus. (**e**, **f**) Retroversio-anteflexio uterus. (**g**, **h**) Retroversio-retroflexio uterus

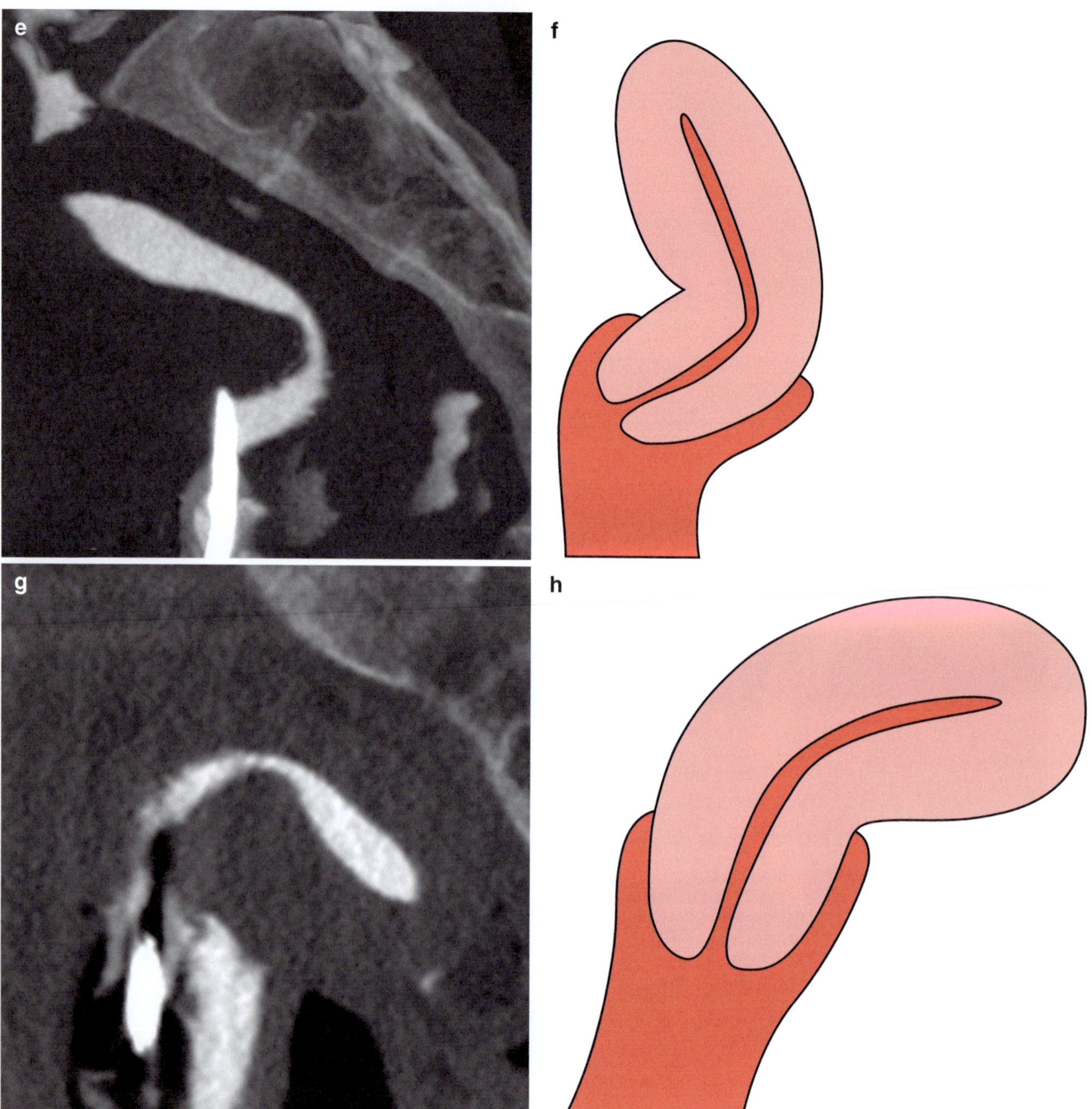

Fig. 4.2 (continued)

reabsorption of the septum that divides the same and that lead to changes in the cavity, give way to the different uterine malformations [3–6, 8, 9]. See Chap. 8.

The lateral distal portion on each side of the uterine fundus is denominated uterine horn or cornual region, place where the Fallopian tubes originate [10].

Predominant longitudinal folds parallel to the larger axis of the endometrial cavity considered as leftovers from the fusion of the Müller ducts during the fetal development can be identified in certain patients [4, 11], not associated to any endometrial pathology (Fig. 4.8).

During the diagnostic procedure venous or lymphatic intravasations of the instilled contrast may occur in patients subject to a VHSG. Although this can occur in healthy patients, there exist a variety of factors that may cause them, like an increase in intrauterine pressure, a recent uterine surgery or excessive pressure in the injection. Intravasation can be appreciated as multiple fine lines forming a reticular

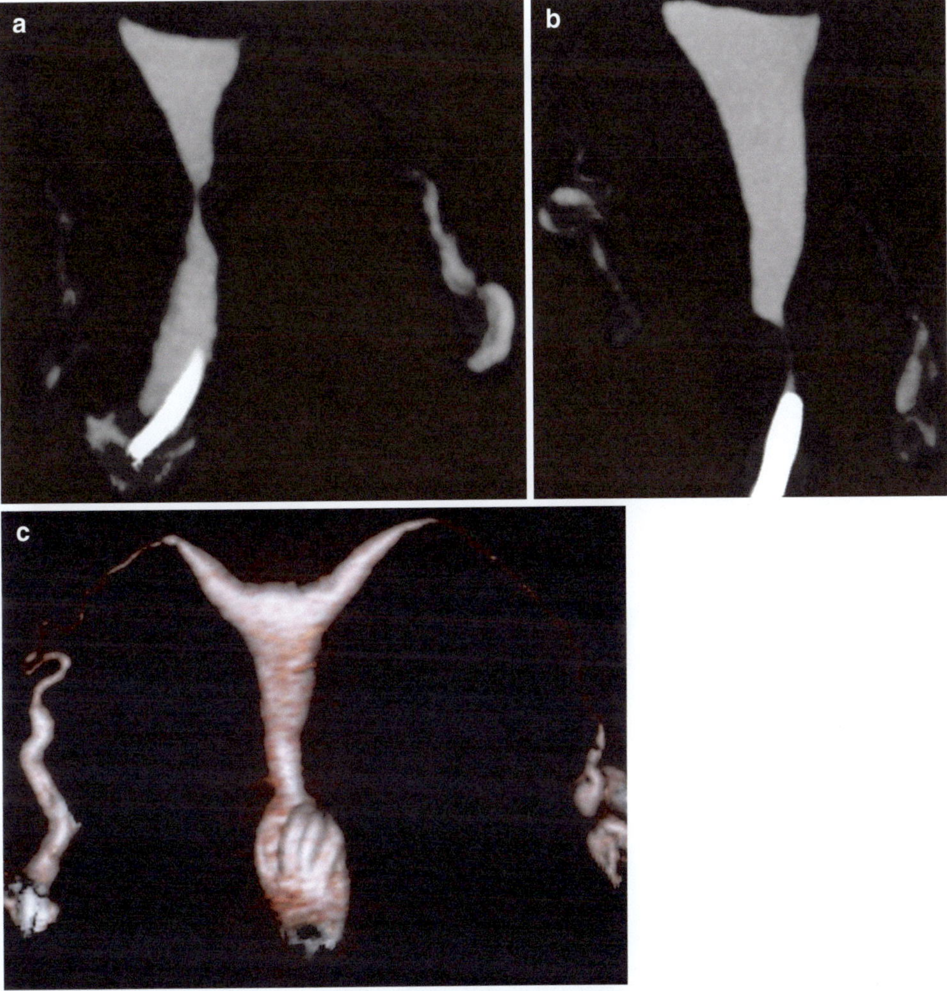

Fig. 4.3 VHSG study. Uterine cervical neck and normal variants. (**a**) Coronal maximum intensity projection (MIP) image which shows a cervical canal of normal caliber and morphology. (**b**) Coronal MIP image which shows a narrow cervical canal. (**c**) 3D volume rendering image which shows a wide cervical canal with normal fold visualization

pattern in the uterine wall and as direct opacification of the pelvic veins (Fig. 4.9).

Fallopian Tubes

Anatomy

In the embryo's development, during the 5th and 6th week of growth, the paramesonephric ducts pairs form from the coelomic epithelium. The cranial pieces turn into the Fallopian tubes, and in the caudal section they fuse to form the uterus. The cranial end of the Fallopian tube remains open, communicating with the peritoneal cavity (coelomic), with multiple invaginations of the free edge that form the fimbria.

At adult age, the Fallopian tubes acquire a tubular configuration with an approximate length of 8–15 cm, and they are located on the top of the wide ligaments. They extend laterally and inferiorly from the cornual region of the uterus up to the ovaries and are divided in three portions: intramural, isthmic and ampullar. On its extreme, the infundible is composed of irregular extensions (fimbriae) that open to the peritoneal cavity and surround the ovary. The ampullar region gradually reduces its caliber from 15 to 4 mm in diameter and joins with the isthmic portion that composes more than half of the Fallopian tube's length (Fig. 4.10). Within the wall of the uterus, the intramural segment presents an extension of 1–2 cm and joins with the endometrial cavity [12].

The wall of the Fallopian tube is composed of three layers: mucosa, muscular and serose. The mucosa presents folds that project towards the lumen and increase in complexity from the medial zone to the lateral zone of the tube. The folds join in the infundible where they continue with the fimbriae. The muscular layer is composed of the circular and longitudinal muscle fibers. The epithelium surrounding the mucosa is formed from ciliated and non ciliated cells. The ciliated epithelium and the mucosa folds push the ovule

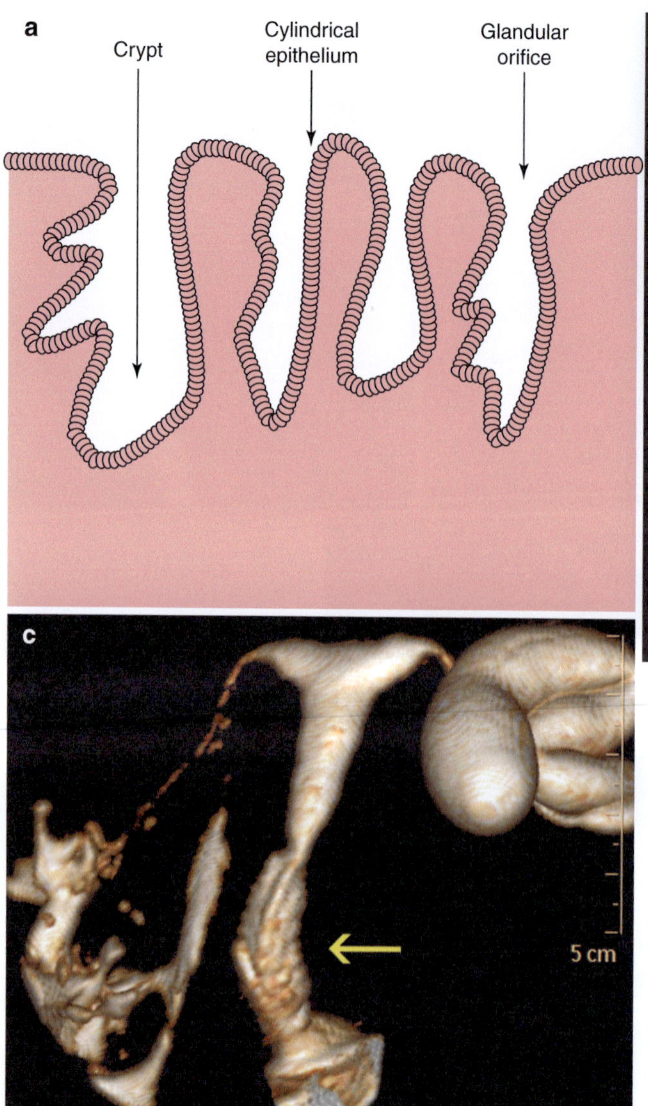

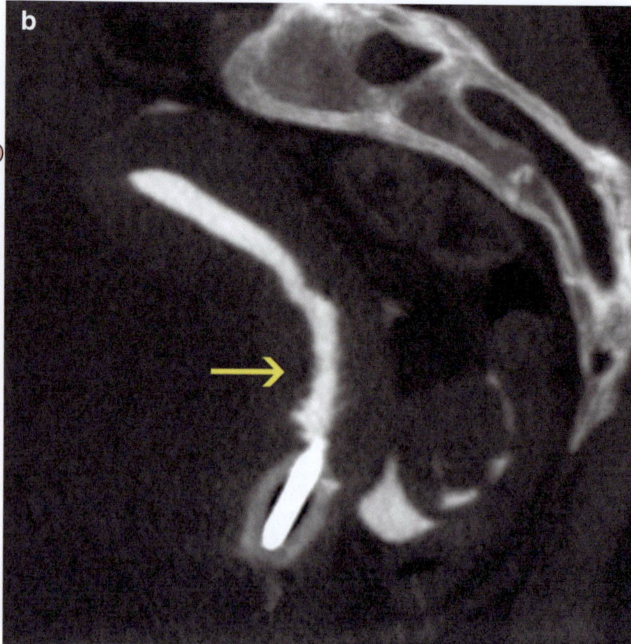

Fig. 4.4 Epithelium lining of the cervical canal. (**a**) Display which shows the epithelial lining of the cervical canal, with longitudinal folds which project towards the lumen and give origin to papillary projec-tions and invaginations or crypts. (**b, c**) Sagittal maximum intensity projection and coronal 3D volume rendering images which show the characteristic longitudinal folds of the cervical canal (*arrows*)

towards the uterine cavity. Unlike the ovule, the secreted liquid of the tubarian epithelium advances towards the fimbria in the tube and is liberated in the peritoneal cavity.

Normal Findings

In the virtual hysterosalpingography studies, the uterine tubes are seen as fine tubular structures that emerge from the cornual region of the uterus and extend towards the lateral region of the pelvic cavity (Figs. 4.11 and 4.12). There exist lots of variations in the course and position of the uterine tubes that can be seen in imaging studies. However, they must be considered as normal variants, unless the existence of a mass that provoques the pathological displacement of them is identified (Figs. 4.13 and 4.14).

The caliber of the tubal lumen that is opacified with the administered contrast is variable. In the intramural segment linear lucencies at the cornual-tubal junction can be observed, it presents an oblique orientation and corresponds to a muscular contraction (Fig. 4.15). The isthmic portion is the most extensive and measures 1–2 mm of diameter, while in the ampullar region the caliber is variable from 2 to 12 mm. Using data processing techniques a spread of the uterine tube in only one plane can be achieved, where one can appreciate and measure the exact caliber of each of the portions (Fig. 4.16). The folds can be observed usually with higher frequency in the ampullar region as lineal and regular filling defects that get more prominent towards the fimbrial region (Fig. 4.17). Here, the infundibulum opens to the peritoneum, but does not present radiological characteristics that differentiate it from the ampullar portion.

When the uterine tubes conserve their normal permeability, the endocavitary contrast administered opacifies all the tubarian portions and passes to the peritoneal cavity through the infundibulum (Fig. 4.18). The dispersion pattern of the contrast depends principally on the quantity administered and the lapse of time between the beginning of the injection and the acquisition of the images.

The incomplete opacification or the lack of passage of the contrast to the peritoneum are not infrequent and do not necessarily indicate a pathologic obstruction. Other situations exist, like the cornual spasm, mucosa stoppages or insufficient quantity of injected contrast can simulate a tubarian obstruction (Fig. 4.19) [11].

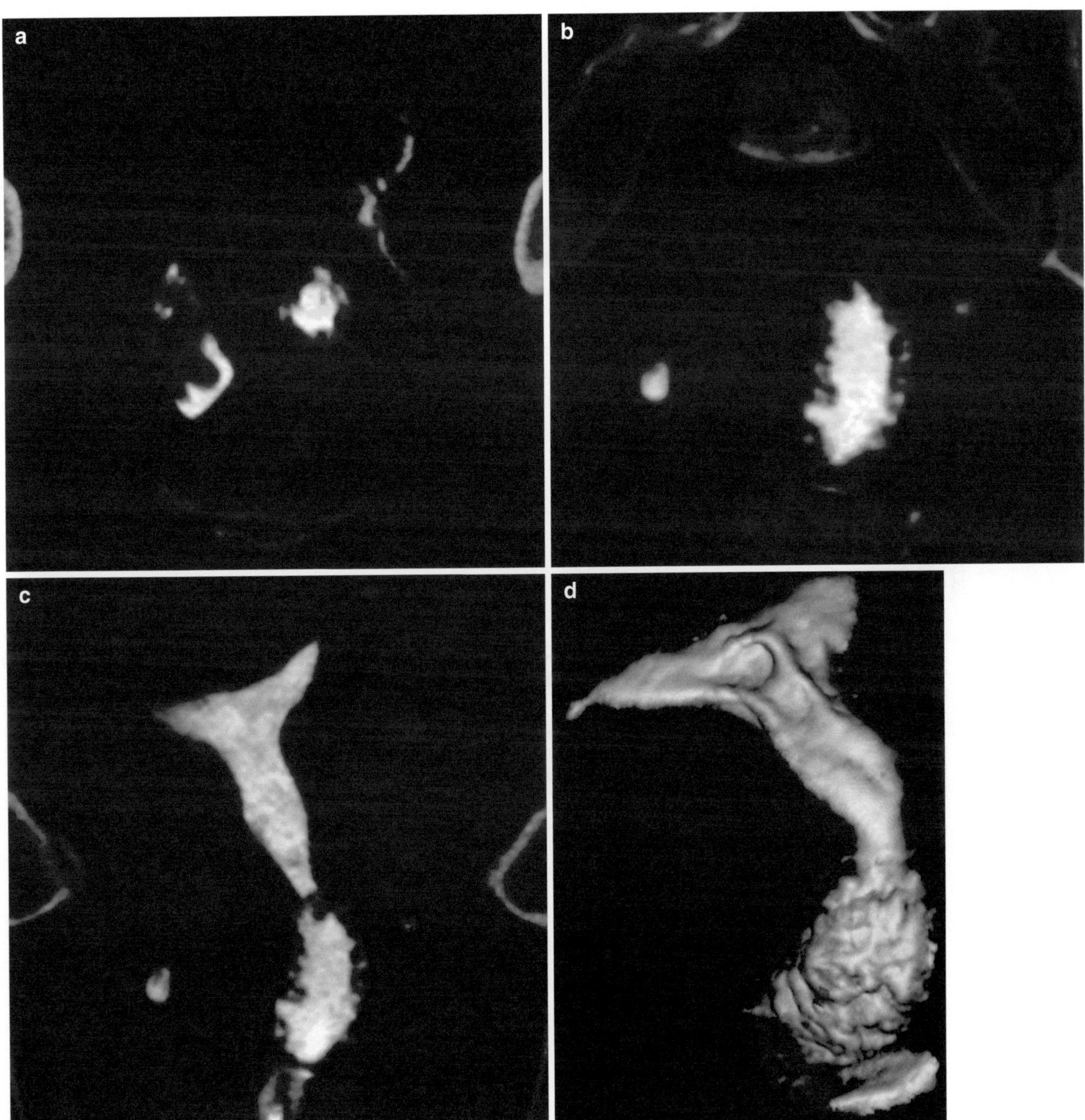

Fig. 4.5 VHSG study. Large cervical canal with prominent glands. (**a**) Axial CT image. (**b**) Coronal multiplanar reconstruction image. (**c**) Coronal maximum intensity projection image. (**d**) Coronal oblique 3D volume rendering image. (**e, f**) Virtual endoscopy images

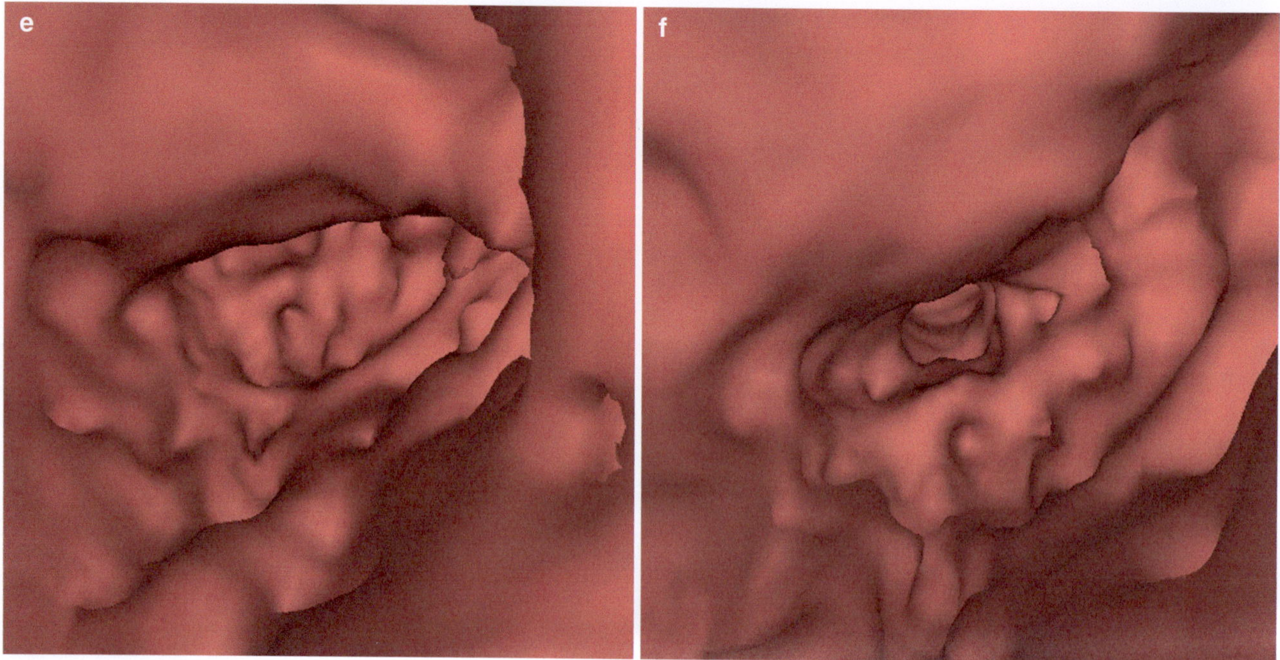

Fig. 4.5 (continued)

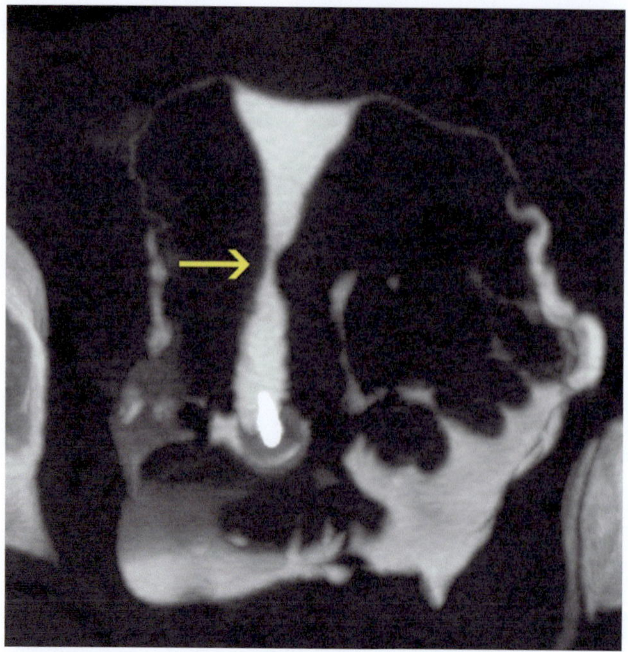

Fig. 4.6 Uterine isthmus (*arrow*). Coronal maximum intensity projection image

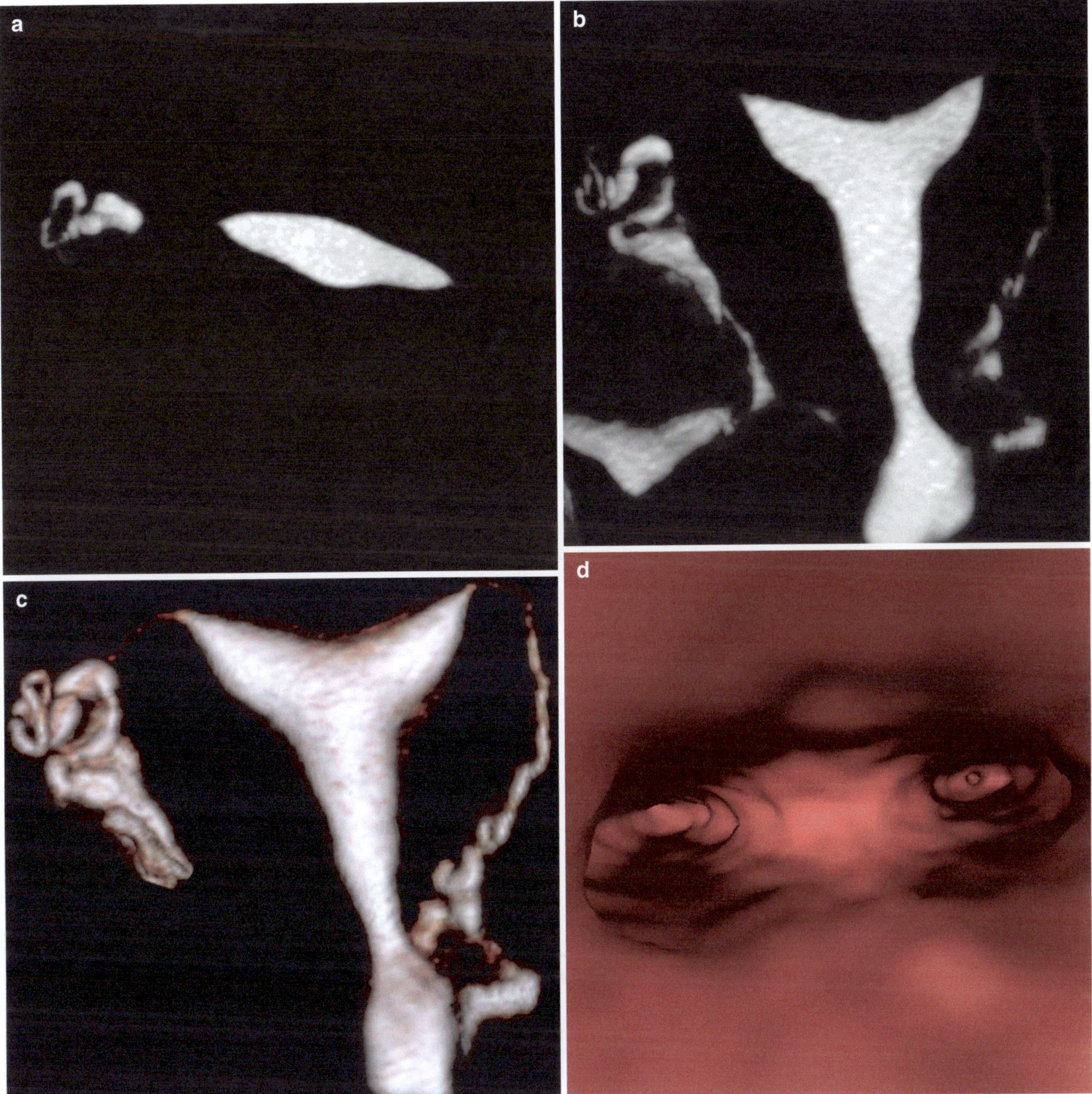

Fig. 4.7 VHSG study. Normal anatomy of the uterine cavity. (**a**) Axial maximum intensity projection (MIP) image. (**b**) Coronal MIP image. (**c**) Coronal 3D volume rendering image. (**d**) Virtual endoscopy image

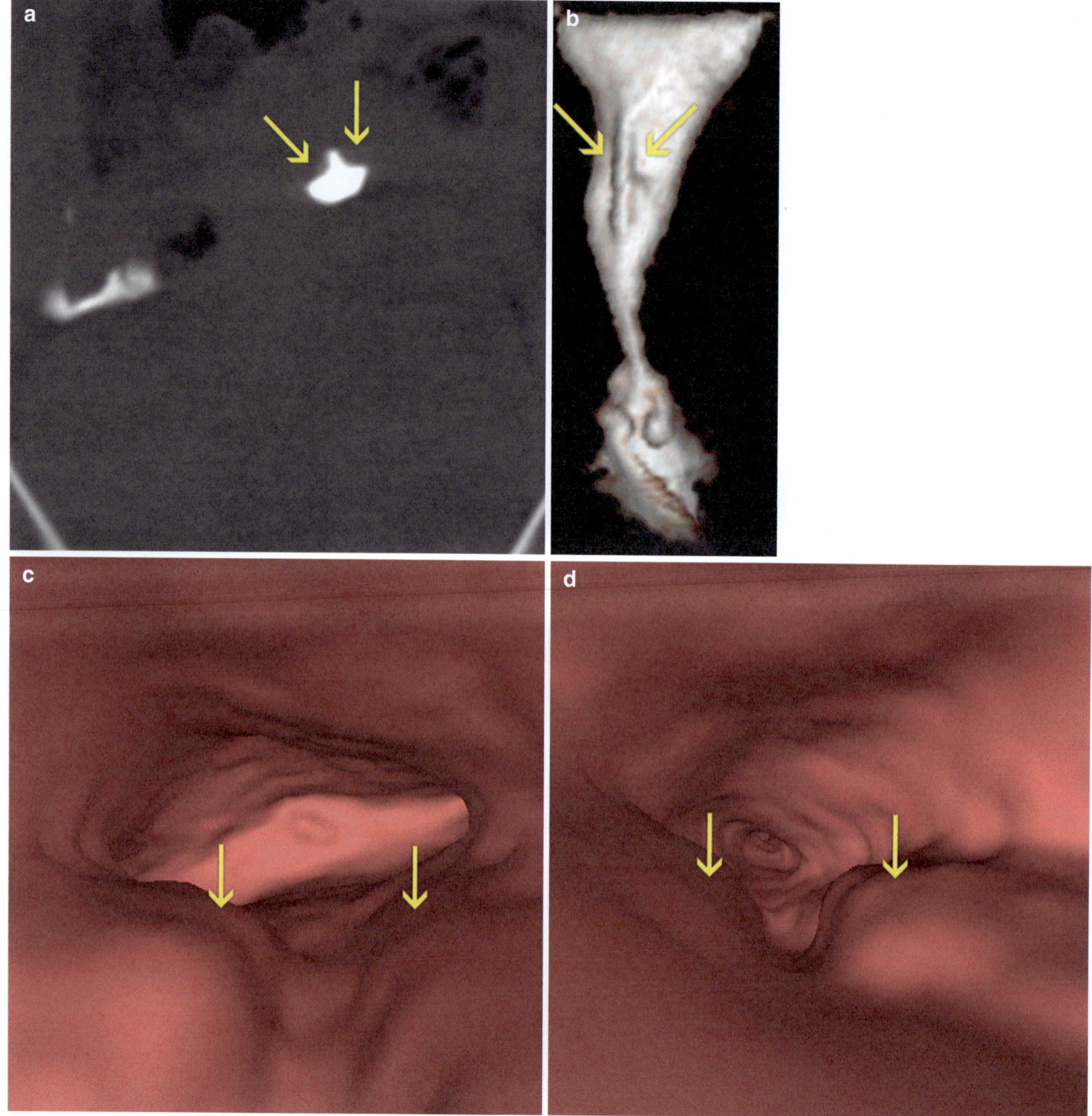

Fig. 4.8 VHSG study. Prominent longitudinal folds (*arrows*) at the level of the endometrial cavity. (**a**) Axial maximum intensity projection (MIP) image. (**b**) Coronal 3D volume rendering image, posterior view. (**c**, **d**) Virtual endoscopy images

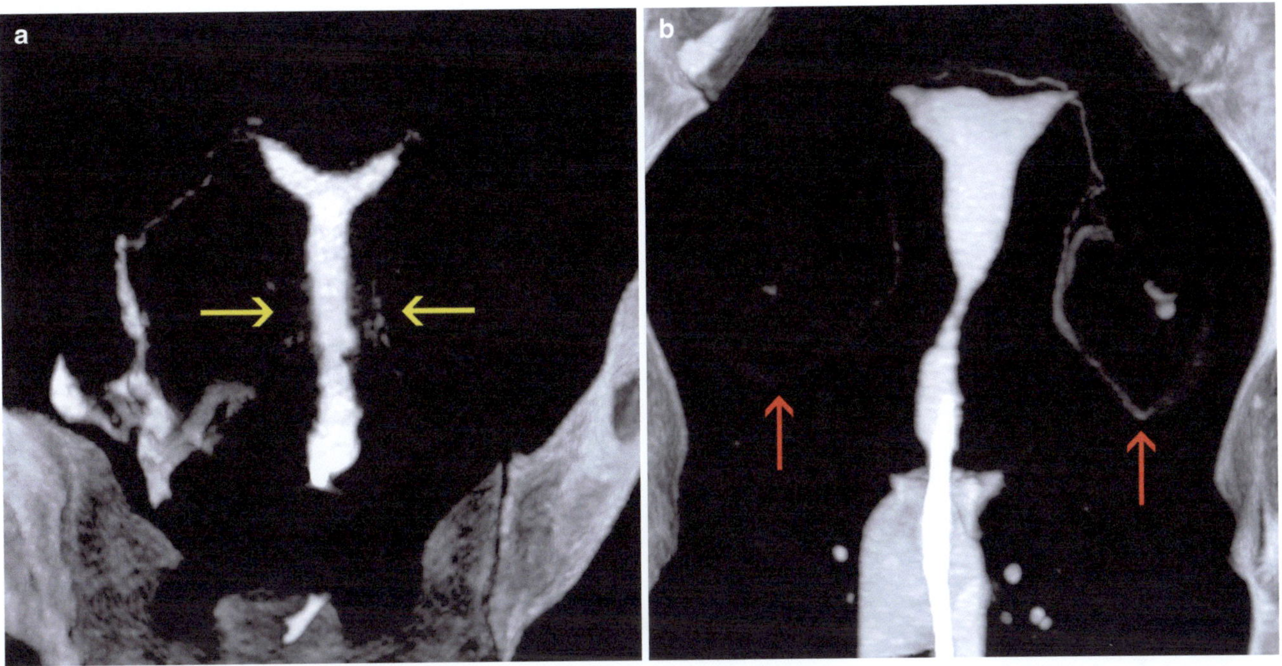

Fig. 4.9 VHSG study. Contrast intravasation to the miometrium and to the periuterine (*yellow arrows*) and pelvic (*red arrows*) venous plexus. (**a**, **b**) Coronal maximum intensity projection images

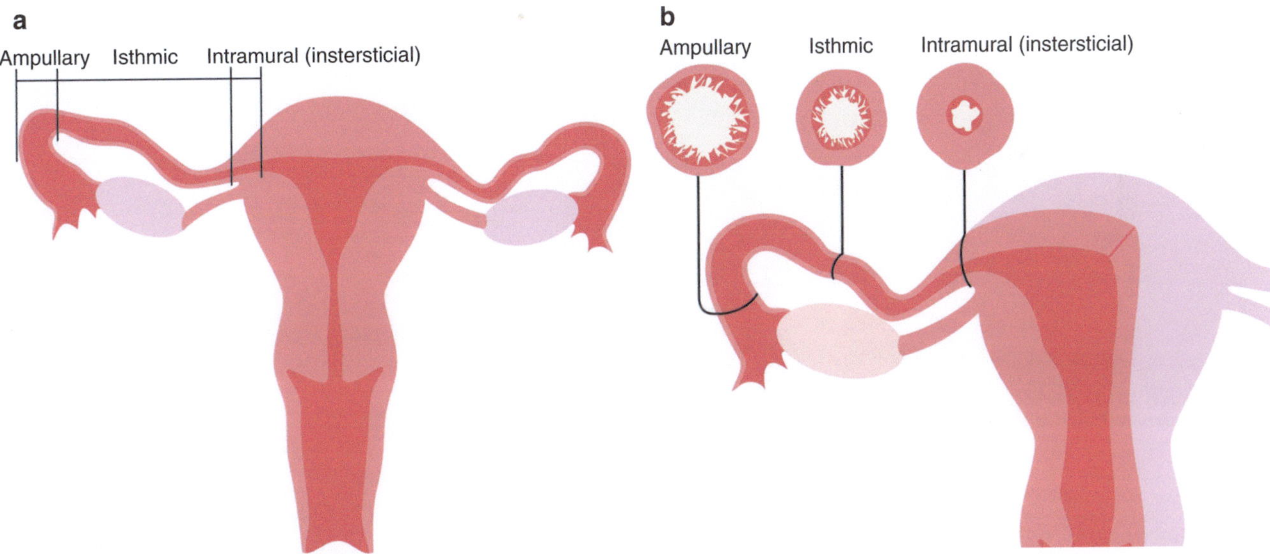

Fig. 4.10 (**a**) Display of the normal anatomy of the uterine tubes. The tubal segments are divided into intramural (interstitial), isthmic and ampullary. (**b**) Display of the structure of the tubal wall in the different segments

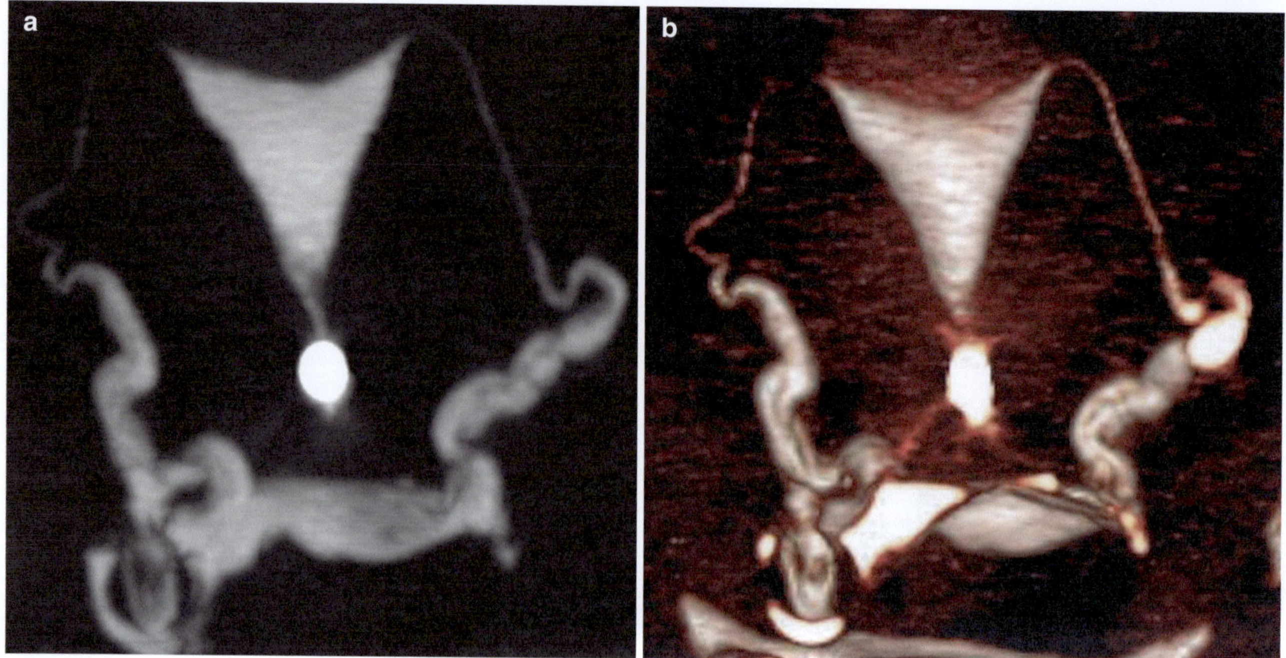

Fig. 4.11 VHSG showing the normal anatomy of the uterus and uterine tubes. (**a**) Coronal maximum intensity projection image. (**b**) Coronal 3D volume rendering image

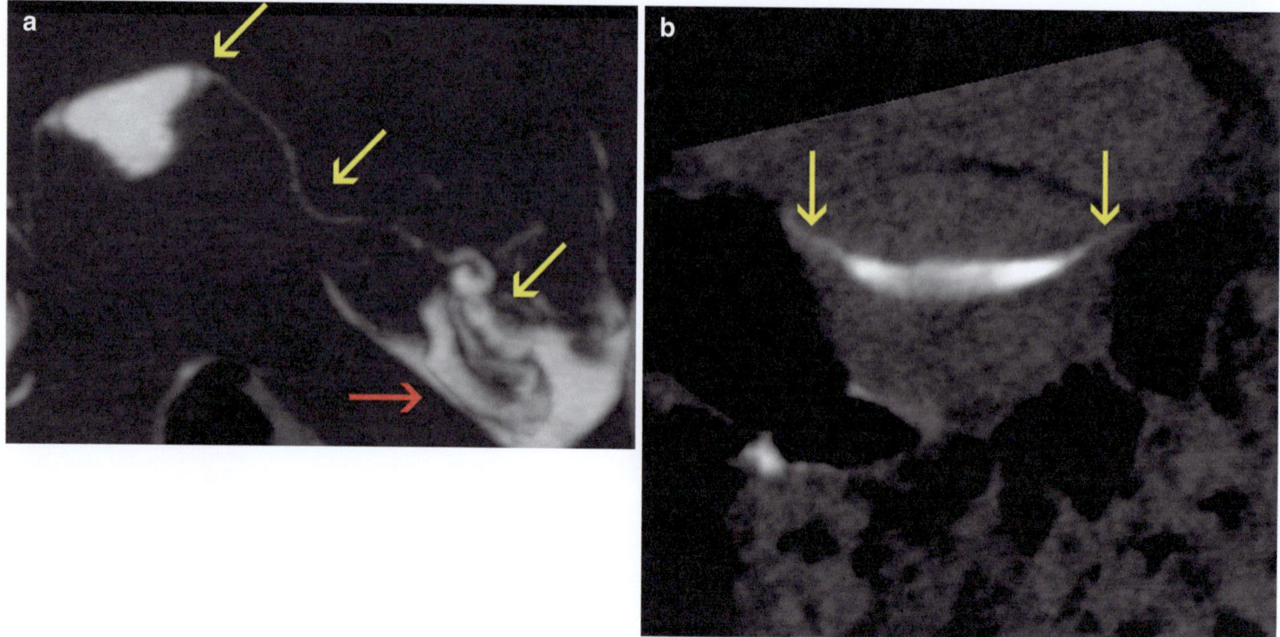

Fig. 4.12 (**a**) VHSG showing a normal left tube displayed with its three portions: intramural, isthmic and ampullary (*yellow arrows*) with abundant spillage of contrast into the peritoneal cavity (*red arrow*). (**b**) Oblique coronal multiplanar reconstruction image showing the intramural portion of both tubes (*arrows*)

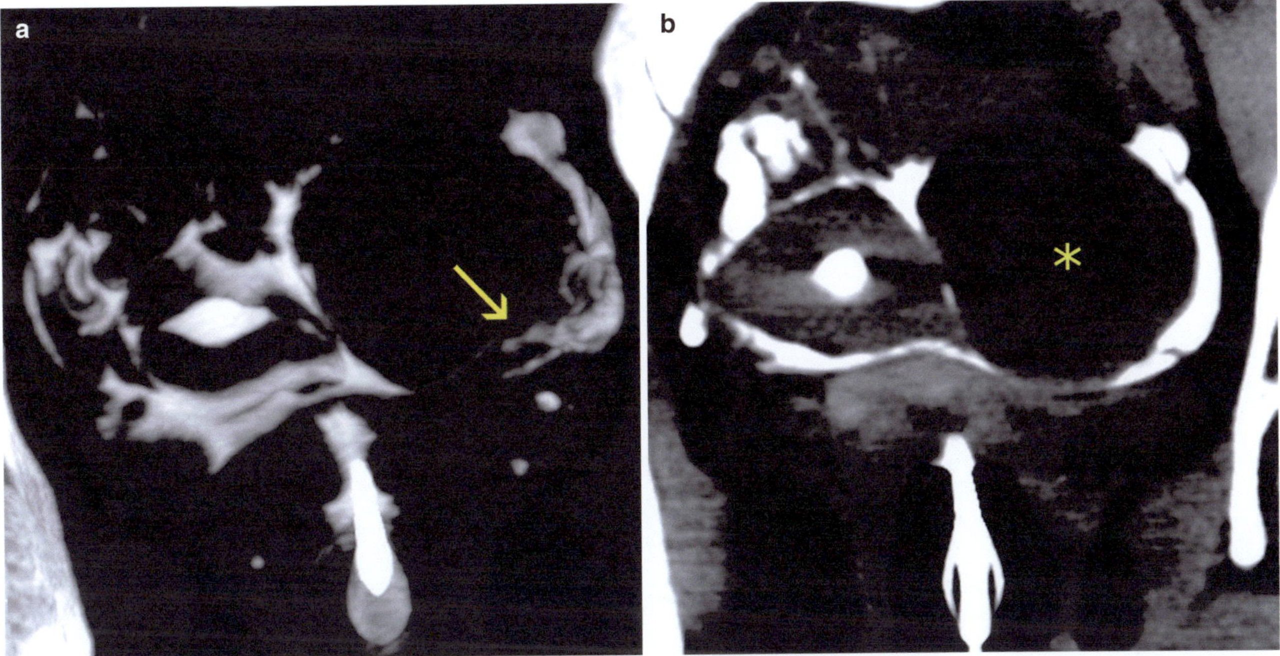

Fig. 4.13 (**a**) VHSG showing that the left uterine tube is displaced downwards (*arrow*). (**b**) Utilizing soft tissue window a heterogeneous adnexal mass (*asterisk*) which caused the tubal displacement was observed

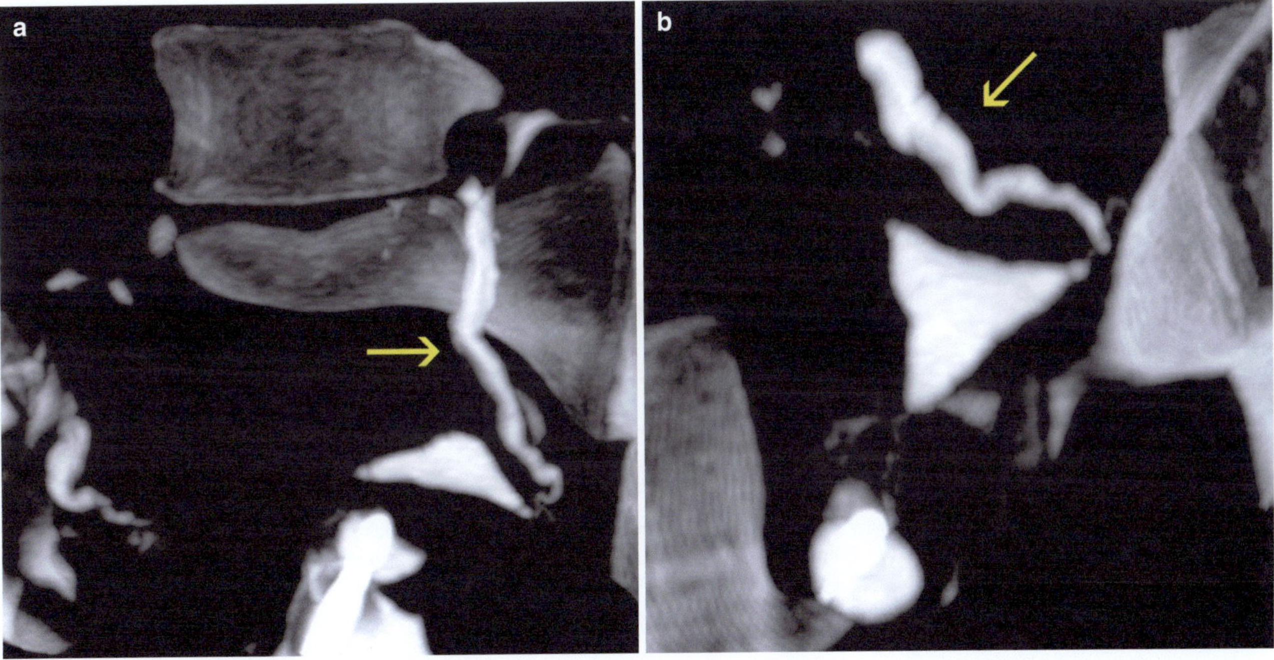

Fig. 4.14 VHSG showing a dilated and displaced upwards left tube (*arrow*), probably due to secondary retraction to sequels of a previous pelvic inflammatory process. (**a**, **b**) Coronal maximum intensity projection images

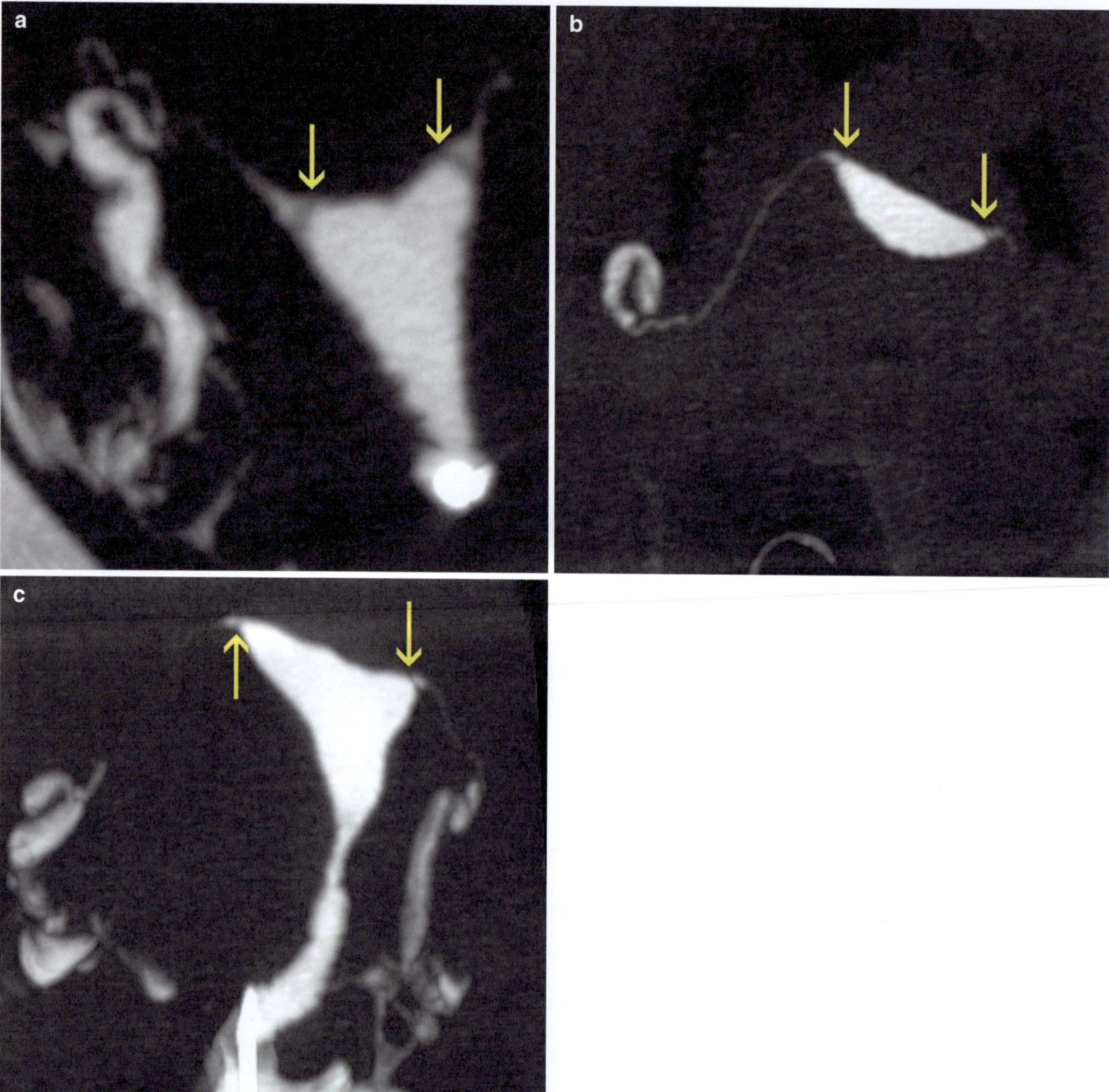

Fig. 4.15 (**a**, **b**) Thin-slab maximum intensity projection images showing circumferential lucencies in the cornual-tubal junctions (*arrows*). Besides, the left uterine tube is obstructed. (**c**) Another normal VHSG study showing similar findings (*arrows*)

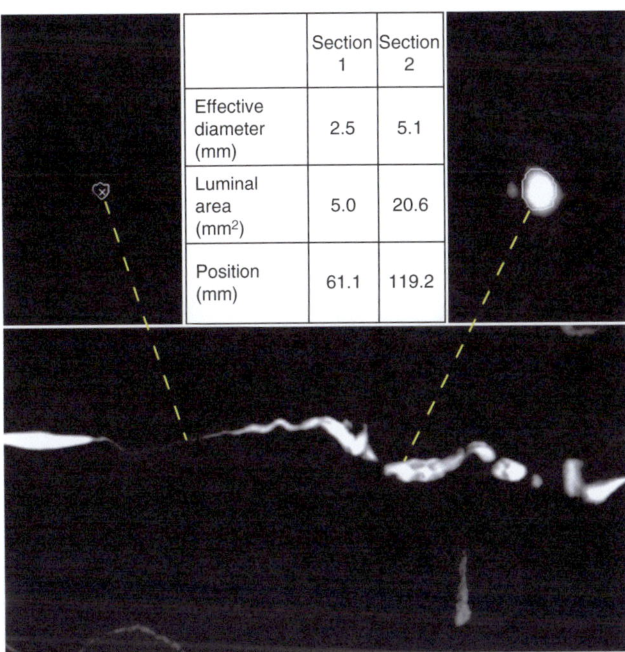

	Section 1	Section 2
Effective diameter (mm)	2.5	5.1
Luminal area (mm^2)	5.0	20.6
Position (mm)	61.1	119.2

Fig. 4.16 Elongated normal tube reconstructed image. Using a vascular post-processing software, the uterine tube can be displayed in one plane. The exact diameter and circumference area of each of its portions can be measured

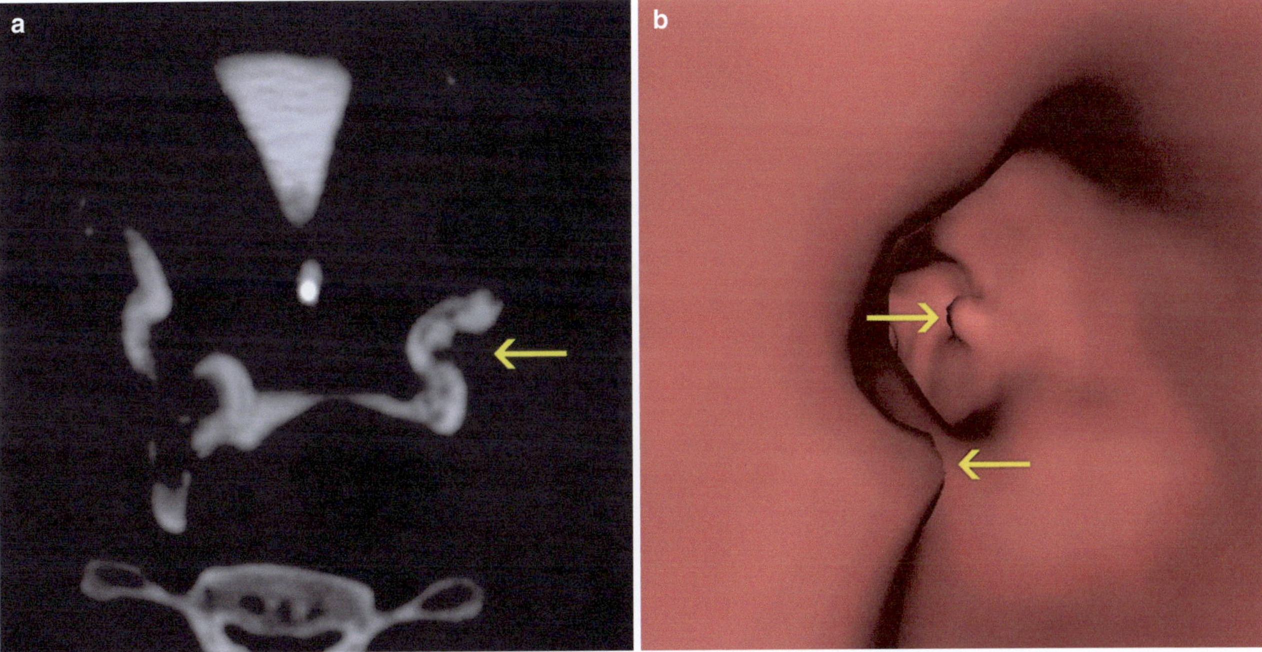

Fig. 4.17 (**a**) Ampullary folds. Axial CT image shows lineal and regular intraluminal defects at the level of the ampullary region of the left tube (*arrow*), compatible with normal folds. (**b**) Virtual endoscopic image where small elevated lesions compatible with tubal folds are visualized (*arrows*)

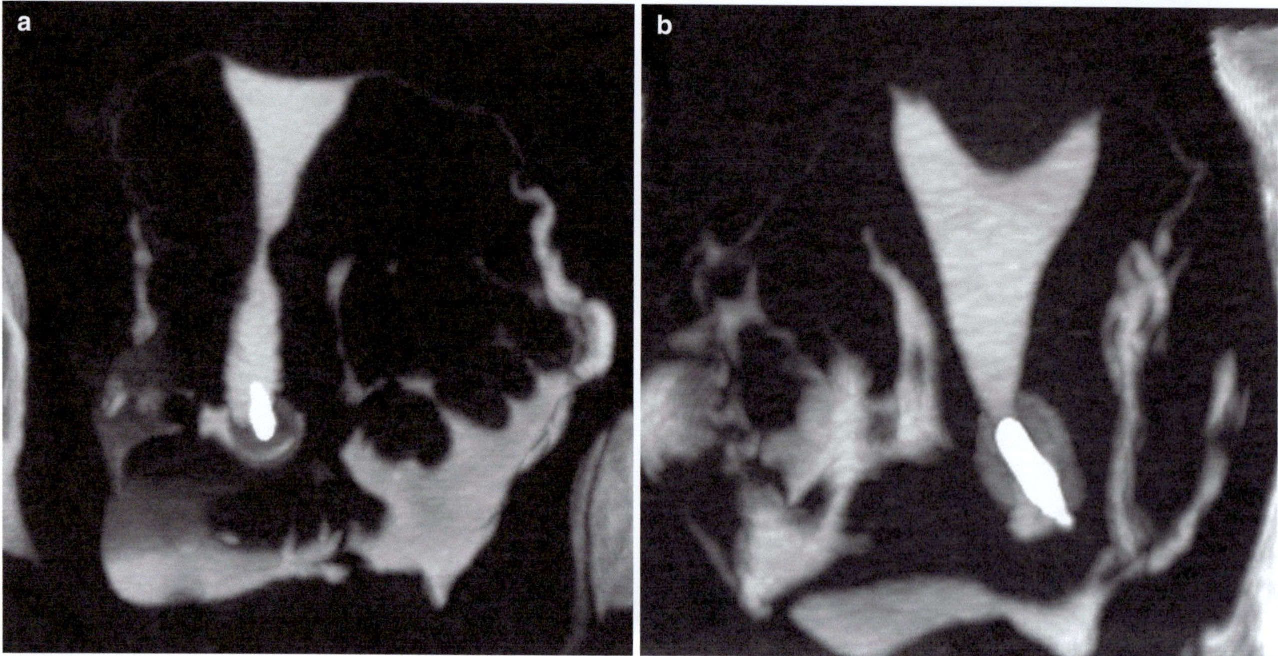

Fig. 4.18 Normal spillage of contrast to the peritoneal cavity. (**a**) Maximum intensity projection image shows normal opacification of the uterine cavity, the tubes and adequate bilateral spillage of contrast to the peritoneal cavity. (**b**) Another case with bilateral tubal permeability and uterus of arcuate morphology

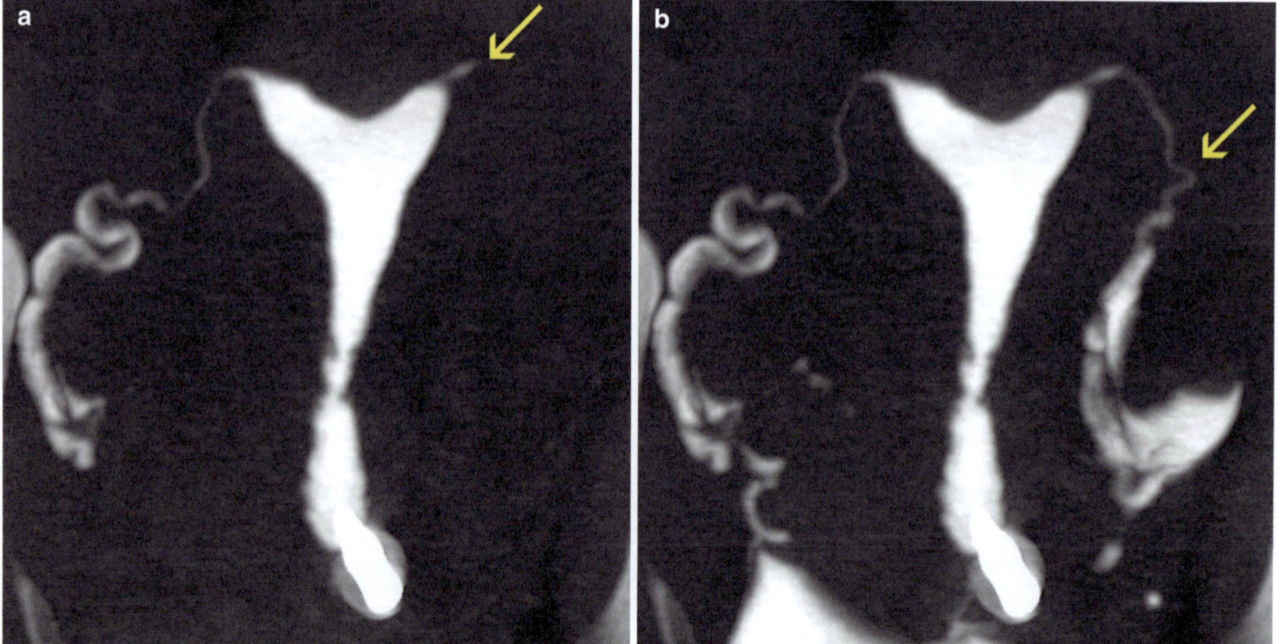

Fig. 4.19 VHSG of 26-year old patient with infertility diagnosis. (**a**) Maximum intensity projection image shows only opacification of the intramural segment of the left uterine tube (*arrow*) during the first CT image acquisition. (**b**) In the second CT image acquisition, normal opacification of the left tube with passage of the contrast to the peritoneal cavity (*arrow*) is observed. It is inferred that the cause of the pseudo-obstruction could be related to spasms or insufficient quantity of administered contrast

Conclusion

Currently, the VHSG is an integral imaging diagnostic method that enhances the diagnostic performance of the conventional radiologic study and adds the advantages of a multislice computed tomography exam. It provides the possibility of evaluating the uterus and the Fallopian tubes bidimensionally and tridimensionally, adding the virtual endoluminal view of the cervical canal, the uterine cavity and eventually the uterine tubes.

References

1. Byrne J, Nussbaum-Blask A, Taylor WS, et al. Prevalence of müllerian duct anomalies detected at ultrasound. Am J Med Genet. 2000;94:9–12.
2. Stampe Sorensen S. Estimated prevalence of mullerian duct anomalies. Acta Obstet Gynecol Scand. 1988;67:441–5.
3. Sarto GE, Simpson JL. Abnormalities of the Mullerian and Wolffian duct systems. Birth Defects Orig Artic Ser. 1978;14:37–54.
4. Troiano RN, McCarthy SM. Müllerian duct anomalies: imaging and clinical issues. Radiology. 2004;233:19–34.
5. Shulman LP. Müllerian anomalies. Clin Obstet Gynecol. 2008;51:214–22.
6. Lin PC, Bhatnagar KP, Nettleton GS, et al. Female genital anomalies affecting reproduction. Fertil Steril. 2002;78:899–915.
7. Rohen JW. Topographische anatomie. Stuttgart: Schattaer; 1999.
8. Toaff ME, Lev-Toaff AS, Toaff R. Communicating uteri: review and classification with introduction of two previously unreported types. Fertil Steril. 1984;41:661–79.
9. Saravelos SH, Cocksedge KA, Li TC. Prevalence and diagnosis of congenital uterine anomalies in women with reproductive failure: a critical appraisal. Hum Reprod Update. 2008;14:415–29.
10. Carrascosa PM, Capuñay C, Vallejos J, et al. Virtual hysterosalpingography: a new multidetector CT technique for evaluating the female reproductive system. Radiographics. 2010;30:643–61.
11. Ubeda B, Paraira M, Alert E, et al. Hysterosalpingography: spectrum of normal variants and nonpathological findings. AJR Am J Roentgenol. 2001;177(1):131–5.
12. Chen MYM, Zagoria RJ. Normal radiographic anatomy. In: Ott DJ, Fayez JA, Zagoria RJ, editors. Hysterosalpingography: a text and atlas. 2nd ed. Baltimore: Williams & Wilkins; 1998. p. 29–30.

Part II

Pathologic Findings of Virtual Hysterosalpingography

Cervical Pathology

The cervical abnormalities, that can be evaluated using virtual hysterosalpingography (VHSG), include diverse types of pathologies such as changes in the cervical diameter, dilatation or stenosis, sinechiae and parietal irregularities with thick folds, polipoyd lesions, diverticules and cesarean scars. All of them constitute benign pathologies. The malignant pathology, as the cervical cancer is, can be detected by VHSG only in advanced stages, and its role is limited [1–5].

Next are described each of the diverse cervical pathologies, including typical images of them through VHSG as well as other complementary diagnostic methods.

Cervix Stenosis

The reduced caliber of the cervix can be a pathological finding, although in certain cases it is just a normal variant.

The causes of pathological cervical stenosis are related to post-surgery synechiae or post-infection causes.

The caliber of the cervix can be reduced focally or diffusely, which can generate changes in patients that require insemination treatments.

The cervix is difficult to evaluate because of the different diagnostic modalities, especially in HSG studies due to its location, angle and superposition with the uterus-cervical region in situations of insufficient traction [6–8] (Fig. 5.1).

VHSG does not require traction because it post-processes the information with 2D and 3D reconstructions and, in this way, permits the evaluation of the cervix without blind spots. VHSG has the ability to angle the gynecologic apparatus in any direction and permits its evaluation from any view (Fig. 5.2) [9, 10].

Maximum intensity projection (MIP) and volume rendering (VR) multiplanar reconstructions are useful in the detection of cervical stenosis. Virtual images complement the diagnosis (Fig. 5.3) [11, 12].

In cases of proximal or distal focal stenosis it is possible to navigate the normal cervical lumen and clearly identify the site of the caliber's reduction (Fig. 5.4).

Synechiae

The cervical adherences are fibrous tissue bands located in the interior of the cervix and thus generating partial or total obliteration of its lumen. They extend from the walls to the center of the cervical lumen.

Methods which detect cervical synechiae are HSG and VHSG.

HSG: shows focal or diffuse lumen filling defects in the cervix (Fig. 5.5). The progressive filling of the cervix with contrast is essential so as not to have false negatives, because the small lesions may not be correctly detected [13–15].

VHSG: can easily see this pathology [16–18]. It identifies endocervical lesions with soft tissue density, of irregular edges, that extend from the cervical wall to the centre of the cervix or else connect the cervical walls, in this way reducing the diameter (Fig. 5.6).

Synechiae can be localized (Fig. 5.7) or diffuse (Fig. 5.8). VHSG evaluates the extension throughout the different reconstructions.

Thick Folds

Thick folds can be a normal finding or constitute an incipient pathology. They are easy to detect through a VHSG study using the multiplanar reconstruction, VR and virtual endoscopy [1–5].

Multiplanar reconstructions show thick cervical folds that extend themselves on the cervix walls. They are observed in coronal and sagittal reconstructions as well as in axial views.

VR reconstructions exhibit the longitudinal trajectory of the folds correlated with the findings seen in the multiplanar reconstruction while endoscopic views confirm previous visualizations (Fig. 5.9).

P. Carrascosa et al., *CT Virtual Hysterosalpingography*,
DOI 10.1007/978-3-319-07560-0_5, © Springer International Publishing Switzerland 2014

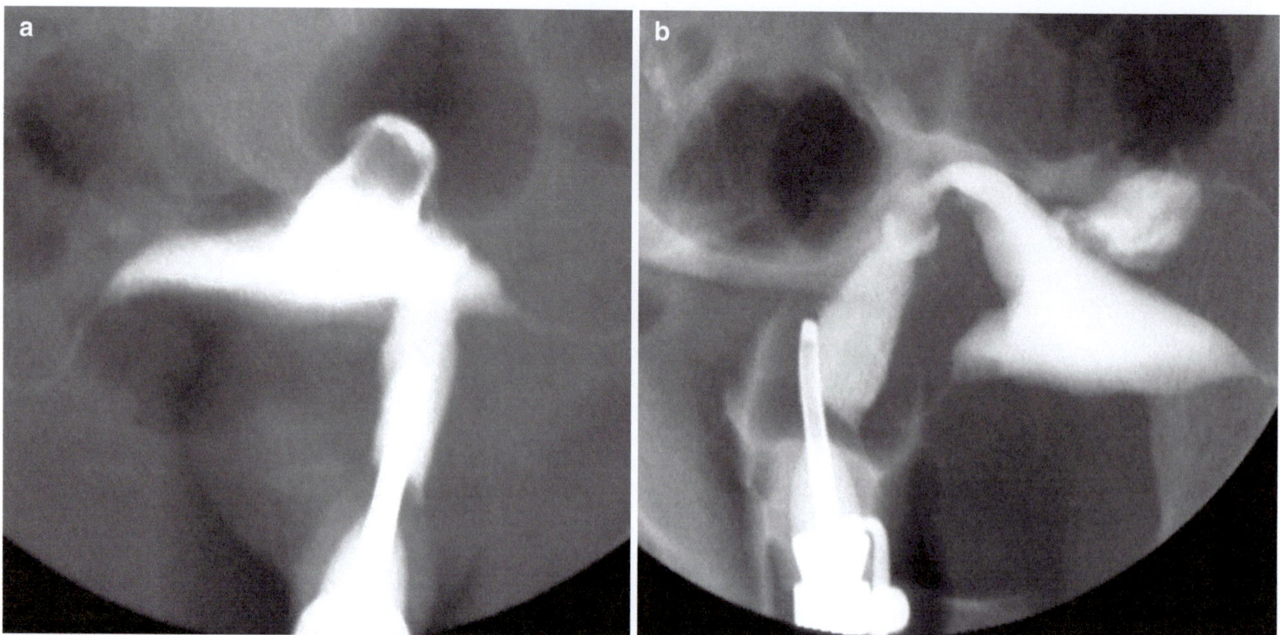

Fig. 5.1 HSG study. (**a**, **b**) Oblique X-ray projections showing partial superposition of the cervix with the proximal sector of the uterine body due to insufficient traction, not allowing a correct evaluation of all of the gynecologic apparatus

Fig. 5.2 VHSG study of normal cervix. (**a**, **b**) 3D volume rendering images that show the cervix from different angles which allow its correct evaluation without the need for traction

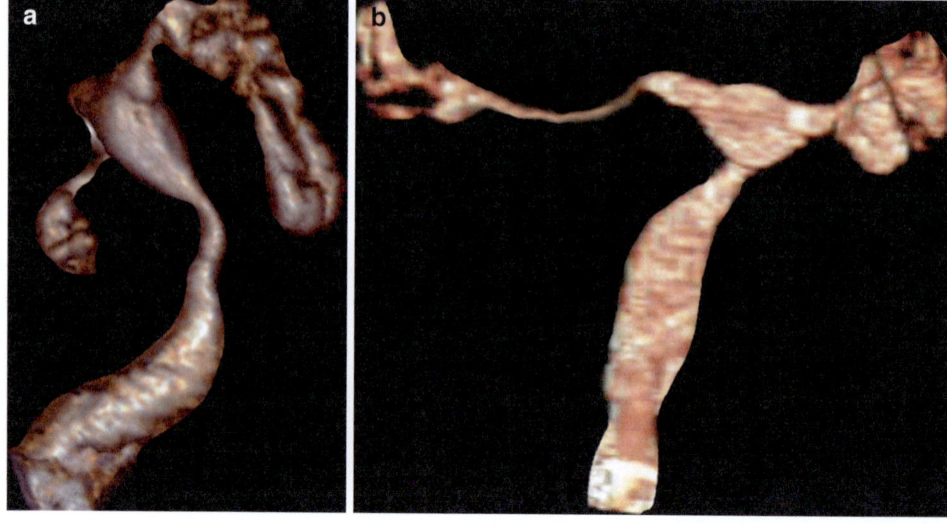

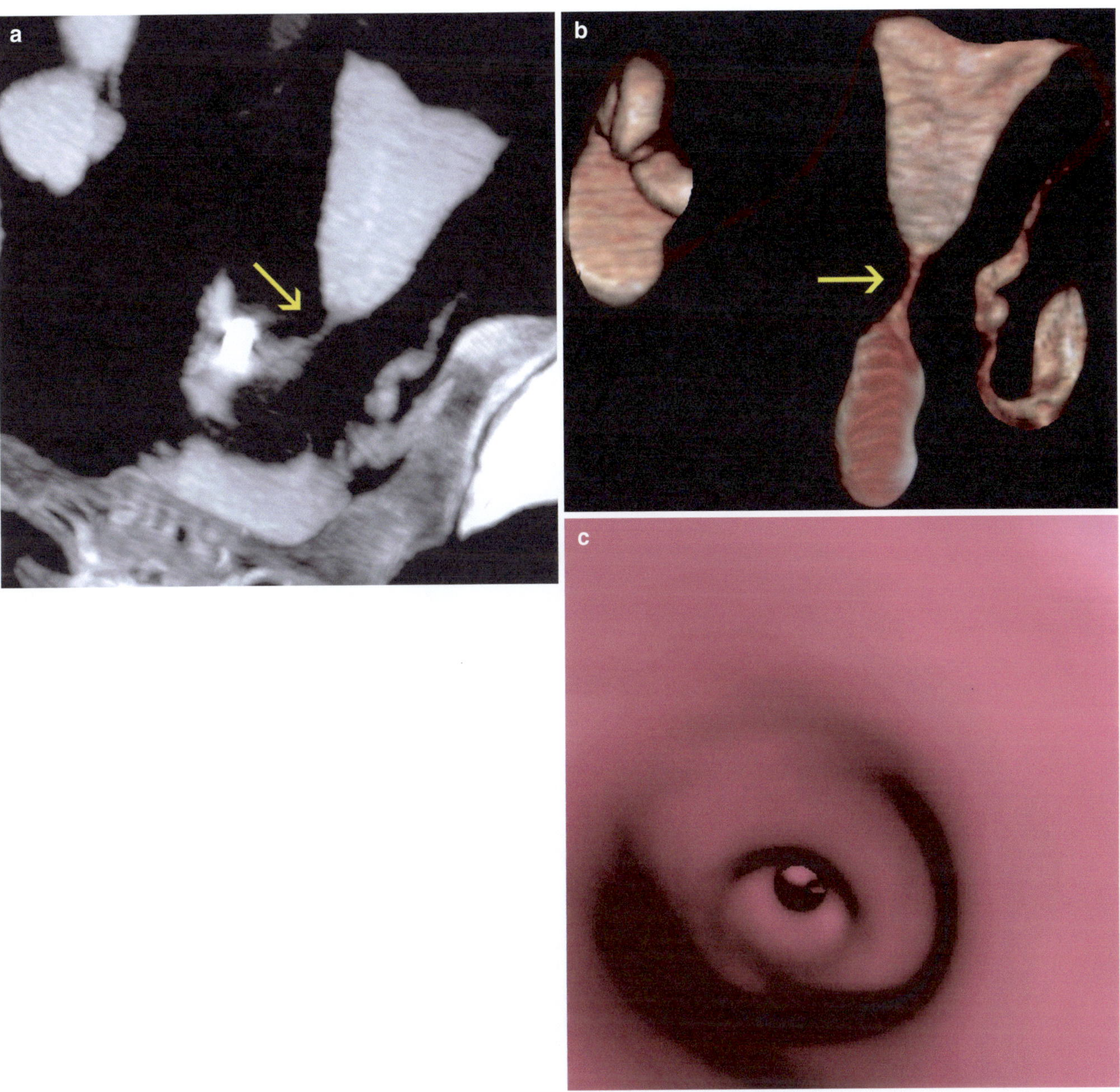

Fig. 5.3 VHSG study which shows cervical stenosis (*arrows*). (**a**) Maximum intensity projection image. (**b**) 3D volume rendering image. (**c**) Virtual endoscopy image

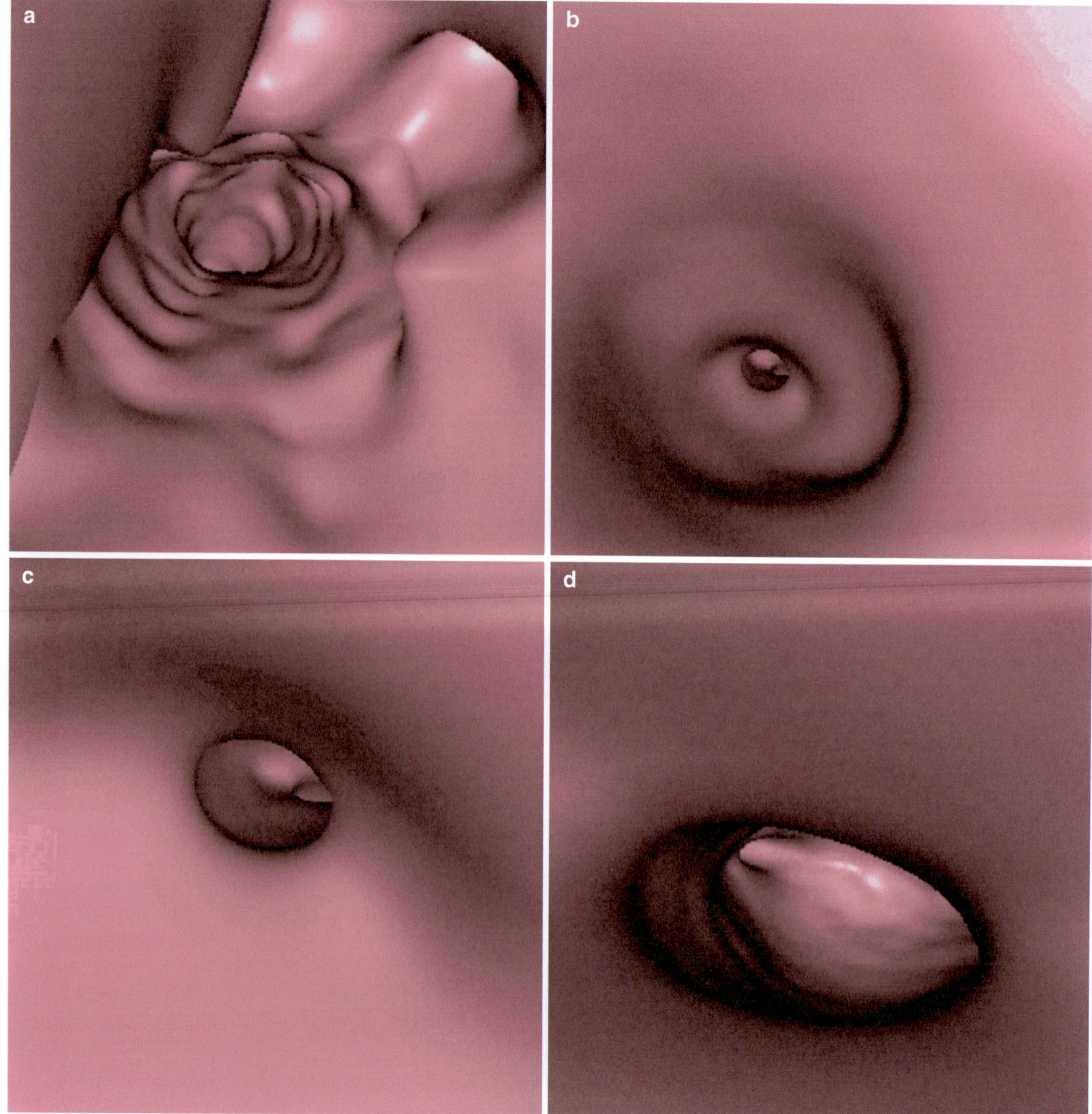

Fig. 5.4 Virtual endoscopy images of a cervical stenosis. (**a**) Pre-stenosis view. (**b**) View at the site of the stenosis. (**c**) Proximal post-stenosis view. (**d**) Distal post-stenosis view

Fig. 5.6 (**a, b**) Maximum intensity projection images which show lineal filling defects in the center of the cervical canal (*arrows*) compatible with synechiae. (**c**) 3D volume rendering image with similar findings (*arrow*). (**d**) Virtual endoscopy image shows irregularities on left lateral wall (*arrow*)

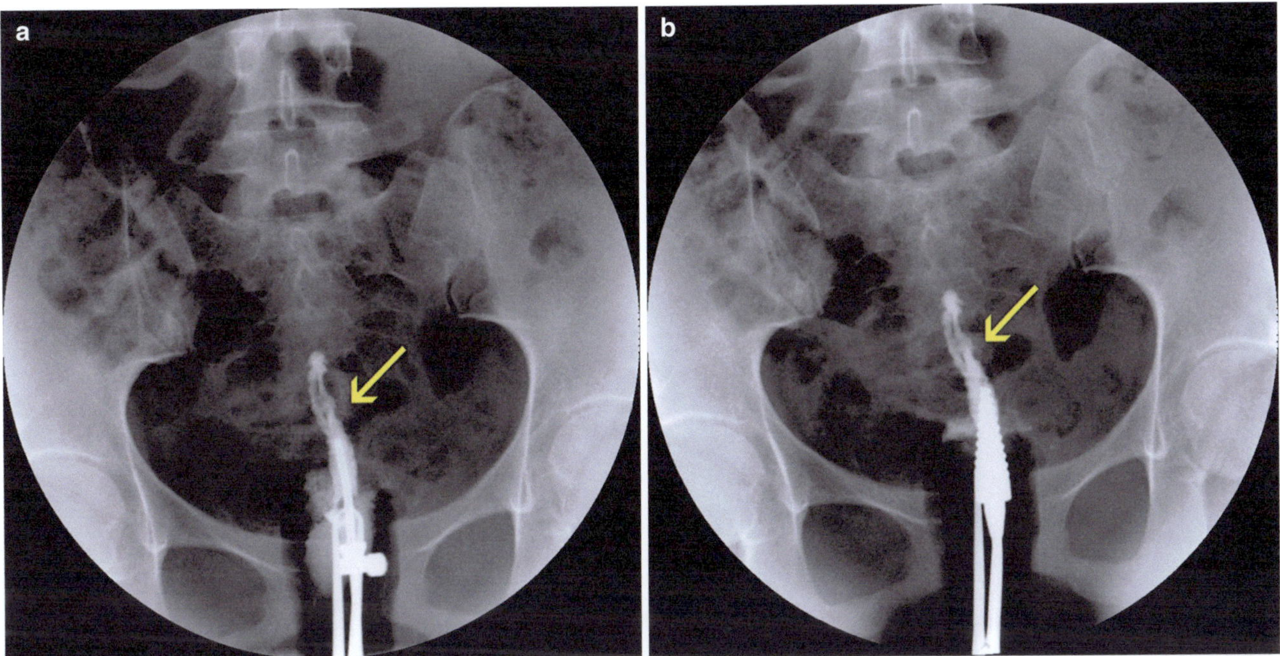

Fig. 5.5 Cervical synechiae in HSG study. (**a**, **b**) Anterioposterior projections with progressive injection of contrast showing filling defects at the level of the cervical lumen compatible with synechiae (*arrows*). Note that the cannulas have been changed to avoid contrast reflux

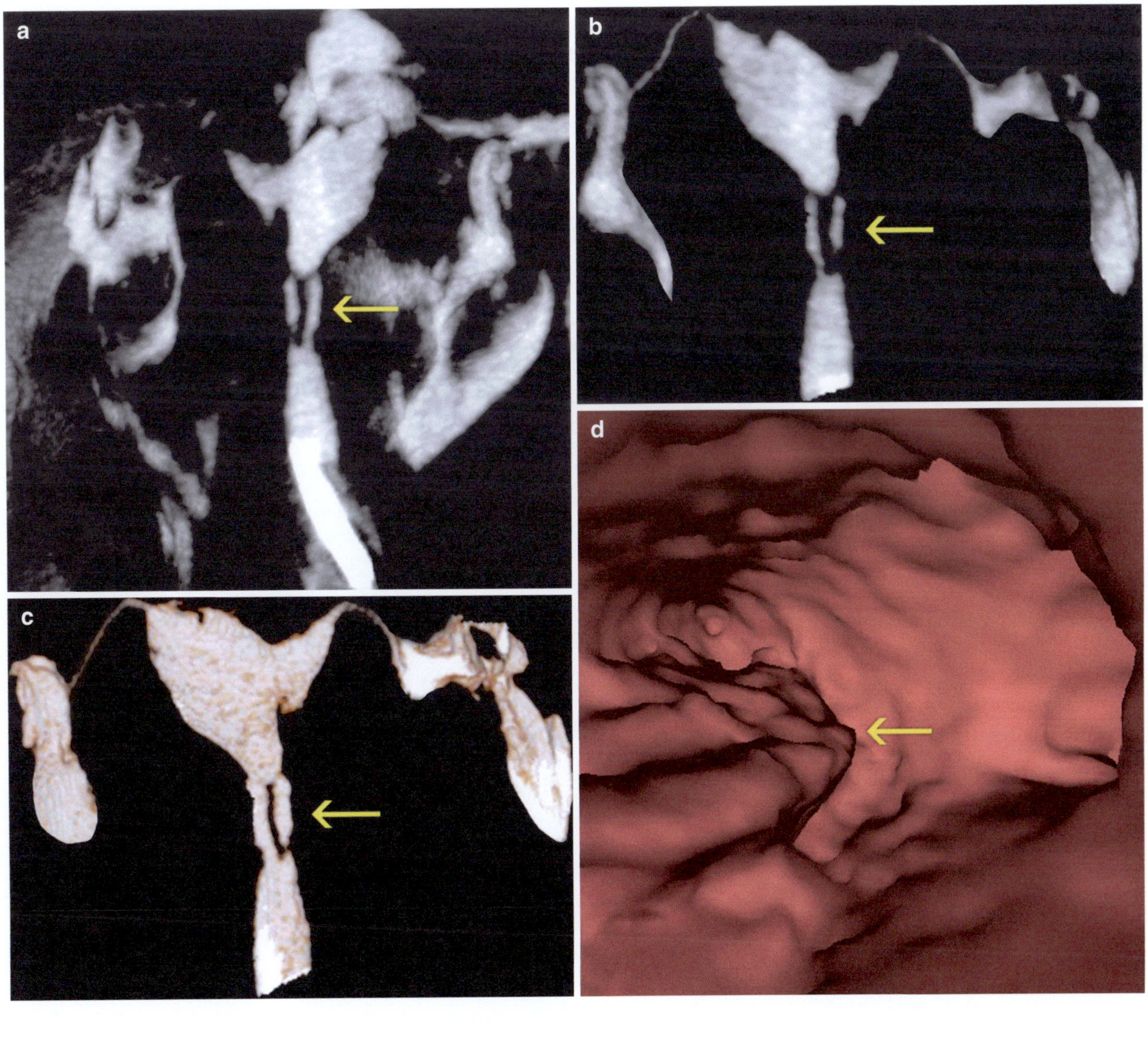

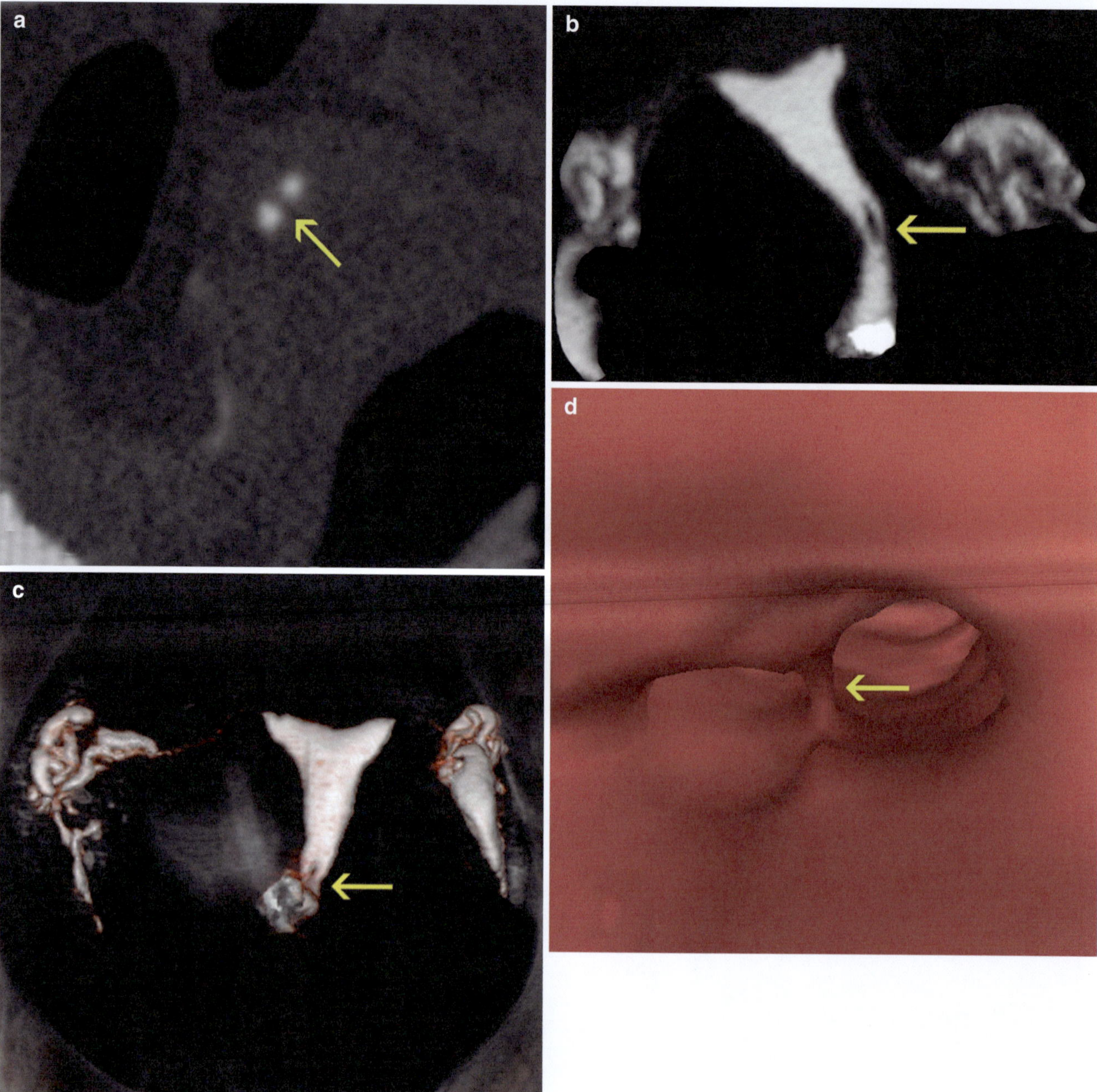

Fig. 5.7 Cervical synechiae in a VHSG study. (**a**) Axial CT image at the level of the distal cervix which shows a soft-tissue, lineal filling defect (*arrow*) corresponding to endocervical synechiae. (**b**) Maximum intensity projection image which shows a filling defect in the cervical lumen, adjacent to the left lateral wall (*arrow*). (**c**) 3D volume rendering image shows similar findings (*arrow*). (**d**) Virtual endoscopy images illustrates a septum that separates the cervical lumen, corresponding to the synechiae (*arrow*)

Polyps

Polyps are elevated lesions which are found with frequency in women older than 20 years old who have had children. It is rare in young women who have not begun menstruating.

Polyps can be single or multiple. Most patients present only one polyp. They have smooth edges and variable size.

These lesions appear as a natural response to the increase in estrogen levels, to chronic inflammation or to obstruction of the blood vessels of the uterine neck. They can be asymptomatic or produce symptoms such as:

- Abnormally abundant periods (menorrhagia).
- Abnormal vaginal bleeding.
- Yellow or white mucus (leucorrhea).

Most of the polyps are benign and easy to remove although in a low percentage of cases can become malignant. It is for this reason that they should be analyzed.

Methods that achieve the capacity to diagnose them are HSG and VHSG.

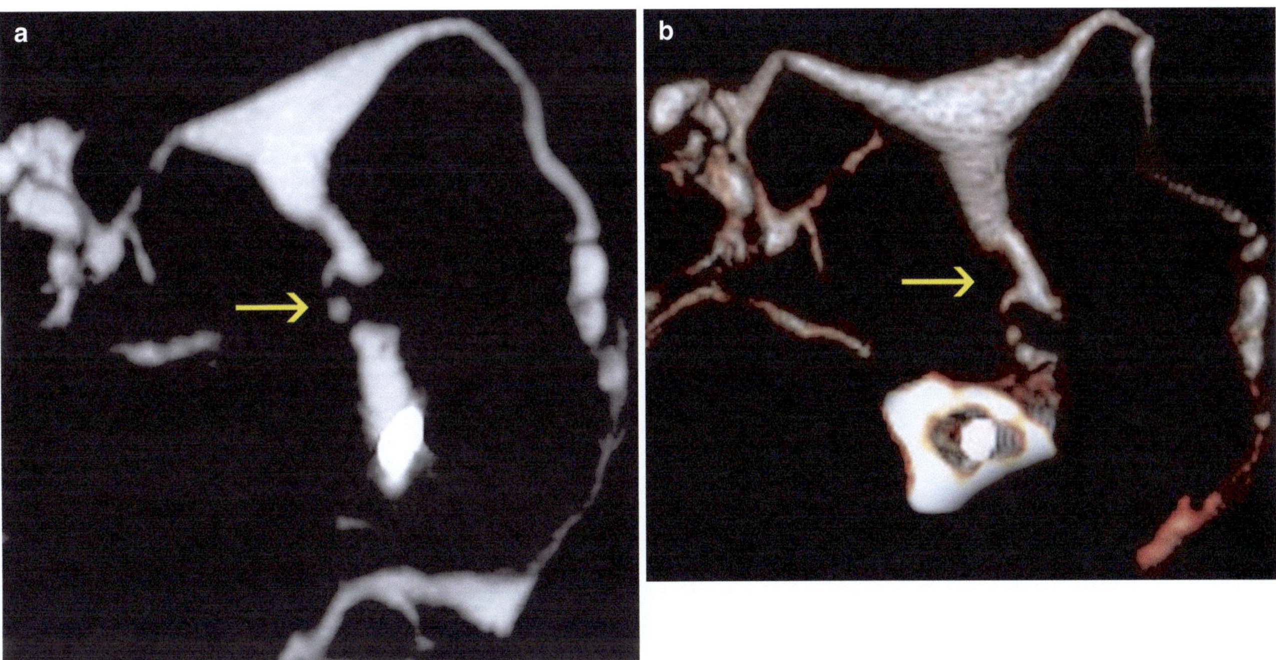

Fig. 5.8 Extensive cervical synechiae in a VHSG study. (**a**) Coronal maximum intensity projection image where an irregular cervix with filling defects compatible with synechiae (*arrow*) is observed. (**b**) Coronal 3D volume rendering image which exhibits similar findings (*arrow*)

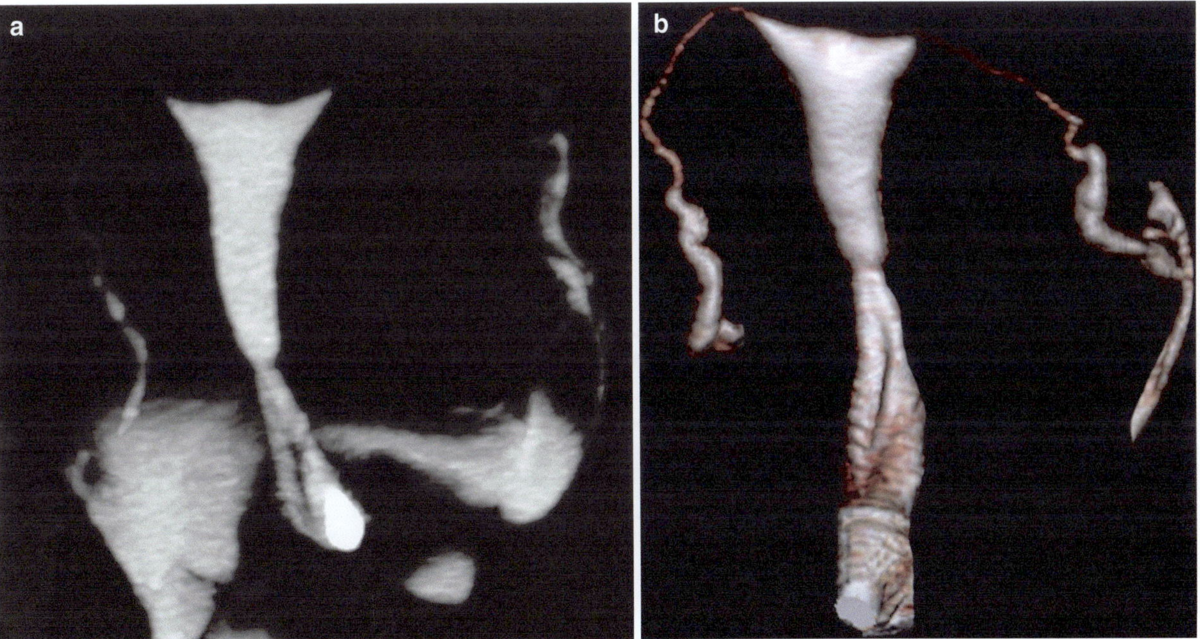

Fig. 5.9 Thick folds in VHSG. (**a**) Coronal maximum intensity projection image which shows a thick fold in the cervix which extends from the proximal to the distal sector. (**b**) Coronal 3D volume rendering image shows similar findings. (**c, d**) Virtual endoscopy images which illustrate the thick fold (*arrow*)

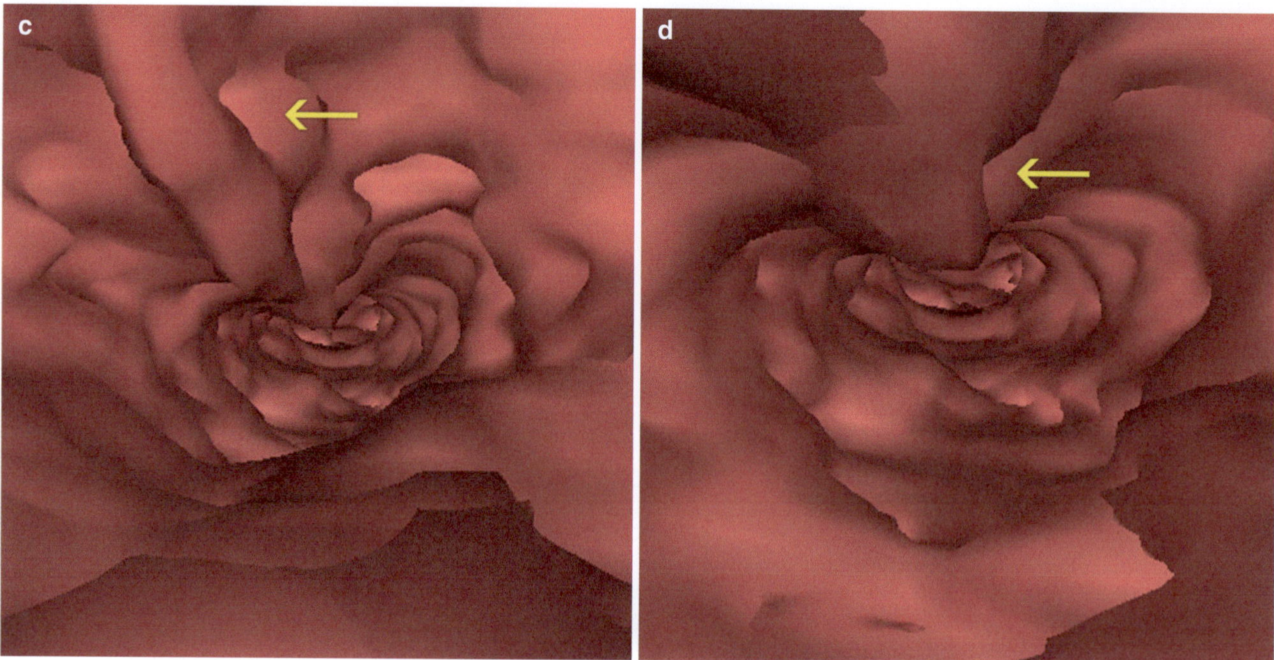

Fig. 5.9 (continued)

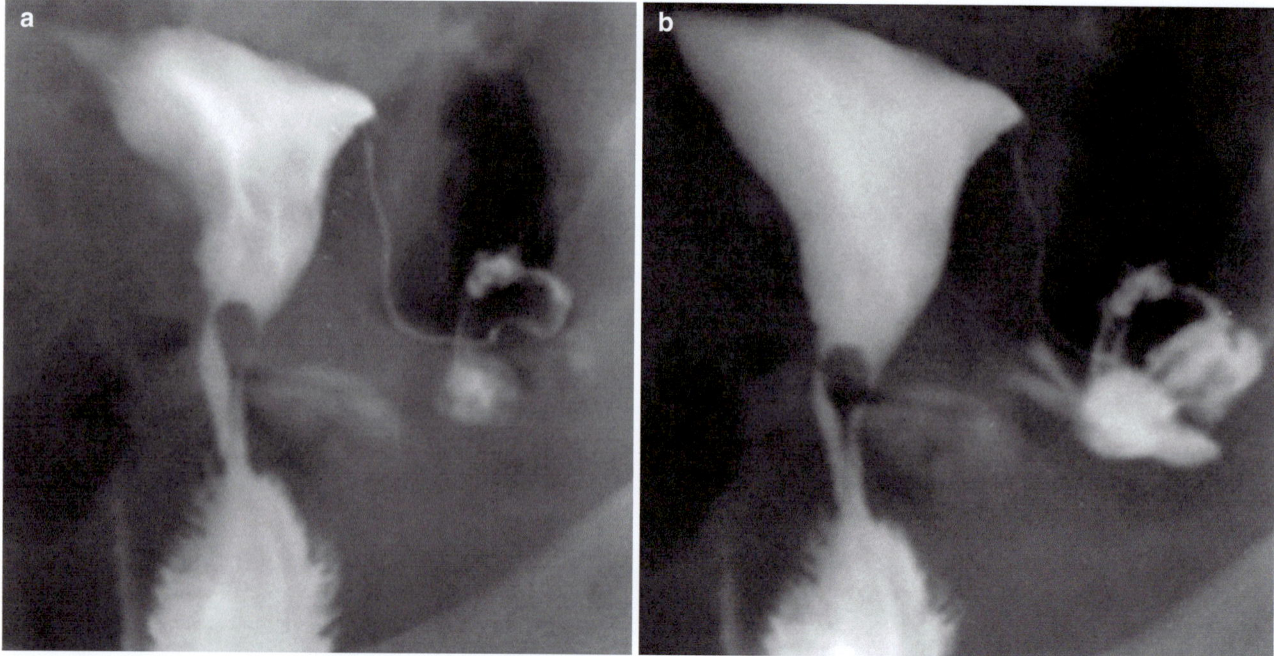

Fig. 5.10 (**a**, **b**) HSG with cervical stalked polyp. The head of the polyp projects towards the cervical isthmic region

HSG: permits the identification of filling defect lesions, if they have a considerable size [19, 20] (Fig. 5.10). These lesions are more difficult to detect if they are small.

VHSG: exhibits the polypoid lesion as an elevated tissue that projects into the cervix lumen [4, 5, 13]. The smaller ones reduce partially the cervical cavity (Fig. 5.11) while the larger ones obliterate it completely (Fig. 5.12).

Multiplanar reconstructions show the densitometry of the polyps (soft tissue). Measurements of polyps size has to be done on them as they provide the most accurate information (Fig. 5.13).

VR reconstructions are also very valuable as they display the filling defect in the location of the polyp.

Endoscopic images exhibit the endoluminal view of the polyp.

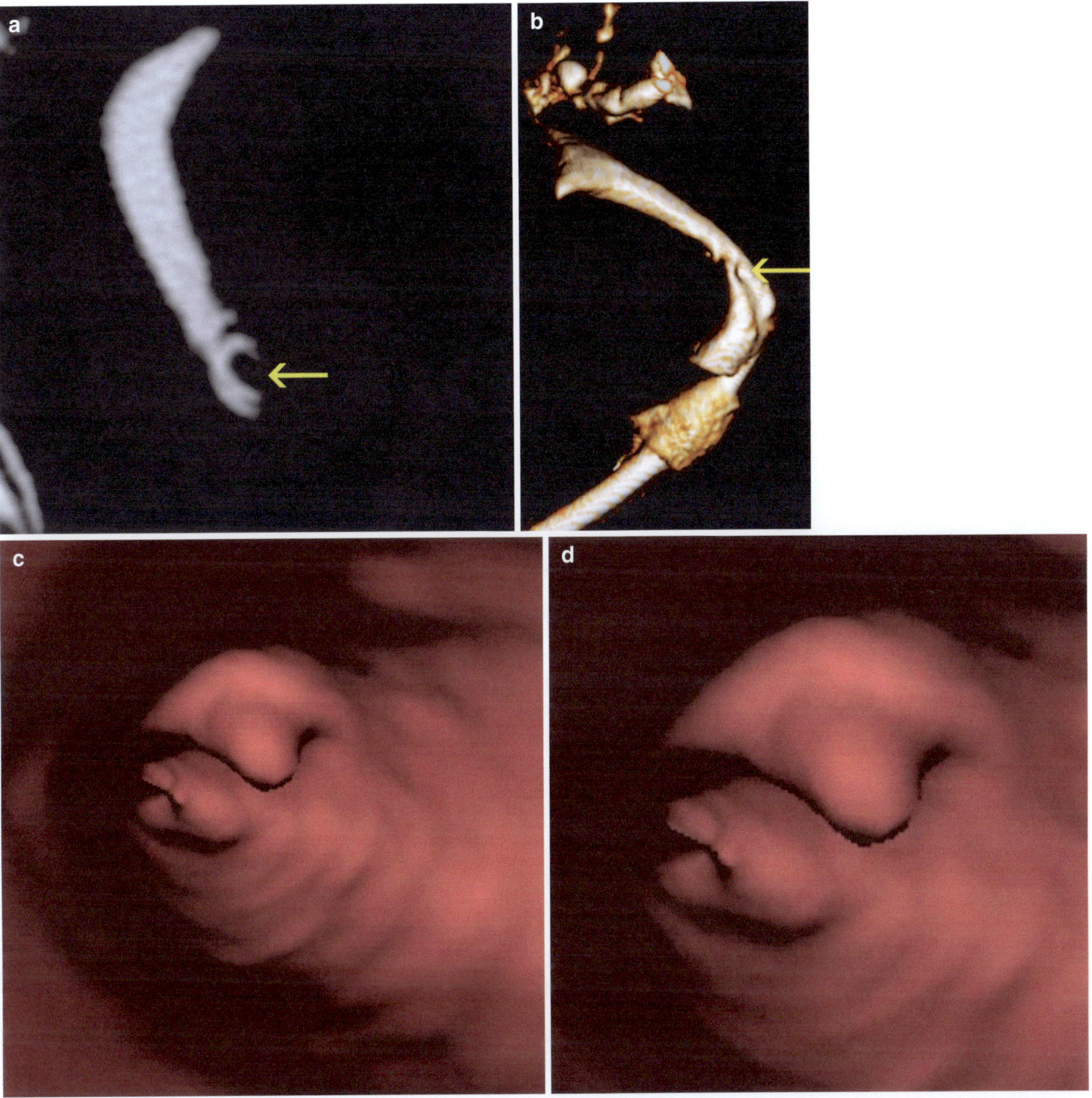

Fig. 5.11 Cervical polyp of great size. (**a**) Multiplanar reconstruction image shows a polyp in the cervix (*arrow*). (**b**) 3D volume rendering image showing a polyp in the cervix (*arrow*). (**c**, **d**) Virtual endoscopy images of the polyp

Diverticles

Diverticles constitute herniations of the cervix wall that project on any of its walls. They do not represent an important finding.

Herniations can be detected by HSG and VHSG [1–3].

HSG: shows the focal dilatation in a cervical wall with defined edges (Fig. 5.14).

VHSG: identifies similar findings to those found in HSG, with the advantage of providing tridimensional and endoscopic images which can detect the neck of the diverticule intra-luminally (Fig. 5.15).

Cesarean Scar

The cesarean scar is located in the isthmic-cervical region and in most of the cases produces an irregularity in the scar section with dilatations of diverse sizes and thinning in the wall at that level (Fig. 5.16). These findings are correctly

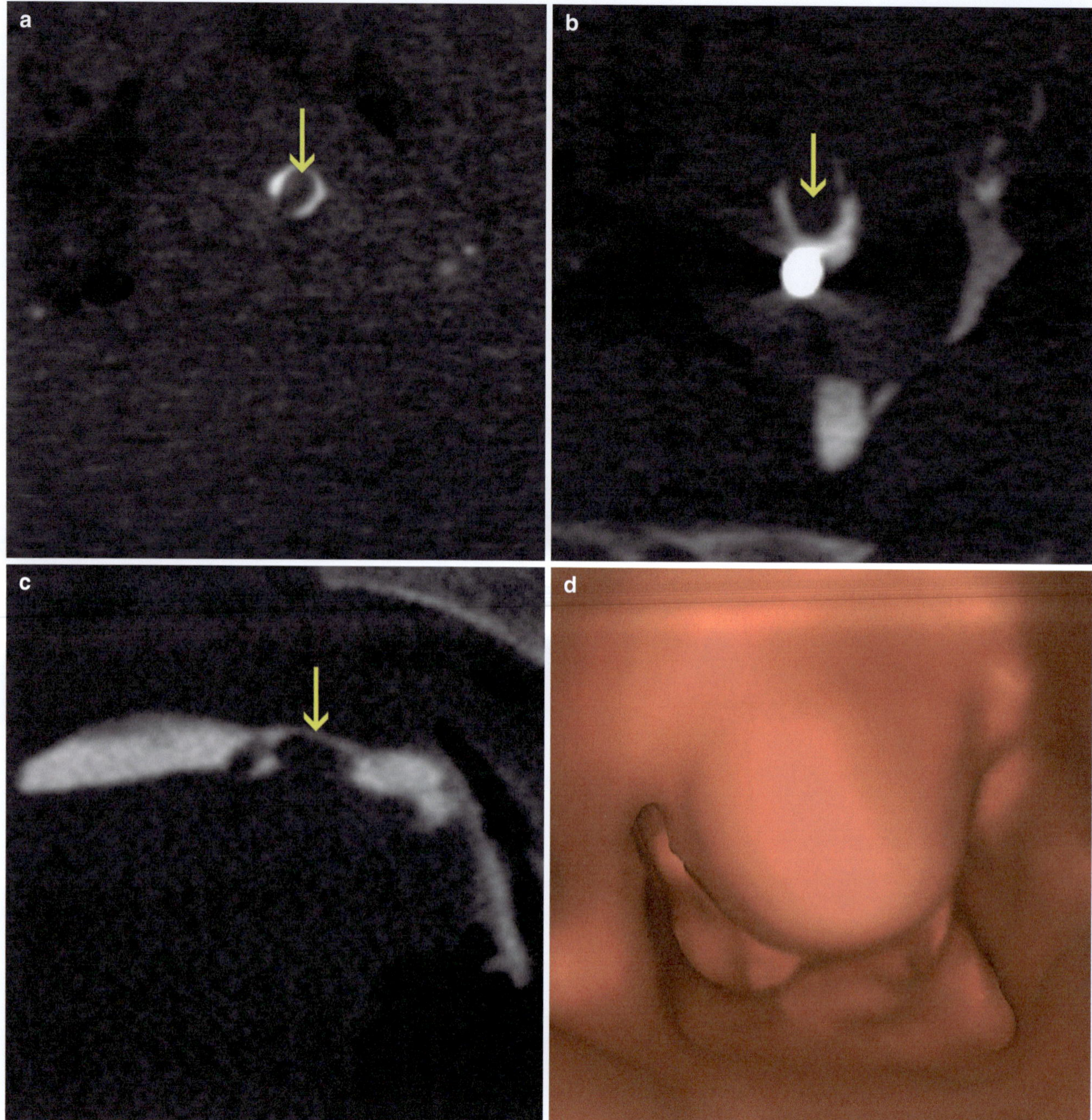

Fig. 5.12 (**a–c**) Coronal, axial and sagittal CT images which show a big cervical polyp that significantly obstructs the lumen (*arrows*). (**d**) Virtual endoscopy image

observed on the sagittal images in the multiplanar reconstruction where one can measure the width of the cervical wall in the site of the scar. VR reconstructions display the post-surgery dilatations and offer volumetric information [1–5].

The information obtained about the width of the wall, as well as the volume of the dilatation could provide useful information to the gynecologist in terms to greater or less risk of complications in future pregnancies.

Cervical Cancer

Cervical cancer constitutes the 4 % of malign diseases and is the eight cancer in frequency in developed countries. It is the gynecological cancer most frequent in women under 50 years of age and the third cause of gynecological tumor in postmenopausal women after the endometrial and ovary cancer.

Approximately 500,000 women are diagnosed with cervical cancer per year worldwide, and 350,000 of them die.

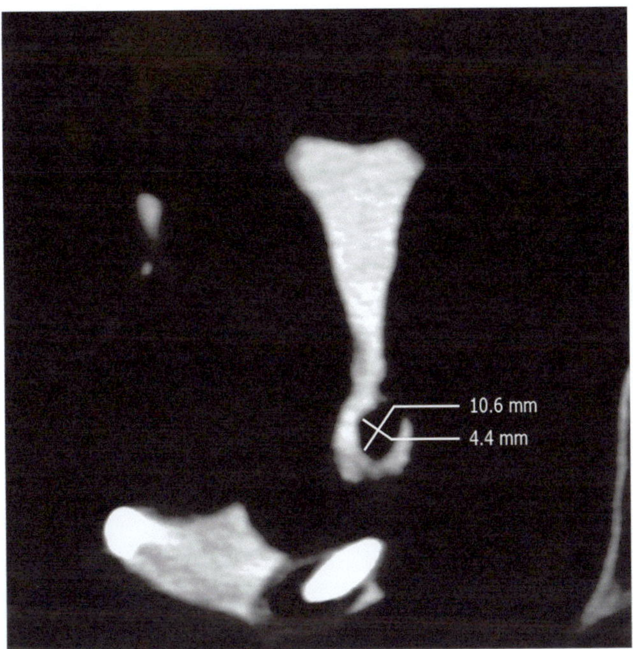

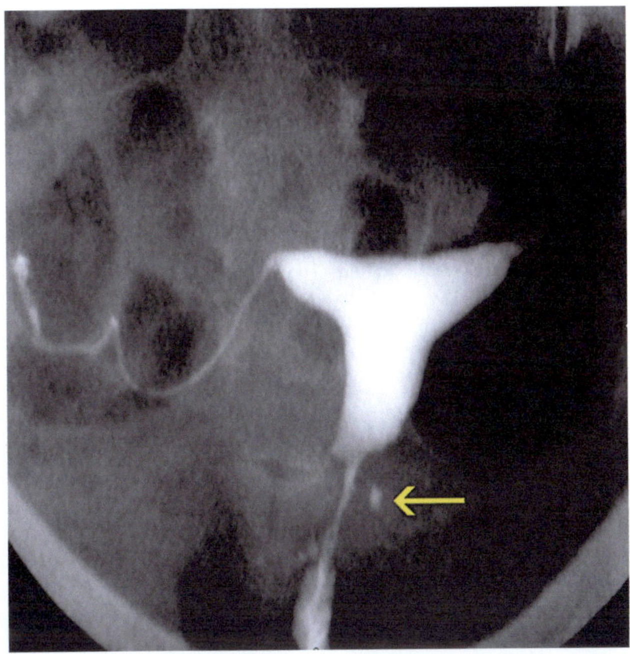

Fig. 5.13 Polyp measurements in multiplanar reconstruction image. An elevated lesion at the level of the lateral wall in the distal cervical region is observed. The transverse and anteroposterior diameters are displayed

Fig. 5.14 Diverticulum seen on HSG exam. A diverticulum is observed on the left lateral wall of the cervix (*arrow*)

The distribution shows a peak between the ages of 35 and 45, and a second peak between 60 and 64 years old. The incidence of cervical cancer has been reduced by a 75 % due to the development of cytological screening programs [21, 22]. The precursor conditions are more frequent in women between the ages of 30 and 40 than invasive cancer. The precursor lesions gradually progress to invasive disease in a period of 10 years [23]. The invasive cervical cancer that occurs before the 35 years of age is typically of a malignant variety. The survival in United States at 5 years is of 70 % and at 10 years of 65 % [24, 25].

The principal cause of cervical cancer is the infection of the epithelium by an oncogenic virus denominated Human Papilloma Virus (HPV). The high risk types include HPV 16, HPV 18, HPV 31, HPV 33, HPV 45, among others. Around three quarters of all uterine neck cancers are caused by HPV 16 and 18 [26–30]. The prevalence of infections by HPV is of 5–20 %, with a peak between 20 and 25 years. Spontaneous regression is frequent However, if the virus is persistent, it associates to epithelium changes in the cervical mucosa, especially in women with other associated risk factors like multiple sexual partners, frequent genital infections, immunosuppression and prolonged use of oral contraceptives [31–33]. Other factors that may influence are the cigarette, vitamin deficiencies and genetic predisposition.

The cervical squamous cancer develops over various stages, from the epithelium proliferation, epithelial changes, dysplasia, to definitive epithelium changes with precancerous lesions. Precancerous stages refer to a cervical intra-epithelial neoplasia (CIN) [34] or a scaly intra-epithelial lesion (SIL) which finally progress to an in situ carcinoma before transforming into an invasive cancer. The early stages of CIN can be observed in women halfway through their second decade. With frequency there are resolved spontaneously but may progress to in situ cancer, between the ages of 25 and 35 and, finally, to cervical cancer.

Early types of cancer do not present symptoms. In more advanced stages vaginal bleeding or pain can be observed after sexual intercourse. In very advanced stages, when the cancer has spread to adjacent structures, it can produce diffuse pelvic pain and pain in the lumbar region, extended to the legs. In cases in which the lymphatic drainage is compromised, a unilateral edema of the leg with increase of the abdominal circumference can be produced. The general symptoms in advanced stages consist in asthenia and loss of weight.

Histologically, 80 % are keratinizing or non keratinizing squamous carcinomas. The second tumor in frequency is the adenocarcinoma in 15 % [35]. Its incidence has increased during the last 5 years. It is associated with chronic cervicitis and estrogens taking The II and III stages of the adenocarcinoma are more disfavorable than the squamous carcinoma [36]. Three percent of the adenocarcinomas have a highly differentiated histological mucinous subtype.

The malignant adenoma, which is actually an adenocarcinoma, has a poor prognosis due to the fact it extends to the abdominal cavity and has an insufficient response to chemotherapy or radiotherapy [37, 38]. It is associated with the Peutz-Jeghers syndrome which is characterized by

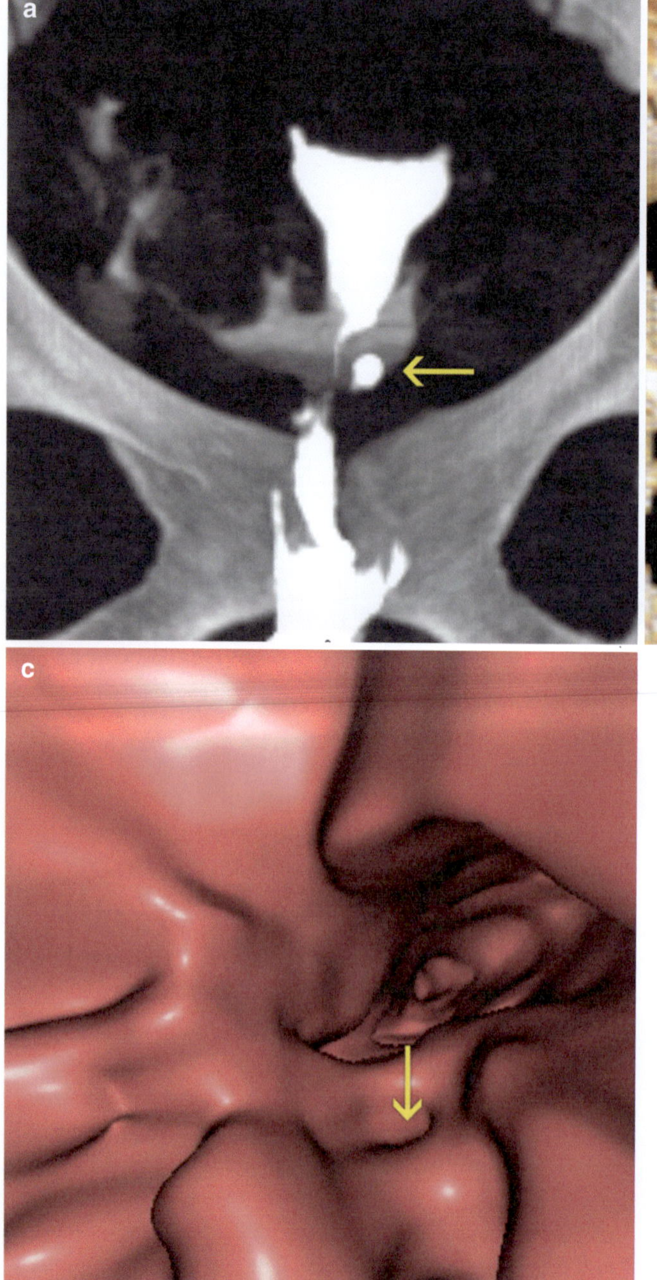

Fig. 5.15 Diverticulum seen on VHSG exam. (**a**) Maximum intensity projection image. A diverticulum is observed on the left lateral wall (*arrow*). (**b**) 3D volume rendering image. Similar findings are identified (*arrow*). (**c**) Virtual endoscopy image. The diverticular neck is visualized (*arrow*)

pigmentation of the skin and mucosa, multiple hamartomas of the gastrointestinal tract and ovary tumors [39].

Other cervical tumors are the neuroendocrine, the adenosquamous tumor and the rhabdomyosarcoma.

The factors which define the prognosis of uterine neck cancer are (i) the tumor size, (ii) the extension of the myocervical invasion (more than half of the myocervical width), (iii) the parametrium invasion, (iv) the extension of the pelvic wall, (v) the affectation of the lymph nodes and (vi) distant metastases [1].

The International Federation of Gynecology and Obstetrics (IFGO) establishes stages of the disease, according to the classification system on which is based the treatment. The correct evaluation of each of these phases is decisive for the therapeutic treatment.

The TNM system of the American Joint Committee on Cancer (AJCC) has been integrated into the accepted stages by the IFGO including the physical exam and imaging diagnosis data [40].

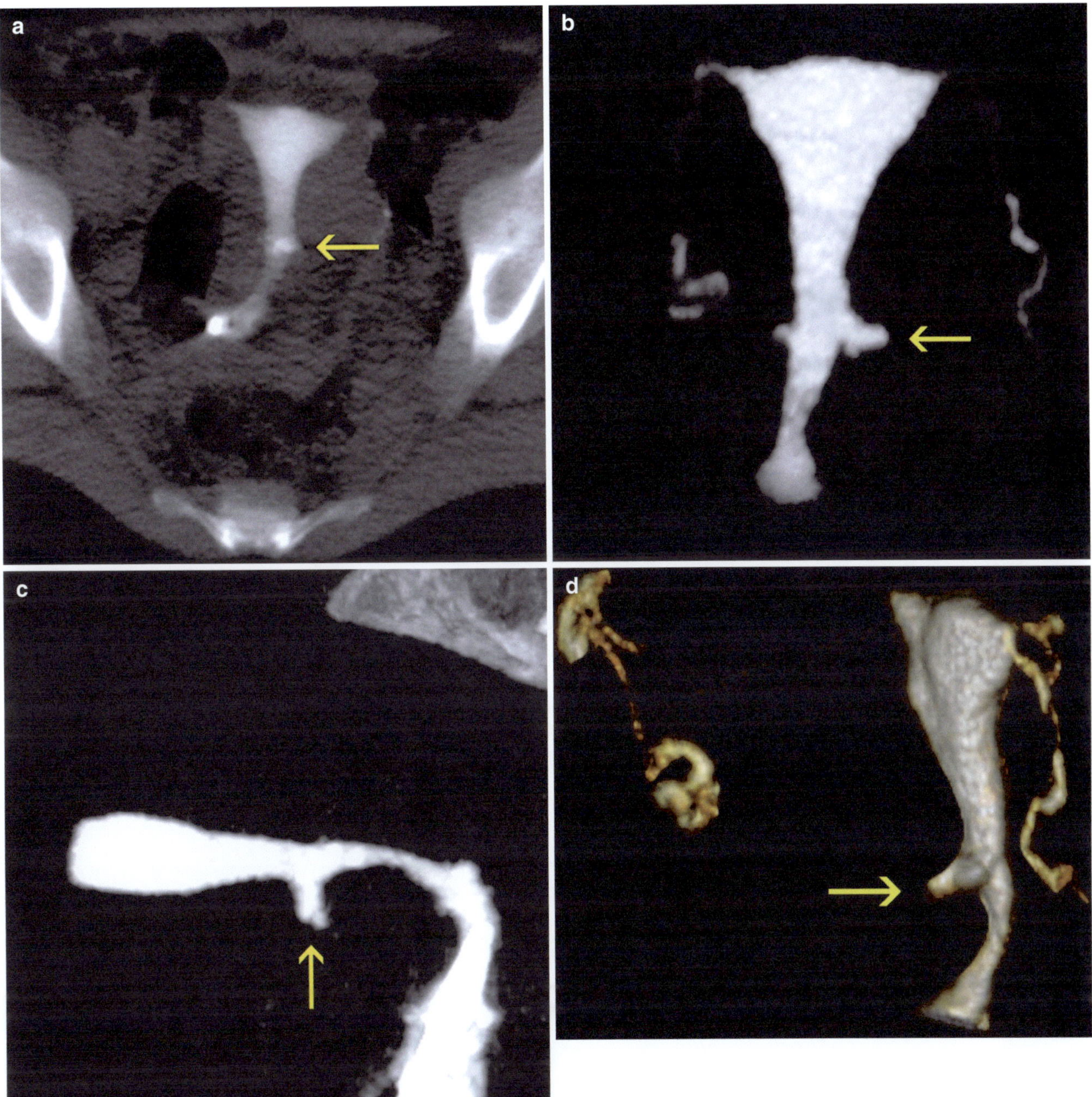

Fig. 5.16 Cesarean scar seen on VHSG exam. (**a**) 10-mm multiplanar reconstruction image which shows a sector of dilatation in the isthmic-cervical region (*arrow*). (**b**) Coronal maximum intensity projection (MIP) image which better displays the dilatation (*arrow*). (**c**) Sagittal MIP image is exhibited in the sector of dilatation towards the anterior wall (*arrow*). (**d**) Oblique sagittal 3D volume rendering image which shows similar findings (*arrow*)

The report of imaging studies must include: (i) tumor size, (ii) depth of the myocervical invasion, (iii) degree of extension of the parametrium invasion (lateral and uterosac parametriums), reporting if it reaches the pelvic wall, (iv) vaginal infiltration, (v) evaluation of pelvic and/or lymphatic nodes from the obturatriz pit, (vi) infiltration of vesical-cervical-vaginal space and/or rectum-vaginal space and (vii) distant metastases.

The definition of TNM and the grouping of the stages have been updated in the 7th edition, reflecting the new staging adopted by the IFGO, which no longer reckons the stage 0 (Tis). Furthermore, the visible macroscopic lesions, even with superficial invasion, are considered like T1b/IB [40].

In Tables 5.1, 5.2, 5.3 and 5.4, the updated and united system for uterine neck cancer is shown.

The IFGO defines the diagnostic procedures which are required for the pre-treatment evaluation like the biopsy, the cervical conization and the hysteroscopy.

Table 5.1 Stages of uterine neck cancer according to the unified criteria of the AJCC and FIGO. Primary tumor (T)

TNM Categories	FIGO Stages	Surgical-pathologic findings
TX		Primary tumor cannot be assessed
T0		No evidence of primary tumor
Tis[a]		Carcinoma in situ (preinvasive carcinoma)
T1	I	Cervical carcinoma confined to the cervix (disregard extension to the corpus)
T1a[b]	IA	Invasive carcinoma diagnosed only by microscopy; stromal invasion with a maximum depth of 5.0 mm measured from the base of the epithelium and a horizontal spread of 7.0 mm or less; vascular space involvement, venous or lymphatic, does not affect classification
T1a1	IA1	Measured stromal invasion ≤3.0 mm in depth and ≤7.0 mm in horizontal spread
T1a2	IA2	Measured stromal invasion >3.0 mm and ≤5.0 mm with a horizontal spread ≤7.0 mm
T1b	IB	Clinically visible lesion confined to the cervix or microscopic lesion greater than T1a/IA2
T1b1	IB1	Clinically visible lesion ≤4.0 cm in greatest dimension
T1b2	IB2	Clinically visible lesion >4.0 cm in greatest dimension
T2	II	Cervical carcinoma invades beyond uterus but not to pelvic wall or to lower third of vagina
T2a	IIA	Tumor without parametrial invasion
T2a1	IIA1	Clinically visible lesion ≤4.0 cm in greatest dimension
T2a2	IIA2	Clinically visible lesion >4.0 cm in greatest dimension
T2b	IIB	Tumor with parametrial invasion
T3	III	Tumor extends to pelvic wall and/or involves lower third of vagina and/or causes hydronephrosis or nonfunctional kidney
T3a	IIIA	Tumor involves lower third of vagina, no extension to pelvic wall
T3b	IIIB	Tumor extends to pelvic wall and/or causes hydronephrosis or nonfunctional kidney
T4	IV	Tumor invades mucosa of bladder or rectum and/or extends beyond true pelvis (bullous edema is not sufficient to classify a tumor as T4)
T4a	IVA	Tumor invades mucosa of bladder or rectum (bullous edema is not sufficient to classify a tumor as T4)
T4b	IVB	Tumor extends beyond true pelvis

[a]FIGO do not consider stage 0 (Tis)
[b]All macroscopically visible lesions, even with superficial invasion, are considered T1b/IB

Table 5.2 Stages of uterine neck cancer according to the unified criteria of the AJCC and FIGO. Regional lymph nodes (N)

TNM Categories	FIGO Stages	Surgical-pathologic findings
NX		Regional lymph nodes cannot be assessed
N0		No regional lymph node metastasis
N1	IIIB	Regional lymph node metastasis

Table 5.3 Stages of uterine neck cancer according to the unified criteria of the AJCC and FIGO. Distant metastases (M)

TNM Categories	FIGO Stages	Surgical-pathologic findings
M0		No distant metastasis
M1	IVb	Distant metastasis (including peritoneal spread; involvement of supraclavicular, mediastinal, or para-aortic lymph nodes; and lung, liver, or bone)

Table 5.4 Stages of uterine neck cancer according to the unified criteria of the AJCC and FIGO

Stage	T	N	M
Stage 0[a]	Tis	N0	M0
Stage I	T1	N0	M0
Stage IA	T1a	N0	M0
Stage IA1	T1a1	N0	M0
Satge IA2	T1a2	N0	M0
Stage IB	T1b	N0	M0
Stage IB1	T1b1	N0	M0
Stage IB2	T1b2	N0	M0
Stage II	T2	N0	M0
Stage IIA	T2a	N0	M0
Stage IIA1	T2a1	N0	M0
Stage IIA2	T2a2	N0	M0
Stage IIB	T2b	N0	M0
Stage III	T3	N0	M0
Stage IIIA	T3a	N0	M0
Stage IIIB	T3b	Any N	M0
	T1-3	N1	M0
Stage IVA	T4	Any N	M0
Stage IVB	Any T	Any N	M1

Anatomical stage – Prognostic groups (FIGO 2008)
[a]FIGO do not consider stage 0 (Tis)

Non invasive imaging methods permit the visualization of the tumor in advanced stages and, simultaneously, observe the compromise of the adjacent structures such as the bladder and the rectum. Hence, Magnetic Resonance (MR) and Multislice Computed Tomography (MSCT) are useful tools

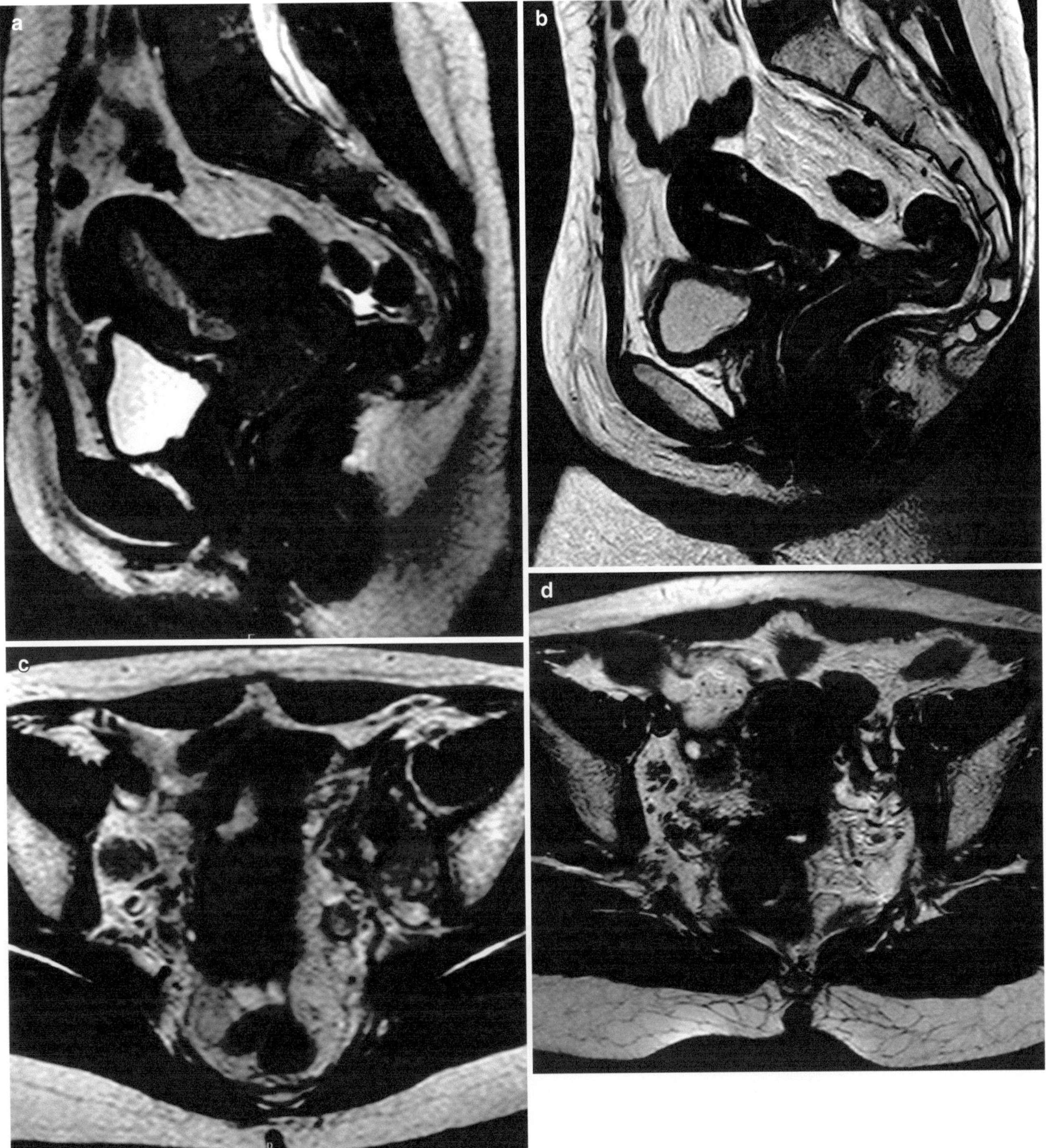

Fig. 5.17 Pelvic MRI. (**a**, **b**) Sagittal T2 weighted MRI images that show a heterogeneous mass in the cervical region which extends towards the posterior adjacent tissue and contacts with the anterior wall of the rectum. (**c**, **d**) Axial T2 weighted MRI images show similar findings

because they allow the visualization of the lesion, and via specific studies like virtual Colonoscopy or Urotomography or Uroresonance, observe the visceral compromise.

MR allows, through high definition studies, the visualization of the tumoral presence, t assessment of its size, and invasion to parametriums as well as the evaluation of the extension at a distance (Fig. 5.17). MR and MSCT are modalities which permit the pre-operative staging [41–43].

The main advantages of the MR and tMSCT are the acquisition speed and the high space resolution. T MR has higher resolution than MSCT but requires the acquisition in multiple planes. MSCT utilizes thin slices of 1 mm width

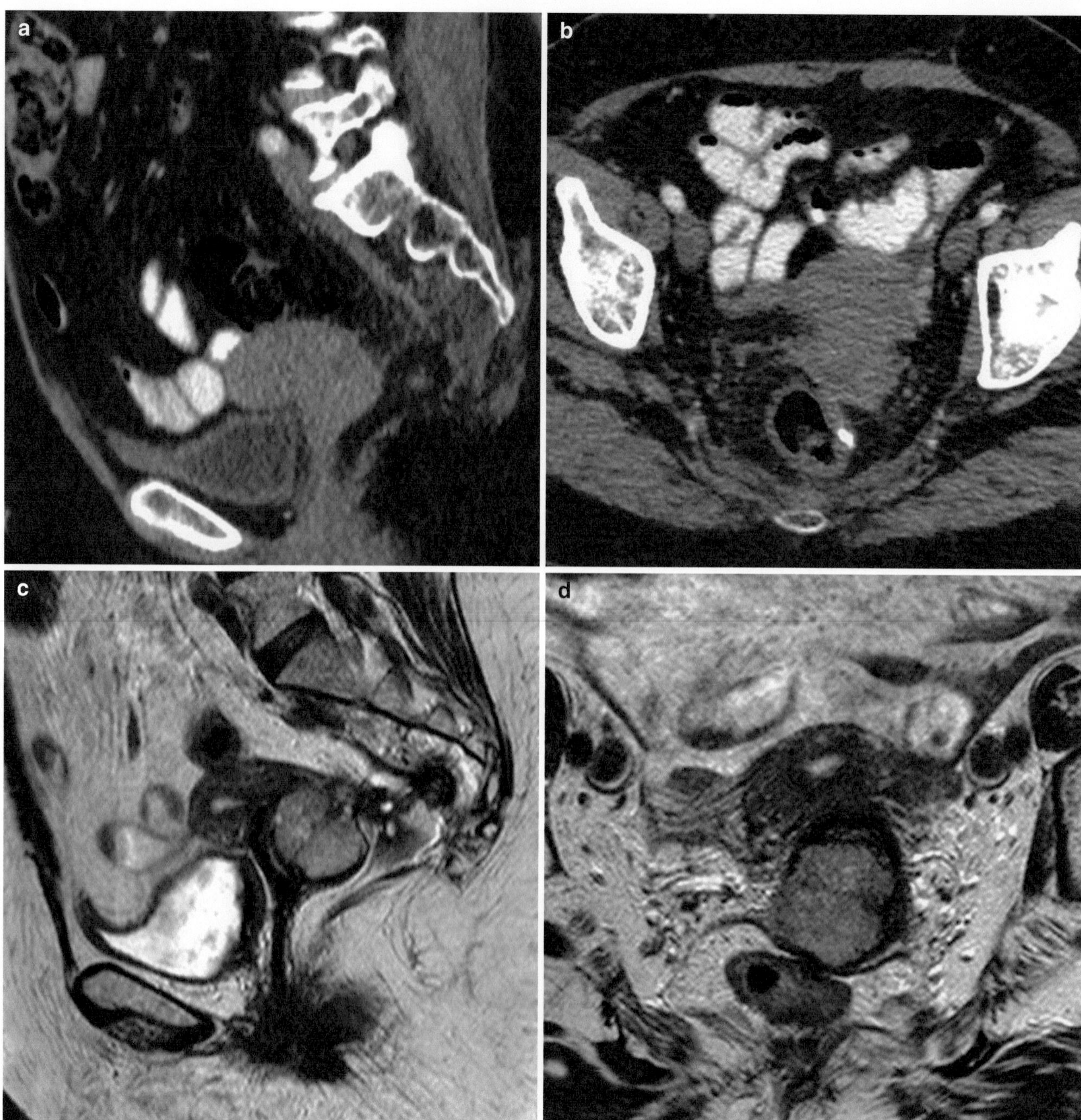

Fig. 5.18 (**a**, **b**) Sagittal and axial CT multiplanar reconstruction images of the pelvis which show an increase in size at the level of the uterine cervical region. (**c**) Sagittal T2 weighted MRI image. A hetero-geneous slightly hyperintense mass with small hyperintense focal areas is observed in the cervix. (**d**) Axial T2 weighted MRI image demon-strates that the cervical contacts with the anterior wall of the rectum

which can then be reconstructed in multiple planes without loss of resolution. Nevertheless, it does not have the same tissue resolution as MR and so the information is much more limited, especially in those high resolution studies (Fig. 5.18).

MR detects small cervical cancers and parametrium inva-sions via high resolution studies [44–56]. MSCT is the method of choice to rule out pulmonary metastases.

VHSG does not have a predominant role in the diagnosis of this type of tumor. It can reveal incidental findings of a patient who undergoes a VHSG study for another reason (Fig. 5.19).

Depending on the tumor stage, it is possible to detect a soft tissue density lesion, which can be associated to the presence of cystic areas at the level of the cervical wall,

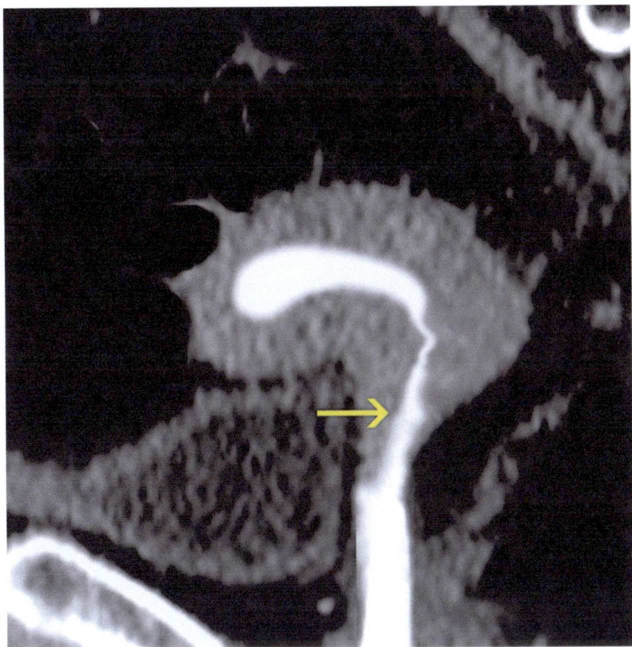

Fig. 5.19 Cervical cancer on VHSG exam. Luminal irregularity is observed in the cervical region (*arrow*)

which can extent towards the vaginal or uterine region, completely or partially obliterating the canal.

In very advanced stages it is possible to observe extension to the bladder or rectum. In these cases, if complimented with endovenose contrast, an urotomography can be performed to show the vesical indemnity or compromise. In the cases where rectal invasion is suspected, virtual colonoscopy would also have a role.

Importance of the VHSG in the Cervical Evaluation in Infertile Patients with Embryo Transfer Treatments

The diverse pathologies previously mentioned at the level of the uterine neck produce partial or total obstruction of the lumen, it is for this reason that their detection, as well as their location and extension would help those patients who must be subject to embryo transfer treatments.

The embryo transfer is a technique where the embryos are deposited in the uterine cavity for their latter implantation and development. It is carried out via a very fine catheter, on which the selected embryos are placed, and is introduced through the vagina across the cervical canal up to the uterine cavity [57]. The evaluation of the neck and endocervix anatomy is fundamental to determine the success and feasibility of the procedure. The cervical transfer test is routinely carried out prior the embryo transfer. It consists in the passing

of a transfer catheter through the cervical canal which is introduced up to the upper third part of the endometrial cavity. It allows knowing the characteristics of the endocervical canal and can be performed via ultrasound to observe the exact location where to place the embryos. There exists a low frequency of error and difficulty during the embryo transfer procedure and a larger rate of successful pregnancy and implantation in patients who underwent the cervical test prior the transfer [58].

An embryo transfer can prove difficult if associated to a traumatic procedure. The causes which may produce this difficulty include the presence of cervical stenosis, endocervical polyps or synechiae, the need of utilizing a traction clamp or the provocation of bleeding when catheterizing. A traumatic transfer is associated with low rates of pregnancy and an increase in ectopic implants. In cases where the cervical test determines that a transfer runs the risk of being troublesome, a hysteroscopy evaluation of the cervical canal and treatment of some solvable causes can be performed, like canal stenosis or cervical polyps [59].

In our center, the usefulness of VHSG in patients who required embryo transfers was evaluated. Hence, the cervical catheter test was compared with VHSG in the evaluation of the cervix prior the embryo transfer.

One hundred patients with a history of infertility were studied. On the day of the exam, a gynecologist performed the cervical canal test with a Wallace catheter. Then, a VHSG was performed with a 256 row multislice CT. Images were evaluated by a radiologist and the permeability of the uterine neck via the passing of contrast to the endometrial cavity, the caliber and length of the cervical canal, the cervical-uterine angle determined by two lines which pass through the longitudinal angle of the cervical and uterine canal, the position of the uterus, and the presence of anatomical variants and of cervical pathologies were determined. VHSG findings were compared with the cervical test and the degree of correlation was calculated via the Cohen's kappa method. Two groups were considered for the analysis: patients with a normal cervical test and permeable cervical canal, and those with a normal cervical test, but not permeable cervical canal, with resistance to the passing of the catheter T Student test was used to calculate the differences between both groups when the distribution of the variable was normal

A good correlation between both methods was observed (n = 0.92) in the evaluation of the permeability of the uterine neck. In 65 % of the patients, the cervical test was successful and non traumatic (normal). Within this group of patients, t VHSG showed a normal cervical canal in 92 % of the cases. The average cervical-uterine angle was 132° (Fig. 5.20); and in 95 % of the patients from this group, the cervical-uterine angle was over 90°. In 8 % of the cases with normal cervical tests, VHSG showed three cervical polyps below 5 mm and two synechiae that did not produce cervical luminal stenosis.

In 35 % of the patients, the cervical test was considered abnormal. In this group, VHSG showed five cervical polyps (Fig. 5.21), six synechiae (Fig. 5.22), and three sinuous cervical canal (Fig. 5.23). The average cervical-uterine angle was of 76° (Fig. 5.24). There were two cases where VHSG was abnormal and no probable cause for the abnormal cervical test could be identified.

There were no significant differences in the caliber nor in the length of the cervical canal between both groups, although a patient with a normal cervical test and cervical stenosis was identified.

It was concluded that a good correlation between the VHSG and the cervical catheter test existed in the evaluation of the permeability of the uterine neck. VHSG also provided useful anatomical information for identifying the probable cause for the failure of the embryo transfer.

Fig. 5.20 Sagittal maximum intensity projection image shows a uterine-cervical angle of 151°

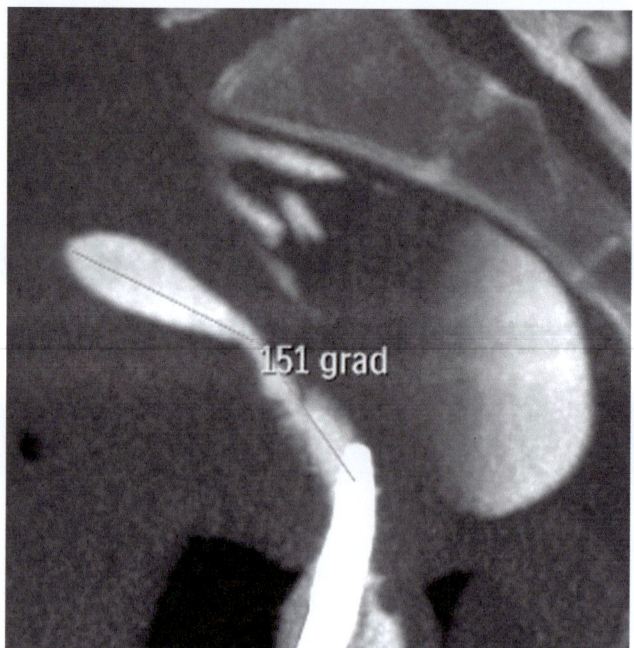

Fig. 5.21 (**a**) Sagittal maximum intensity projection image shows a filling defect compatible with a polyp in the cervix (*arrow*). (**b**) Coronal 3D volume rendering image. The polyp is clearly identified (*arrow*)

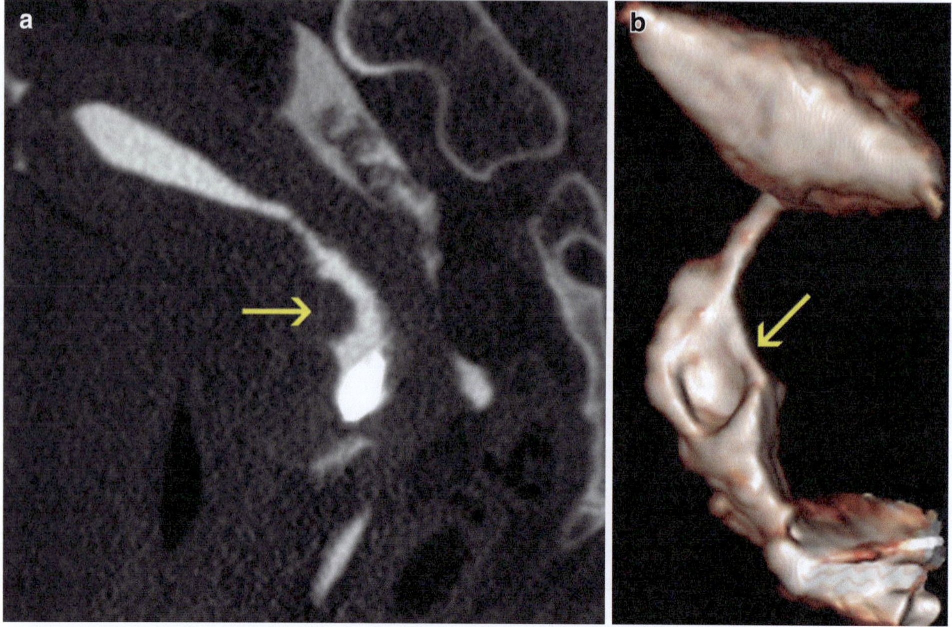

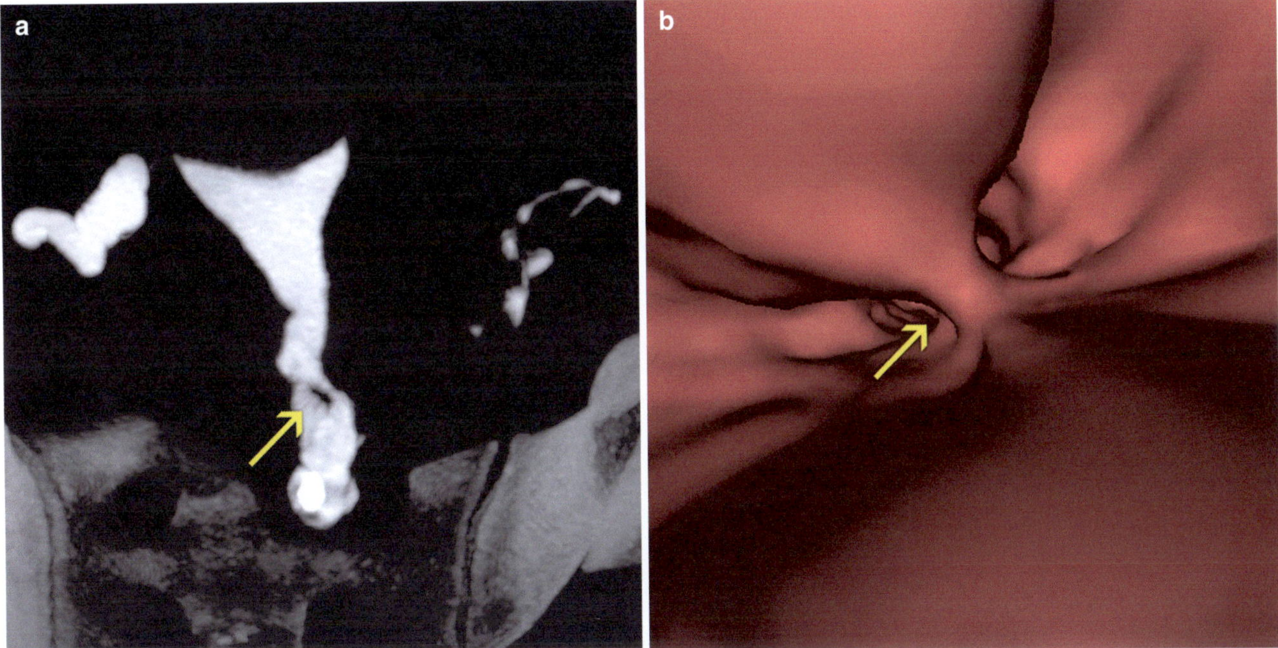

Fig. 5.22 (**a**) Coronal maximum intensity projection image. An irregularity in the cervix is observed with a hypodense lineal image compatible with synechiae (*arrow*). (**b**) Virtual endoscopy image shows a filling defect that extends from the anterior to the posterior wall of the cervical canal (*arrow*)

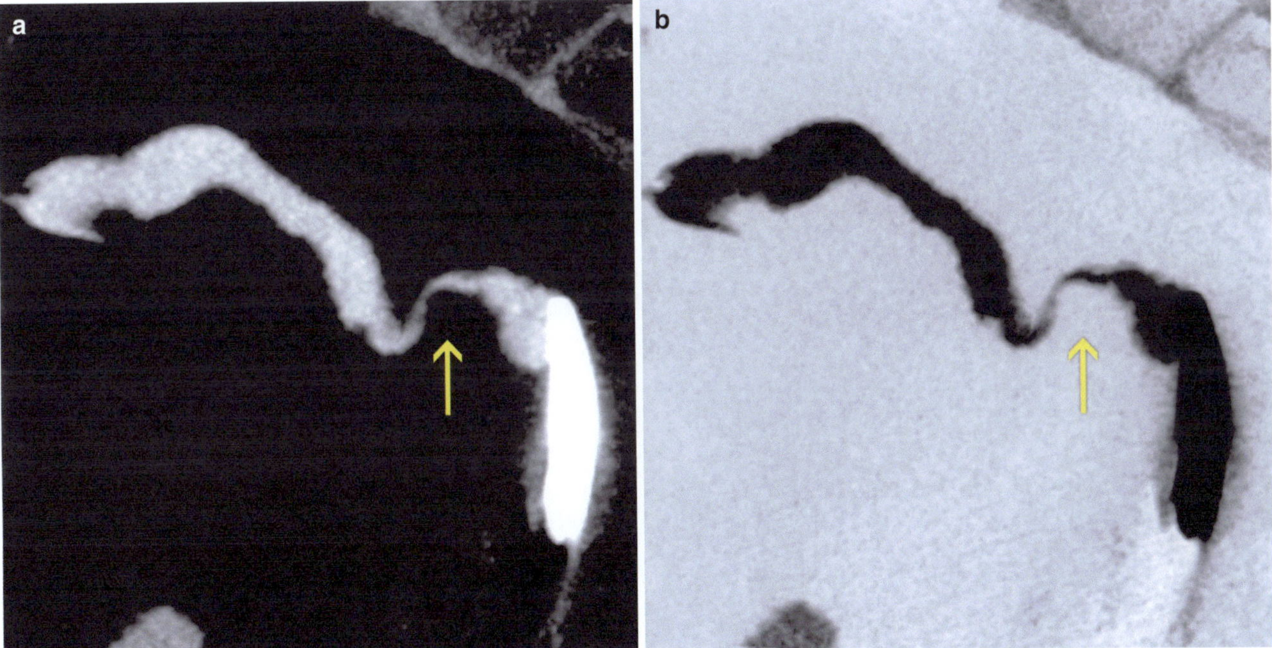

Fig. 5.23 Sinuous cervix (*arrows*). (**a**) Sagittal maximum intensity projection (MIP) image. (**b**) Sagittal MIP image with inverted window

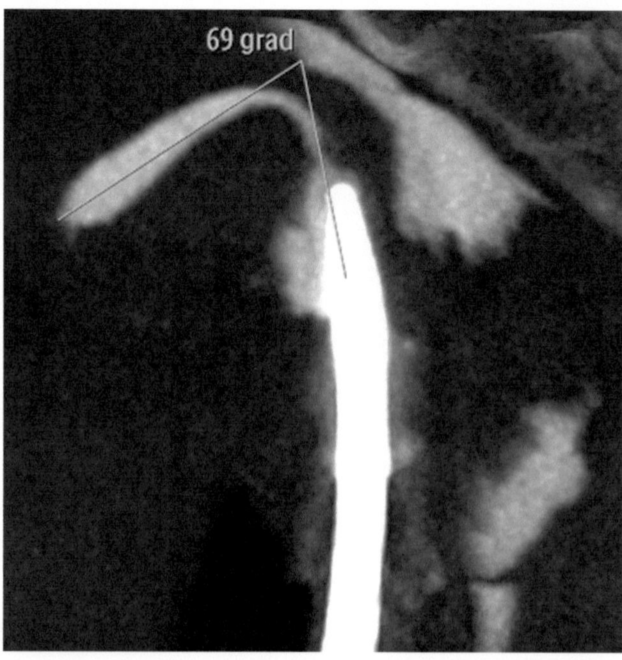

Fig. 5.24 Sagittal multiplanar reconstruction image showing a narrow cervical isthmic angle

Conclusion

Different types of pathological findings exist at the cervical level. Said findings can be diagnosed via multiple imaging methods. VHSG is a new non invasive diagnostic tool which permits the clear identification of each one of the possible cervical pathologies. Their identification is of the utmost importance, especially in infertile patients who require the use of embryo transfer methods to obtain successful treatments.

References

1. Carrascosa P, Baronio M, Capuñay C, et al. Multidetector computed tomography virtual hysterosalpingography in the investigation of the uterus and fallopian tubes. Clinical Imaging. 2009;33:165.
2. Carrascosa P, Capuñay C, Mariano B, et al. Virtual hysteroscopy by multidetector computed tomography. Abdom Imaging. 2008;33(4):381–7.
3. Carrascosa P, Capuñay C, Baronio M, et al. 64- Row multidetector CT virtual hysterosalpingography. Abdom Imaging. 2009;34:121–33.
4. Carrascosa P, Capuñay C, Vallejos J, et al. Virtual Hysterosalpingography: a new multidetector CT technique for evaluating the female reproductive system. Radiographics. 2010;30:643–61.
5. Carrascosa P, Capuñay C, Vallejos J, et al. Virtual hysterosalpingography: experience with over 1000 consecutive patients. Abdom Imaging. 2011;36(1):1–14.
6. Ott DJ, Fayez JA. Tubal and adnexal abnormalities. In: Ott DJ, Fayez JA, Zagoria RJ, editors. Hysterosalpingography: a text and atlas. 2nd ed. Baltimore: Williams & Wilkins; 1998. p. 90–3.
7. Simpson Jr WL, Beitia LG, Mester J. Hysterosalpingography: a reemerging study. Radiographics. 2006;26(2):419–31.
8. Vardhana PA, Silberzweig JE, Guarnaccia M, et al. Hysterosalpingography with selective salpingography. J Reprod Med. 2009;54(3):126–32.
9. Carrascosa P, Capuñay C, Baronio M, et al. 64- Row multidetector CT virtual hysterosalpingography. Abdom Imaging. 2009;34:133–7.
10. Carrascosa P, Baronio M, Capuñay C, et al. Multidetector computed tomography virtual hysterosalpingography in the investigation of the uterus and fallopian tubes. Eur J Radiol. 2008;67:531–5.
11. Sebastian S, Kalra MK, Mittal P, et al. Can independent coronal multiplanar reformatted images obtained using state-of-the-art MDCT scanners be used for primary interpretation of MDCT of the abdomen and pelvis? A feasibility study. Eur J Radiol. 2007;64(3):439–46.
12. Kirchgeorg MA, Prokop M. Increasing spiral CT benefits with postprocessing applications. Eur J Radiol. 1998;28(1):39–54. Review.
13. Baronio M, Carrascosa P, Capuñay C, et al. Diagnostic performance of CT virtual hysteroscopy in 69 consecutive patients. Fertil Steril. 2010;94(Suppl):S77.
14. Capuñay C, Baronio M, Carrascosa P, et al. CT virtual hysterosalpingography in the evaluation of uterine myomas. Fertil Steril. 2010;94(Suppl):S211.
15. Carrascosa P, Baronio JM, Borghi M, et al. Histerosalpingoscopía virtual. Una técnica novedosa y no invasiva para diagnosticar patología intrauterina. Reproduccion. 2006;21:19–26.
16. Chalazonitis A, Tzovara I, Laspas F, et al. Hysterosalpingography: technique and applications. Curr Probl Diagn Radiol. 2009;38(5):199–205.
17. Lee A, Ying YK, Novy MJ. Hysteroscopy, hysterosalpingography and tubal ostial polyps in infertility patients. J Reprod Med. 1997;42(6):337–41.
18. Radić V, Canić T, Valetić J, et al. Advantages and disadvantages of hysterosonosalpingography in the assessment of the reproductive status of uterine cavity and fallopian tubes. Eur J Radiol. 2005;53(2):268–73.
19. Roma Dalfó A, Ubeda B, Ubeda A, et al. Diagnostic value of hysterosalpingography in the detection of intrauterine abnormalities: a comparison with hysteroscopy. AJR Am J Roentgenol. 2004;183(5):1405–9.
20. López Navarrete JA, Herrera Otero JM, Quiroga Feuchter G, et al. Comparison between hysterosonography and hysterosalpinography in the study of endometrial abnormalities in infertility patients. Ginecol Obstet Mex. 2003;71:277–83.
21. Gustafsson L, Ponten J, Bergstrom R, et al. International incidence rates of invasive cervical cancer before cytological screening. Int J Cancer. 1997;71:159–65.
22. Womack C, Warren AY. The cervical screening muddle. Lancet. 1998;351:1129.
23. Plaxe SC, Saltzstein SL. Estimation of the duration of the preclinical phase of cervical adenocarcinoma suggests that there is ample opportunity for screening. Gynecol Oncol. 1999;75:55–61.
24. Green JA, Kirwan JM, Tierney JF, et al. Survival and recurrence after concomitant chemotherapy and radiotherapy for cancer of the uterine cervix: a systematic review and meta-analysis. Lancet. 2001;358:781–6.
25. Brenner H. Long-term survival rates of cancer patients achieved by the end of the 20th century: a period analysis. Lancet. 2002;360:1131–5.
26. Castle PE, Wacholder S, Lorincz AT, et al. A prospective study of high-grade cervical neoplasia risk among human papillomavirus-infected women. J Natl Cancer Inst. 2002;94:1406–14.
27. Lorincz AT, Castle PE, Sherman ME, et al. Viral load of human papillomavirus and risk of CIN3 or cervical cancer. Lancet. 2002;360:228–9.
28. Walboomers JM, Jacobs MV, Manos MM, et al. Human papillomavirus is a necessary cause of invasive cervical cancer worldwide. J Pathol. 1999;189:12–9.

29. Yamada T, Manos MM, Peto J, et al. Human papillomavirus type 16 sequence variation in cervical cancers: a worldwide perspective. J Virol. 1997;71:2463–72.

30. Bosch FX, Manos MM, Munoz N, et al. Prevalence of human papillomavirus in cervical cancer: a worldwide perspective. International biological study on cervical cancer (IBSCC) Study Group. J Natl Cancer Inst. 1995;87:796–802.

31. Munoz N, Franceschi S, Bosetti C, et al. Role of parity and human papillomavirus in cervical cancer: the IARC multicentric case–control study. Lancet. 2002;359:1093–101.

32. Smith JS, Herrero R, Bosetti C, et al. Herpes simplex virus-2 as a human papillomavirus cofactor in the etiology of invasive cervical cancer. J Natl Cancer Inst. 2002;94:1604–13.

33. Smith JS, Munoz N, Herrero R, et al. Evidence for Chlamydia trachomatis as a human papillomavirus cofactor in the etiology of invasive cervical cancer in Brazil and the Philippines. J Infect Dis. 2002;185:324–31.

34. Richart RM. Cervical intraepithelial neoplasia. Pathol Annu. 1973;8:301–28.

35. Vizcaino AP, Moreno V, Bosch FX, et al. International trends in incidence of cervical cancer: II. Squamous-cell carcinoma. Int J Cancer. 2000;86:429–35.

36. Davidson SE, Symonds RP, Lamont D, et al. Does adenocarcinoma of uterine cervix have a worse prognosis than squamous carcinoma when treated by radiotherapy? Gynecol Oncol. 1989;33:23–6.

37. Kaminski PF, Norris HJ. Minimal deviation carcinoma (adenoma malignum) of the cervix. Int J Gynecol Pathol. 1983;2:141–52.

38. Fu YS, Reagan JW, Fu AS, et al. Adenocarcinoma and mixed carcinoma of the uterine cervix. II. Prognostic value of nuclear DNA analysis. Cancer. 1982;49:2571–7.

39. Chen KT. Female genital tract tumors in Peutz-Jeghers syndrome. Hum Pathol. 1986;17:858–61.

40. American Joint Committee on Cancer. Cervix uteri cancer staging. 7th ed. Disponible en: http://www.cancerstaging.org/staging/posters/cervix24x30.pdf. Accedido 17 enero 2012.

41. Ho CM, Chien TY, Jeng CM, et al. Staging of cervical cancer: comparison between magnetic resonance imaging, computed tomography and pelvic examination under anesthesia. J Formos Med Assoc. 1992;91:982–90.

42. Scheidler J, Hricak H, Yu KK, et al. Radiological evaluation of lymph node metastases in patients with cervical cancer. A meta-analysis. JAMA. 1997;278:1096–101.

43. Grigsby PW, Dehdashti F, Siegel BA. FDG-PET evaluation of carcinoma of the cervix. Clin Positron Imaging. 1999;2:105–9.

44. Brenner DE, Whitley NO, Prempree T, et al. An evaluation of the computed tomographic scanner for the staging of carcinoma of the cervix. Cancer. 1982;50:2323–8.

45. Villasanta U, Whitley NO, Haney PJ, et al. Computed tomography in invasive carcinoma of the cervix: an appraisal. Obstet Gynecol. 1983;62:218–24.

46. Hricak H, Lacey CG, Sandles LG, et al. Invasive cervical carcinoma: comparison of MR imaging and surgical findings. Radiology. 1988;166:623–31.

47. Kim SH, Han MC. Invasion of the urinary bladder by uterine cervical carcinoma: evaluation with MR imaging. AJR Am J Roentgenol. 1997;168:393–7.

48. Kim SH, Choi BI, Han JK, et al. Preoperative staging of uterine cervical carcinoma: comparison of CT and MRI in 99 patients. J Comput Assist Tomogr. 1993;17:633–40.

49. Brodman M, Friedman Jr F, Dottino P, et al. A comparative study of computerized tomography, magnetic resonance imaging, and clinical staging for the detection of early cervix cancer. Gynecol Oncol. 1990;36:409–12.

50. Togashi K, Nishimura K, Sagoh T, et al. Carcinoma of the cervix: staging with MR imaging. Radiology. 1989;171:245–51.

51. Preidler KW, Tamussino K, Szolar DM, et al. Staging of cervical carcinomas. Comparison of body-coil magnetic resonance imaging and endorectal surface coil magnetic resonance imaging with histopathologic correlation. Invest Radiol. 1996;31:458–62.

52. Ebner F, Tamussino K, Kressel HY. Magnetic resonance imaging in cervical carcinoma: diagnosis, staging, and follow-up. Magn Reson Q. 1994;10:22–42.

53. Yamashita Y, Harada M, Torashima M, et al. Dynamic MR imaging of recurrent postoperative cervical cancer. J Magn Reson Imaging. 1996;6:167–71.

54. Brown JJ, Gutierrez ED, Lee JK. MR appearance of the normal and abnormal vagina after hysterectomy. AJR Am J Roentgenol. 1992;158:95–9.

55. Hricak H, Powell CB, Yu KK, et al. Invasive cervical carcinoma: role of MR imaging in pretreatment workup-cost minimization and diagnostic efficacy analysis. Radiology. 1996;198:403–9.

56. Heron CW, Husband JE, Williams MP, et al. The value of CT in the diagnosis of recurrent carcinoma of the cervix. Clin Radiol. 1988;39:496–501.

57. Schoolcraft WB, Surrey ES, Gardner DK. Embryo transfer: techniques and variables affecting success. Fertility and Sterility. 2001;76:863–70.

58. Mansour RT, Aboulghar MA. Optimizing the embryo transfer technique. Hum. Reprod. 2002;17:1149–53.

59. Oliveira FG, Abdelmassih VG, Diamond MP, et al. Uterine cavity findings and hysteroscopic interventions in patients undergoing in vitro fertilization-embryo transfer who repeatedly cannot conceive. Fertil Steril. 2003;80:1371–5.

Causes of infertility by uterine factors have a prevalence of a 10 %.

The uterus participates in key processes of the reproductive system that involve the transport of spermatozoids, embryo implantation and fetal nutrition. It is for this reason that congenital uterine anomalies (unicornuate, bicornuate, septate uterus, etc.) and acquired pathologies (endometrial polyps, intrauterine synechiae and fibroids) can negatively influence fertility [1–7].

Uterine pathology is classified in intraluminal pathology and mural pathology. The intraluminal pathologies include alterations that may be found in the interior of the uterine cavity. In the present chapter these topics are focused on exclusively intraluminal findings.

There are various diagnostic methods for the evaluation of the uterine cavity such as conventional hysterosalpingography (HSG) [8–11], sonohysterography [12–14], magnetic resonance imaging [15, 16] and hysteroscopy [17, 18]. The first three are exclusively diagnostic modalities while the hysteroscopy is a diagnostic and therapeutic study.

HSG is the method most commonly used in the study of infertile patients because it is easy to perform and has low costs. Nevertheless, this modality is relatively invasive because it requires clamping of the uterine neck in order to place a cannula in the external cervical os to instill contrast into the uterine cavity [19, 20]. HSG also requires traction of the cervical neck to avoid the overlapping of structures of the gynecologic apparatus that may impede the visualization and detection of the pathology. The invasiveness of this procedure can be associated with complications such as bleeding, infections and vasovagal reactions due to the intra-study discomfort.

Sonohysterography is a less invasive exam compared to the HSG which permits the adequate evaluation of the uterine cavity via the instillation of physiologic solution [21]. However, this imaging technique is not widely used because it does not provide information on the cervix or of the fallopian tubes. So other diagnostic methods are necessary to complement this information.

Magnetic resonance imaging is a study that is carried out principally for the diagnosis of uterine malformations [15, 22, 23]. However, it does not allow detecting all associated intra-luminal pathology and does not offer information of the fallopian tubes.

Hysteroscopy is a diagnostic and therapeutic method and is considered the gold standard modality for the evaluation of the uterus, with the disadvantage that it requires anesthesia [24]. This technique is most commonly utilized to confirm suspicious findings in other diagnostic methods [25].

Currently, a new non invasive diagnostic tool is available, the virtual hysterosalpingography (VHSG) [2, 5]. This new modality provides, in few seconds and with a very low radiation dose, excellent information on the uterus and offers, simultaneously, the evaluation of the cervix, the fallopian tubes and the associated intrapelvic pathology.

Within the intra-luminal pathology there exist diverse alterations that may be found in the interior of the uterus:

- Synechiae
- Endometrial infections sequelae.
- Other endometrial processes: hypoplasia, endometrial polyps, adenomyosis.
- Neoplasias: submucous myomas, endometrial carcinoma.
- Intrauterine devices.
- Post surgery changes.

Intrauterine Synechiae

They are fibrous bands of conjunctive tissue that stick to the uterine walls between themselves. Their prevalence in the general population is of 1.5 % and this percentage increases to 13 % if a history of infertility and repeated abortions exists [26–28]. Intrauterine synechiae represent a scar in the uterine cavity and are the result of an infection or trauma, frequently after a birth or post-abortion curettage. Trauma on the uterine wall induces the scarring and causes fibrosis. Fibrosis can be minor and involve a small section of the uterine wall or be extensive with a diffuse commitment and obliteration of various sectors of the cavity.

The clinical manifestations are commonly menstrual problems like amenorrhea, oligomenorrhea, repeated abortions, infertility or premature births.

The American Society of Fertility and Reproductive Medicine classifies the synechiae according to observed findings in radiologic and hysteroscopy studies, and in menstrual changes determining their severity.

Patients present themselves with menstrual dysfunction, infertility, repeated abortions or post-pregnancy complications. The association of infertility and synechiae is known as the Asherman Syndrome [29].

Synechiae can be located anywhere in the uterus. When they involve the cervical region they produce, in certain cases, stenosis of the internal cervical orifice. They can also generate stenosis of the tubarian ostium.

The useful diagnostic methods for its diagnosis are the HSG, VHSG and hysteroscopy [30–36].

HSG: the uterine synechiae are observed as filling defects which distort the morphology of the uterine cavity. They acquire an irregular and angular shape and do not present mobility (Fig. 6.1). They are easily differentiated from endometrial polyps because these have regular edges [37] (Fig. 6.2).

To make a correct diagnosis, the progressive filling of the uterine cavity is essential.

VHSG: this modality identifies the uterine synechiae in the different postprocessing techniques [38, 39].

Multiplanar reconstructions show irregular elevated lesions with soft tissue density which extend from the uterine walls. They can also be located in the isthmus-cervical region, center or fundus of the uterine cavity or adjacent to cornual regions (Figs. 6.3, 6.4, and 6.5). If they comprise various regions simultaneously, findings can be diffuse. (Figs. 6.6 and 6.7).

Maximum intensity projection images (MIP) may exhibit sections of irregularities on the uterine wall, although they constitute the reconstruction format which offers reduced information in the evaluation of this pathology (Fig. 6.8).

Volume rendering reconstructions show filling defect where the synechiae are located (Fig. 6.9).

Virtual endoscopy images expose endoluminal lesions that project towards the uterine lumen reducing its size. The level of compromise depends on the extension of the synechiae (Fig. 6.10).

Hysteroscopy: is a diagnostic and therapeutic method at the same time because it permits the extraction of the adhesions once confirmed. A Foley catheter is introduced which is placed in the uterine cavity and a balloon is insufflated to keep the walls separated.

The synechiae are extracted and, later, antibiotics are administered post-operatively for a week. In the post-surgery, estrogen is supplied twice a day during 30 days and then medroxyprogesterone for 7 consecutive days. In general, after a month of treatment, an improvement of the symptoms

and uterine morphology is observed, although the rate of infertility is not significantly modified [40, 41].

Endometrial Infections

Endometrial infections can be acute or chronic. The acute infections are in general of bacterium etiology, being Chlamydia trachomatis and Ureaplasma urealyticum the most frequent agents. The most common causes of the chronic infections are due to intrauterine devices, tuberculosis or gonococcia [42–44].

Frequently, origin is the post-delivery infection, due to instrumentation in the uterine cavity or because of the propagation of adjacent infections of the genital tract.

Acute infections can progress to chronic and end up generating extensive uterine synechiae with severe cavity deformation (Fig. 6.11)

Other Endometrial Processes

- Hypoplasia
- Hyperplasia
- Endometrial polyps
- Adenomyosis

Endometrial Hypoplasia

This pathology is frequently observed in old women with premature menopause. It can also be seen in young patients due to an ovary dysfunction or because of the use of oral contraceptives.

Atrophic endometrium produces a diffuse irregularity in the uterine walls.

Available methods for its diagnosis are HSG and VHSG.

HSG: shows uterus with diffuse parietal irregularities and spiculated aspect [45, 46] (Fig. 6.12).

VHSG: shows diverse forms of two-dimensional and tridimensional reconstructions show a uterus with diffuse irregular walls [38, 39] (Fig. 6.13). These irregularities can also be identified endoluminally at the level of all of the walls.

Hyperlapsia

Constituted by a proliferation of the glands. The patients may have metrorrhagia.

Useful diagnostic methods are pelvic and transvaginal ultrasound, VSHG and hysteroscopy [47].

- **Ultrasound**: shows a bigger and wider endometrium of 10 mm (Fig. 6.14). Ovary tumors can be observed.

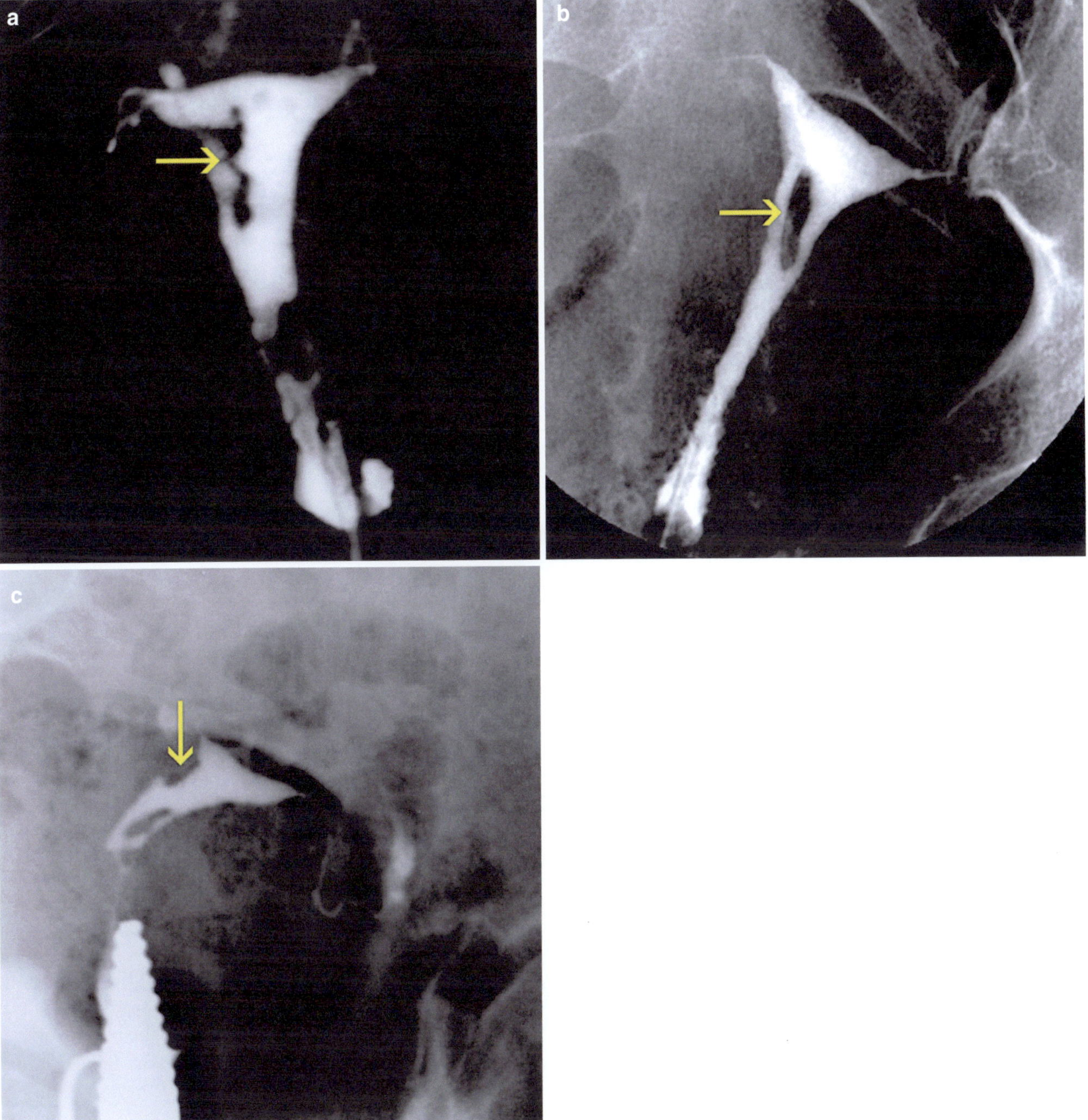

Fig. 6.1 (**a–c**) Uterine synechiae seen on HSG images. Multiple filling defects are observed in the uterine cavity with irregular edges (*arrows*) compatible with synechiae

- **VHSG**: shows an irregular endometrium that can be appreciated in multiplanar reconstructions, volume rendering and virtual endoscopy images.

  Multiplanar reconstructions: irregular margins of the lumen can be observed. They show an endometrium with diffuse multiple elevated pseudopolyps that project into the lumen with no preponderant lesion (Fig. 6.15).

  Volume rendering: exhibits irregular uterine margins, frequently associated with a reduced cavity due to endometrial hypertrophy (Fig. 6.16).

Virtual endoscopy: shows a small uterine cavity with irregular hypertrophic mucosal folds with polypoid appearance (Fig. 6.17).

Endometrial Polyps

They constitute focal overgrowths of tissue in the endometrium. They contain glands, fibrous stroma and vessels. They occur more frequently in the fifth decade. Their growth is

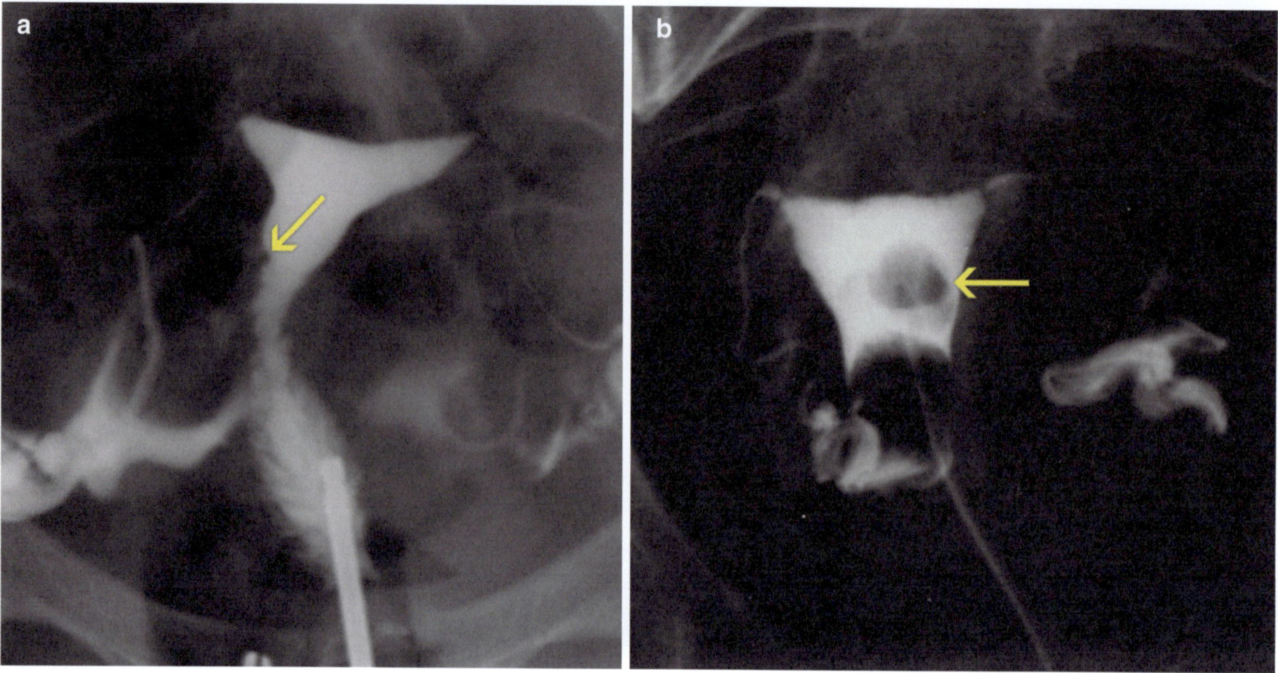

Fig. 6.2 Uterine polyps seen on HSG images. (**a**) Small polyp on the right lateral wall of the uterine silhouette (*arrow*). (**b**) Large polyp in the medial aspect of the uterine cavity (*arrow*)

sensitive to the hormone levels. It is estimated that they affect 11–24 % of infertile women [48].

Risk factors include age, arterial hypertension, diabetes and hormonal tamoxifen treatment among others.

Polyps can be asymptomatic or be associated to uterine bleeding. They are benign lesions and rarely become malignant. Only 0.5 % of cases correspond to an endometrial carcinoma [49–51].

Morphologically they are sessile (Fig. 6.18) or pedunculated (Fig. 6.19). Pedunculated polyps can even pass through the internal cervical orifice (Fig. 6.24).

They can be solitary (Fig. 6.20) or in groups (Fig. 6.21). In 75 % of cases they are alone.

Their size is variable, from scarce millimeters (Fig. 6.22) to a couple of centimeters (Fig. 6.23).

The diagnosis of this pathology can be carried out with one of the following diagnostic methods: ultrasound, HSG, VHSG and hysteroscopy [18].

- **Ultrasound**: polyps show an unspecific thickening or a single, or multiple, intracavitary mass surrounded by liquid or normal endometrium (Fig. 6.24).
- **HSG**: exhibits singular (Fig. 6.25) or multiple (Fig. 6.26) filling defects. It is fundamental to carry out a progressive filling of the uterine cavity to avoid losing the visualization of small lesions [10, 52, 53]

In certain cases another diagnostic method is required to define if that filling defect corresponds to a polyp or a myoma with a submucous projection. HSG does not provide information on the uterine wall, only of the lumen

- **VHSG**: this modality allows diverse forms of reconstruction (two-dimensional, tridimensional and endoscopic)

that permit not only to visualize an intrauterine lesion but also to characterize it [33–35].

- Multiplanar reconstructions with soft tissue window show polyps as elevated lesions of the uterine wall that project toward the cavity with soft part density (Fig. 6.27). In certain cases intrauterine areal bubbles can be observed that also project toward the endometrial cavity but do not possess a real density, which facilitates its differential diagnosis (Fig. 6.28).

MIP reconstructions are not very useful in the evaluation of the intraluminal uterine pathology due to the fact that, in most cases they do not show intrauterine lesions (Fig. 6.29). They are most frequently used to evaluate the uterine tubes.

Volume Rendering reconstructions are of utmost utility to diagnose endometrial polyps because they show filling defects where they are located, this allows the confirmation of the identified findings in the multiplanar reconstruction (Fig. 6.30).

Lastly, virtual endoscopic images show the polyps with endoluminal views. They can have an orientation from the cervix towards the uterine fundus (Fig. 6.31) or vice versa. Virtual images can evaluate the size and morphology of the polyps.

Prognosis

When referring to the reproductive prognosis, it is unknown the mechanism through which endometrial polyps influence fertility. It is believed that they could interfere in the sperm transport and embryo implantation.

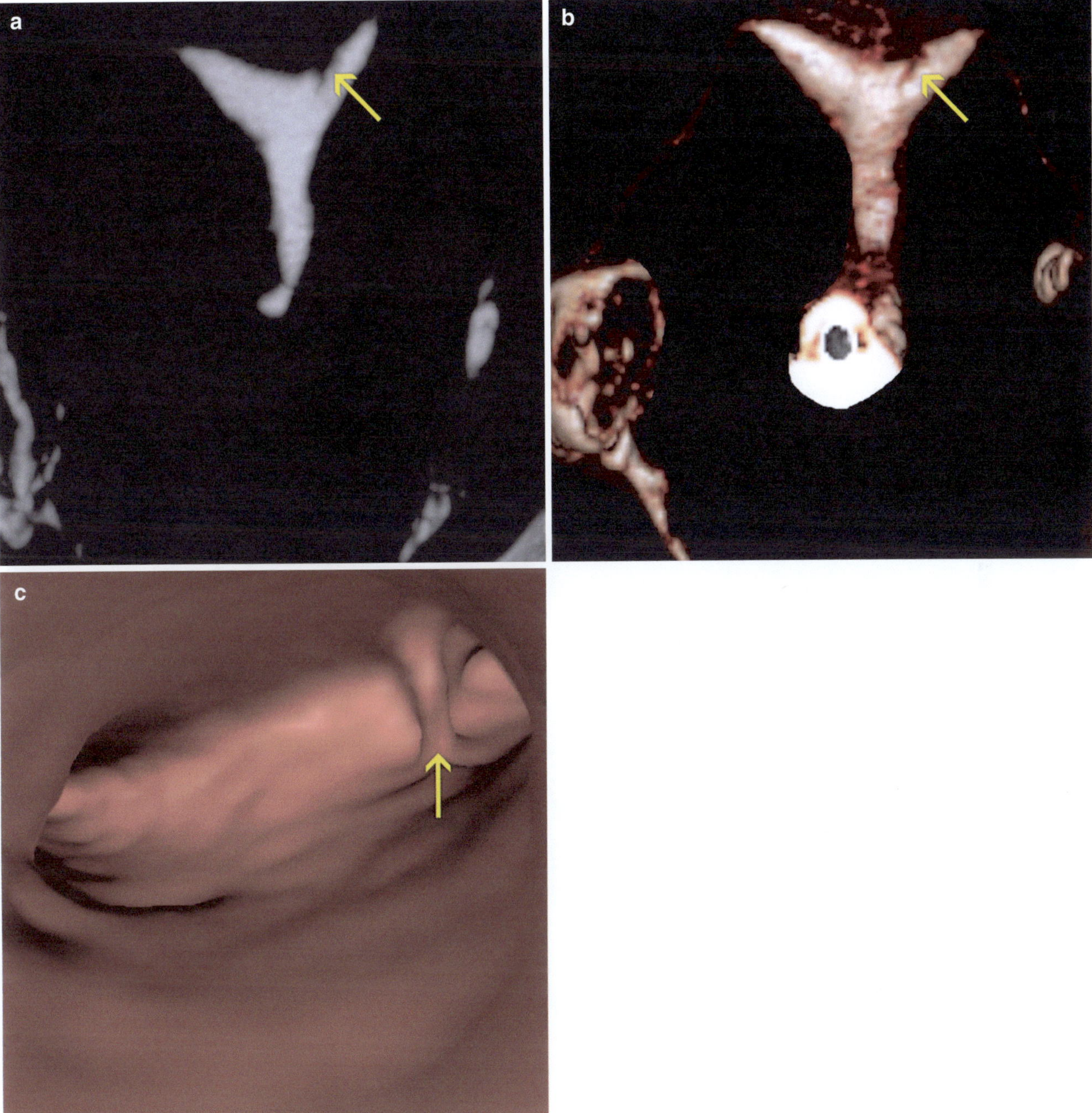

Fig. 6.3 Synechiae in uterine fundus adjacent to left horn. (**a**) Coronal maximum intensity projection image which shows a lineal image (*arrow*) at the level of the uterine fundus compatible with synechiae. (**b**) 3D vol-ume rendering image which illustrates similar findings (*arrow*). (**c**) Virtual endoscopy image of the uterine fundus which exhibits a lineal band that joins the anterior and posterior walls of the uterus (synechiae) (*arrow*)

Retrospective studies have demonstrated an increase in the rate of pregnancy of up to 76 % in patients who were subject to a polypectomy.

In another randomized prospective study, "Pérez-Medina y cols." [54] evaluated the effect of polypectomy on infertile patients prior to an intrauterine insemination (IUI). They observed that the rate of pregnancy was of 64 % in the group with a polypectomy, compared to 28.8 % in the control group (p<0.0001). Sixty five percent of the pregnancies which occurred in the first 3 months post-surgery were spontaneous before beginning the IUI, hence it was concluded that the polyps exert a negative influence over fertility.

Treatment generally consists in the removal of the polyp, usually done via a hysteroscopy.

Another way of eliminating the polyps, of small size, is scraping the uterine cavity (curettage).

Hysteroscopy: this method shows the lesion directly, allowing the precise evaluation of the polyp size, morphol-

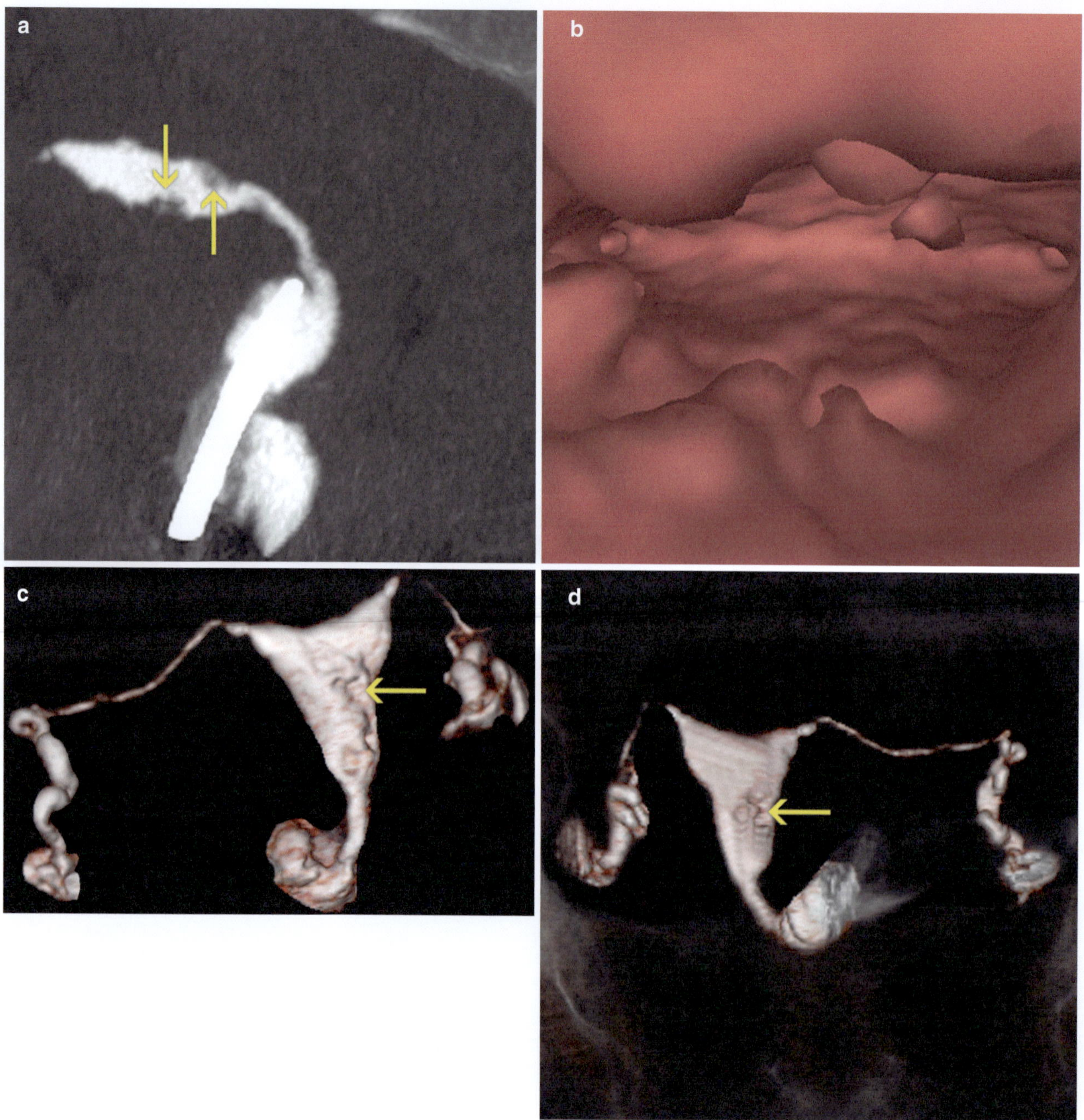

Fig. 6.4 Uterine synechiae. (**a**) Sagittal maximum intensity projection image that shows an anteverted uterus, which presents multiple filling defects compatible with synechiae (*arrows*). (**b**) Virtual endoscopy image which illustrates endoluminal lesions. (**c, d**) 3D volume rendering images which exhibit irregularities on the wall corresponding to synechiae (*arrows*)

ogy and location (Fig. 6.32). It can also removes the polyp being a diagnostic and therapeutic modality [17].

Adenomyosis

Adenomyosis is a pathology which affects women who are in their late reproductive stage. It presents itself as abnormal uterine bleeding, dysmenorrhea and infertility [5].

Singular or multiple focal cavities are produced by glandular dilatation in the uterine walls. The most frequent loca-tions are in fundus of the uterus. If these findings are located on the inferior uterine borders or closer to the cervical region they are of another etiology.

Imaging methods which offer information on this pathology are the HSG and VHSG [4, 55, 56].

- **<u>HSG</u>**: shows irregular uterine walls and sectors of glandular dilatation that are located on the fundus (Fig. 6.33).
- **<u>VHSG</u>**: different reconstruction formats offer valuable information for the diagnosis of the adenomyosis. VHSG allows better evaluation of this pathology, due

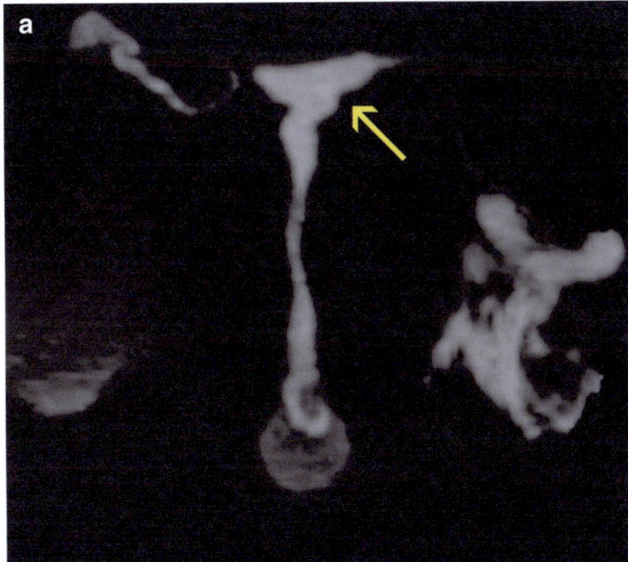

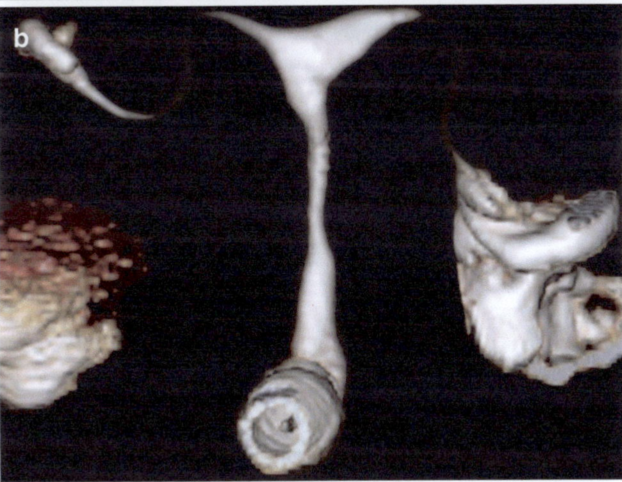

Fig. 6.5 Uterine synechiae. (**a**) Coronal maximum intensity projection image which shows a uterus with irregular edges (*arrow*) due to the presence of synechiae. (**b**) 3D volume rendering image which illustrates similar findings

to the fact that, besides possessing glandular dilatations that project towards the miometrium, they have associated myometrial hypertrophia, which is clearly identified in the multiplanar reconstructions with soft tissue window. MIP and VR reconstructions illustrate typical dilatation of the adenomyosis that appear as saccular herniations.

Endoscopic views exhibit endoluminal neck dilatations (Fig. 6.34).

Malignancies

- Submucous myomas (see Chap. 7).
- Endometrial carcinoma.

Endometrial Carcinoma

Endometrial carcinoma is the most frequent gynecologic cancer in developed countries. The mean age is 60 [57, 58]. 75 % of cases present themselves in post-menopausal periods and 25 % in peri-menopausal periods (5 % in younger than 40 years old).

The most common risk factors are: nulliparity, late menopause, obesity, diabetes and estrogen treatment with no opposition.

Diagnostic methods are: pelvic ultrasound, HSG and VHSG.

- **Ultrasound**: an unspecific thickening, with mixed or heterogeneous echogenicity, can be observed in patients with endometrial carcinoma.
- **HSG**: depending on the size of the tumor, a focal or diffuse irregular filling defect can be observed in advanced carcinoma cases.
- **VHSG**: shows a mass with variable size and irregular margins that protrudes towards the uterine cavity. Since necrosis and hemorrhage can be a feature, VHSG shows an heterogeneous soft tissue density mass.

Intrauterine Devices

Intrauterine devices (IUD) are utilized to prevent pregnancies. A variety of them exist, some of which possess hormonal medication which reduces the rate of menstrual bleeding. Its use can be associated to complications such as intrauterine retention, bleeding, endometritis, salpingitis and uterine perforation [59, 60].

Endometritis and salpingitis can produce adherences and later be associated with infertility.

In cases where there could have been IUD displacement with posterior location, it is necessary to achieve the exact placement of the devices for its secure extraction.

Methods which provide this information are: ultrasound, HSG and VHSG. These allow evaluation of the exact location and determine IUD integrity that is observed with high density within the uterine light (Fig. 6.35). The distance to uterine fundus can be measured

Hysteroscopy is utilized for the IUD extraction of the migrated devices towards the miometrium. If there is a perforation of the uterine wall, a laparoscopy is preferred for its removal.

Post-surgery Changes

Post-surgery changes can be due to multiple causes:
- Cesarean scar
- Synechiae correction
- Myoma removal

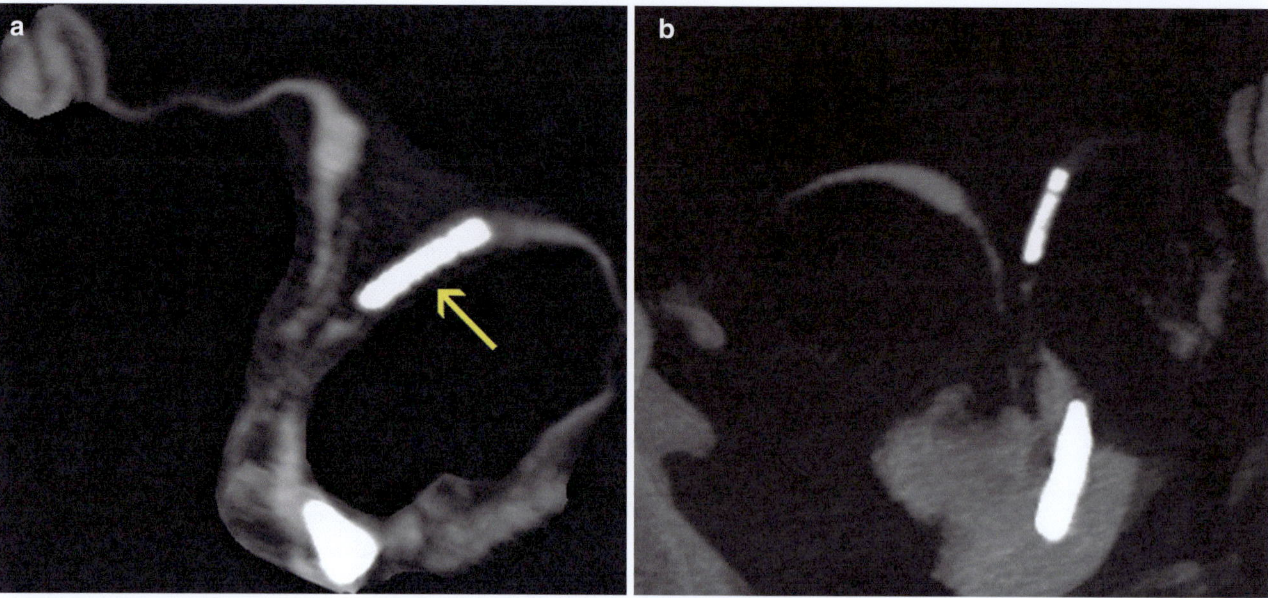

Fig. 6.6 Diffuse uterine synechiae. (**a**, **b**) Maximum intensity projection images that show a bicornuate uterus with intrauterine contraceptive device in the left horn (*arrow*). Multiple intraluminal filling defects are observed in the corpus and proximal sector of both uterine horns compatible with diffuse synechiae

Cesarean Scar

Cesarean scar is the most frequent post-surgery finding. A symmetric or asymmetric irregularity is observed in the cesarean incision site (isthmus-cervical region).

Methods which exhibit the normal typical findings and possible associated complications are HSG and VHSG.

- **HSG**: cesarean scar looks like a symmetric or asymmetric dilatation in the site of the scar, of different size. Its evaluation requires visualizations in diverse projections to value the real size of the operated area (Fig. 6.36).
- **VHSG**: this modality shows this typical finding in patients subject to a prior cesarean operation.

Two-dimensional and tridimensional reconstructions offer integral information of the cesarean scar (Figs. 6.37, 6.38, and 6.39).

Multiplanar reconstructions allow the visualization of the saccular dilatations in the region of the scar and at the same time provide information with respect to the width of the wall in the site of the operation. It is possible to measure the width in the sagittal plane, in this way being able to determine the possibility of a pregnancy without risk of uterine rupture (Fig. 6.40).

A normal parietal width is of approximately 8 mm, while in patients who have had cesarean operations it is reduced. The objective of carrying out a precise measurement of the width of the wall in the site of the surgery is to provide the gynecologist with this information and know if there is a risk of possible uterine rupture in cases of severe parietal thinning.

VR reconstructions: the section of the saccular dilatations is located and their volumes are quantified (Fig. 6.41).

EV: shows the neck of the dilatations virtually. Our research group carried out a study with 100 patients, 50 with a history of cesarean surgery and 50 as control group; they were all subject to the previously mentioned measurements.

It was observed that the patients with previous cesarean surgery possessed a parietal width of 5.3 mm, while the width of the control group was of 11.5 mm.

There was one case of a patient with a post-surgery complication, where a uterine fistula was identified. That patient presented a miometrial width of 2 mm and a discontinuity section of 1 mm through which filtration of the contrast towards the peritoneal cavity was observed. After a VHSG study, the patient underwent surgery in which the diagnosis was confirmed and the fistula fixed.

It is worth mentioning that the importance of a precise diagnosis in this type of patients allows knowing exactly the integrity of the scar area, the width of the wall and the probability of a safe future pregnancy. See also Chap. 10.

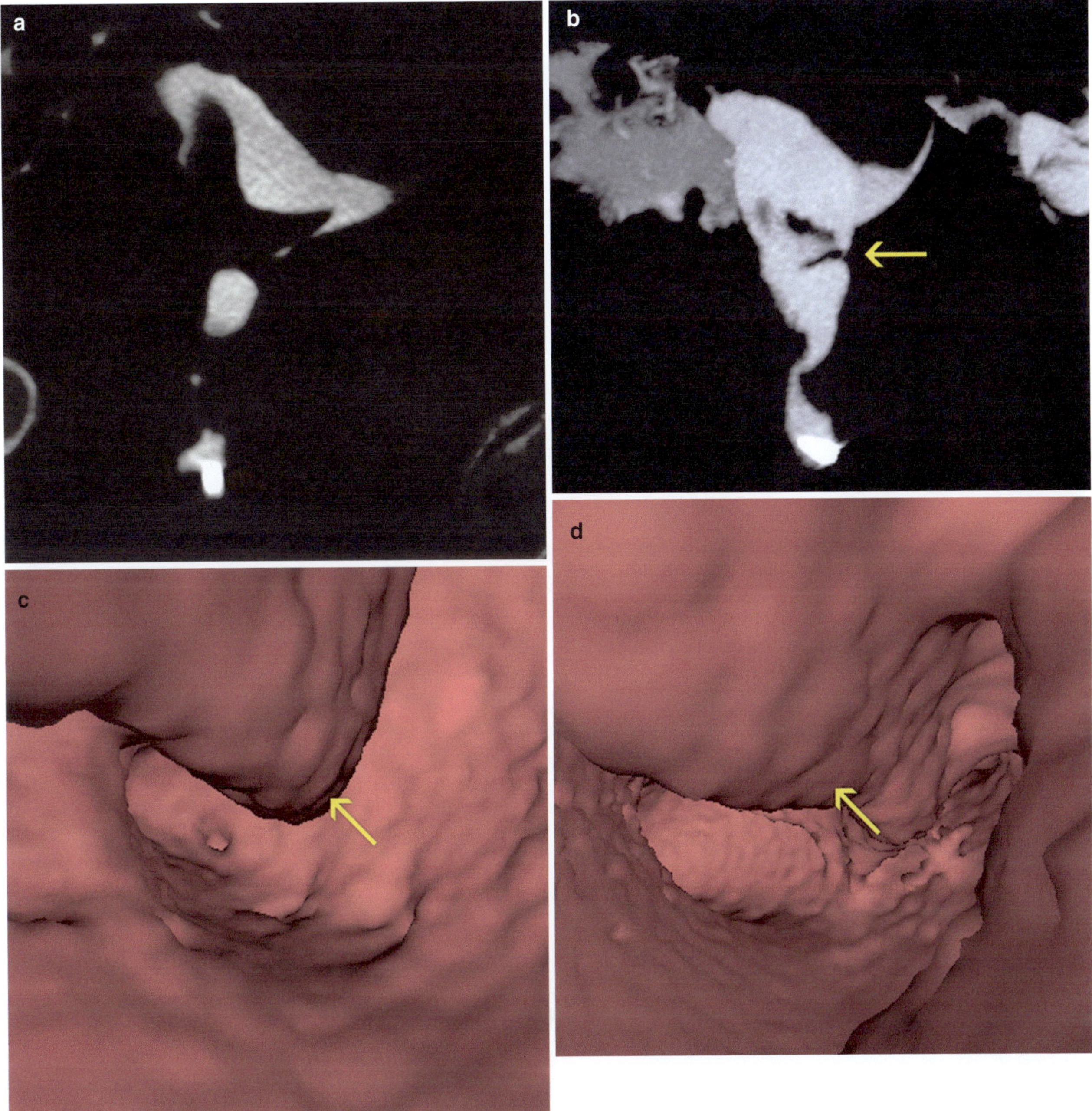

Fig. 6.7 Diffuse uterine synechiae. (**a**) Coronal multiplanar reconstruction image which shows a uterus multiple filling defects in the proximal and medial aspects of the uterine cavity compatible with synechiae. (**b**) Coronal maximum intensity projection image which exhibits an irregular uterus with intraluminal filling defects (*arrow*). (**c**, **d**) Virtual endoscopy images that illustrate a uterus with irregular walls due to diffuse synechiae (*arrows*)

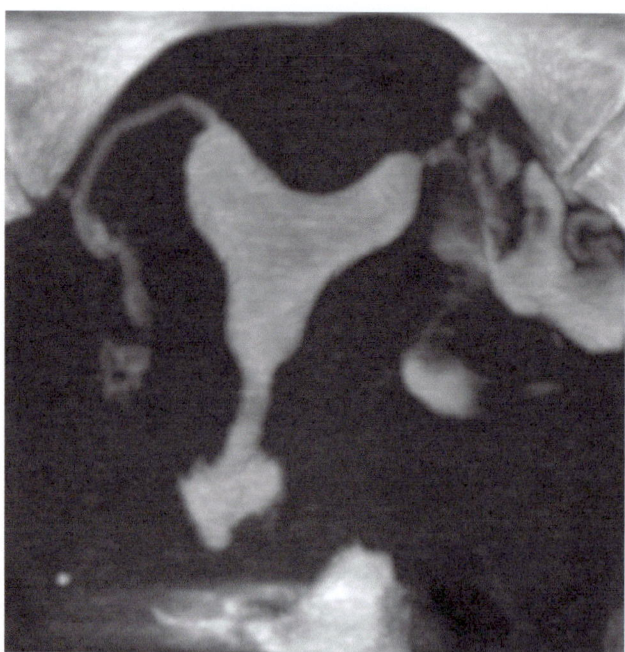

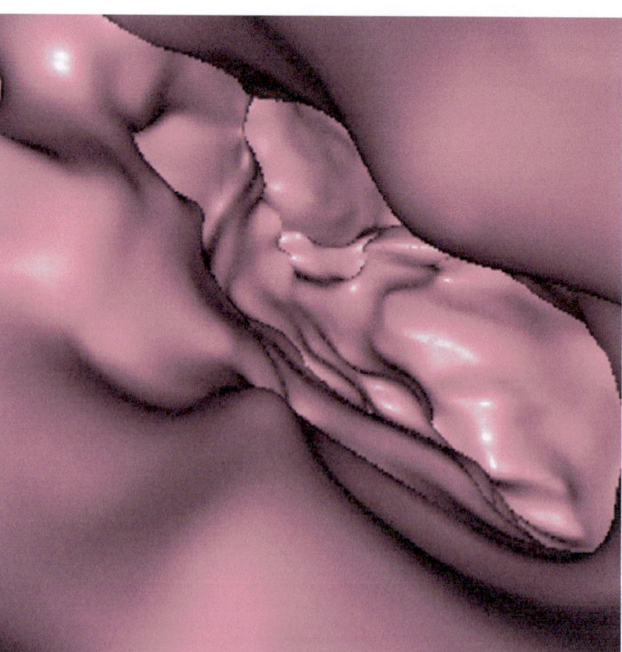

Fig. 6.8 Maximum intensity projection (MIP) images for the evaluation of synechiae. The MIP images possess limitations in the identification of intraluminal pathologies such as synechiae and polyps. Its main utility is for the evaluation of the Fallopian tubes

Fig. 6.10 Virtual endoscopy images for the evaluation of synechiae. These images offer intraluminal views which provide the location, extension and compromise of synechiae

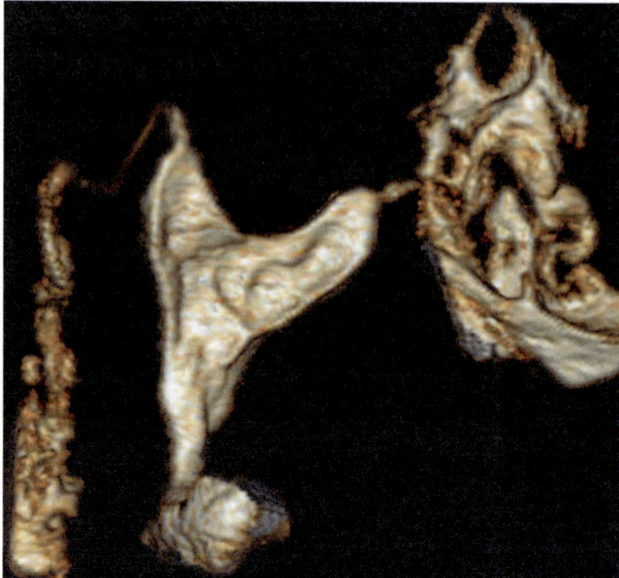

Fig. 6.9 3D volume rendering images for the evaluation of synechiae. These 3D images are ideal in the evaluation of this pathology, showing filling defect areas. The appearance of the uterine morphology contributes to a precise diagnosis

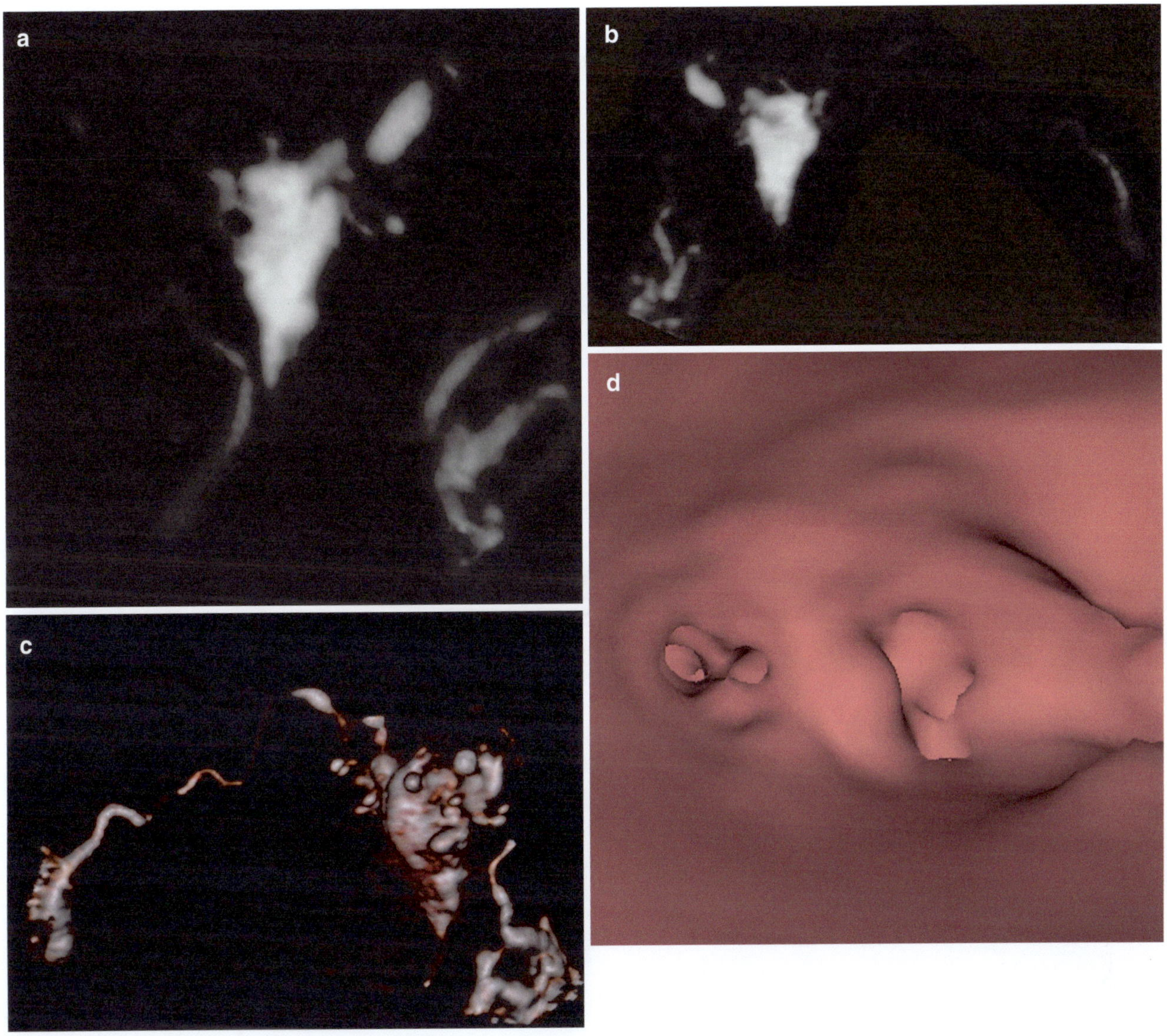

Fig. 6.11 (**a**, **b**) Maximum intensity projection images showing a totally deformed uterus with irregular edges due to extensive synechiae. (**c**) 3D volume rendering image illustrating similar findings. (**d**) Virtual endoscopy image showing a small uterine cavity due to extensive synechiae

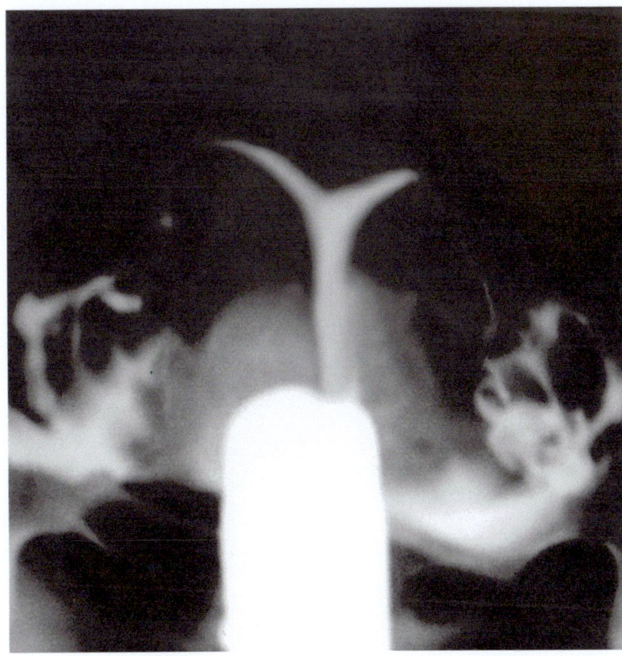

Fig. 6.12 Hypoplasia of the uterus seen on HSG exam

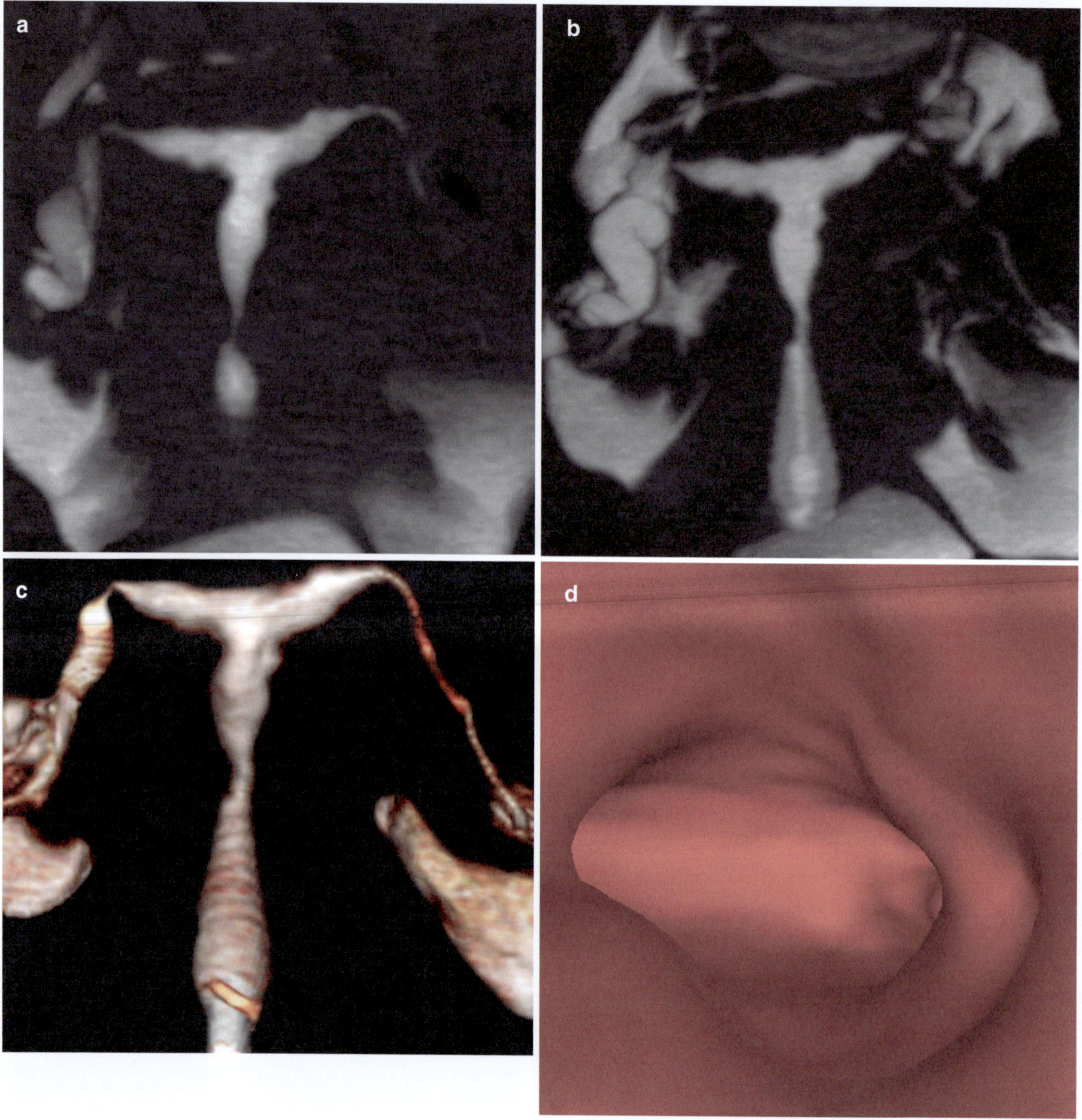

Fig. 6.13 Hypoplasia of the uterus seen on VHSG exam. (**a, b**) Maximum intensity projection images showing a small uterus of irregular edges. (**c**) 3D volume rendering image illustrating similar findings. (**d**) Virtual endoscopy image showing irregular endoluminal edges

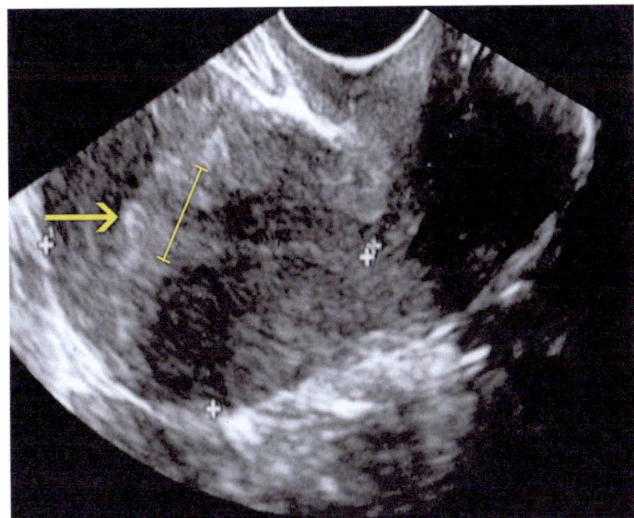

Fig. 6.14 Endometrial hyperplasia seen on transvaginal ultrasound. Longitudinal image of the uterus showing an abnormally thickened endometrium of 14 mm (*arrow*)

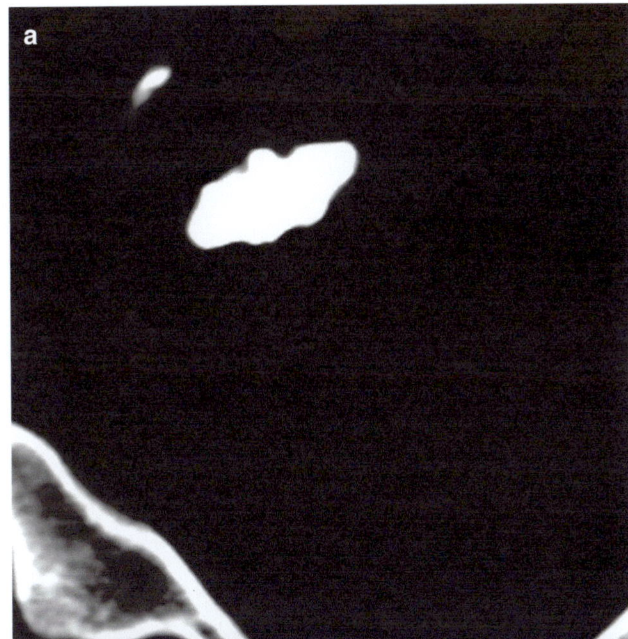

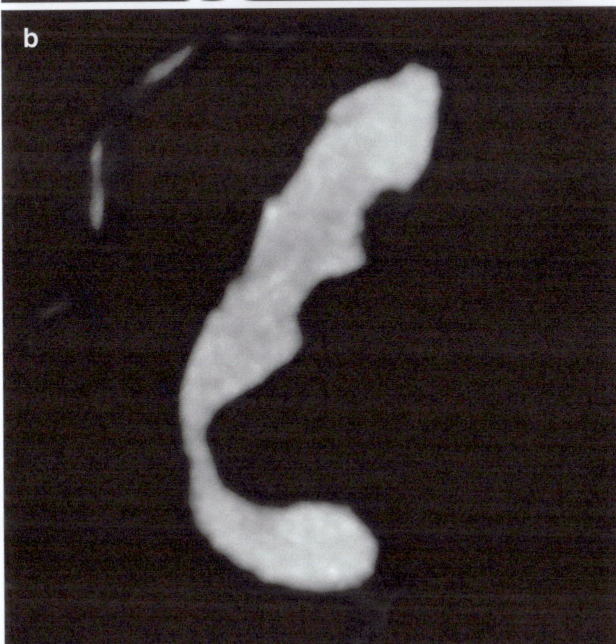

Fig. 6.15 CT multiplanar reconstruction (MPR) image of endometrial hyperplasia. (**a**) Coronal MPR image with soft tissue window. (**b**) Sagittal MPR image with soft tissue window showing an irregular uterine cavity

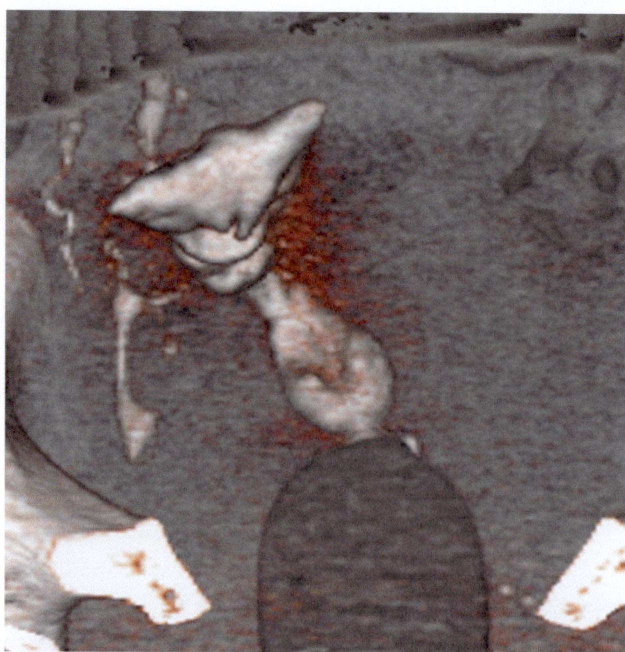

Fig. 6.16 3D volume rendering image of endometrial hyperplasia. Uterus with irregular edges and walls due to an abnormally thickened endometrium

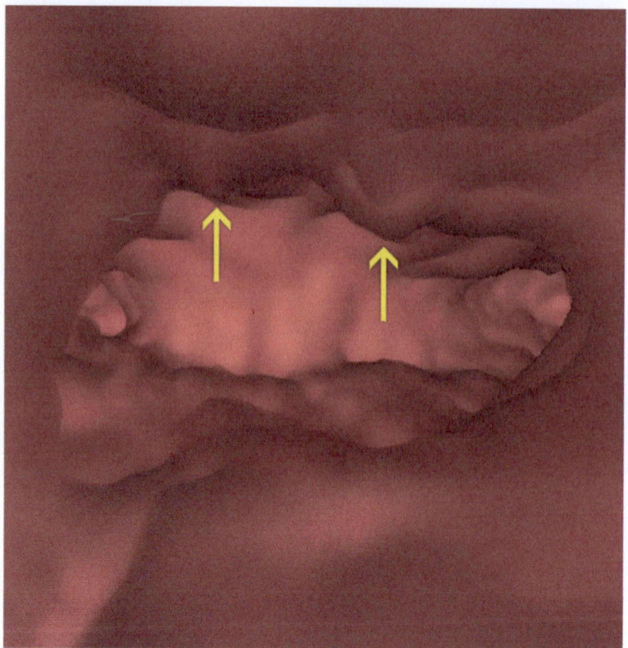

Fig. 6.17 Virtual endoscopy image of an abnormally thickened endometrium. An irregular cavity due to hypertrophic mucosal folds with polypoid appearance is observed (*arrows*)

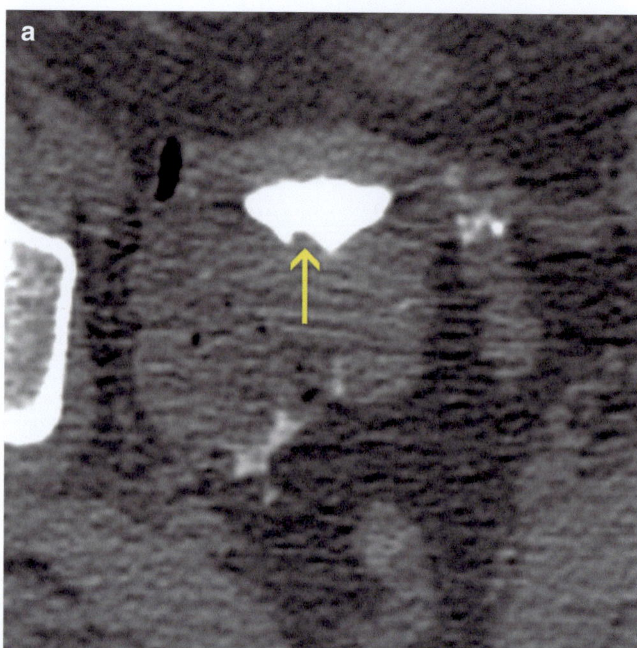

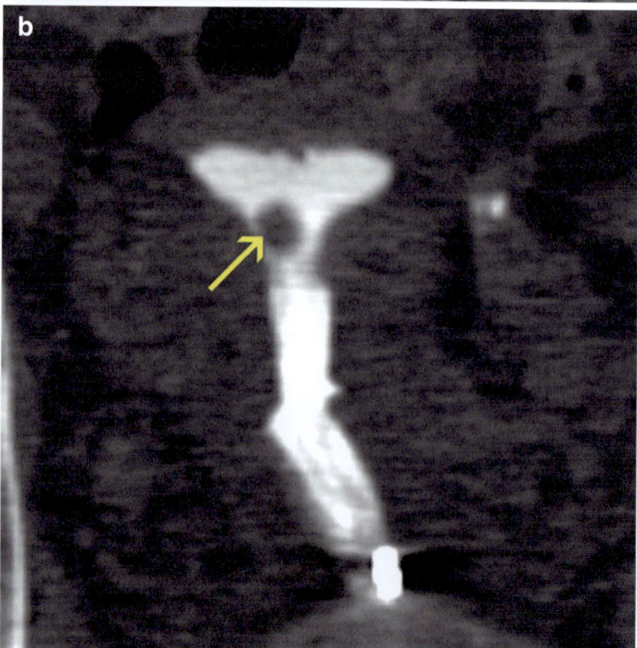

Fig. 6.18 Endometrial sessile polyp. (**a**) Axial CT image with soft tissue window which shows an elevated lesion in the anterior wall of the uterine cavity compatible with a sessile polyp (*arrow*). (**b, c**) Coronal and sagittal multiplanar reconstruction images with soft tissue window that illustrate a polyp lesion at the level of the uterine cavity (*arrow*). (**d**) Virtual endoscopy image which exhibits the polyp (*arrow*)

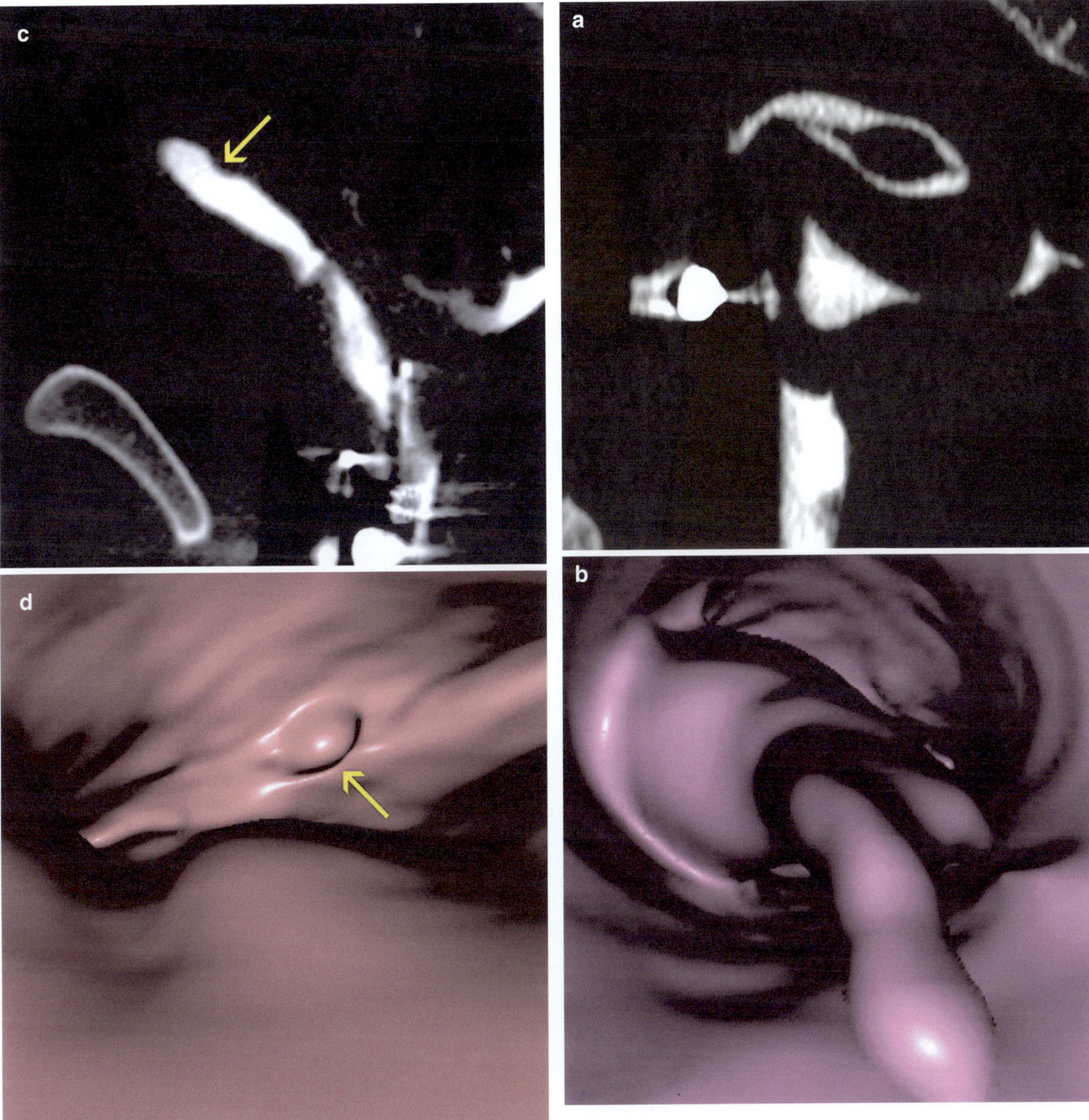

Fig. 6.18 (continued)

Fig. 6.19 Endometrial pedunculated polyp. (a) Sagittal multiplanar reconstruction image with soft tissue window which shows a pedunculated polyp. The head of the polyp projects towards the uterine fundus. (b) Virtual endoscopy images which shows the polyp from the cervical region

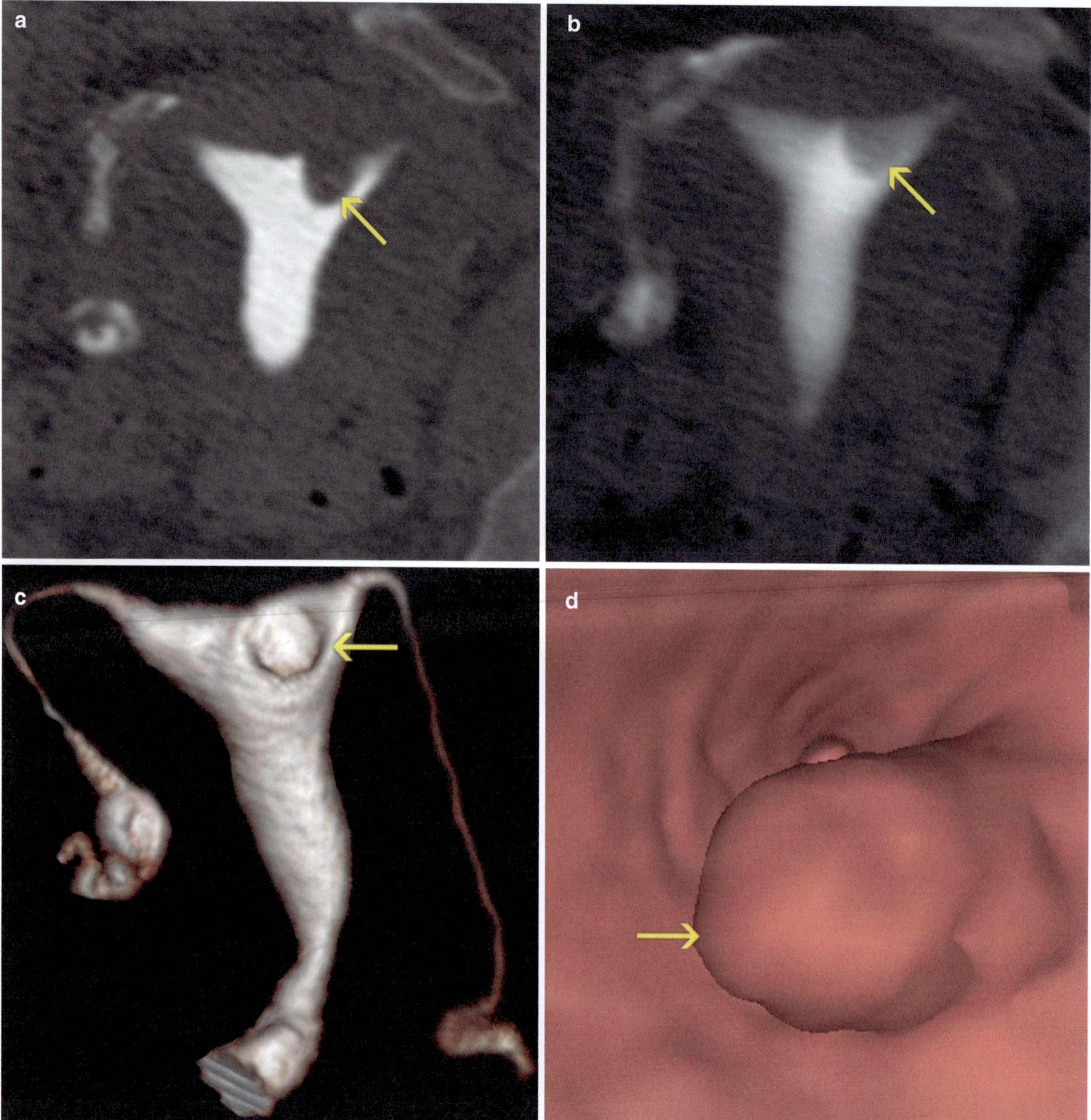

Fig. 6.20 Isolated endometrial polyp (*arrows*). (**a**) Coronal multiplanar reconstruction (MPR) image with soft tissue window which shows an isolated elevated lesion at the level of the uterine fundus adjacent to the left horn compatible with polyp. (**b**) 10-mm coronal MPR image with soft tissue window illustrates similar findings. (**c**) 3D volume rendering image that illustrates similar findings. (**d**) Virtual endoscopy image. The endoluminal elevated lesion can be clearly observed

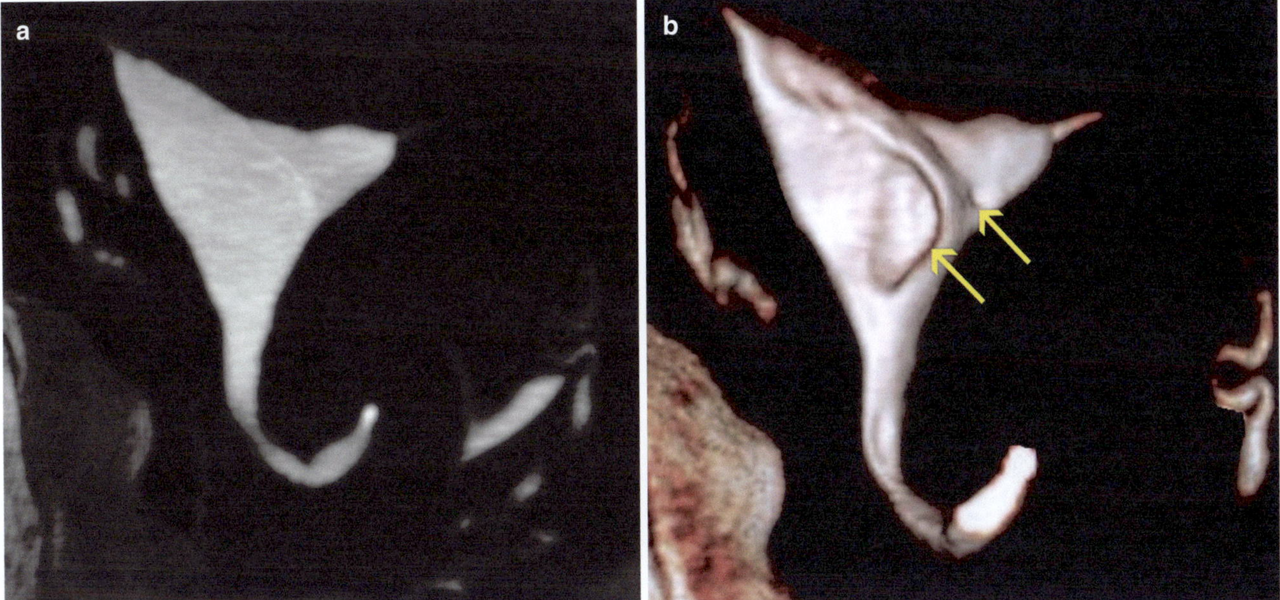

Fig. 6.21 Multiple endometrial polyps. (**a**) Maximum intensity projection image which shows a normal uterine cavity with no evidence of further findings. This type of image reconstruction does not correctly visualize the endoluminal lesions. (**b**) 3D volume rendering image which illustrates the presence of two elevated lesion: a small one and a large one (*arrows*) near the right uterine horn

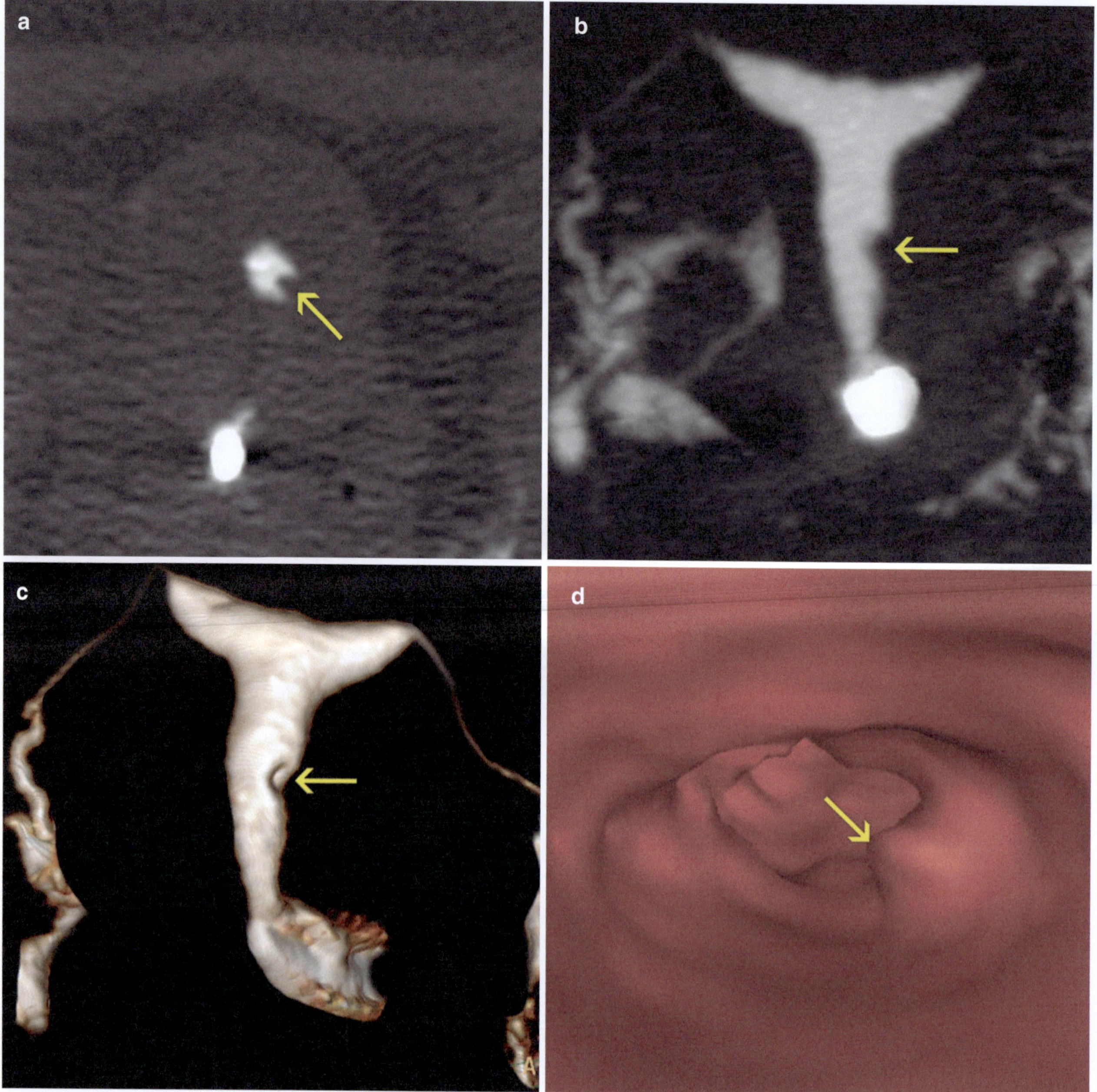

Fig. 6.22 Millimetric endometrial polyp. (**a**) Axial CT image with soft tissue window which shows an elevated lesion in the left lateral wall of the uterus (*arrow*) compatible with a polyp. (**b**, **c**) Coronal maximum intensity projection and 3D volume rendering images showing a small filling defect in the left lateral wall (*arrow*). (**d**) Virtual endoscopy image which shows the polyp (*arrow*)

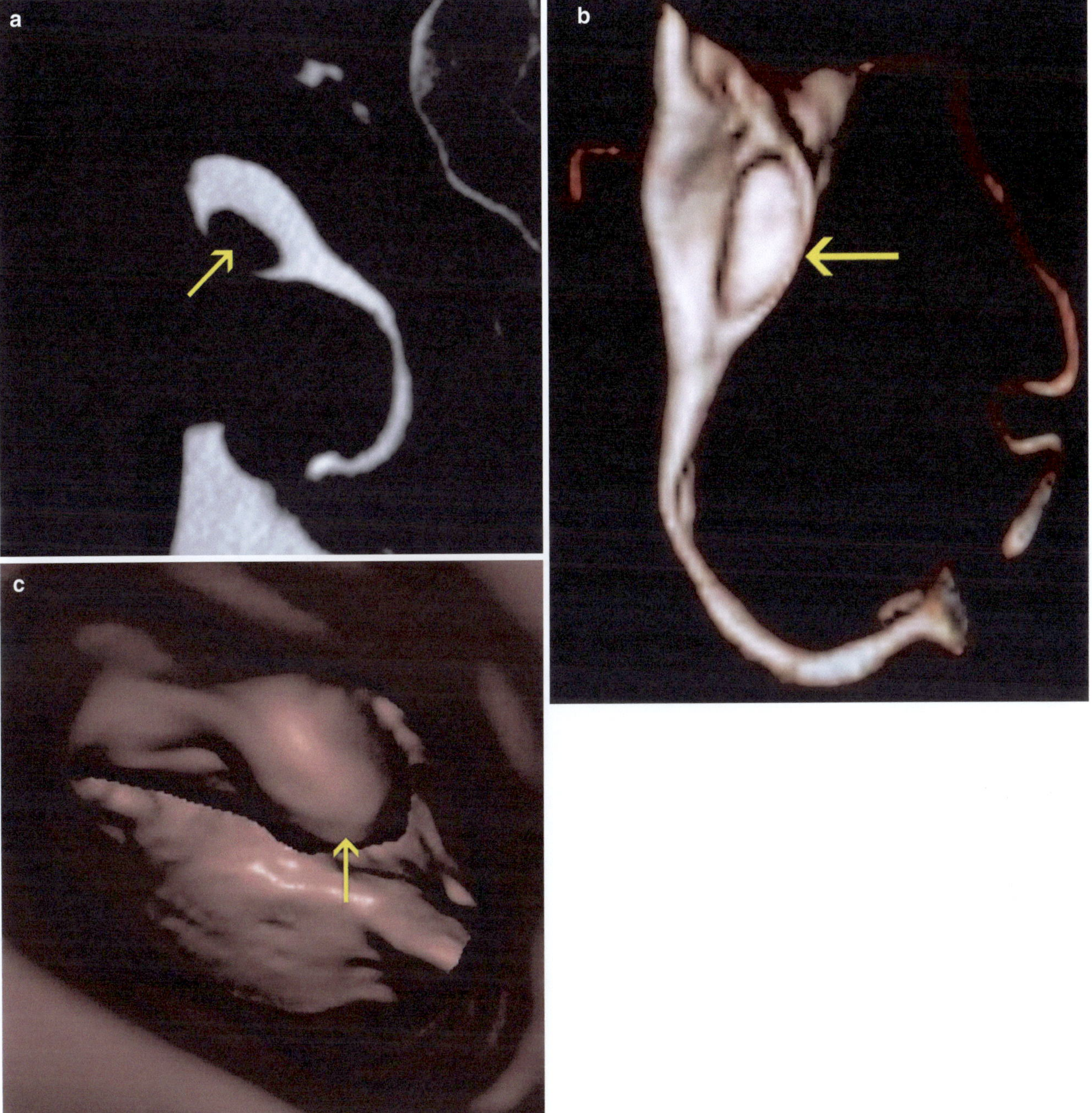

Fig. 6.23 Large endometrial polyp. (**a**) Sagittal multiplanar reconstruction image with soft tissue window that shows a large elevated lesion on the anterior wall (*arrow*) compatible with a polyp. (**b**) Oblique sagittal 3D volume rendering image which illustrates a large filling defect on the anterior wall (*arrow*). (**c**) Virtual endoscopy image that illustrates the polyp (*arrow*)

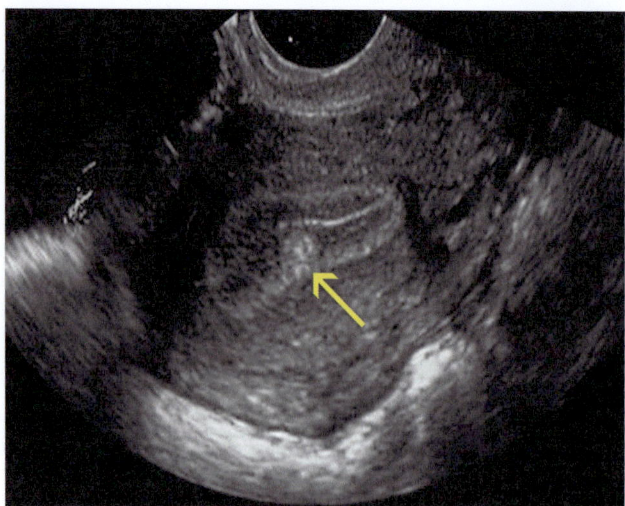

Fig. 6.24 Endometrial polyp seen on ultrasound exam. Hyperechoic round lesion in the medial aspect of the endometrial cavity (*arrow*)

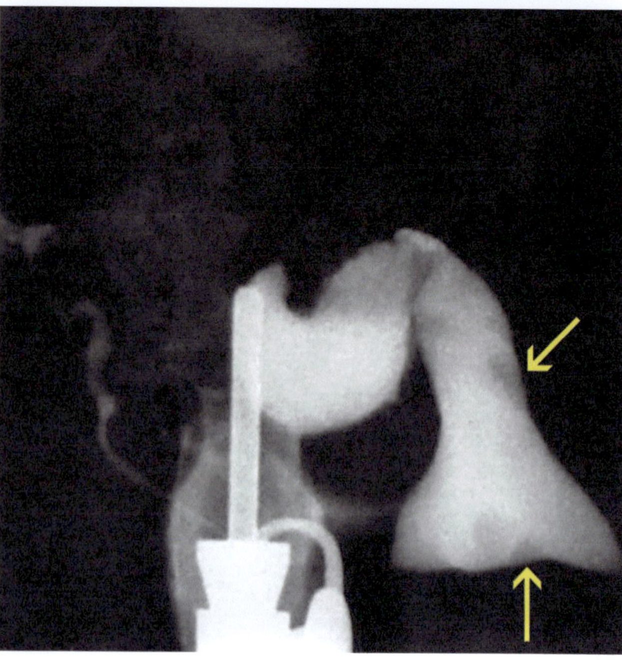

Fig. 6.26 Endometrial polyps seen on HSG exam. Multiple filling defects of different sizes are observed at the level of the uterine cavity compatible with uterine polyps (*arrows*)

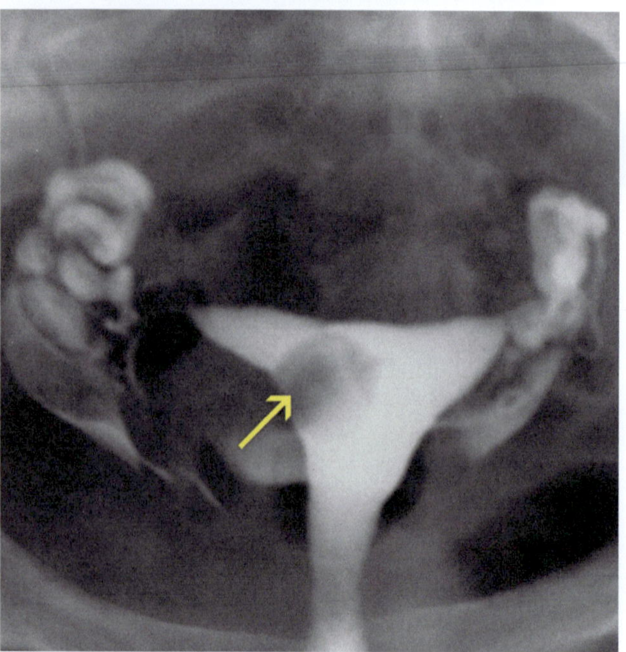

Fig. 6.25 Endometrial polyp seen on HSG exam. A rounded filling defect is observed at the level of the uterine cavity adjacent to the fundus and near the right horn compatible with a polyp (*arrow*)

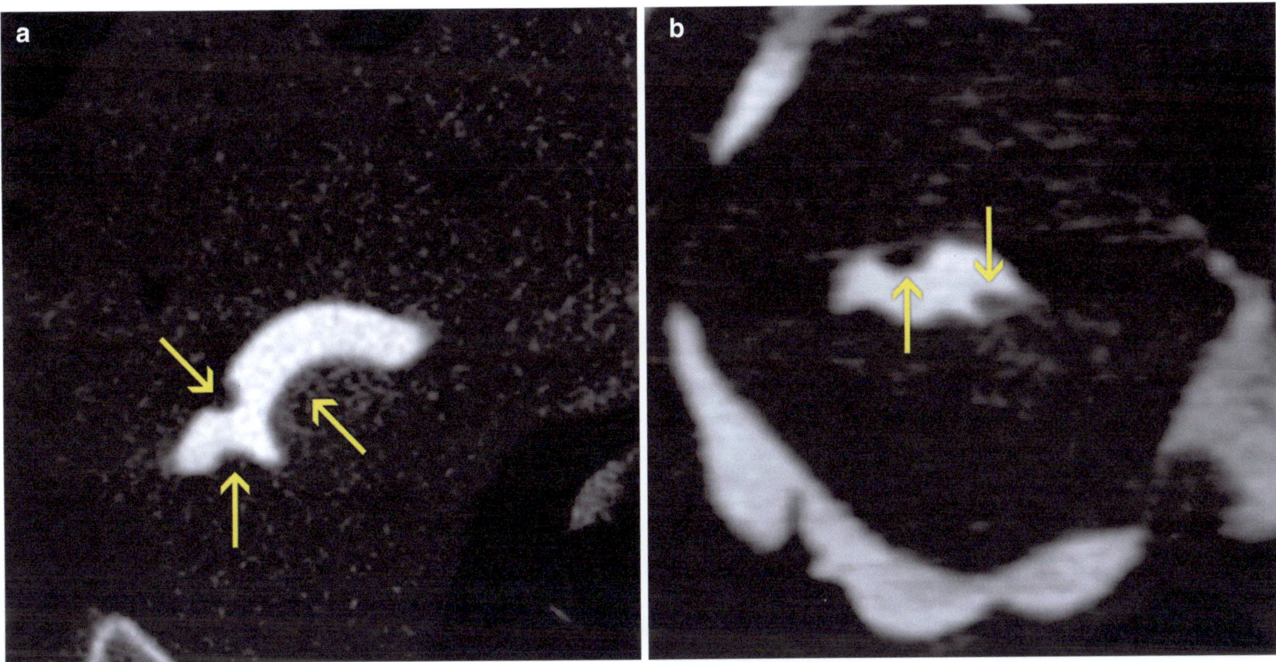

Fig. 6.27 Endometrial polyps seen on VHSG exam. (**a, b**) Sagittal and coronal multiplanar reconstruction images with soft tissue window that show elevated lesions of different sizes (*arrows*) compatible with endometrial polyps

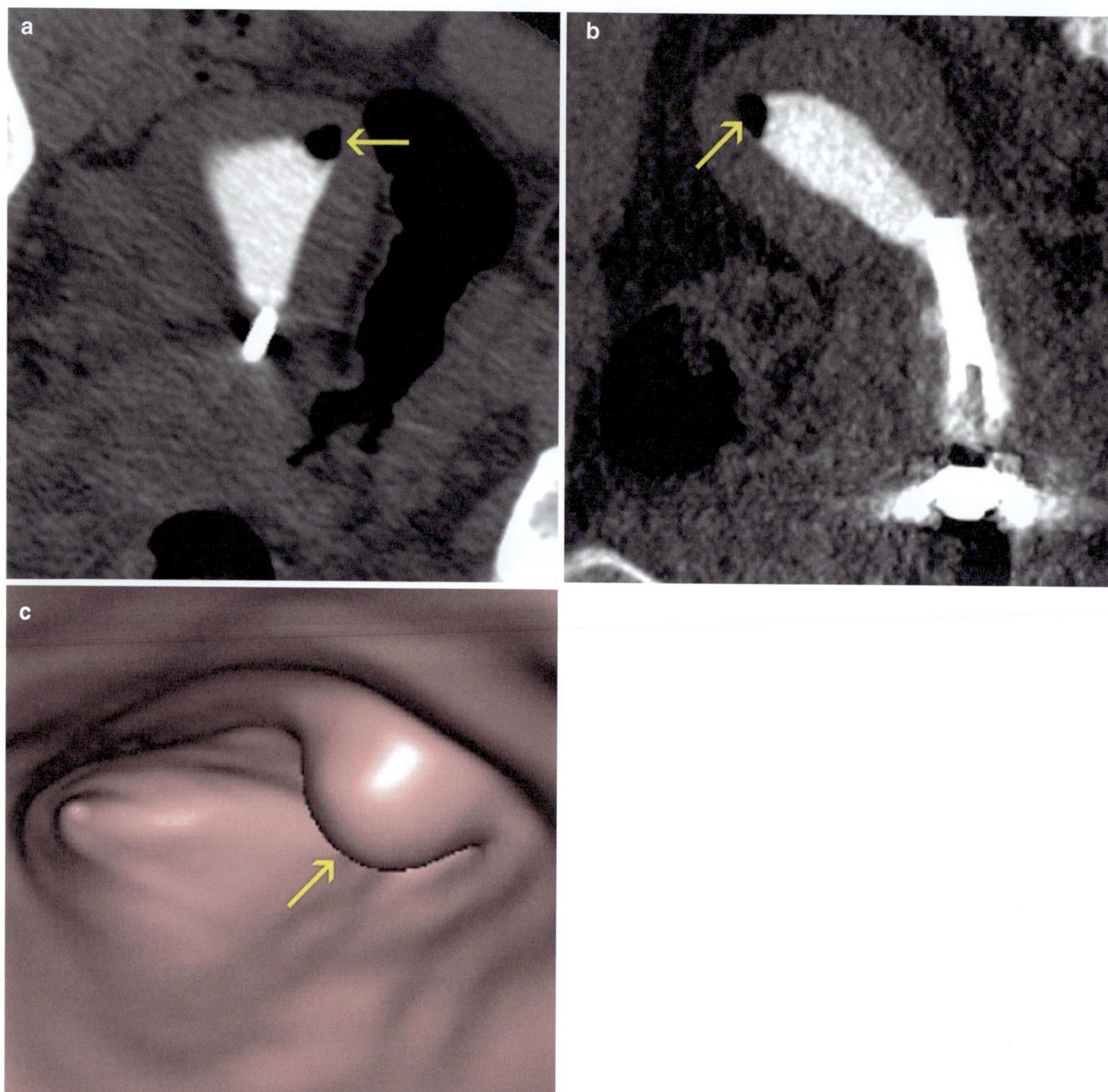

Fig. 6.28 Air bubble. (**a, b**) Coronal and sagittal multiplanar reconstruction images which show an air bubble in the left uterine horn (*arrow*). The CT density of the air bubble is characteristic, and permits to clearly differentiate it from a uterine polyp. (**c**) Virtual endoscopy image illustrates an elevated lesion that can be misdiagnosed as a polyp (*arrow*). For this reason evaluation with different types of image reconstructions is required

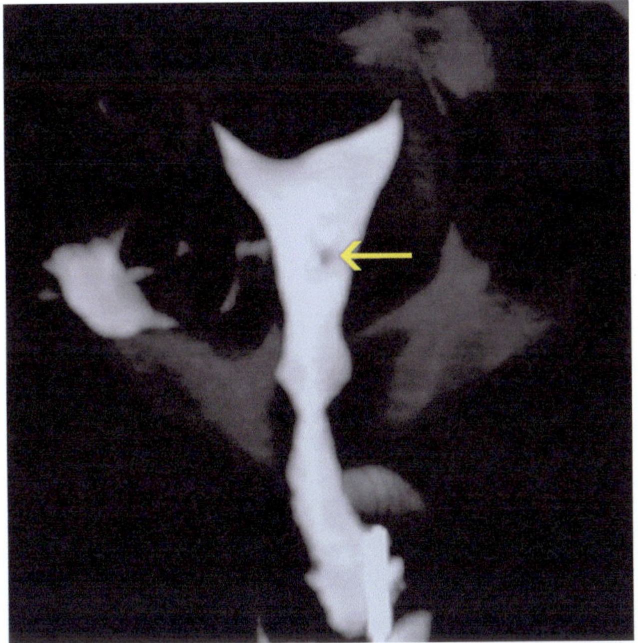

Fig. 6.29 Maximum intensity projection image. A filling defect in the uterine cavity can be observed with difficulty (*arrow*)

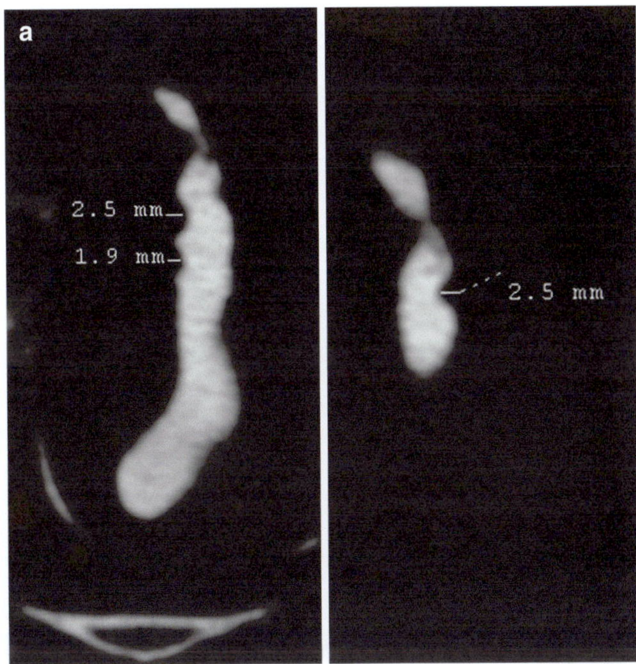

Fig. 6.30 Endometrial polyps. (**a**) CT multiplanar reconstruction images. (**b**) 3D volume rendering image. (**c**) Virtual endoscopy image

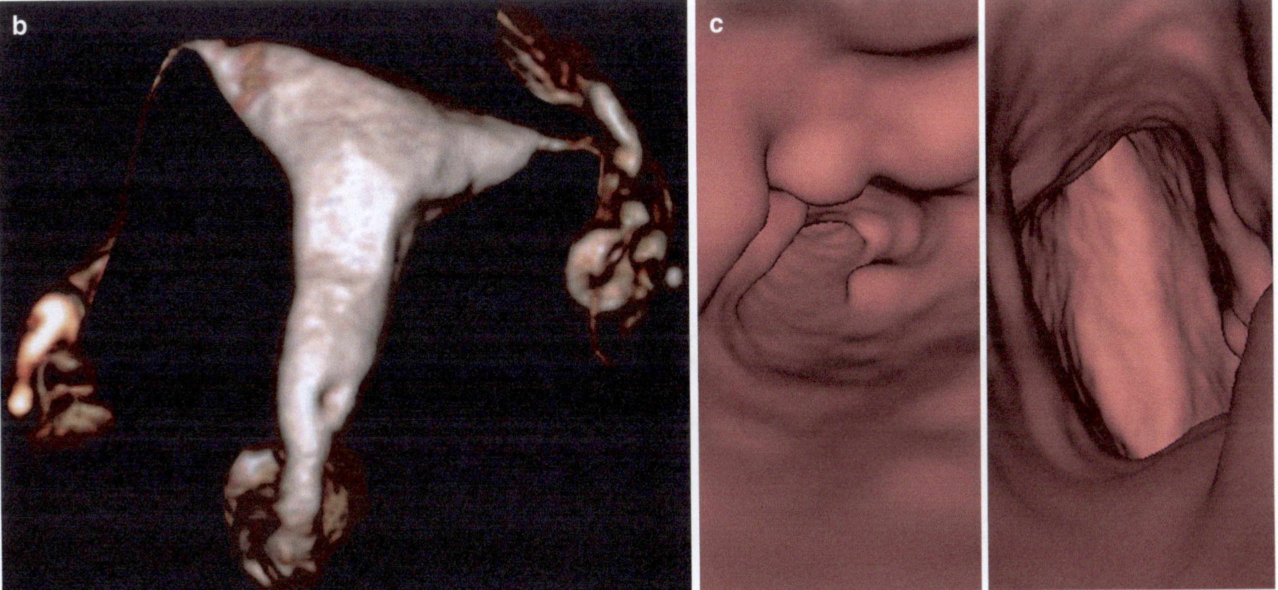

Fig. 6.30 (continued)

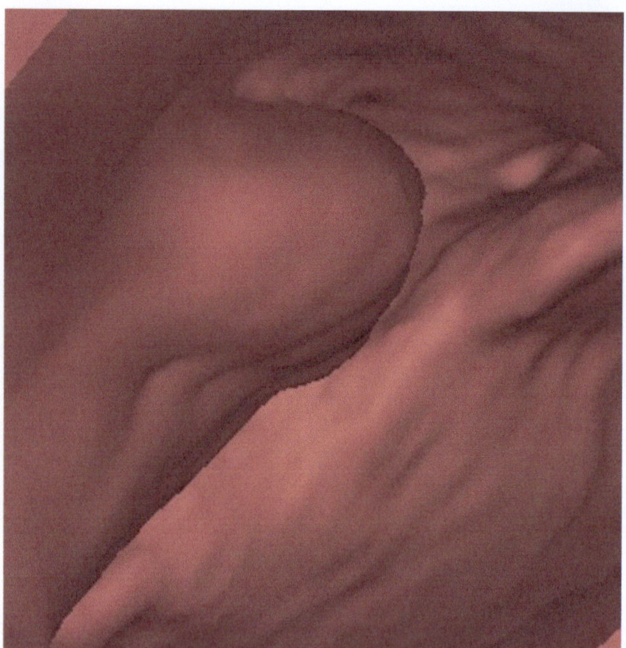

Fig. 6.31 Virtual endoscopy image. An elevated endoluminal lesion compatible with a polyp is observed

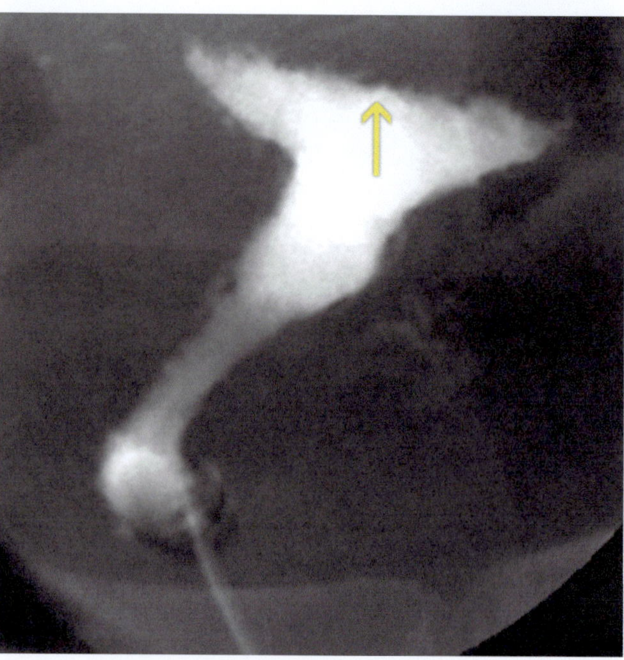

Fig. 6.33 Adenomyosis seen on HSG exam. The X-ray image shows a uterus with speculated edges, predominantly in the fundus, representing glandular projections towards the myometrial wall (*arrow*)

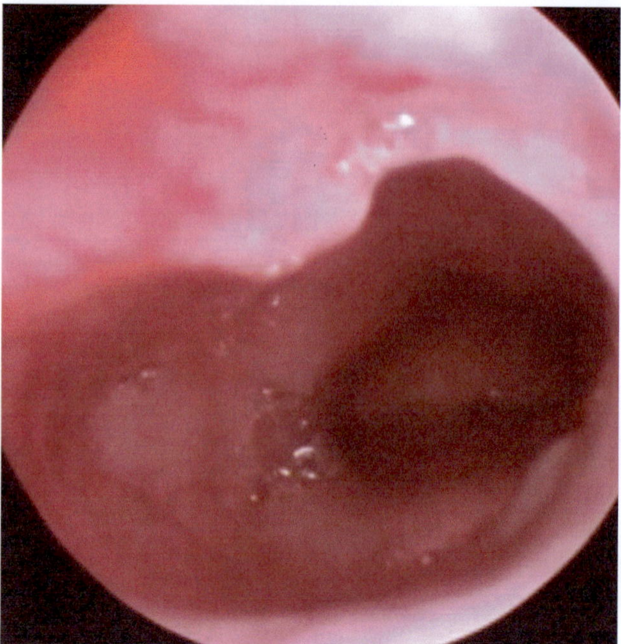

Fig. 6.32 Conventional hysteroscopy. An endometrial polyp is observed

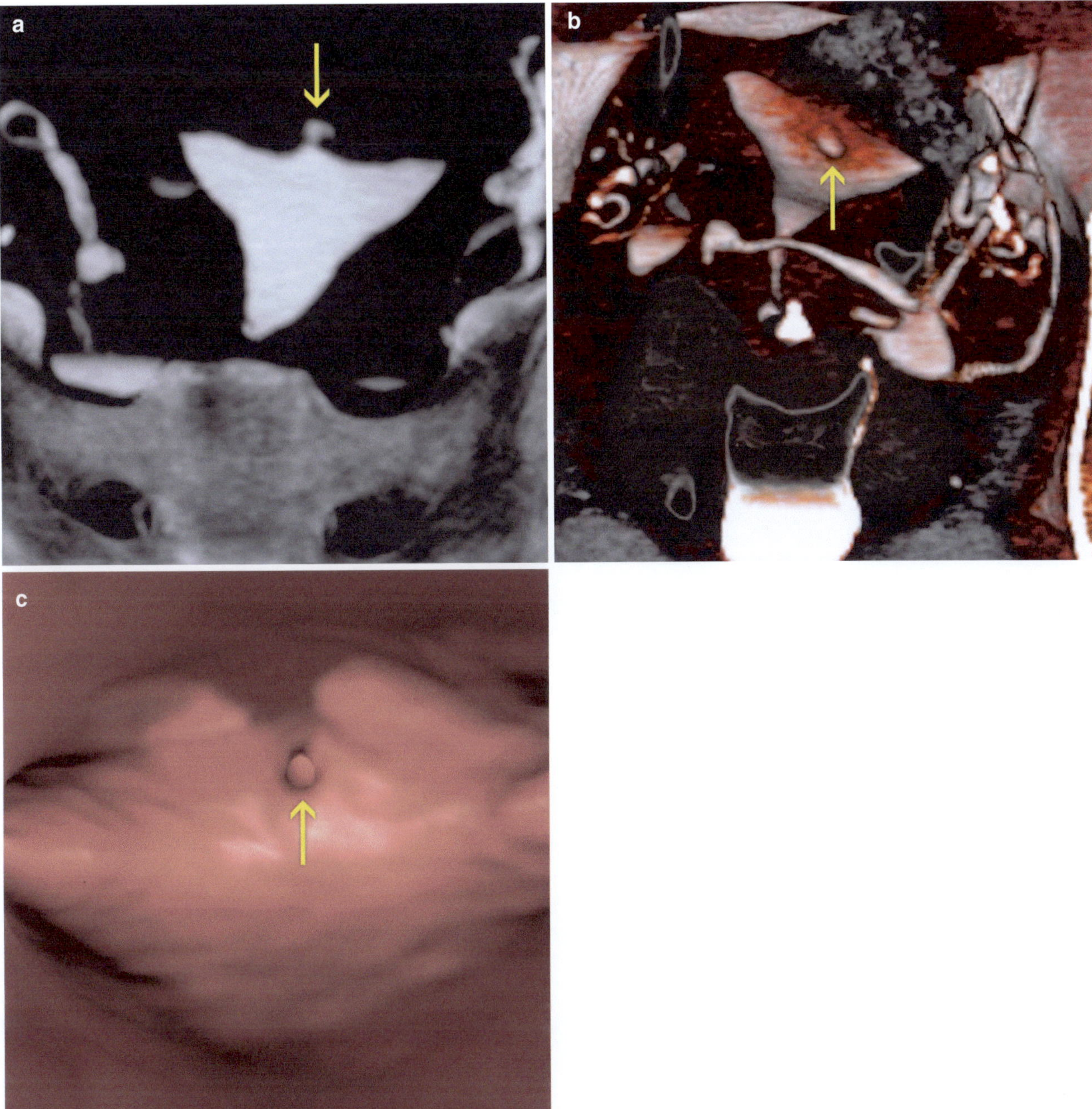

Fig. 6.34 Adenomyosis seen on VHSG exam. (**a**) Maximum intensity projection image which shows unique glandular dilatation at the level of the medial aspect of the uterine fundus compatible with adenomyosis (*arrow*). (**b**) 3D volume rendering image which shows similar findings (*arrow*). (**c**) Virtual endoscopy image. The diverticular neck is observed in the uterine fundus (*arrow*)

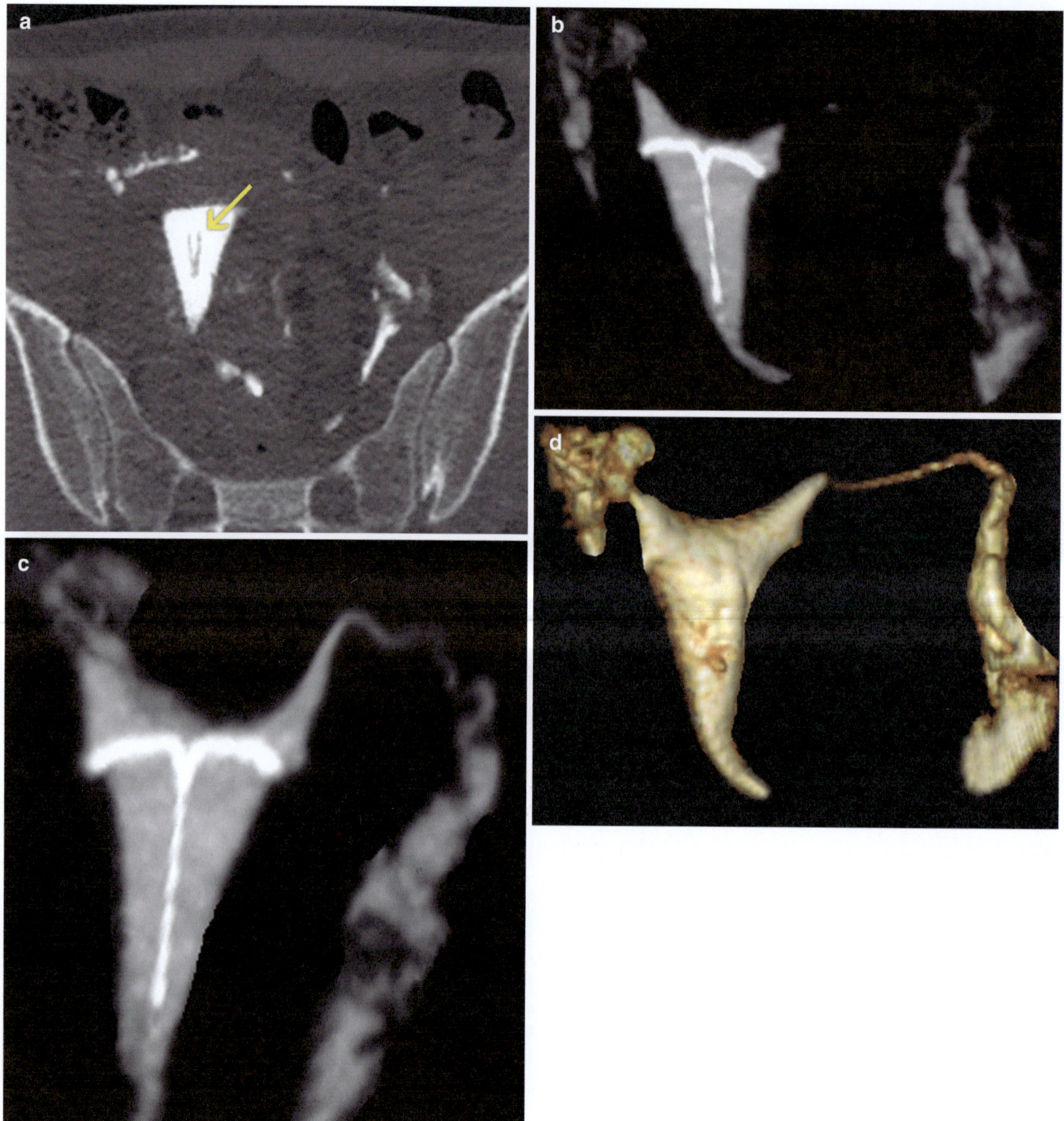

Fig. 6.35 Intrauterine contraceptive device (IUCD). (**a**) Axial CT image with soft tissue window which shows an IUCD (*arrow*). (**b**, **c**) Maximum intensity projection images in different projections which show the IUCD. (**d**) In the 3D volume rendering image the IUCD cannot be identified

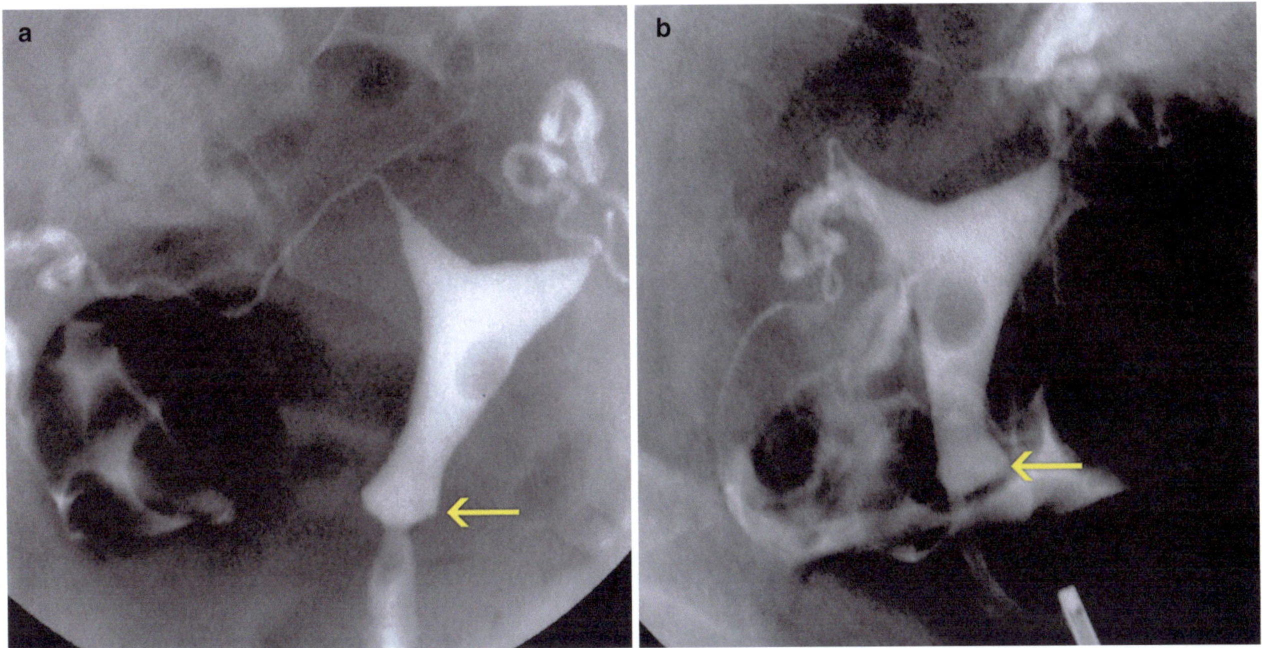

Fig. 6.36 Cesarean scar seen on HSG exam. (**a, b**) A focal dilatation in the isthmic-cervical region compatible with a cesarean scar can be observed in different views (*arrows*)

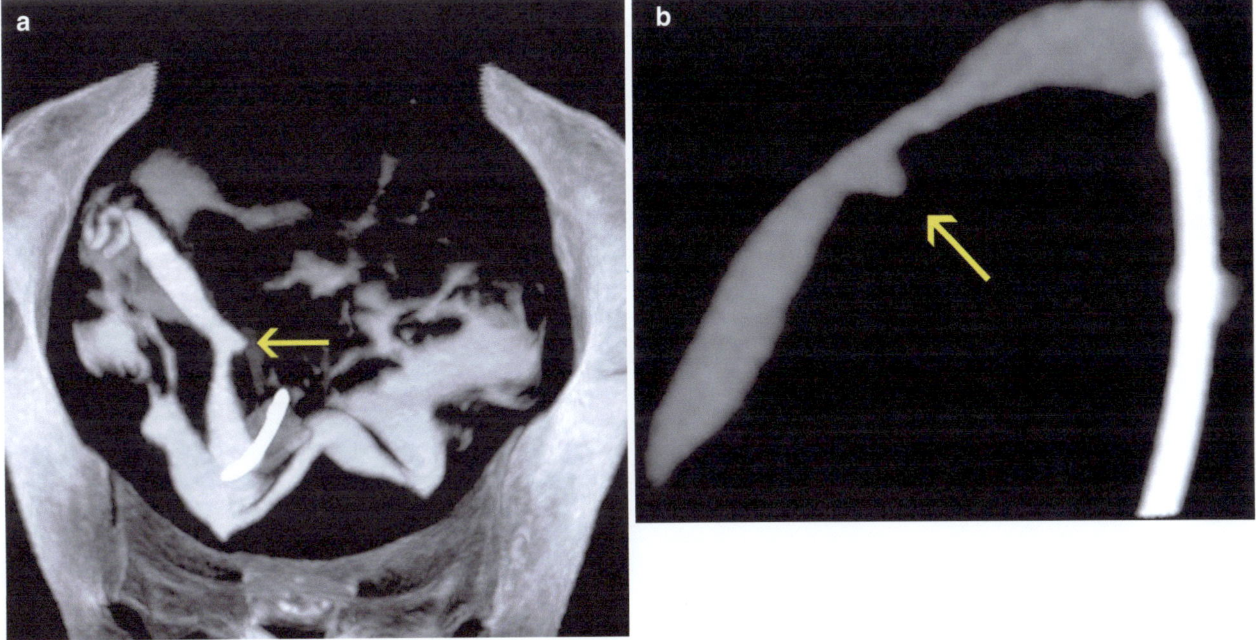

Fig. 6.37 Unicornuate uterus with cesarean scar. (**a, b**) Axial and sagittal maximum intensity projection images which illustrate a unicornuate uterus with cesarean scar (*arrows*). (**c**) Sagittal 3D volume rendering image which exhibits similar findings (*arrow*)

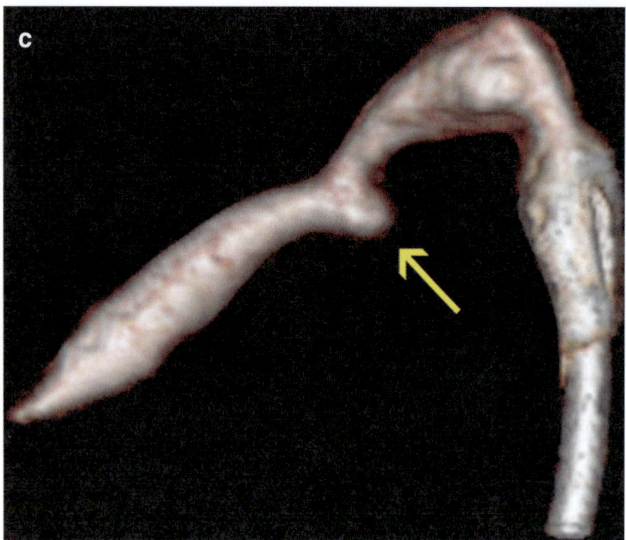

Fig. 6.37 (continued)

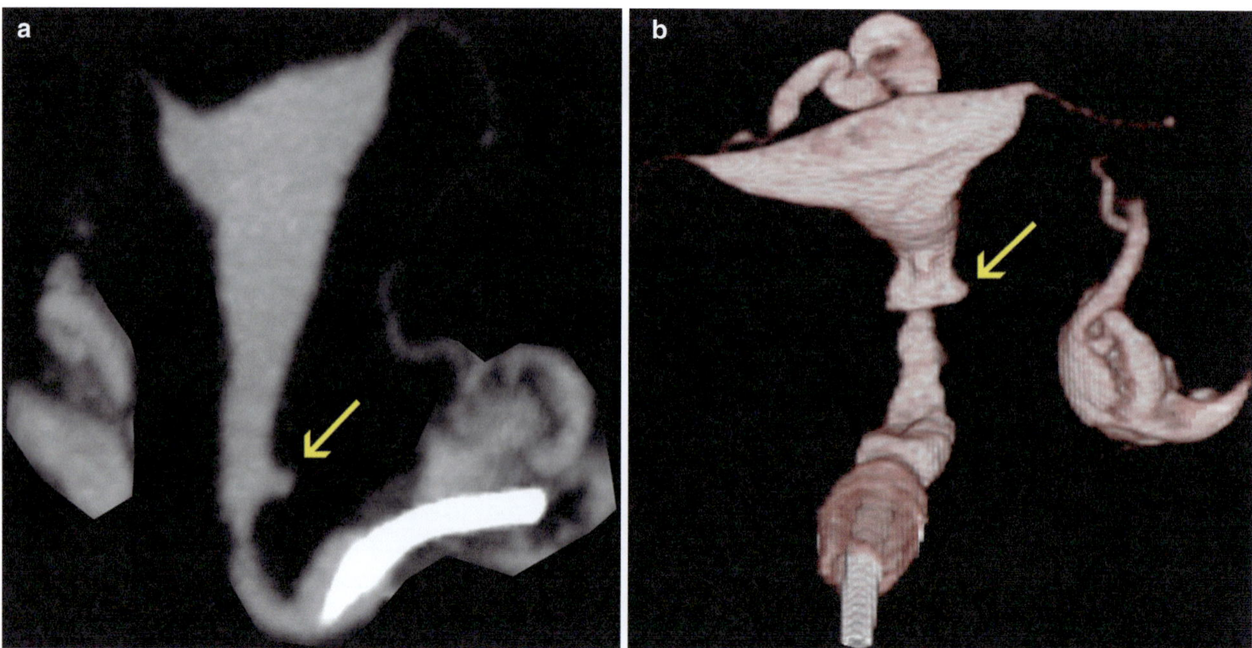

Fig. 6.38 Uterus with cesarean scar (*arrows*). (**a**) Coronal maximum intensity projection image which shows cesarean scar. (**b**) Coronal 3D volume rendering image which exhibits similar findings

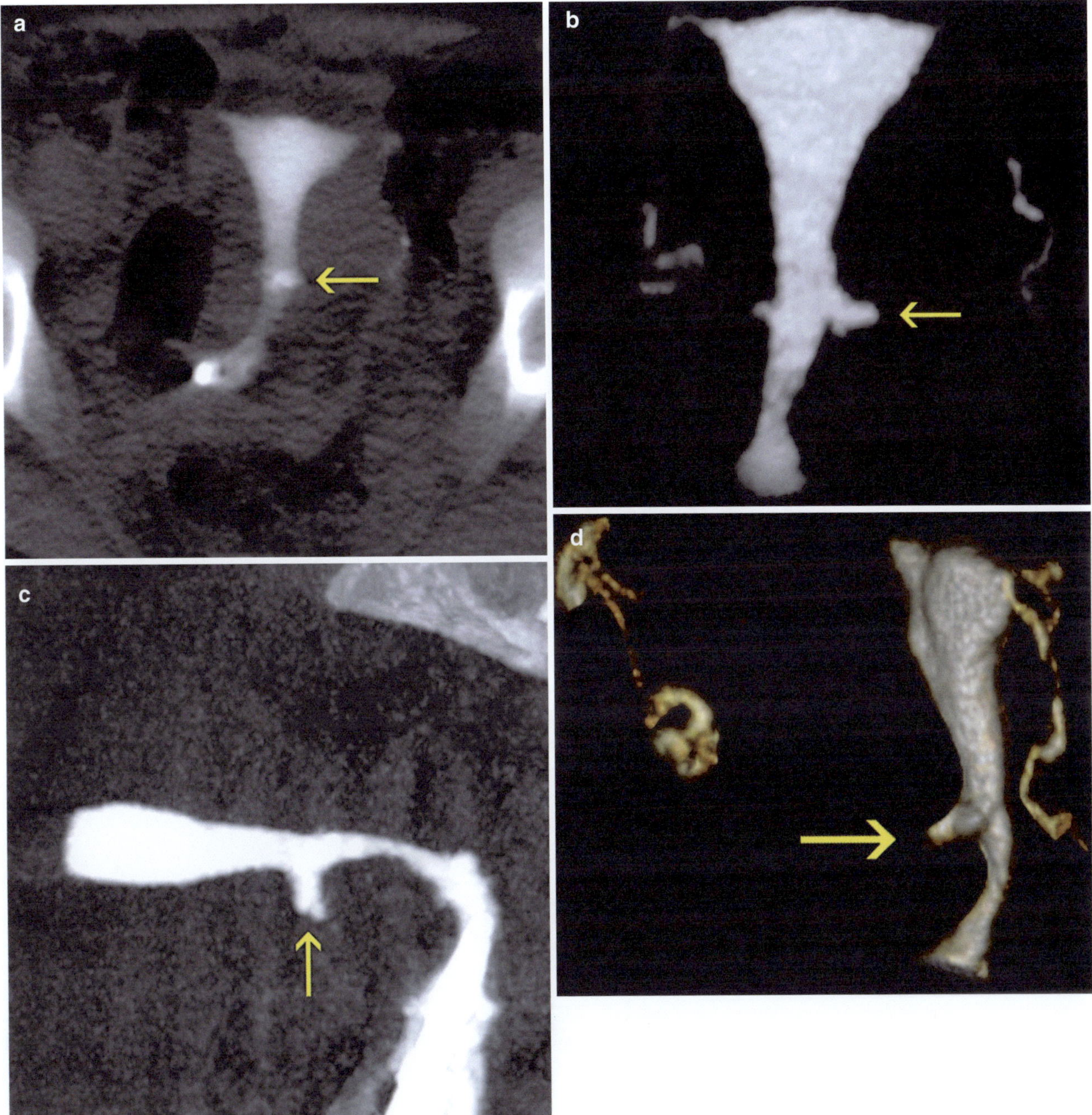

Fig. 6.39 Uterus with cesarean scar (*arrows*). (**a**) Axial CT image with soft tissue window. (**b**, **c**) Maximum intensity projection images in different projections. (**d**) Oblique sagittal 3D volume rendering image which illustrates similar findings

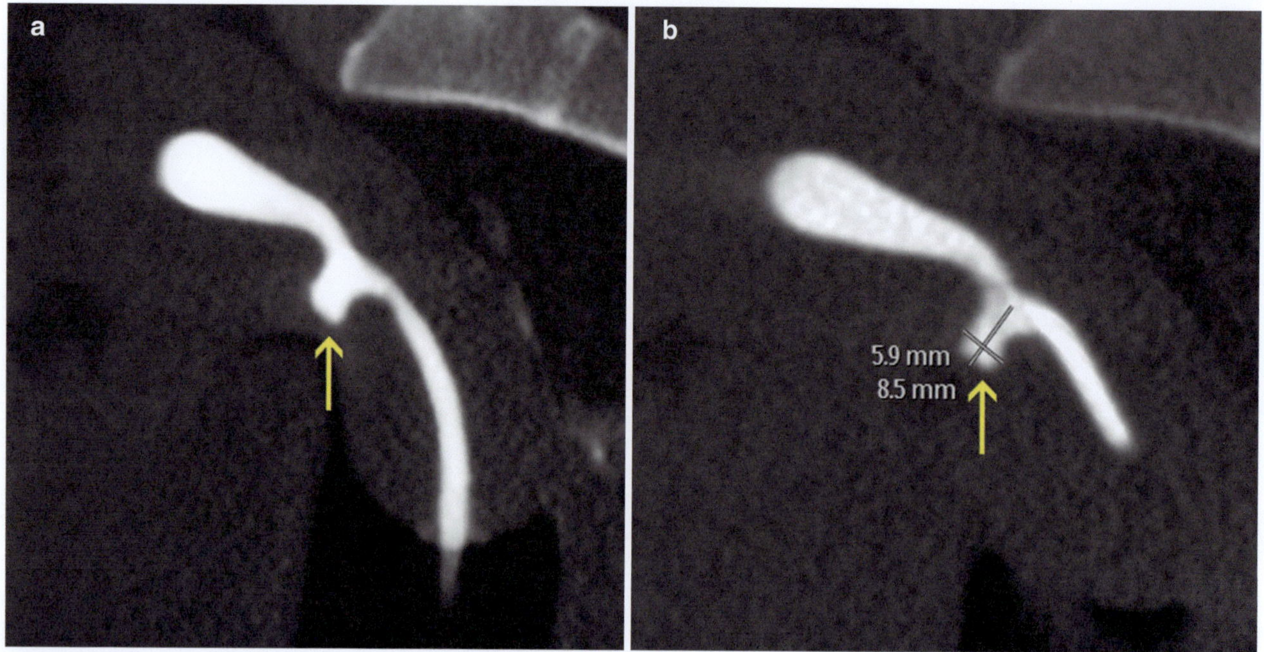

Fig. 6.40 Uterus with cesarean scar. (**a, b**) Sagittal maximum intensity projection images which show cesarean scar and its diameters (*arrows*)

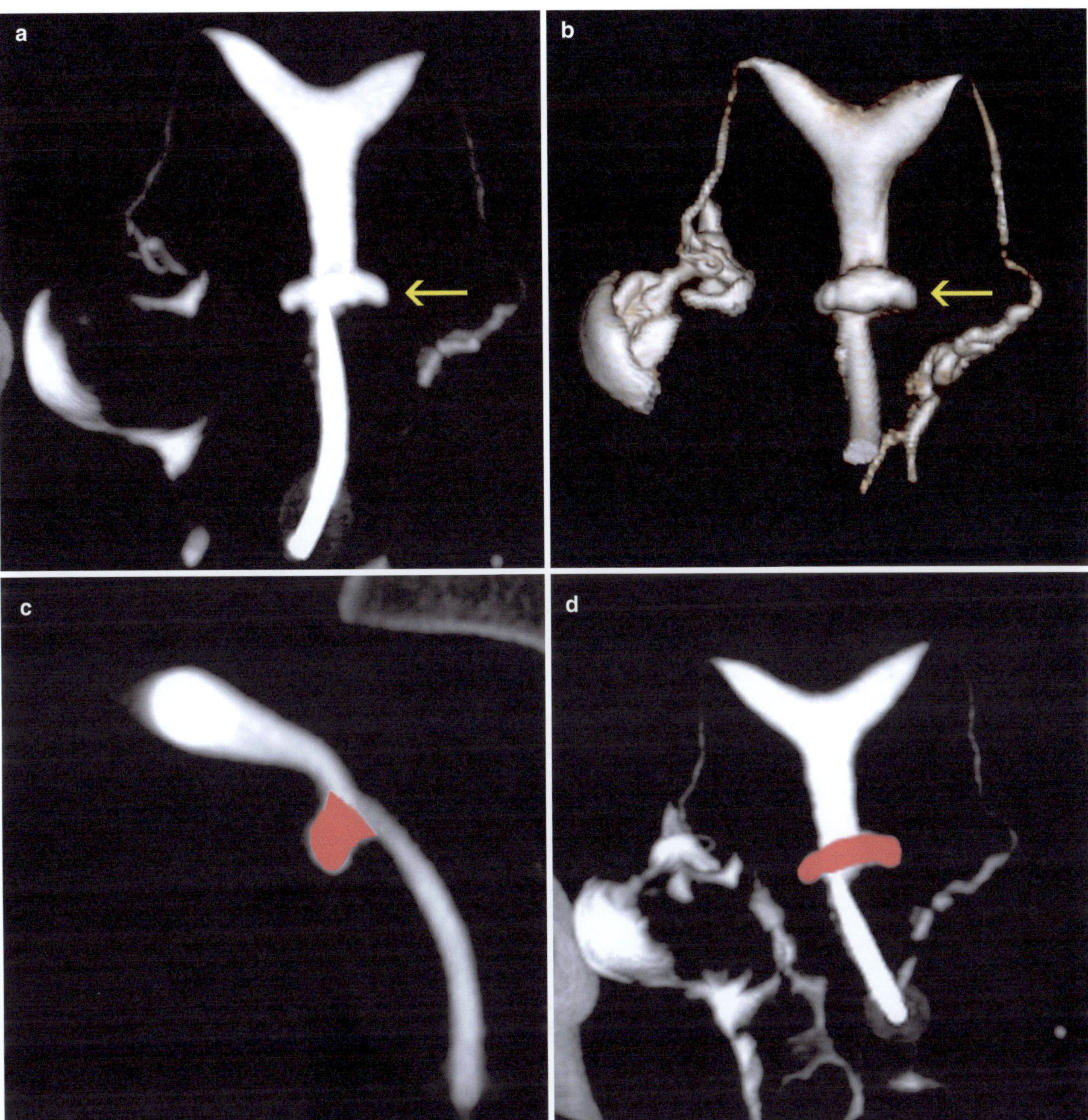

Fig. 6.41 Uterus with cesarean scar. Measurement of its volume. (**a**) Coronal MIP reconstruction which displays the cesarean scar (*arrow*). (**b**) Coronal VR reconstruction which illustrates similar findings (*arrow*). (**c**, **d**) MIP reconstruction in different projections which display the measurement of the volume of the cesarean scar (*red color*)

Conclusion

There exist diverse intrauterine pathologies like polyps, synechiae, etc. which can be evaluated via different diagnostic methods.

VHSG allows the quick and safe detection of the different pathologies which may be present in the uterus. It offers comfort to the patient and provides greater diagnostic information to the referring physician.

References

1. Hunt JE, Wallach EE. Uterine factors in infertility an overview. Clin Obstet Gynecol. 1974;17:44–64.
2. Donnez J, Jadoul P. What are the implications of myomas on fertility? A need for a debate? Hum Reprod. 2002;17:1424–30.
3. Karasick S, Goldfarb AF. Peritubal adhesions in infertile women: diagnosis with hysterosalpingography. AJR Am J Roentgenol. 1989;152(4):777–9.
4. Kunz G, Beil D, Huppert P, et al. Adenomyosis in endometriosis – prevalence and impact on fertility. Evidence from magnetic resonance imaging. Hum Reprod. 2005;20:2309–16.
5. Matalliotakis IM, Katsikis IK, Panidis DK. Adenomyosis: what is the impact on fertility? Curr Opin Obstet Gynecol. 2005;17:261–4.
6. Lin PC, Bhatnagar KP, Nettleton GS, et al. Female genital anomalies affecting reproduction. Fertil Steril. 2002;78:899–915.
7. Saravelos SH, Cocksedge KA, Li TC. Prevalence and diagnosis of congenital uterine anomalies in women with reproductive failure: a critical appraisal. Hum Reprod Update. 2008;14:415–29.
8. Mendoza Aguilar M, Herrera Flores I, Viramontes Trejo G, et al. Incidencia de patología de útero y anexos diagnosticada por histerosalpingografía en el Hospital General de México. An Radiol Méx. 2009;3:201–9.
9. Ott DJ, Fayez JA. Tubal and adnexal abnormalities. In: Ott DJ, Fayez JA, Zagoria RJ, editors. Hysterosalpingography: a text and atlas. 2nd ed. Baltimore: Williams & Wilkins; 1998. p. 90–3.
10. Simpson Jr WL, Beitia LG, Mester J. Hysterosalpingography: a reemerging study. Radiographics. 2006;26(2):419–31.
11. Vardhana PA, Silberzweig JE, Guarnaccia M, et al. Hysterosalpingography with selective salpingography. J Reprod Med. 2009;54(3):126–32.
12. Sankpal RS, Confino E, Matzel A, et al. Investigation of the uterine cavity and fallopian tubes using three-dimensional saline sonohysterosalpingography. Int J Gynaecol Obstet. 2001;73(2):125–9.
13. American Institute of Ultrasound in Medicine; American College of Radiology; American College of Obstetricians and Gynecologists; Society of Radiologists in Ultrasound. AIUM practice guideline for the performance of sonohysterography. J Ultrasound Med. 2012; 31(1):165–72.
14. Bhaduri M, Khalifa M, Tomlinson G, et al. Sonohysterography: the utility of diagnostic criteria sets. AJR Am J Roentgenol. 2012; 198(1):W83–8.
15. Winter L, Glücker T, Steimann S, et al. Feasibility of dynamic MR-hysterosalpingography for the diagnostic work-up of infertile women. Acta Radiol. 2010;51(6):693–701.
16. Fujii S, Matsusue E, Kigawa J, et al. Diagnostic accuracy of the apparent diffusion coefficient in differentiating benign from malignant uterine endometrial cavity lesions: initial results. Eur Radiol. 2008;18(2):384–9.
17. Dexeus S, Labastida R, Marqués L. Hysteroscopy in daily gynaecologic practice. Acta Eur Fertil. 1986;17:423–5.
18. Lee A, Ying YK, Novy MJ. Hysteroscopy, hysterosalpingography and tubal ostial polyps in infertility patients. J Reprod Med. 1997;42(6):337–41.
19. Chalazonitis A, Tzovara I, Laspas F, et al. Hysterosalpingography: technique and applications. Curr Probl Diagn Radiol. 2009;38(5):199–205.
20. Roma A, Ubeda B, Nin Garaizabal P. Hysterosalpingography: how, when, what for? Radiologia. 2007;49(1):5–18.
21. Elsayes KM, Pandya A, Platt JF, et al. Technique and diagnostic utility of saline infusion sonohysterography. Int J Gynaecol Obstet. 2009;105(1):5–9.
22. Tello R, Tempany CM, Chai J, et al. MR hysterography using axial long TR imaging with threedimensional projections of the uterus. Comput Med Imaging Graph. 1997;21(2):117–23.
23. Unterweger M, De Geyter C, Fröhlich JM, et al. Three-dimensional dynamic MR-hysterosalpingography; a new, low invasive, radiation-free and less painful radiological approach to female infertility. Hum Reprod. 2002;17(12):3138–41.
24. Florio P, Puzzutiello R, Filippeschi M, et al. Lowdose spinal anesthesia with hyperbaric bupivacaine with intrathecal fentanyl for operative hysteroscopy: a case series study. J Minim Invasive Gynecol. 2012;19(1):107–12.
25. Evangelista A, Oliveira MA, Crispi CP, et al. Diagnostic hysteroscopy using liquid distention medium: comparison of pain with warmed saline solution vs room-temperature saline solution. J Minim Invasive Gynecol. 2011;18(1):104–7.
26. Heinonen PK. Intrauterine adhesions-Asherman's syndrome. Duodecim. 2010;126(21):2486–91.
27. Rathat G, Do Trinh P, Mercier G, et al. Synechia after uterine compression sutures. Fertil Steril. 2011;95(1):405–9.
28. Deans R, Abbott J. Review of intrauterine adhesions. J Minim Invasive Gynecol. 2010;17(5):555–69.
29. Berman JM. Intrauterine adhesions. Semin Reprod Med. 2008; 26(4):349–55.
30. Ceccaldi PF, Nguyen T, Mandelbrot L. Unusual synechia at hysterosalpingography: intrauterine fallopian tube after surgical abortion. Fertil Steril. 2011;95(6):2078–9.
31. Yasmin H, Nasir A, Noorani KJ. Hystroscopic management of Ashermans syndrome. J Pak Med Assoc. 2007;57(11):553–5.
32. Carrascosa P, Baronio M, Capuñay C, et al. Multidetector computed tomography virtual hysterosalpingography in the investigation of the uterus and fallopian tubes. Eur J Radiol. 2008;67:531–5.
33. Carrascosa P, Capuñay C, Mariano B, et al. Virtual hysteroscopy by multidetector computed tomography. Abdom Imaging. 2008;33:381–7.
34. Carrascosa P, Capuñay C, Baronio M, et al. 64-Row multidetector CT virtual hysterosalpingography. Abdom Imaging. 2009;34(1):121–33.
35. Carrascosa P, Baronio JM, Borghi M, et al. Histerosalpingoscopía virtual. Una técnica novedosa y no invasiva para diagnosticar patología intrauterina. Reproduccion. 2006;21:19–26.
36. Baronio M, Carrascosa P, Capuñay C, et al. Diagnostic performance of CT virtual hysteroscopy in 69 consecutive patients. Fertil Steril. 2010;94(Suppl):S77.
37. Sharma JB, Pushpraj M, Roy KK, et al. Hyster osalpingographic findings in infertile women with genital tuberculosis. Int J Gynaecol Obstet. 2008;101(2):150–5.
38. Carrascosa P, Capuñay C, Vallejos J, et al. Virtual hysterosalpingography: a new multidetector CT technique for evaluating the female reproductive system. Radiographics. 2010;30:643–61.
39. Carrascosa P, Capuñay C, Vallejos J, et al. Virtual hysterosalpingography: experience with over 1000 consecutive patients. Abdom Imaging. 2011;36(1):1–14.
40. Thomson AJ, Abbott JA, Deans R, et al. The management of intrauterine synechiae. Curr Opin Obstet Gynecol. 2009;21(4):335–41.
41. AAGL Advancing Minimally Invasive Gynecology Worldwide. AAGL practice report: practice guidelines for management of intrauterine synechiae. J Minim Invasive Gynecol. 2010;17(1):1–7.
42. Elbahraoui H, Elmazghi A, Bouziane H, et al. Postmenopausal tuberculous endometritis simulating endometrial cancer: report of a case. Pan Afr Med J. 2012;11:7.

43. Iovenitti P, Ruggeri G, Tatangelo R, et al. Endometrial tuberculosis: a clinical case. Clin Exp Obstet Gynecol. 2011;38(2):186–7.

44. Larosa M, Facchini F, Pozzoli G, et al. Endometriosis: aetiopathogenetic basis. Urologia. 2010;77 Suppl 17:1–11.

45. Roma Dalfó A, Ubeda B, Ubeda A, et al. Diagnostic value of hysterosalpingography in the detection of intrauterine abnormalities: a comparison with hysteroscopy. AJR Am J Roentgenol. 2004; 183(5):1405–9.

46. López Navarrete JA, Herrera Otero JM, Quiroga Feuchter G, et al. Comparison between hysterosonography and hysterosalpinography in the study of endometrial abnormalities in infertility patients. Ginecol Obstet Mex. 2003;71:277–83.

47. Sindi O, Saleh A, Rouzi AA. Diagnosis of simple endometrial hyperplasia in a woman with polycystic ovary syndrome with use of hysterosalpingography. Fertil Steril. 2002;77(5):1069–70.

48. Golan A, Cohen-Sahar B, Keidar R, et al. Endometrial polyps: symptomatology, menopausal status and malignancy. Gynecol Obstet Invest. 2010;70(2):107–12.

49. Tabrizi AD, Vahedi A, Esmaily HA. Malignant endometrial polyps: report of two cases and review of literature with emphasize on recent advances. J Res Med Sci. 2011;16(4):574–9.

50. Costa-Paiva L, Godoy Jr CE, Antunes Jr A, et al. Risk of malignancy in endometrial polyps in premenopausal and postmenopausal women according to clinicopathologic characteristics. Menopause. 2011;18(12):1278–82.

51. Growdon WB. Age and postmenopausal bleeding risk factors for malignant changes in endometrial polyps. Menopause. 2011; 18(12):1267.

52. Ubeda B, Paraira M, Alert E, et al. Hysterosalpingography: spectrum of normal variants and nonpathological findings. AJR Am J Roentgenol. 2001;177(1):131–5.

53. Preutthipan S, Linasmita V. A prospective comparative study between hysterosalpingography and hysteroscopy in the detection of intrauterine pathology in patients with infertility. J Obstet Gynaecol Res. 2003;29:33–7.

54. Pérez-Medina T, Bajo-Arenas J, Salazar F, et al. Endometrial polyps and their implication in the pregnancy rates of patients undergoing inrauterine inseination: a prospective, randomized study. Hum Reprod. 2005;20:1632–5.

55. Bohlman ME, Ensor RE, Sanders RC. Sonographic findings in adenomyosis of the uterus. AJR Am J Roentgenol. 1987;148:756–66.

56. Reinhold C, Tafazoli F, Mehio A, et al. Uterine adenomyosis: endovaginal US and MR imaging features with histopathologic correlation. Radiographics. 1999;19:S147–60.

57. Juhasz-Böss I, Haggag H, Baum S, et al. Laparoscopic and laparotomic approaches for endometrial cancer treatment: a comprehensive review. Arch Gynecol Obstet. 2012;286(1):167–72.

58. Karimi-Zarchi M, Mousavi AS, Behtash N, et al. Conservative management of young women with endometrial carcinoma or complex atypical hyperplasia: report of three cases and literature review. Eur J Gynaecol Oncol. 2011;32(6):695–8.

59. Ikeda S, Kato T. A case of pelvic actinomycosis unrelated to an intrauterine device. Jpn J Clin Oncol. 2012;42(3):237–8.

60. Berisavac M, Sparić R, Argirović R, et al. Application of a hormonal intrauterine device causing uterine perforation: a case report. Srp Arh Celok Lek. 2011;139(11–12):815–8.

The uterus plays a primordial role in the transport of spermatozoids. In the evaluation of the infertile patient, the uterine pathology does not occupy a principal place. As a unique factor, the uterine disorders represent only 5 % of the causes of infertility; nevertheless it can be linked to other alterations and represent an important cause in patients with frequent abortions.

In the present, however, the influence of the uterine factor is increasing. The maternity at a later age is associated in the nullipara woman with a tendency to develop pathology in the wall of the uterus, in particular with the apparition of myomas. This does not influence only natural conception. The uterus has a fundamental role in the success of different techniques of assisted reproduction, in which the process of the implantation of the embryo in the endometrium is the event that limits the success of the procedure [1]. The mechanisms involved are not completely determined; a chronic inflammation of the endometrium, alteration in the vascularization, an increase in the uterine contraction and local endocrine alterations are causes that may potentially interfere in the process and outcome of the conception [2–4].

The uterus is principally a muscular organ, whose parietal structure can be divided into three components: (i) the inner layer or endometrium; (ii) the middle layer, muscular or myometrium; (iii) the external or serose layer. The pathological processes that have origin in the endometrium can manifest themselves as lesions that protrude to the cavity (polyps, endometrial hyperplasia; see Chap. 6) or extend themselves towards the muscular layer and act as complications on the uterine wall. Nevertheless, most of the processes that compromise the uterine wall originate from the myometrium, and are represented by the myomas.

Myomas

The myomas, also called leiomyomas, fibromas or fibroids constitute the most frequent neoplasia during and after the reproductive age, with a prevalence of between 20 and 40 %

in women older than 30, which variates with age, race and diagnostic modality. In a study published by Baird and cols [5] the accumulative incidence of the myomas in American women over 50 was greater than 80 % in black women and close to 70 % in white women. European studies have shown a minor prevalence of myomas in the population of the old continent. Heinemann and cols [6] reported that 10.7 % of German women with an average age of 40 had one or more myomas. Following the same steps, Marino and cols [7] in a population of Italian women showed a rate of 21.4 % in women of 30 years of age studied with ultrasound, and Borgfelt and cols [8] in Swedish women found only an incidence of 7.8 % in patients between the ages of 33 and 40.

The myomas are benign tumors of the smooth muscle, unique or multiple (more frequently) and of variable size [9, 10]. They constitute round masses of defined edges that displace the normal myometrium, which forms a pseudocapsule that delimits them. The most frequent location is at the fundus of the uterus, on the middle line. The locations at the level of the cervix are infrequent, and are rare on the round ligaments. In Table 7.1 the macroscopic classification of the myomas is detailed.

Frequently asymptomatic, these tumors can be associated with metrorrhagia, pelvic pain, intestinal or vesical dysfunction, infertility and recurrent abortions. Approximately 5–10 % of the infertile women have at least one myoma, while that as the only cause is found in only 1–2.4 % of the patients [2]. In its evolution, the myomas can suffer different changes that alter its habitual structure, which are enumerated in Table 7.2. The hyaline degeneration is the most frequent and is present in almost all the myomas. It is characterized by the replacement of muscular fibers for poorly delimited collagen bands that confer an extra soft appearance. In certain circumstances, the hyaline areas can liquate and give place to the formation of cysts. In other cases the presence of amorphous calcifications is frequent, in occasions of very high density (Fig. 7.1). When the blood supply is insufficient, in particular if the myoma acquires a considerable size, necrosis is produced (Fig. 7.2). Grease and sarcomatose transformations in myomas are rare.

P. Carrascosa et al., *CT Virtual Hysterosalpingography*,
DOI 10.1007/978-3-319-07560-0_7, © Springer International Publishing Switzerland 2014

Table 7.1 Classification of myomas

Based on uterine location

  Body

  Isthmic

  Cervical

  Round ligament and tubes

Based on uterine wall location

  Submucous

  Intramural

  Subserous

Based on the number

  Unique

  Multiple

Based on its disposition

  Sessile

  Pedunculated

Based on its size

  Microscopic

  Giant (>10 kg)

Table 7.2 Degenerative processes of the myomas

Hyaline degeneration

Cystic degeneration

Calcifications

Myxomatous and mucoid degeneration

Red degeneration

Necrosis

Infection

Suppuration

Fat degeneration

Sarcomatous degeneration

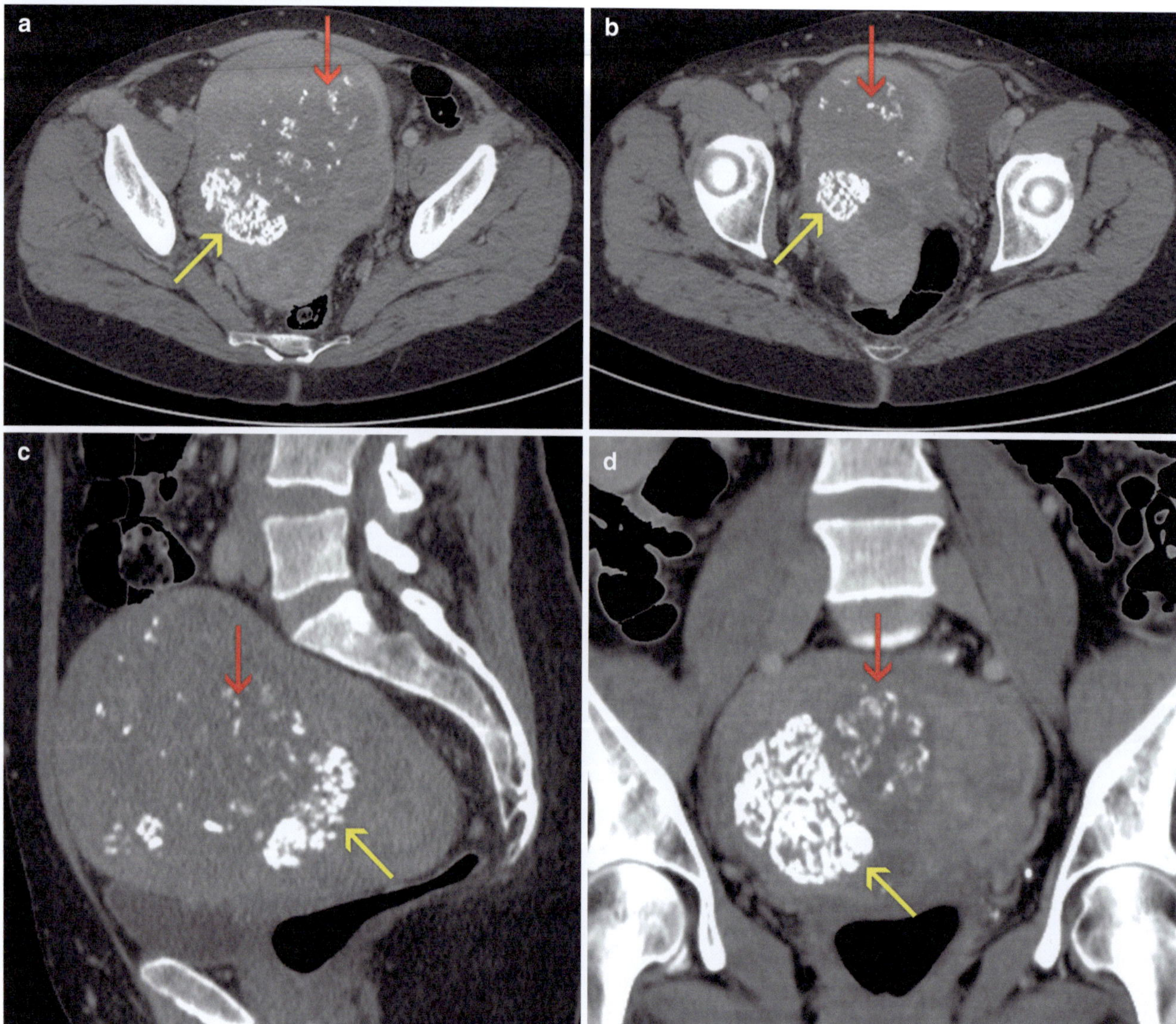

Fig. 7.1 Uterine myomas. Enlarged, globular uterus, with focal calcifications (*yellow arrows*) and signs of hyaline degeneration (*red arrows*). (**a, b**) Axial CT images. (**c**) Sagittal multiplanar reconstruction (MPR) image. (**d**) Coronal MPR image

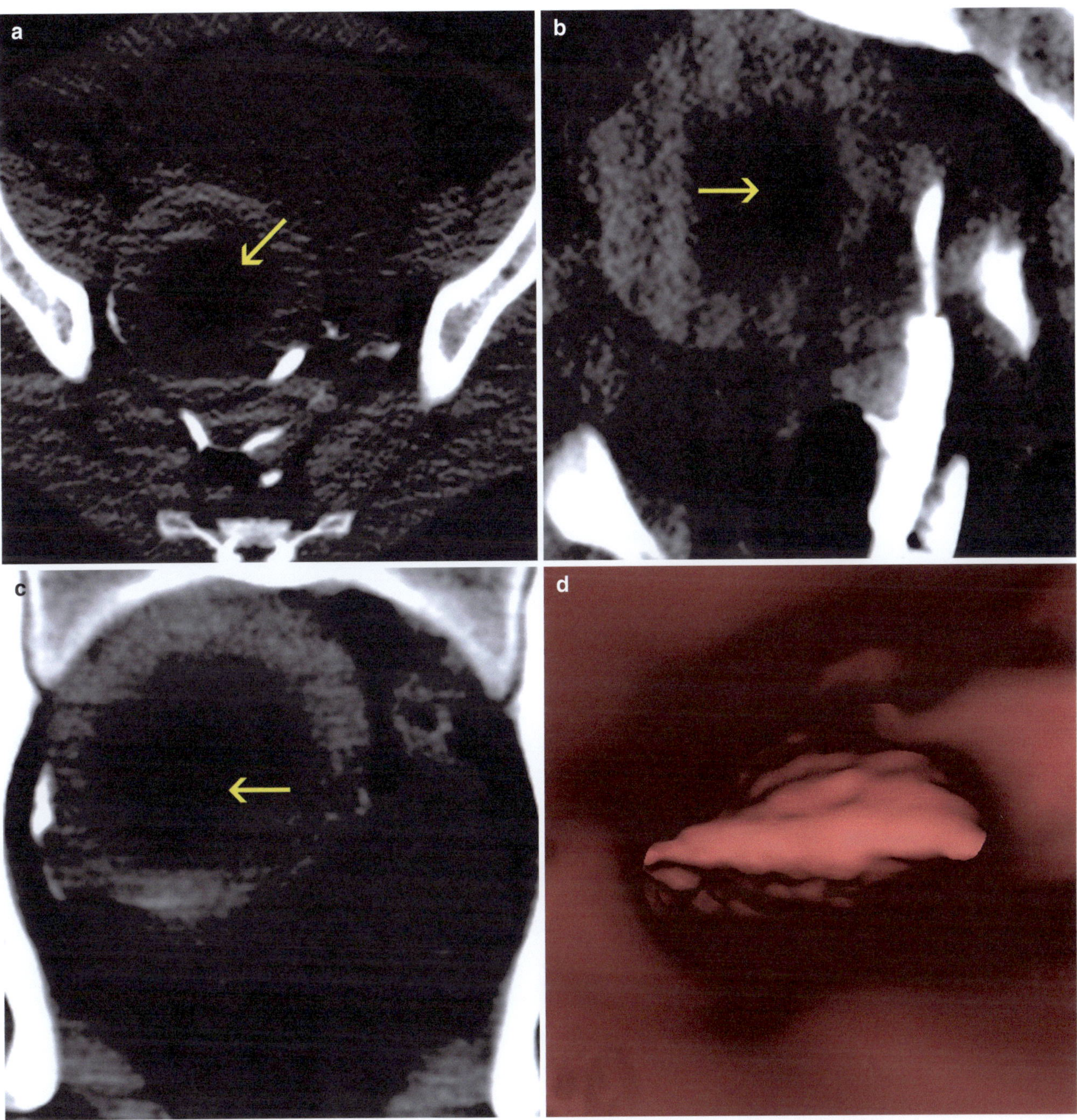

Fig. 7.2 Subserous myoma at the anterior wall of the uterus, with signs of necrosis (*arrows*). VHSG study. (**a**) Axial maximum intensity projection (MIP) image. (**b**) Sagittal MIP image. (**c**) Coronal MIP image. (**d**) Virtual endoscopy image. Due to the subserous location, the uterine cavity does not show alterations

Classification

The traditional classification of the myomas is based on the location of the tumor in the width of the uterine wall and they are divided in submucosal, intramural and subserosal (Fig. 7.3).

Submucosal Myomas

Submucosal myomas, the least common, are the ones that most frequently generate symptoms. They grow under the endometrium and push it, distorting the uterine cavity. In Table 7.3 the two proposed classifications for the

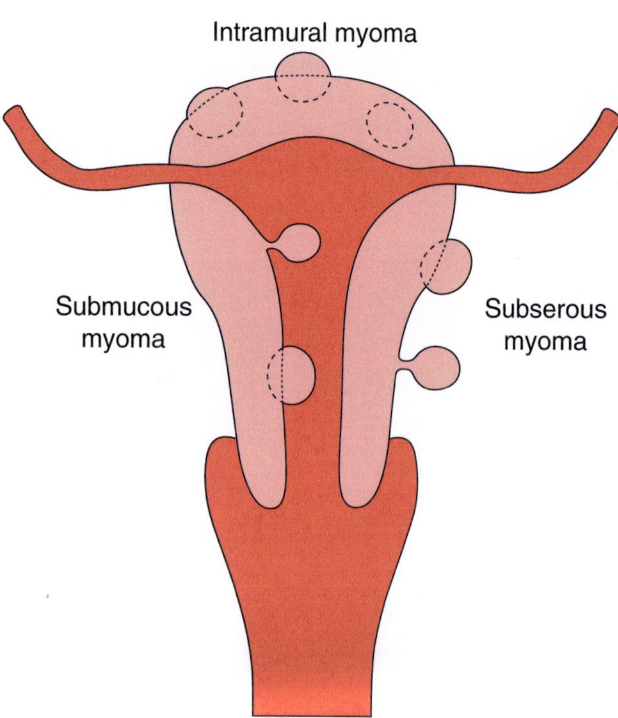

Fig. 7.3 Classification of myomas according to their location on the uterine wall

Table 7.3 Submucosal myoma classification

Wamsteker classification [11]
G0: Myoma totally located in the endometrial cavity, without intramural extension (pedunculated or sessile)
GI: Sessile myoma with intvramural extension <50 % (more than 50 % in cavity)
GII: Sessile myoma with intramural extension >50 % (less than 50 % in cavity)
Labastida classification [12]
Type I: Pedunculated myoma
Type II: Sessile myoma
Type III: Myoma with intramural extension <1/3
Type IV: Myoma with intramural extension of 50 %
Type V: Myoma with intramural extension <2/3

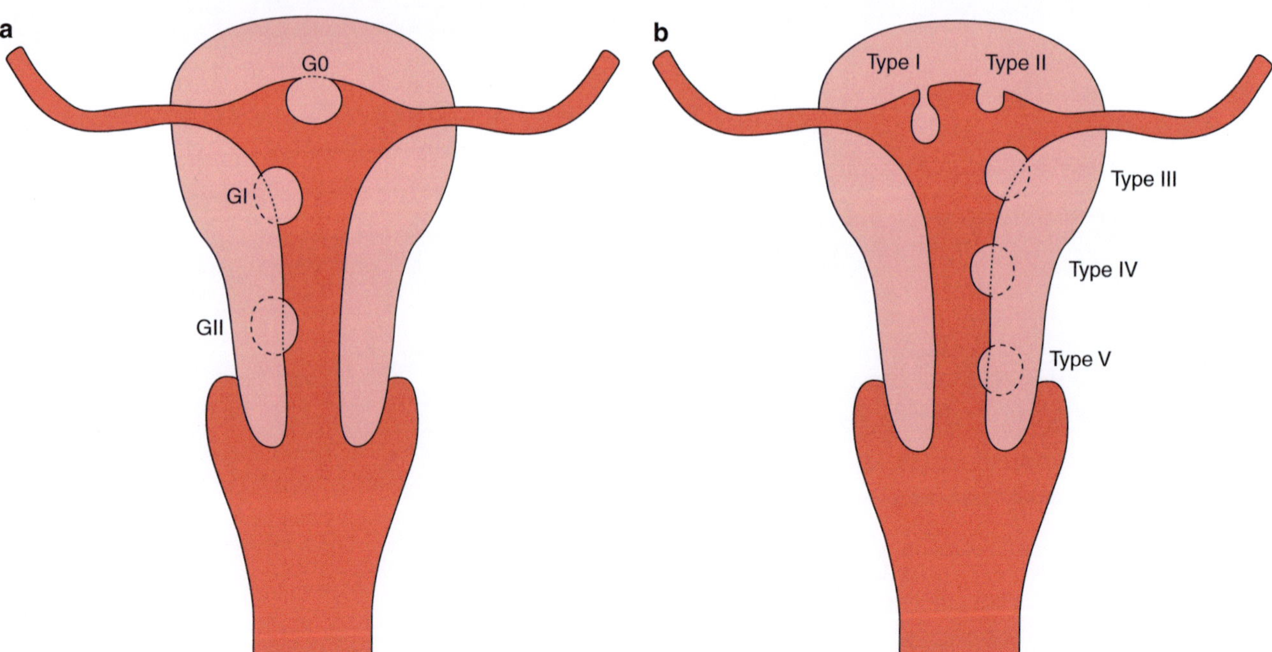

Fig. 7.4 Submucous myomas. (**a**) Wamsteker classification. (**b**) Labastida classification

differentiation of the submucosal leiomyomas in respect to the intramural component of the tumor are mentioned, which is important at the moment of deciding the surgical technique and of foreseeing the success of the procedure (Fig. 7.4) [11, 12].

Intramural Myomas

The intramural or interstitial myomas are located in the width of the myometrium and do not distort the endometrial cavity. They can however deform the external uterine outlines, but the projection on the serose surface must be less than 50 % of its volume. When they are of great size they generate an important increase of the uterus, which acquires a lobulated and globulated aspect, with distortion of its morphology [13].

Subserosal Myomas

The subserosal myomas grow towards the external surface of the uterus, and more than 50 % of the volume of the myoma must stick out of the serose surface. They can adopt a sessile or pedunculated configuration.

Diagnosis

From the point of view of the imaging diagnosis, the ultrasound is the method most frequently used, because of its availability as well as for its low cost and relatively good diagnostic accuracy. The assessment of the endometrium-myometrial interface permits the establishment of the differential diagnosis between intracavitary submucosal myomas and the endometrial polyps. This discrimination is possible in the ultrasound as well as in the magnetic resonance imaging (MRI), but cannot be precisely established in the conventional hysterosalpingography studies (HSG) or in the virtual hysterosalpingography (VHSG). The submucosal myomas with intramural extensions are harder to differentiate from the polyps with an echography, having the MRI or the hysteroscopy a larger diagnostic importance (Fig. 7.5). In the echography or hysteroscopy, the grade of the intramural extension is determined taking into account the angle formed by the myoma and the endometrium (Fig. 7.6). Also, on occasions, the echography can clearly discriminate a tumor in the width of the healthy myometrium and determine its depth. The HSG does not provide this information. On the other hand, the VHSG allows the estimation of the intramural component of the submucosal myomas in relation to the angle that is formed with the wall of the endometrium, also of the density of the myomatose nucleus when this one is different to the rest of the myometrium that surrounds it (Fig. 7.7). The MRI is the most trustful and sensible method for the classification of the different types and grades of intramural extension, thanks to its great tissular discrimination that permits the clear identification of the endometrial-myometrial interface and of the signal changes of the leiomyomas, different to the signal of the normally organized myometrium (Fig. 7.8).

The echography evaluates the different layers of the uterus wall and its widths, as well as the endometrial-myometrial interface [14]. The characteristic finding in the myomas is the presence of a solid hipoechoic mass,

on occasions heterogeneous depending on the calcium content or type of associated degeneration (Fig. 7.9). When the number is great and the lesions voluminous, they distort the uterine silhouette. The sensitivity of the transvaginal ultrasound (TVU) for the diagnosis of the myomas is of 80–90 % specificity and a positive predictive value of 90 %. The sonohysterography that distends the endometrial cavity with physiological solution notably enhances the diagnostic capacity of the TVU (Fig. 7.10). It is one of the best methods to classify the submucosal myomas, and in this way decide the surgical approach for the treatment. These myomas are visualized as subendometrial masses, of low echogenicity and wide base, which displace the endometrium alterating the endometrial-myometrial interface. The grade of protrusion in the cavity is variable. When the line of the endometrium is distinguished on the surface of the mass, the submucose nature of the lesion is documented; nevertheless this finding is not always present (Fig. 7.11) [15].

The HSG possesses limitations for the diagnosis of uterine myomatosis. One of the most important is the incapacity to differentiate in between the different types of submucosal myomas, or with voluminous sessile polyps. In general, the myomas are normally bigger, unique and are visualized as filling defects of smooth edges, of diverse sizes and locations (Fig. 7.12).

The HSG has proven to be a better imaging evaluation for images of partial filling, with the particularity of persisting the defect in the images of maximum filling (Fig. 7.13). The intramural leiomyomas of great size distort the shape and size of the uterus; but this is difficult to appreciate if the uterine cavity is not involved. On occasions the liquid in the peritoneal cavity can delimit the uterine silhouette and indirectly demonstrate a globulose and greatened uterus [2, 4]. After different revisions, the method has shown specificity of 97 %, but with a very low sensitivity, of only 9 % [4].

The assessment and characterization of the myomas by VHSG is a great challenge. Although similitudes with the traditional radiological method exist, the capacity of the procedure is superior. With respect to the identification of submucosal myomas, their measuring is easier, and it is possible on occasions to determine the percentage of the intramural extension, allowing the discrimination between type I and type II myomas (Figs. 7.14 and 7.15). Nevertheless, because of not being able to identify the myo-endometrial line, it is not factible to distinguish between sessile and submucosal myomas with the same ease as in the ecographic study. The identification of the intramural myomas is not simple and many times impossible. Pure intramural myomas cannot be diagnosed unless they show changes in their density secondary to the intratumoral degeneration. The fibrosis or calcification phenomenon generates a higher density in the myoma, while the hyaline degeneration, grease or necrosis produce lower density. These modifications in density help to

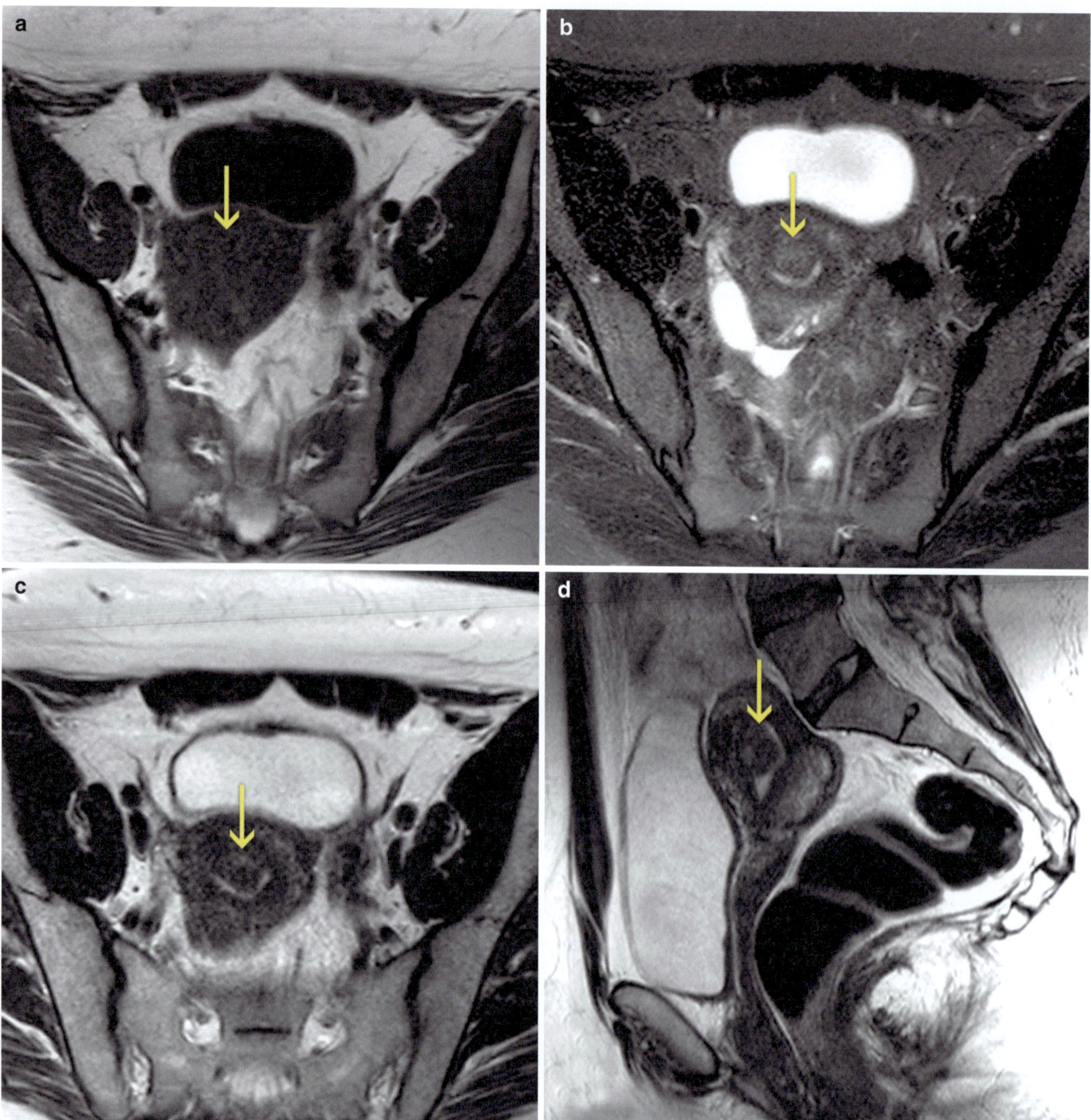

Fig. 7.5 MRI of the female pelvis which shows a submucous myoma (*arrows*). (**a**) Axial T1 weighted image. (**b**) Axial T2 weighted image with fat suppression. (**c**) Axial T2 weighted image. (**d**) Sagittal T2 weighted image

differentiate them from the rest of the normal myometrium (Fig. 7.16). When the intramural myoma deforms the external outline or acts like a subserosal myoma, the identification is simpler. The method allows the visualization of all the parietal width and adjacent regions to the uterus, which along with the use of the different imaging post-processing tools, in particular the multiplanar reformats with a width of 4–5 mm and a soft tissue window, offers an enhanced vision of the wall, of its changes in density and of the deformation

of the edges of the uterine silhouette (Figs. 7.17, 7.18 and 7.19). The sensitivity and specificity in the detection of submucosal myomas is of 91.7 and 100 %; for subserosal myomas: 81.8 and 97.4 %; and for the intramural ones: 65.4 and 92.6 % respectively [16].

The pelvic MR is the imaging modality of most specificity for the evaluation of the size, location, and number of the leiomyomas. Based on its great tissue discrimination, the MR allows to clearly distinguish the endometrial-myometral

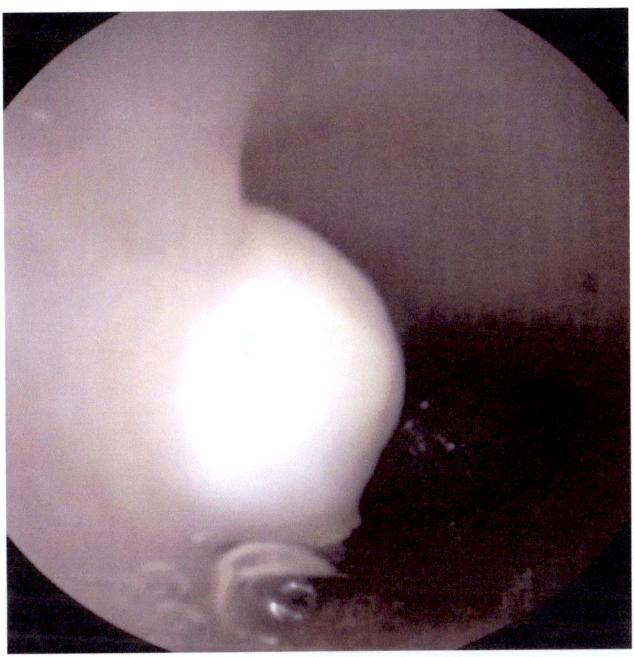

Fig. 7.6 Submucous myoma. Conventional CO_2 hysteroscopy

line, exactly locate the myoma and its relation with the endometrial cavity, and differentiate the submucosal myomas from endometrial polyps. In MR, the myomatose uterus generally appears increased in size, bigger and lobulated. The myomas are appreciated as focal masses, with hypointense signals with respect of the myometrium in the T2 weighted images (Figs. 7.20 and 7.21). The MR clearly differentiates a bigger uterus because of adenomyosis, which manifests itself as a badly defined area, hypointense with hyperintense areas in its interior, from one larger in size because of multiple myomas. Its utility in the valorization of the answer to the treatment in GnRH analogues has been postulated [17].

Adenomyosis

The adenomyosis is a benign pathologic process relatively frequent in the uterus, fundamentally in women between the ages of 30 and 50. It is characterized by the ectopic location of the glands and the endometrial stroma in the thick of the myometrium associated to the hypertrophy and hyperplasia of the uterine muscle [18–20]. In 60–80 % the cases can be linked to other pelvic pathologies, the most frequent are the leiomyomas. In young women, there exists a strong association with the pelvic endometriosis, present in 90 % of these patients [21].

The endometrial stroma is a layer of highly cellular connective tissue that contains multiple blood vessels, which show cyclic changes related to menstruation. The adenomyosis depends on the estrogen and, between the predisposed

factors the multiparity and a history of previous uterine surgeries are found (cesarean section, curettages, hysteroscopies). Macroscopically, an increase in the width of the uterine musculature and interstitial fibrosis associated to the presence of multiple endometrial or hemorrhagic nuclei are observed. These alterations determine the increase in volume and the uterine consistency.

The adenomyosis can compromise the uterus diffusely or focally (adenomyoma or adenoma of Cullen). The diffuse form, the most frequent, is characterized by a uterus increased in size and the identification of multiple small glandular crypts, of 2–8 mm, that infiltrate the myometrium. If it is focal, it presents itself as endometrial fibroglandular macronodules in the thick of the myometrium, badly delimited and without a capsule, which can orientate in the differential diagnosis with an intramural myoma.

Diagnosis

The clinical diagnosis of the adenomyosis is hard due to the fact that most of the signs and symptoms are similar to other benign uterine pathologies. In symptomatic patients, the most frequent is the secondary dysmenorrhea, with a progressive increase in intensity, while the menorrhea and pelvic pains are less constant. In other women it is associated to infertility, due to the alteration that the infiltration of the myometrium generates on the contractibility necessary for the transport of spermatozoids in their uterine trajectory [21].

The most precise noninvasive imaging modality for the diagnosis of adenomyosis is MR, being the modality by choice for the cases of hard resolution. Its sensitivity oscillates between 78 and 88 %, with a specificity of 67–93 %. The characteristic sign is an increase in the width of the Z line or an endometrial-myometrial union zone larger than 12 mm, along with a hypointense area of ill-defined edges (Fig. 7.22) [22, 23]. A union zone below the 8 mm in general excludes an adenomyosis diagnosis with a negative predictive value of 99 %, while when the thickness of the endometrial-myometrial union is between 8 and 12 mm the diagnosis is not excluding and must complement itself with other studies. Another frequent finding in MR exams is the presence of hyperintense nodular nuclei in T1 and T2 weighted images located in the thick of the myometrium (Fig. 7.23) [23]. In daily clinical practice, the transvaginal echography is the initial imaging method that is used upon a clinical suspicion, or better yet it is the method that suggests its diagnosis in a woman studied with suspicion of another pathology. The ultrasound is a method of ample availability, easy access, simple, relatively cheap and with good diagnostic credit. The sensitivity of the method varies between 53 and 89 %, with a specificity between 67 and 98 % [23].

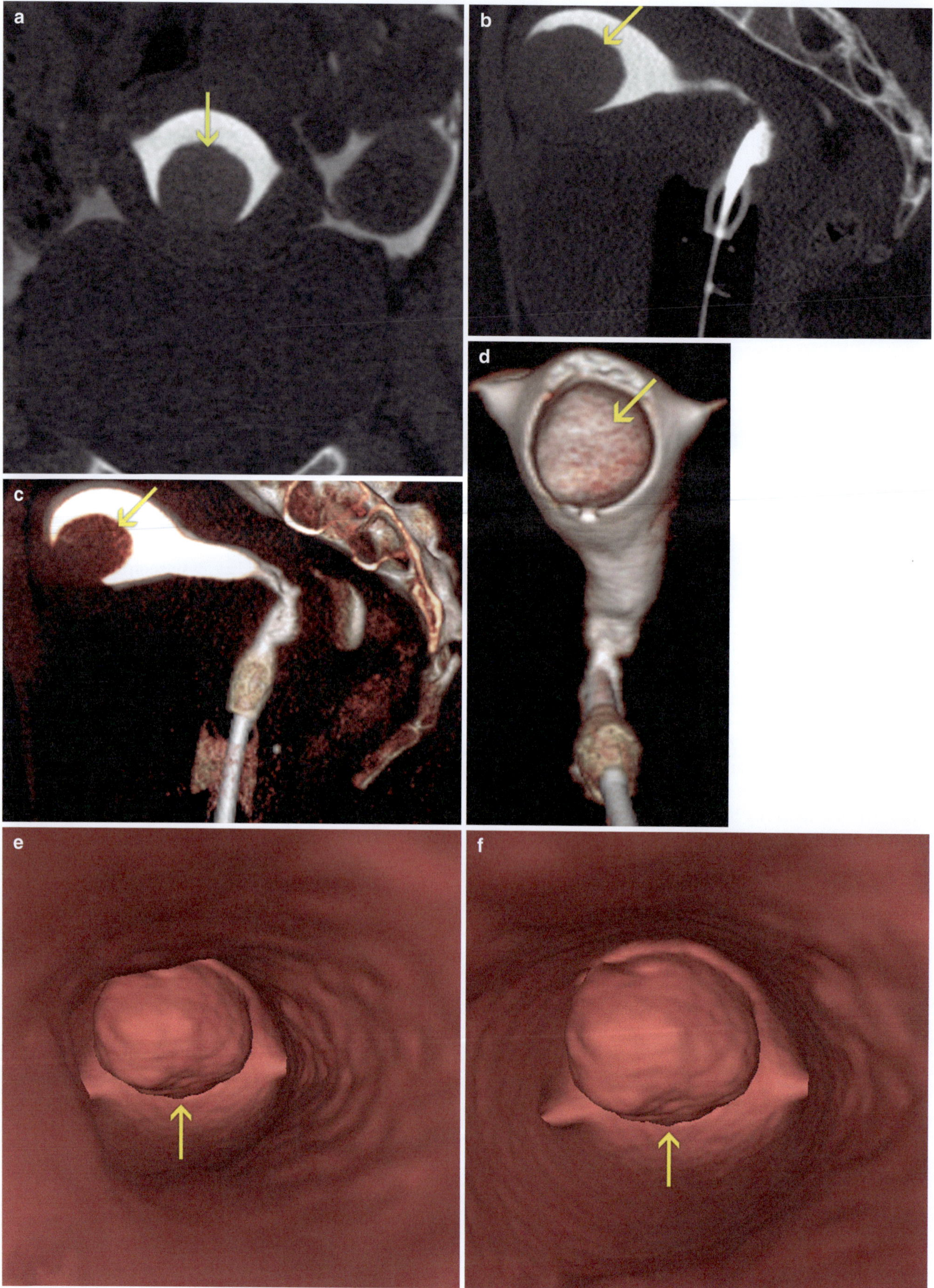

Fig. 7.7 Submucous myoma at the level of the anterior wall of the uterus (*arrows*). VHSG exam. (**a**) Coronal maximum intensity projection (MIP) image. (**b**) Sagittal MIP image. (**c**) Sagittal 3D volume rendering image. (**d**) Coronal 3D volume rendering image, anterior view. (**e**, **f**) Virtual endoscopy images

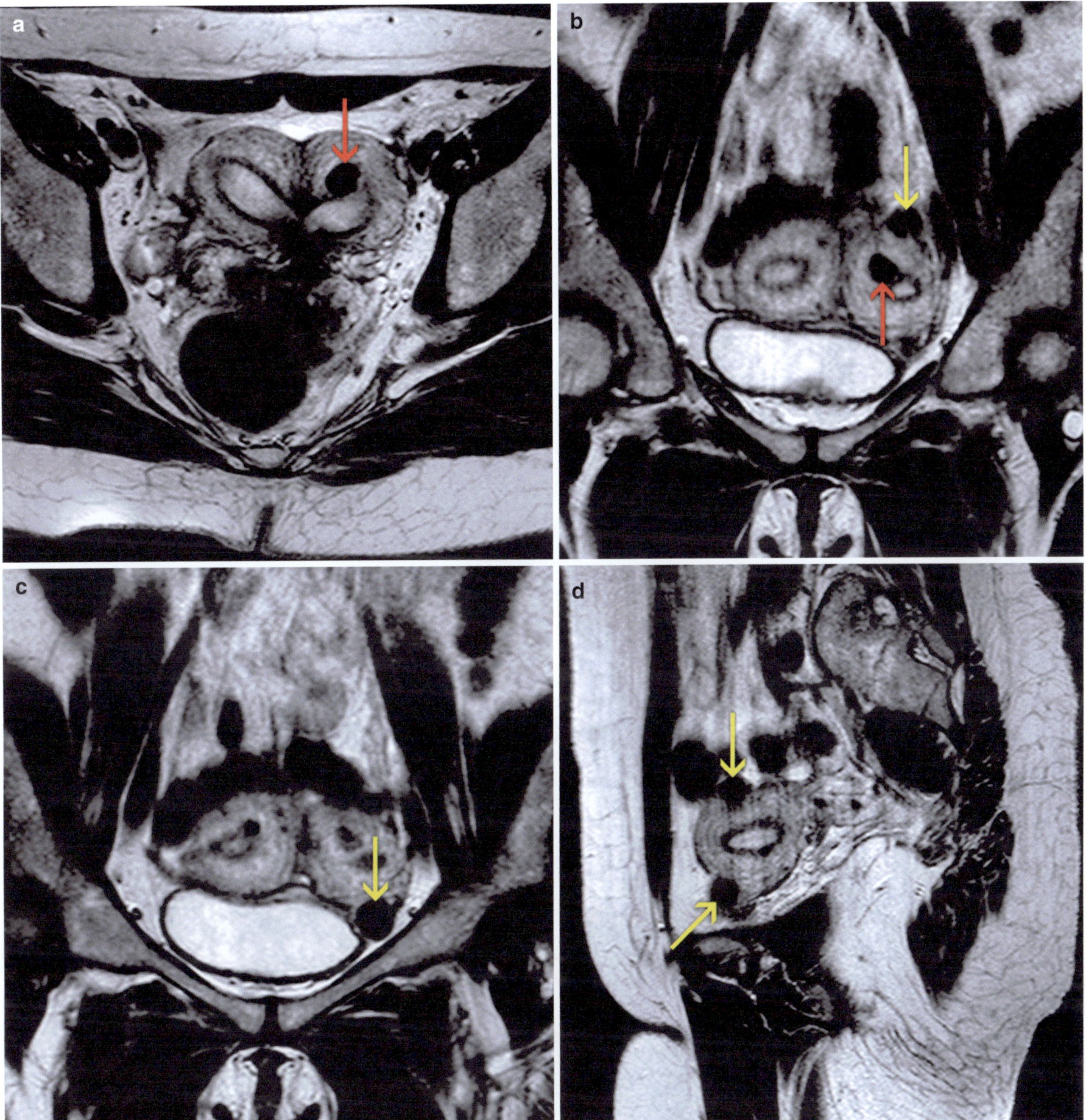

Fig. 7.8 MRI of the female pelvis. Bicornuate uterus, with presence of small subserous (*yellow arrows*) and intramural (*red arrows*) myomas. (**a**) Axial T2 weighted image. (**b**, **c**) Coronal T2 weighted images. (**d**) Sagittal T2 weighted image

The most common finding is an increase in the size of the uterus, of a globulous aspect. A marked asymmetric increase in the width of the myometrium is observed, which shows a diminished and heterogeneous echogenicity (Fig. 7.24). Myometrial cysts, hypoechoic nodules or lineal striations located in the subendometrium, and the loss of the endometrial-myometrial interface can be identified [24–26].

In the HSG, a diagnosis is only possible when the remains of the endometrial stroma located in the interior of the uterine muscle have a communication with the uterine cavity. In these cases lineal and saccular projections that are dyed with the injected contrast and project through the myometrium width, beyond the normal outline of the endometrial cavity can be identified. Another finding is a uterine silhouette increased in size, as well as a bigger and deformed uterine cavity (Fig. 7.25) [18, 19].

The manifestations of the adenomyosis in VHSG are characterized by a combination of findings previously

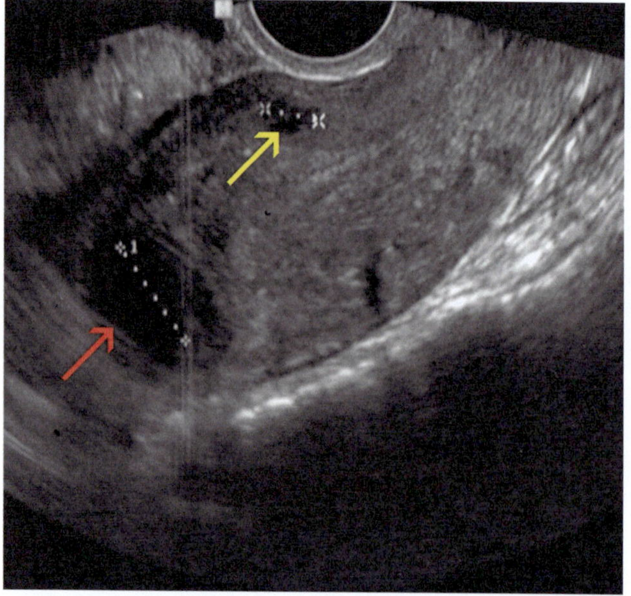

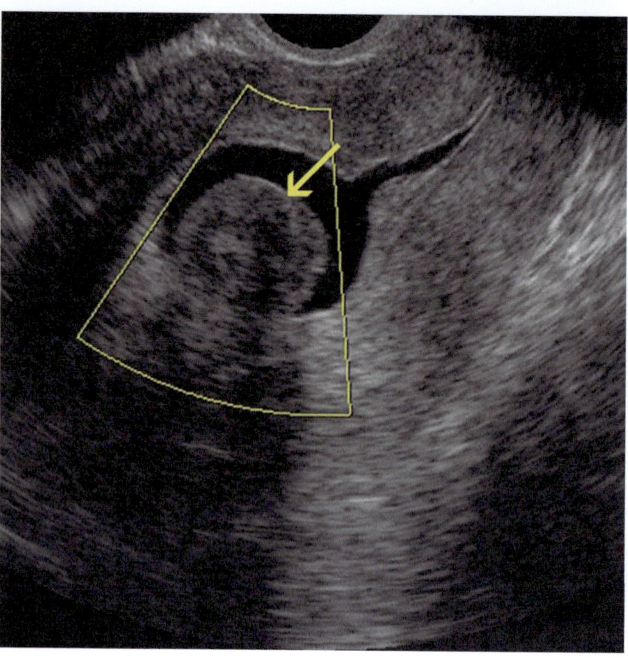

Fig. 7.9 Sagittal transvaginal ultrasound image where a small intra-mural anterior myoma (*yellow arrow*) and an intramural myoma that makes contact with the serosa at the level of the uterine fundus (*red arrow*) can be appreciated

Fig. 7.10 Sagittal sonohysterography image where an intracavitary extension of a submucosal myoma can be appreciated (*arrow*)

Fig. 7.11 Transvaginal ultrasound showing a submucosal myoma (*yellow arrows*). Note the displacement of the endome-trium-myometrial interface (*red arrow*). (**a**) Coronal image. (**b**) Sagittal image

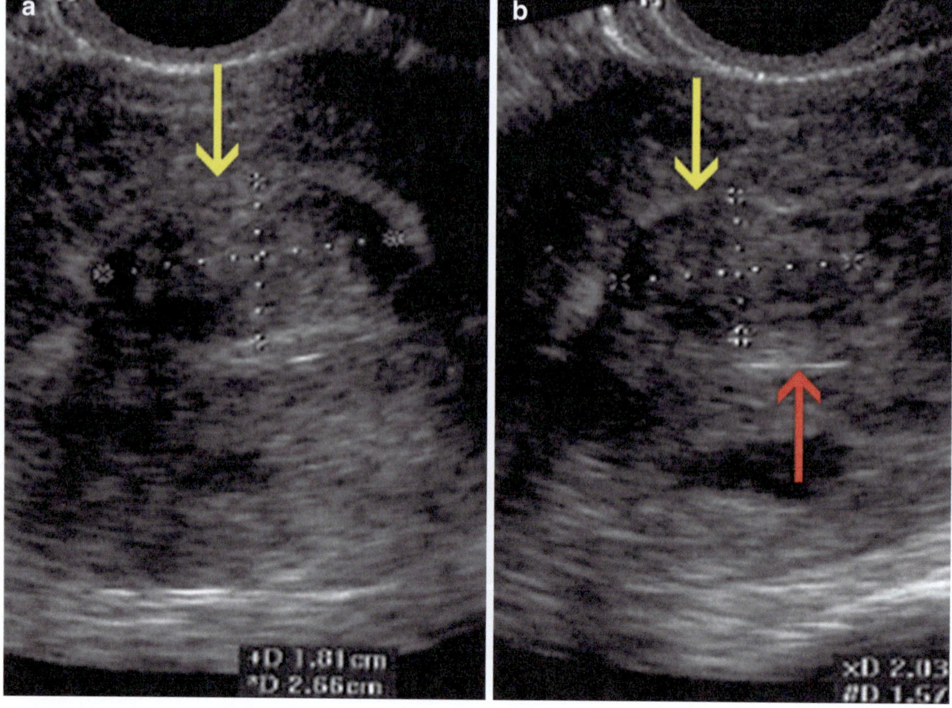

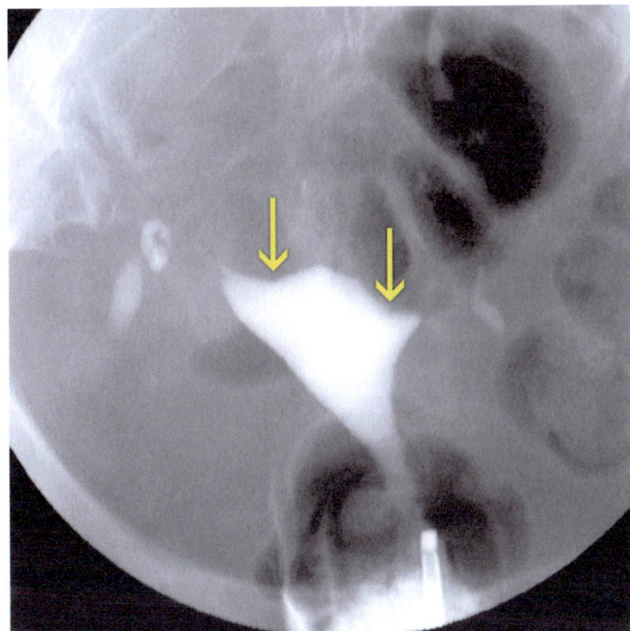

Fig. 7.12 HSG that shows two submucous myomas at the level of the uterine fundus (*arrows*)

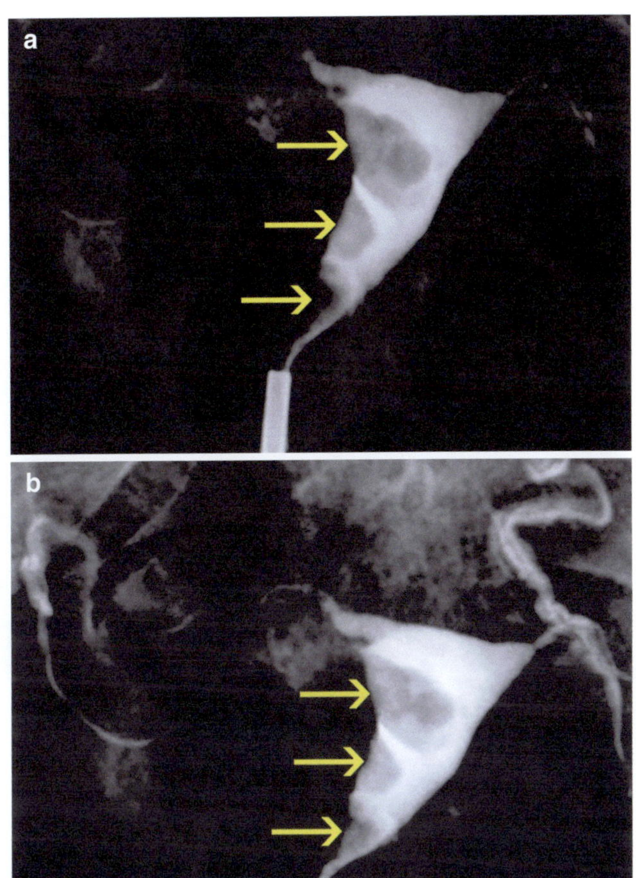

Fig. 7.13 HSG with progressive filling. (**a**, **b**) Endocavitary filling defects can be appreciated in both x-ray spots on the right uterine margin secondary to the presence of submucous myomas (*arrows*)

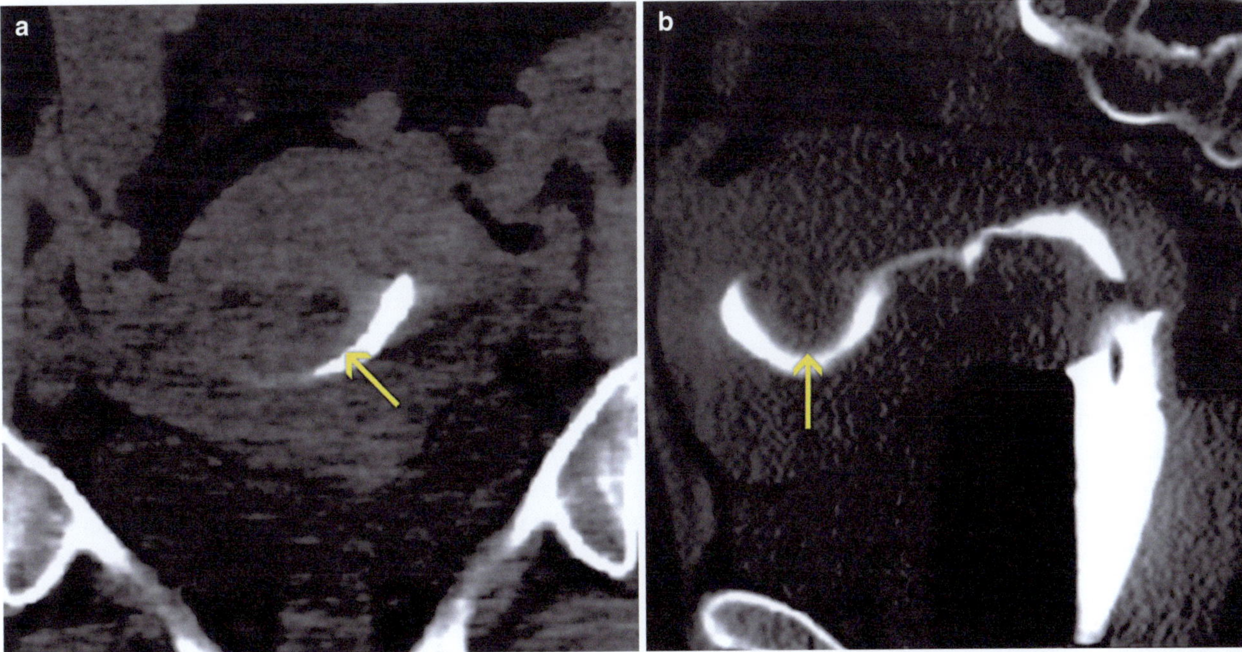

Fig. 7.14 Type II submucous myoma (*arrows*). VHSG study. (**a**) Coronal maximum intensity projection (MIP) image. (**b**) Sagittal MIP image. (**c**) Coronal 3D volume rendering image, anterior view. (**d**) Coronal 3D volume rendering image, left oblique anterior view. (**e**) Virtual endoscopy image. (**f**) Transvaginal ultrasound image, coronal view

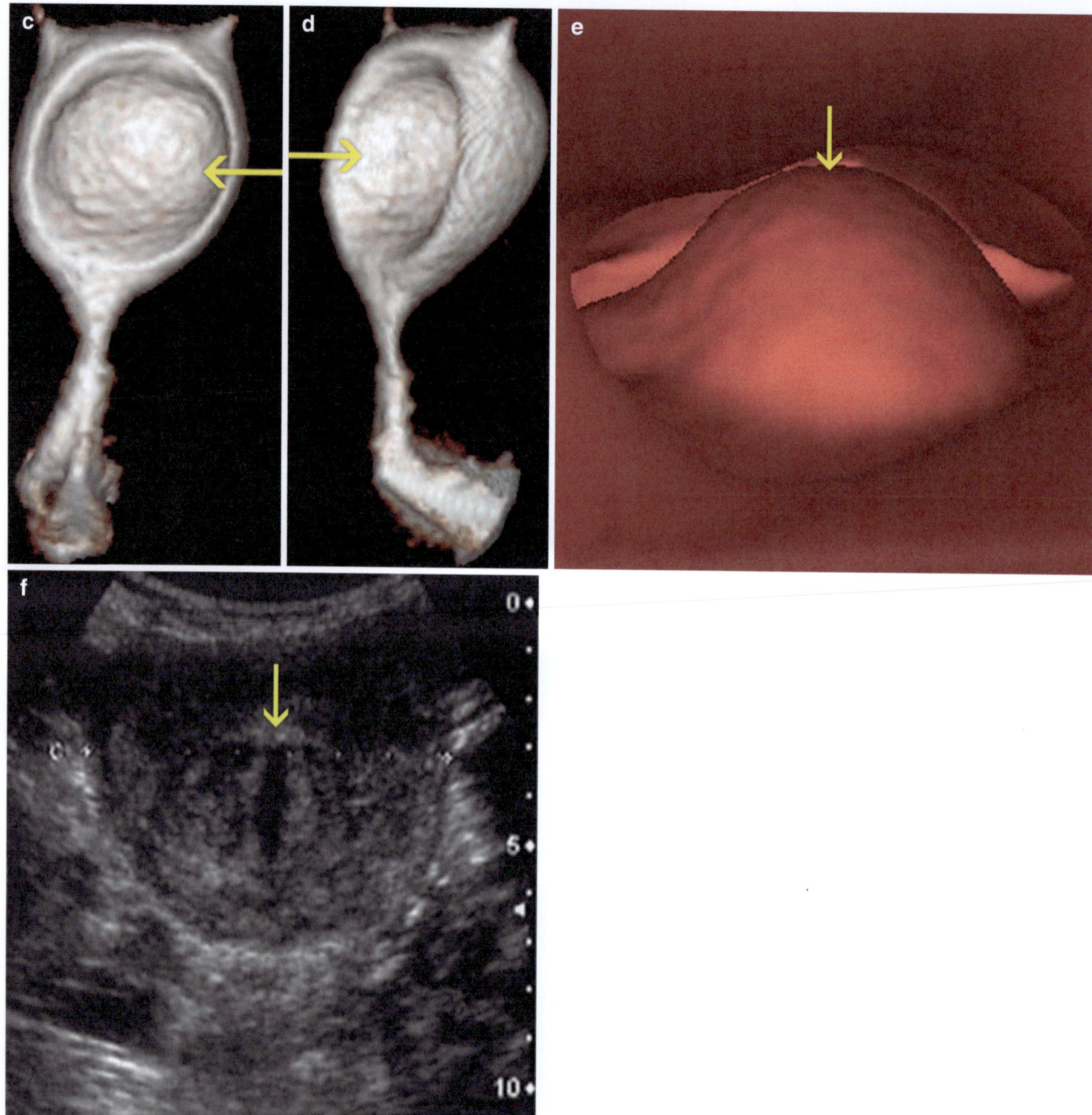

Fig. 7.14 (continued)

mentioned for other imaging methods. Similar to what occurs in the HSG studies, the findings in VHSG will depend on if the ectopic endometrial tissue in the uterine muscle is found with a connection to the endometrial cavity or not. When a communication exists, the most representative finding of the adenomyosis is the identification of lineal and saccular images of pseudodiverticular aspect, that opacificate with the instilled contrast and project into the myometrium, beyond the normal outline of the endometrial cavity (Figs. 7.26, 7.27 and 7.28) [18, 27]. A uterine cavity increased in size and/or deformed can also be identified. When visualizing the wall, the VHSG can show asymmetric and heterogeneous thickening of the myometrium, with ill-defined limits with the normal myometrium (Figs. 7.29 and 7.30) [28]. The method does not allow the visualization of the endometrial-myometrial interface.

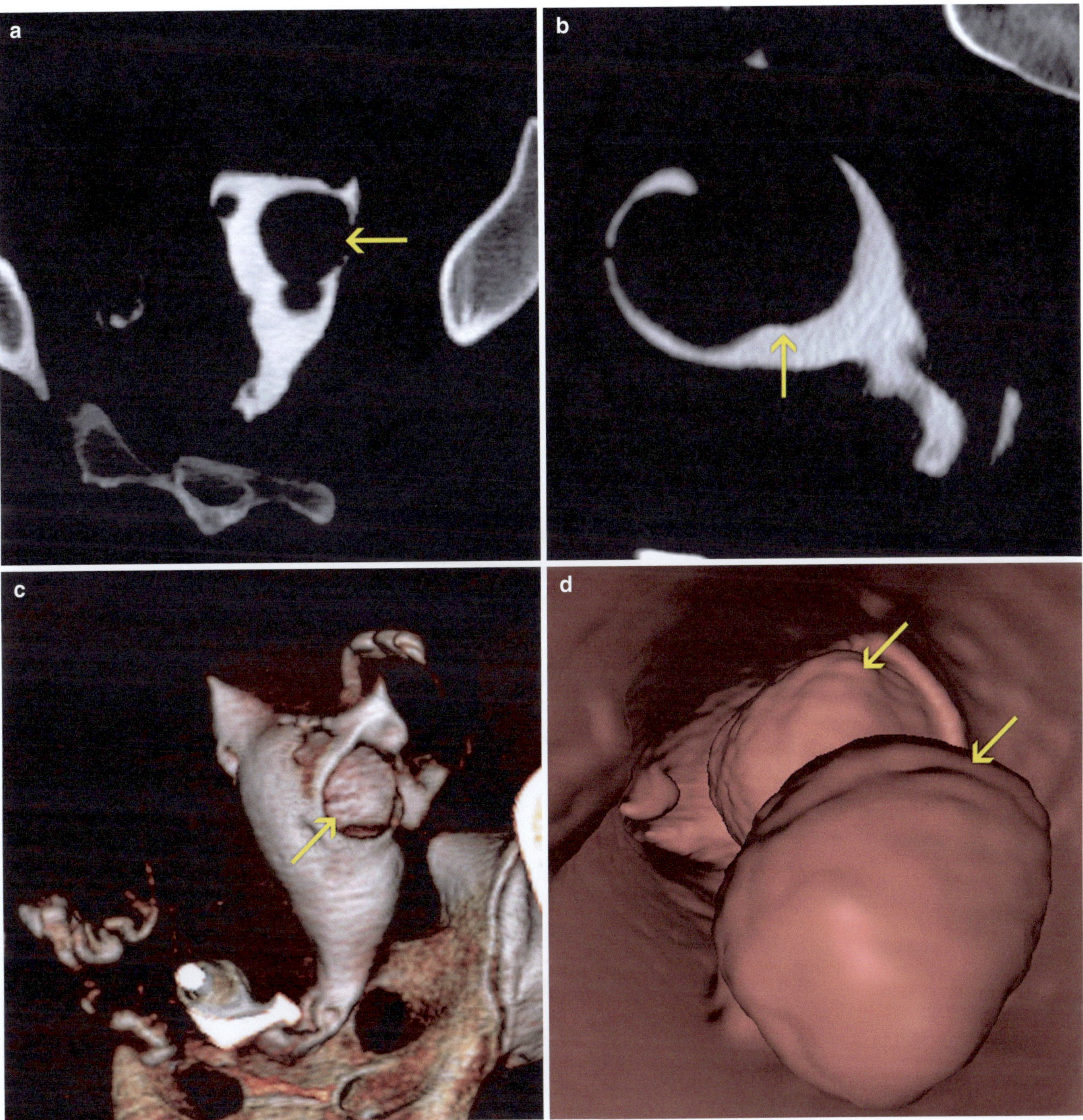

Fig. 7.15 Type III submucous myomas (*arrows*). VHSG study. (**a**) Axial maximum intensity projection (MIP) image. (**b**) Sagittal MIP image. (**c**) Coronal 3D volume rendering image, left oblique posterior view. (**d**) Virtual endoscopy image. (**e**) Conventional CO_2 hysteroscopy image

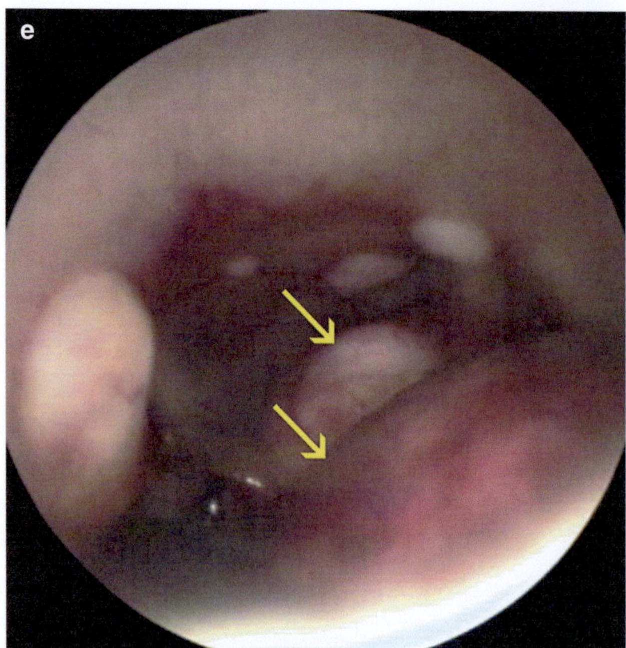

Fig. 7.15 (continued)

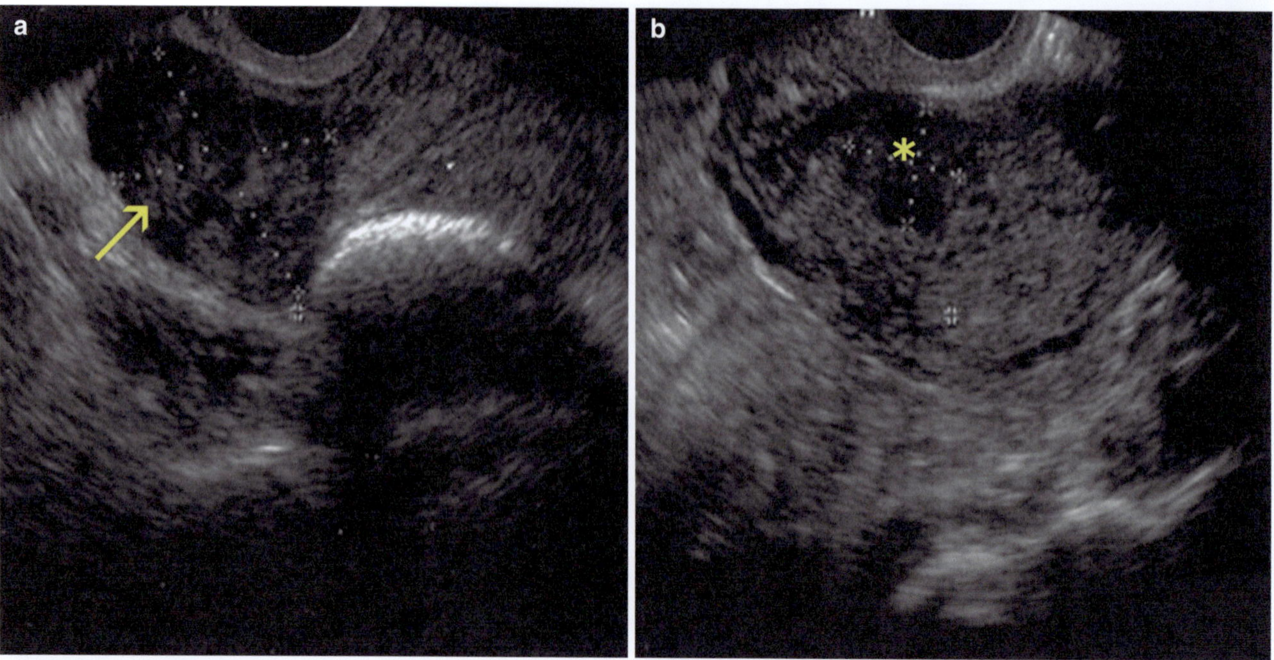

Fig. 7.16 Uterine myomas. A subserous myoma (*yellow arrows*), a calcified intramural myoma (*red arrows*) and an intramural myoma (*asterisk*) only visible in an ultrasound exam can be appreciated. (**a**) Sagittal transvaginal ultrasound image. (**b**) Coronal transvaginal ultrasound image. (**c**) Coronal maximum intensity projection (MIP) image. (**d**) Sagittal MIP image. (**e**) Axial 3D volume rendering images, superior view. (**f**) Virtual endoscopy image. Due to the location of the myomas, the uterine cavity does not present alterations

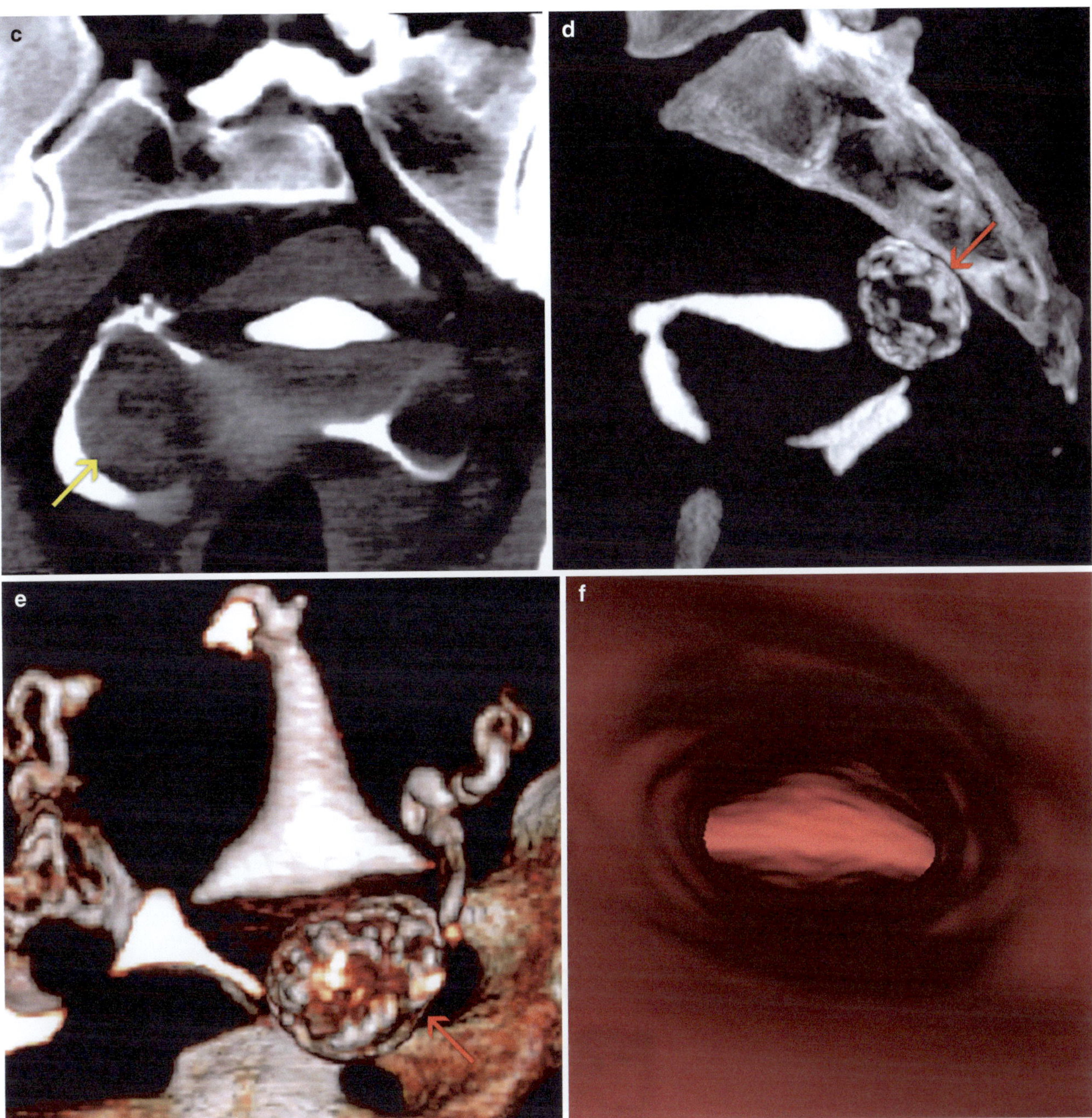

Fig. 7.16 (continued)

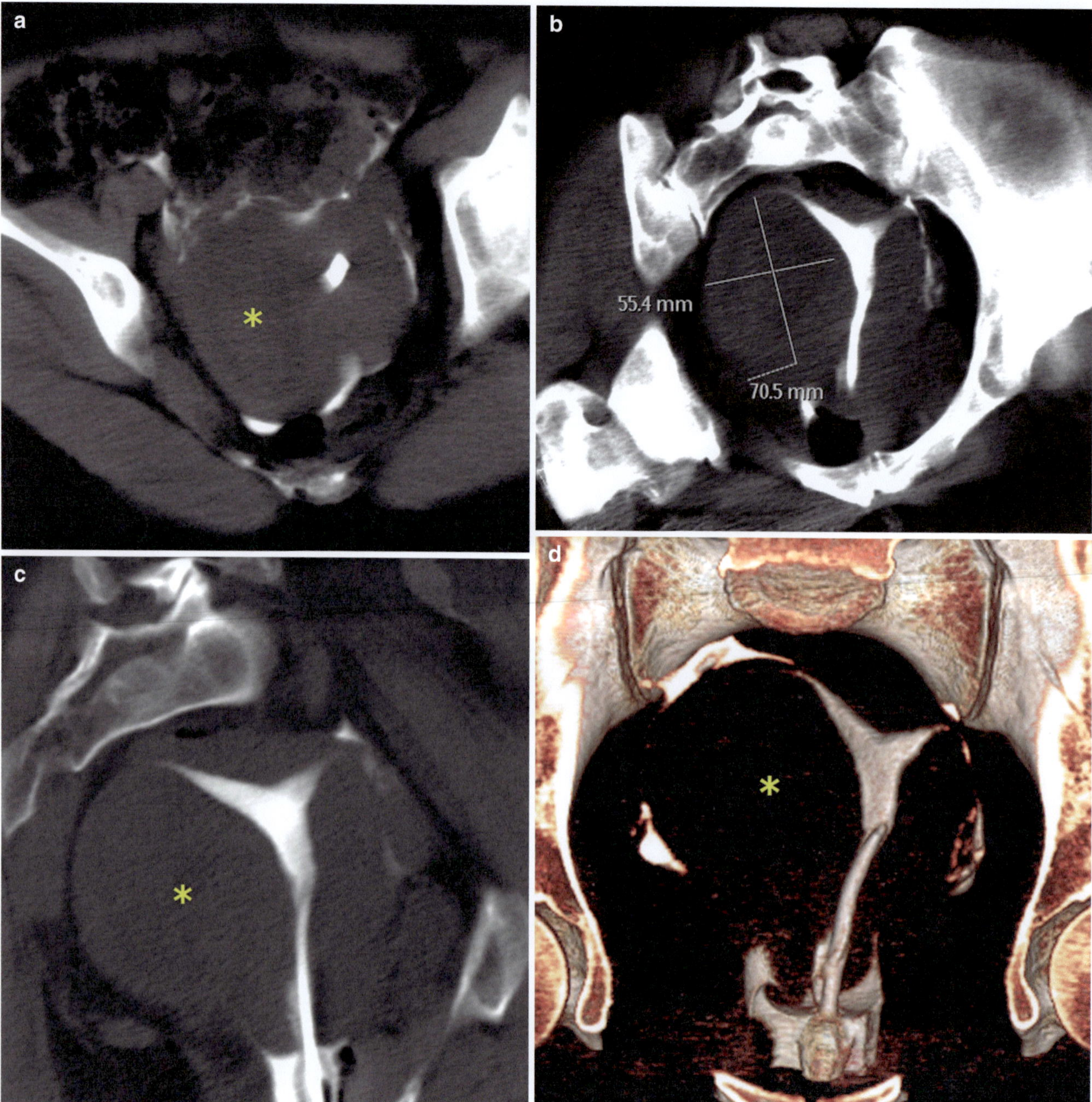

Fig. 7.17 Intramural myoma on the right uterine wall, which increases the size of the uterine silhouette and deforms its contour (*asterisk*). VHSG study. (**a**) Axial multiplanar reconstruction (MPR) image with soft tissue window. (**b**) Coronal MPR image with soft tissue window. (**c**) Coronal maximum intensity projection image. (**d**) Coronal 3D volume rendering image, superior view. The left displacement of the uterine cavity can be appreciated. (**e**, **f**) Virtual endoscopy images. Due to the location of the myomas, the uterine cavity presents no alterations

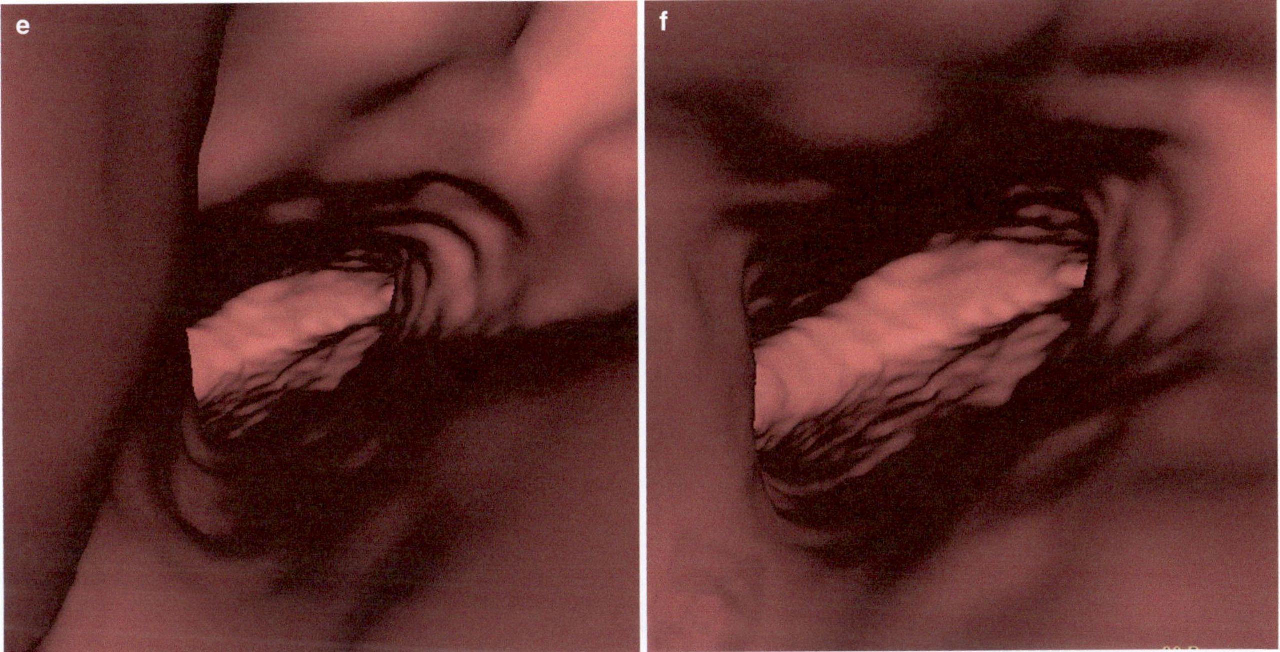

Fig. 7.17 (continued)

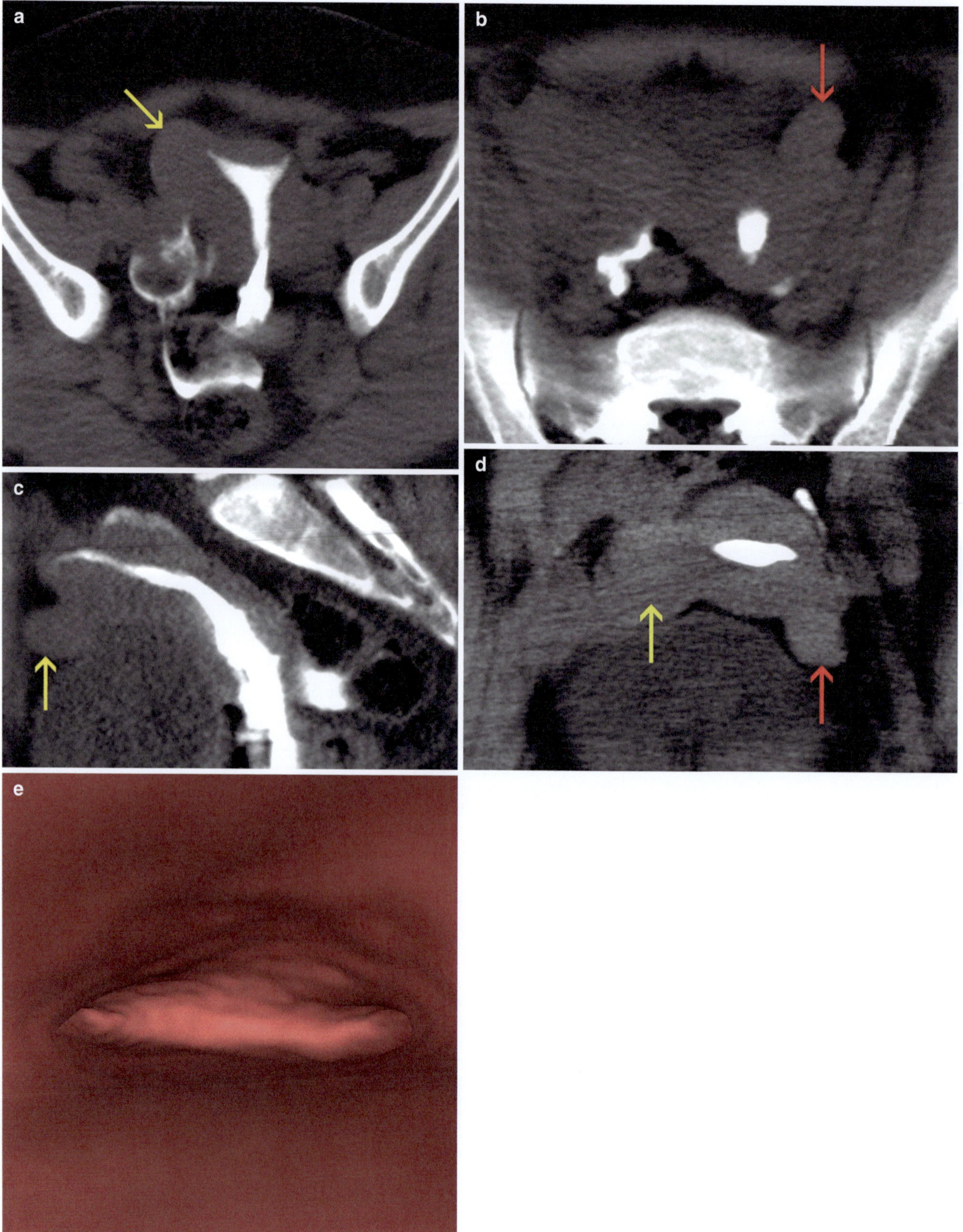

Fig. 7.18 Subserous myoma. A sessile subserous myoma can be appreciated on the right uterine margin (*yellow arrows*), and another pedunculated subserous myoma on the left margin (*red arrows*). VHSG study. (**a**, **b**) Axial multiplanar reconstruction (MPR) images with soft tissue window. (**c**) Sagittal MPR image, with soft tissue window. (**d**) Coronal MPR image, with soft tissue window. (**e**) Virtual endoscopy image. Due to the location of the myomas, the uterine cavity presents no alterations

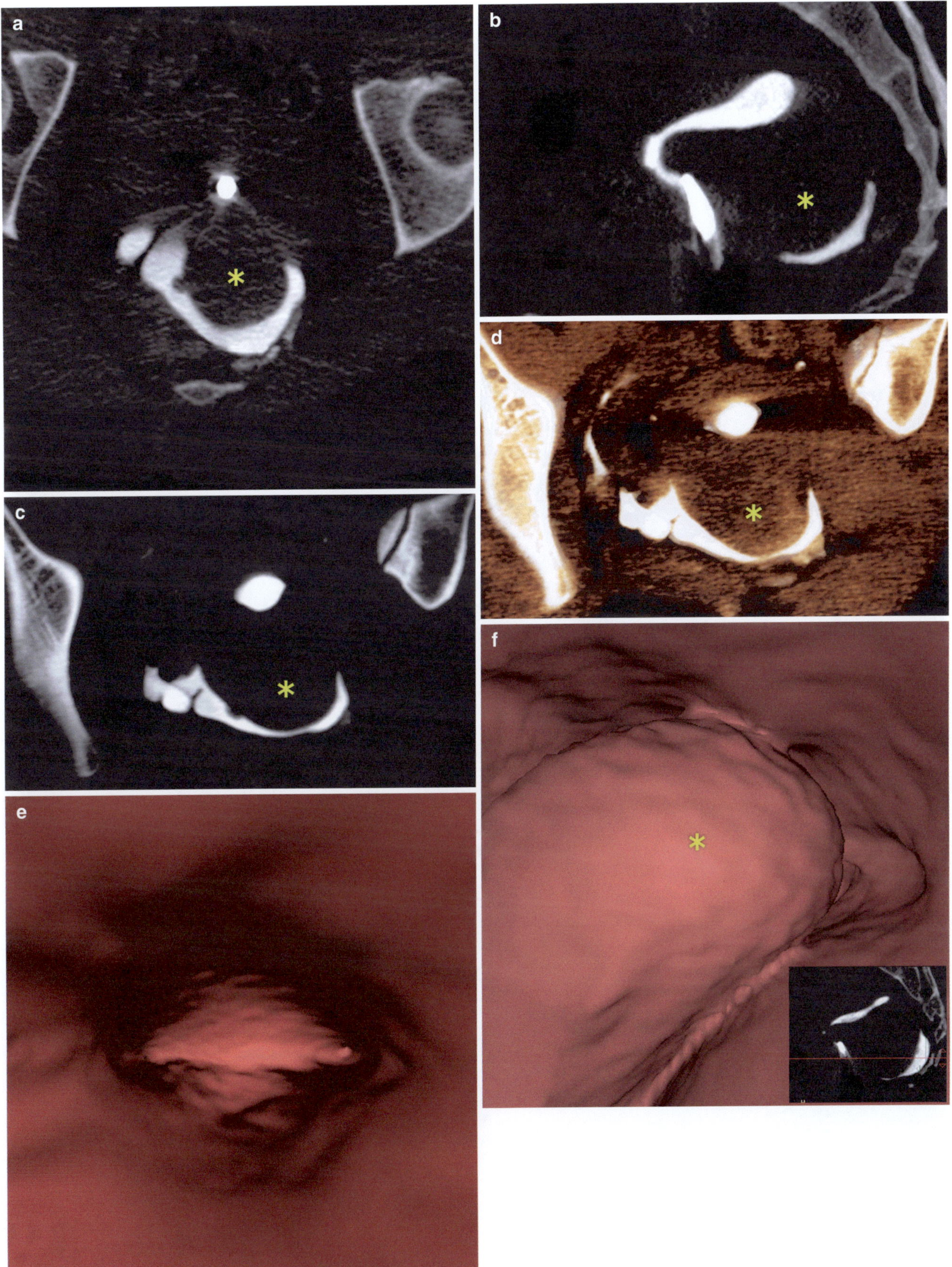

Fig. 7.19 Increase in the size of the uterus secondary to the presence of a posterior subserous myoma (*asterisk*). VHSG study. (**a**) Axial multiplanar reconstruction (MPR) image. (**b**) Sagittal MPR image. (**c**) Coronal MPR image. (**d**) Coronal 3D volume rendering image. (**e**) Virtual endoscopy image. Due to the location of the myoma, the uterine cavity presents no alterations. (**f**) Virtual endoscopy image of the peritoneal cavity showing the subserous myoma

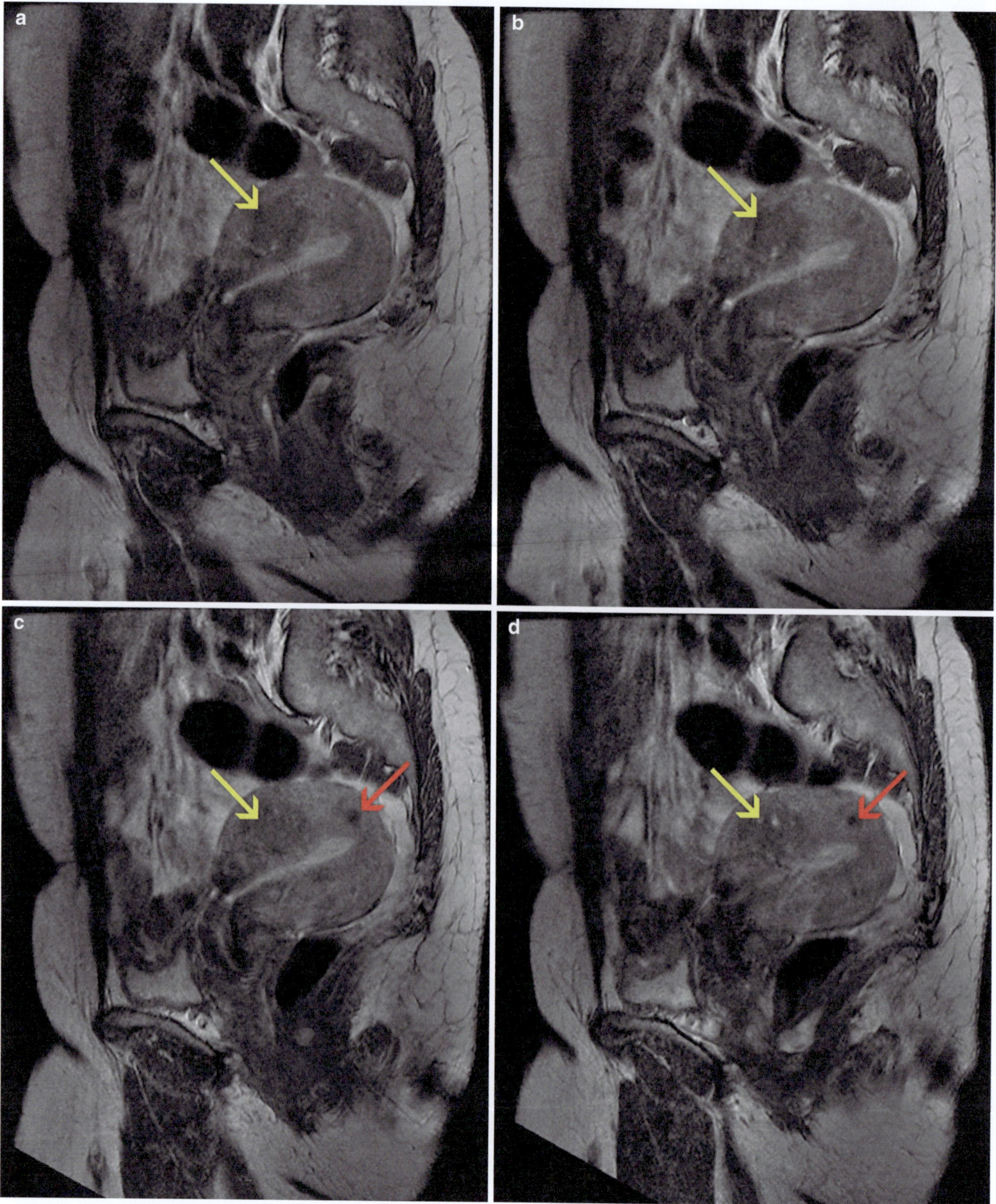

Fig. 7.20 MRI of the female pelvis which shows intramural myomas at the level of the anterior wall of the miometrium. The larger one (*yellow arrows*) appears on the Z line, while the smaller one is purely intra-mural (*red arrows*). (**a–d**) Sagittal weighted MR images. (**e, f**) Nonenhanced coronal T1 weighted MR images with fat suppression

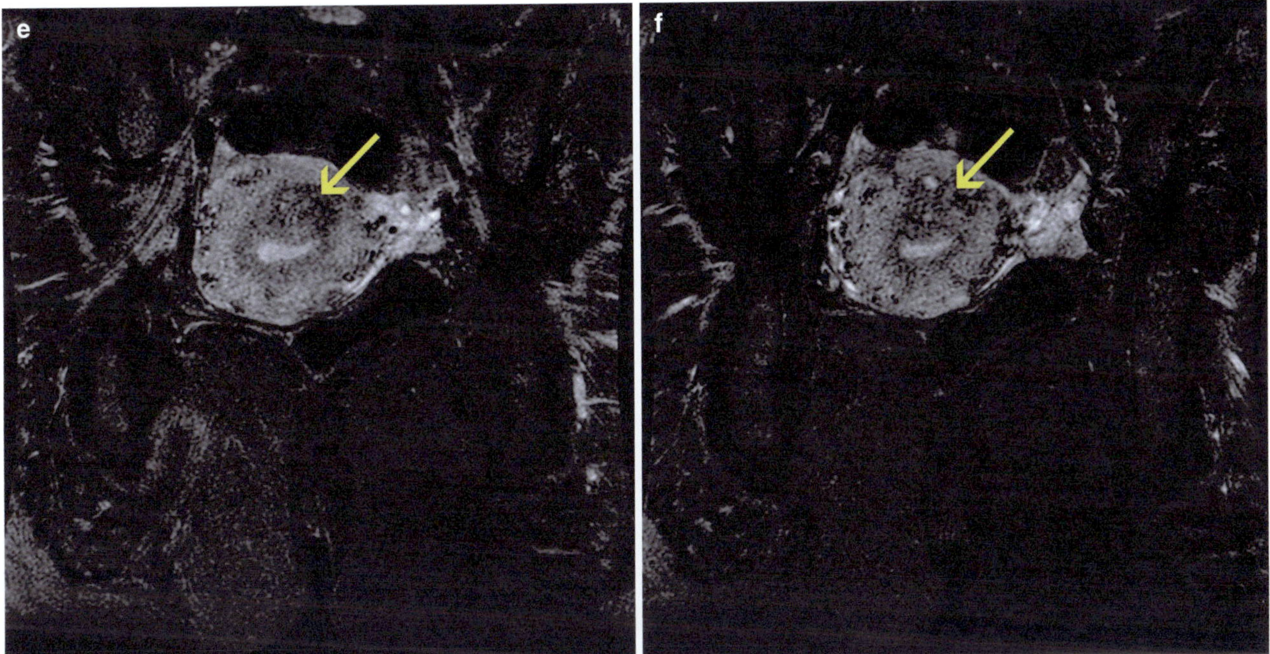

Fig. 7.20 (continued)

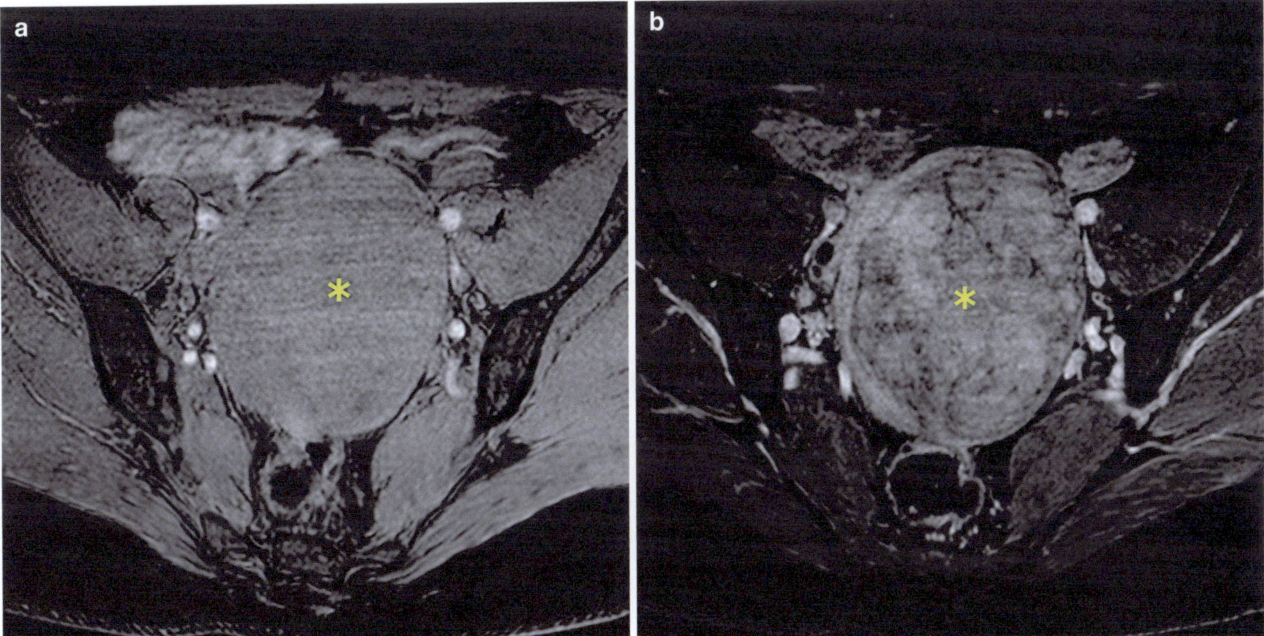

Fig. 7.21 MRI of the female pelvis which shows a subserous myoma on the left uterine wall, which increases in size and deforms the uterine silhouette (*asterisk*). A well delimited outline is appreciated, with heterogeneous signal and enhancement. (**a**) Nonenhanced axial T1 weighted MR image with fat suppression. (**b**) Enhanced axial T1 weighted MR image with fat suppression. (**c**) Enhanced coronal T1 weighted MR image. (**d–f**) Coronal T2 weighted MR images

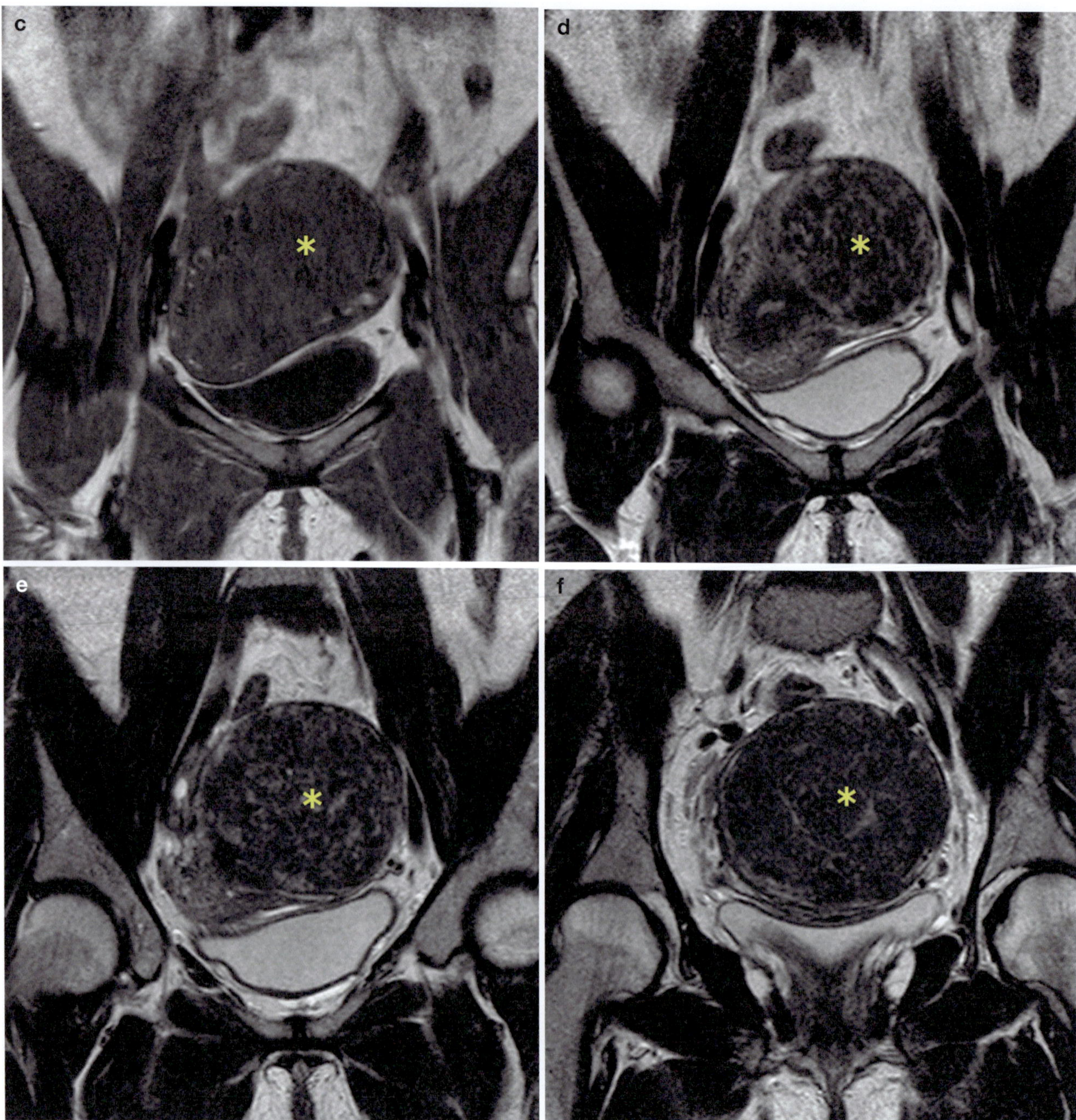

Fig. 7.21 (continued)

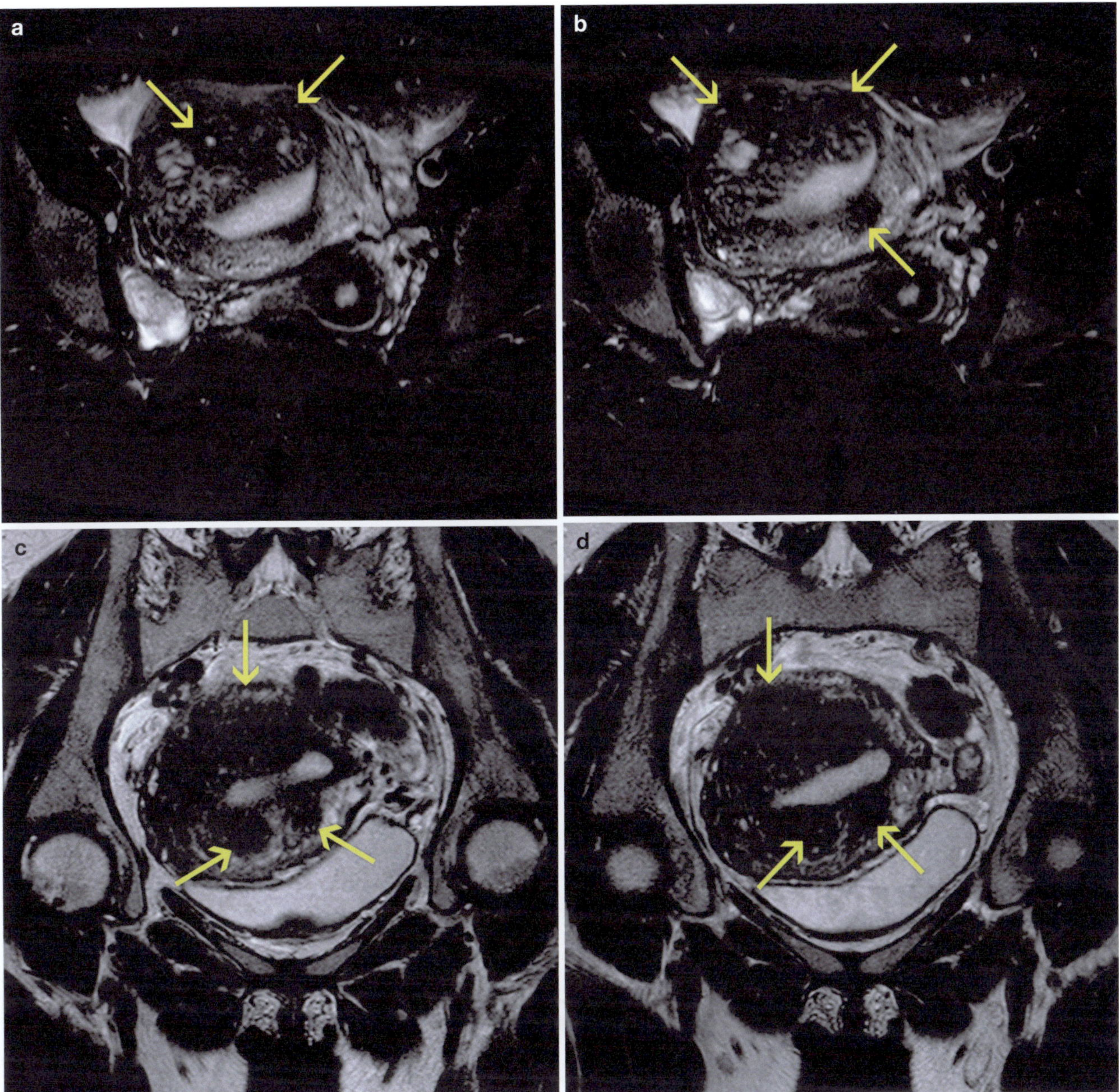

Fig. 7.22 MRI of the female pelvis which shows multiple myomas (*arrows*). Marked asymmetric abnormal thickening of the myometrium. A Z line >12 mm can be appreciated. (**a**, **b**) Axial STIR weighted MR images. (**c**, **d**) Coronal T2 weighted MR images. (**e**, **f**) Sagittal T2 weighted MR images

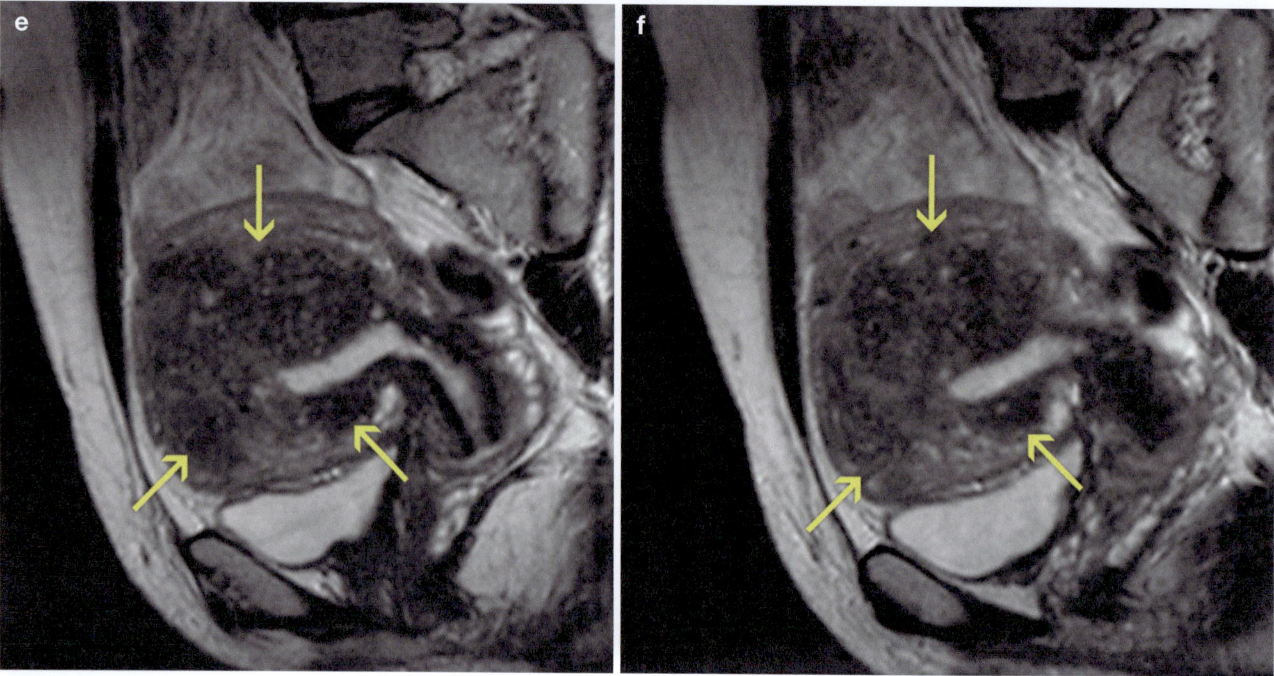

Fig. 7.22 (continued)

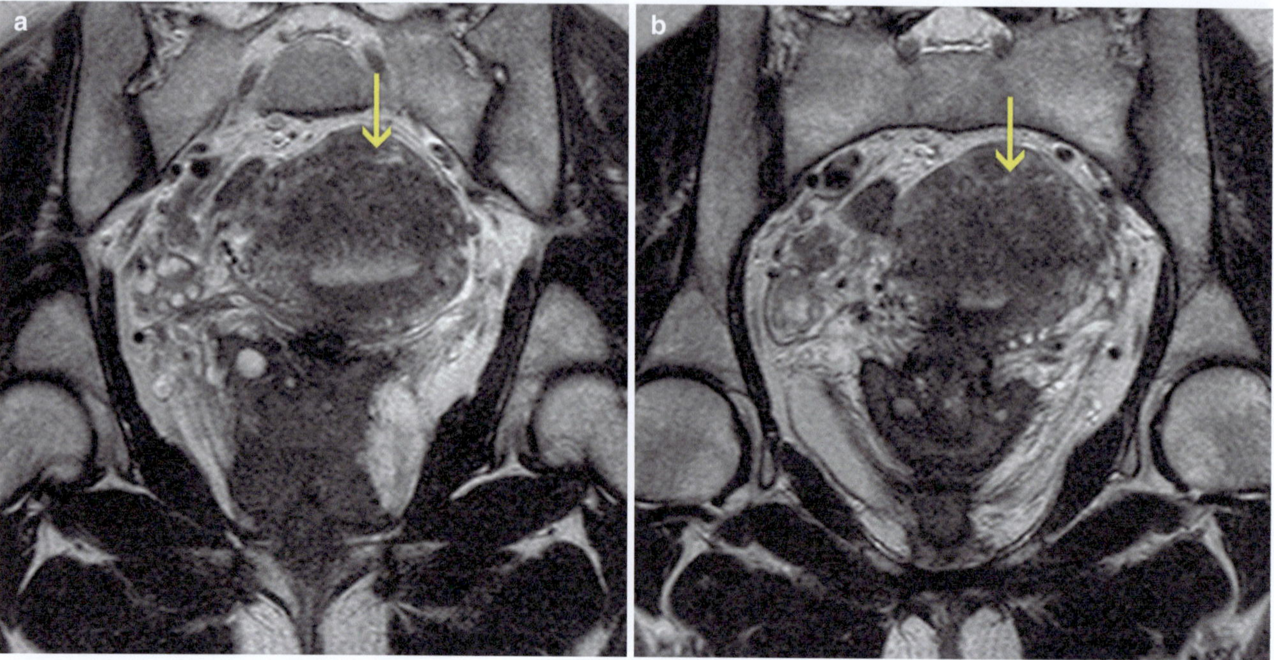

Fig. 7.23 MRI of the female pelvis in a patient with uterine myomas. Marked asymmetric abnormal thickening of the anterior myometrial wall. A Z line >12 mm can be appreciated (*arrows*). (**a**, **b**) Coronal T2 weighted MR images. (**c–f**) Sagittal T2 weighted MR images

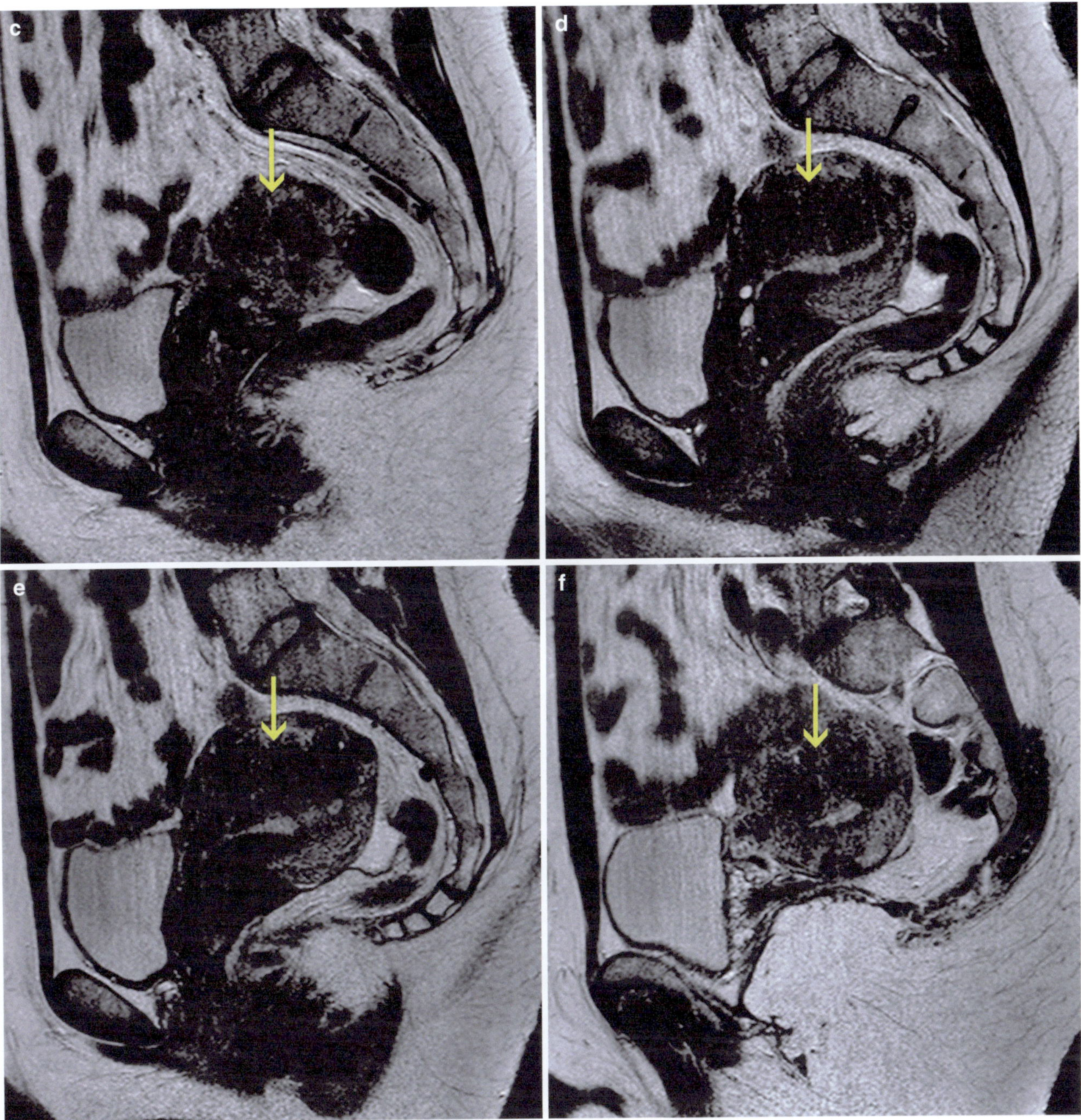

Fig. 7.23 (continued)

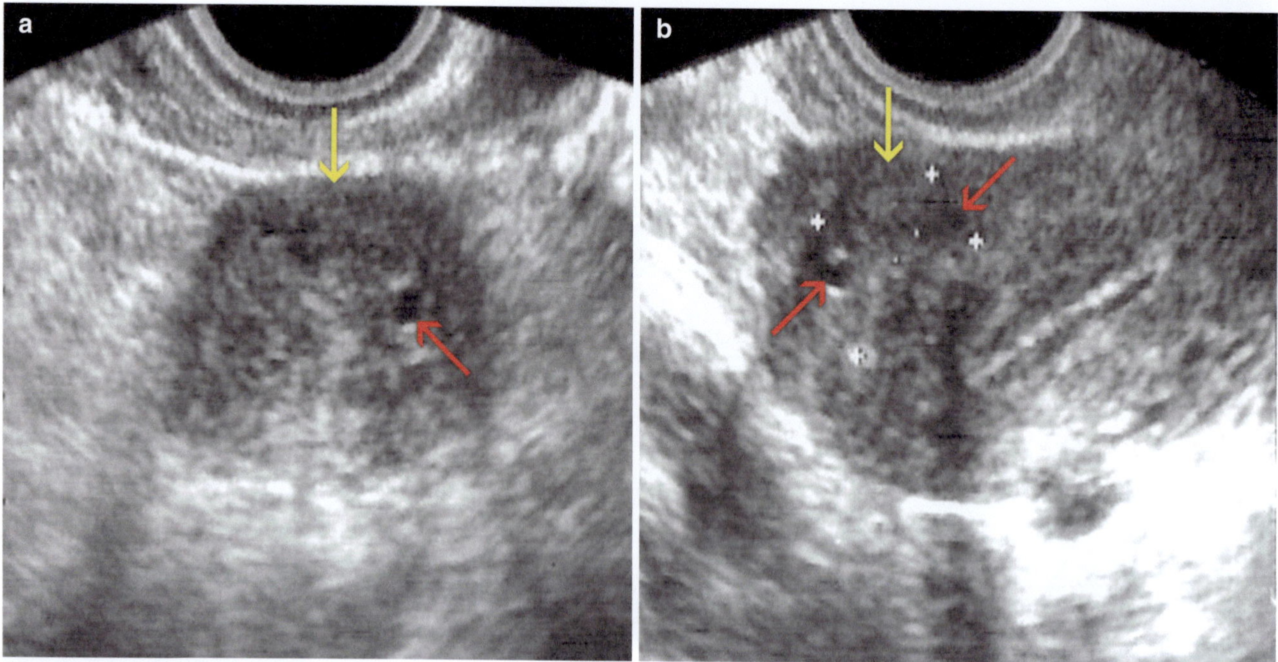

Fig. 7.24 Focal adenomyosis on transvaginal ultrasound images. A focal and asymmetric increase in the myometrial thickness at the uterine fundus (*yellow arrows*), which shows heterogeneous echo-genicity and small myometrial cysts (*red arrows*) can be appreciated. (**a**) Sagittal image. (**b**) Coronal image

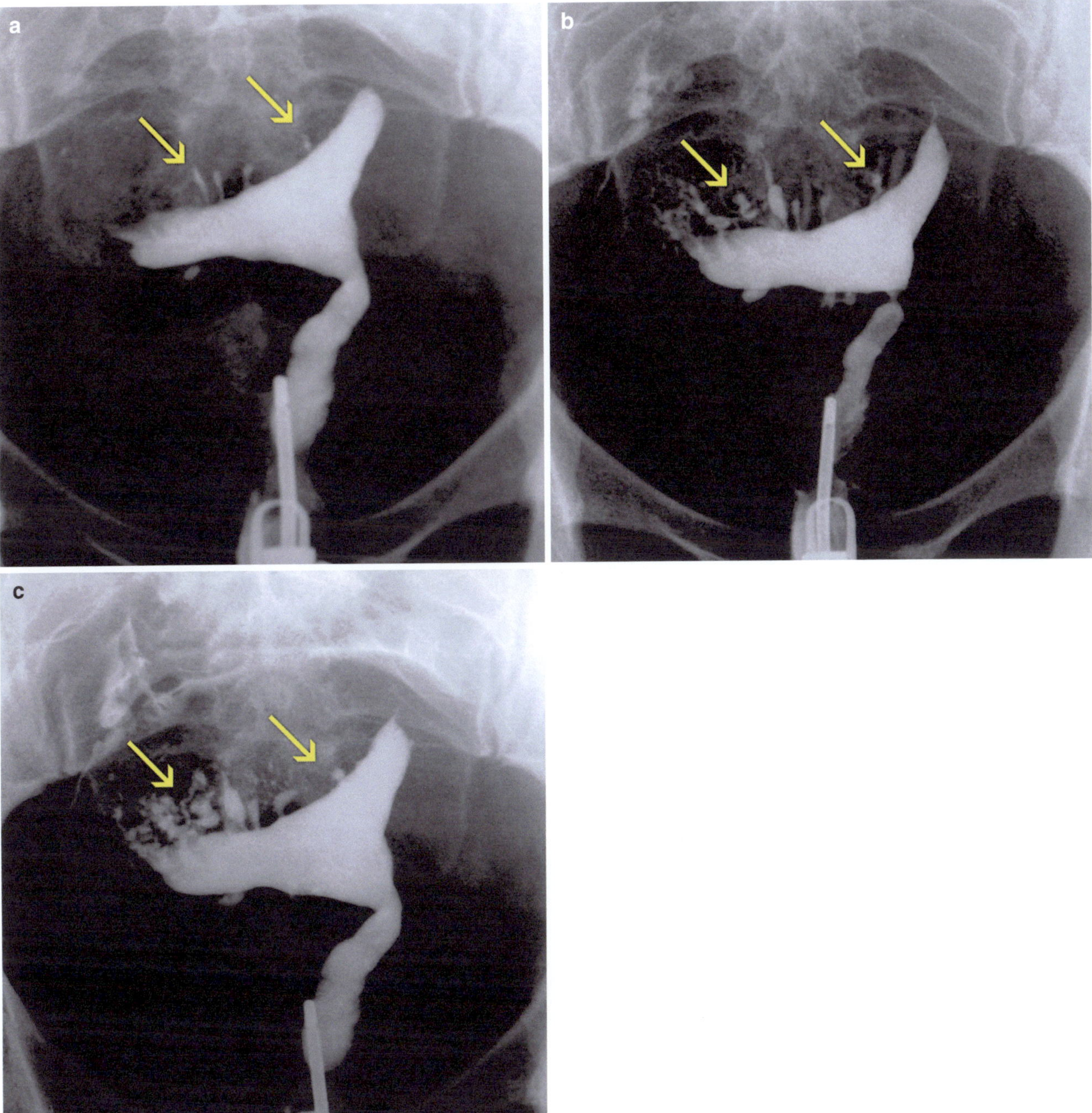

Fig. 7.25 Typical adenomyosis findings seen on HSG exam. (**a–c**) In the successive X-ray spots, multiple lineal and saccular projections into the myometrium beyond the normal outline of the endometrial cavity are appreciated with the injected contrast material (*arrows*)

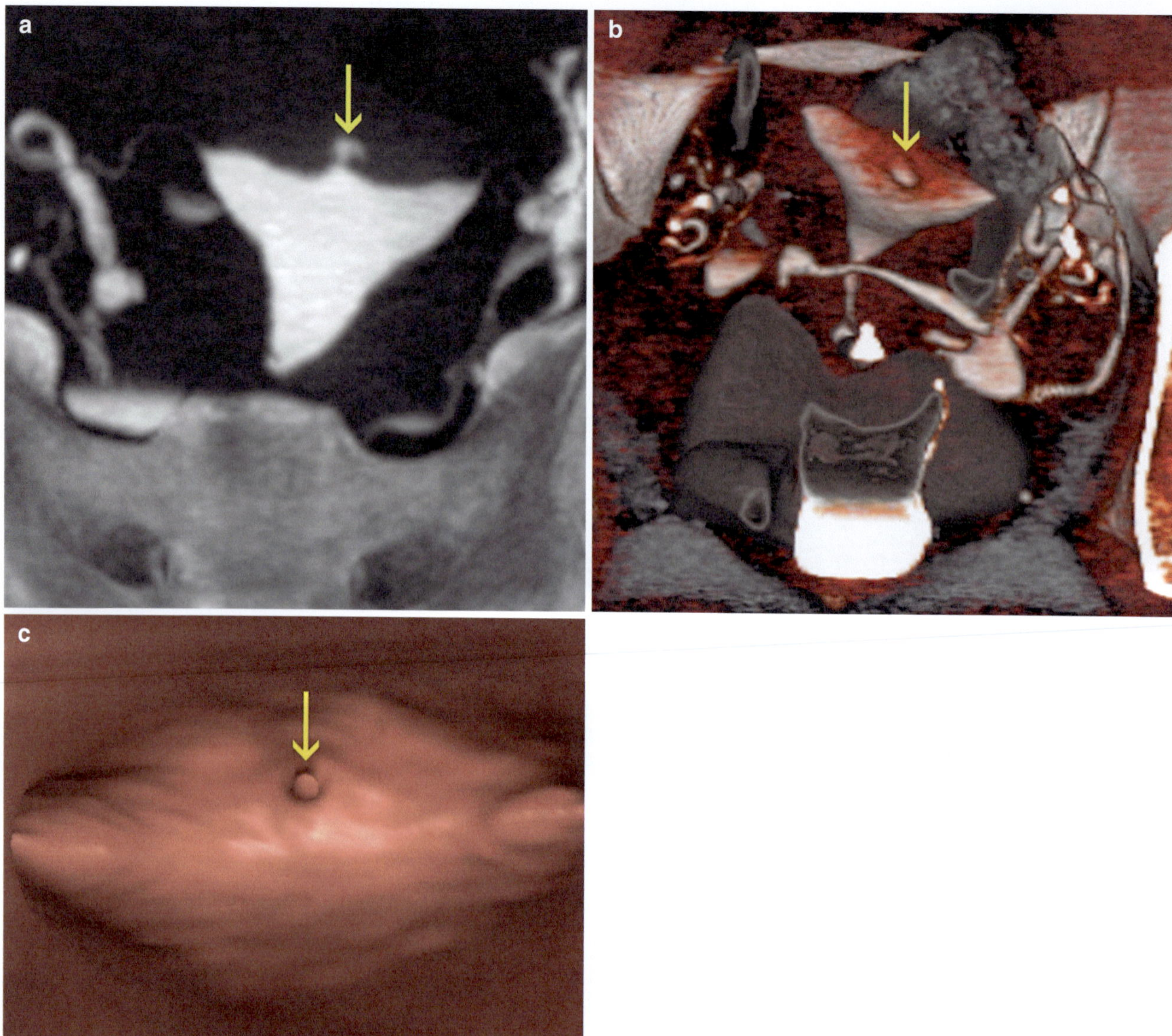

Fig. 7.26 Focal adenomyosis at the level of the uterine fundus (*arrow*) on VHSG study. Saccular projections into the myometrium beyond the normal outline of the endometrial cavity are appreciated with the injected contrast material. (**a**) Coronal maximum intensity projection image. (**b**) Coronal 3D volume rendering image, superior view. (**c**) Virtual endoscopy image

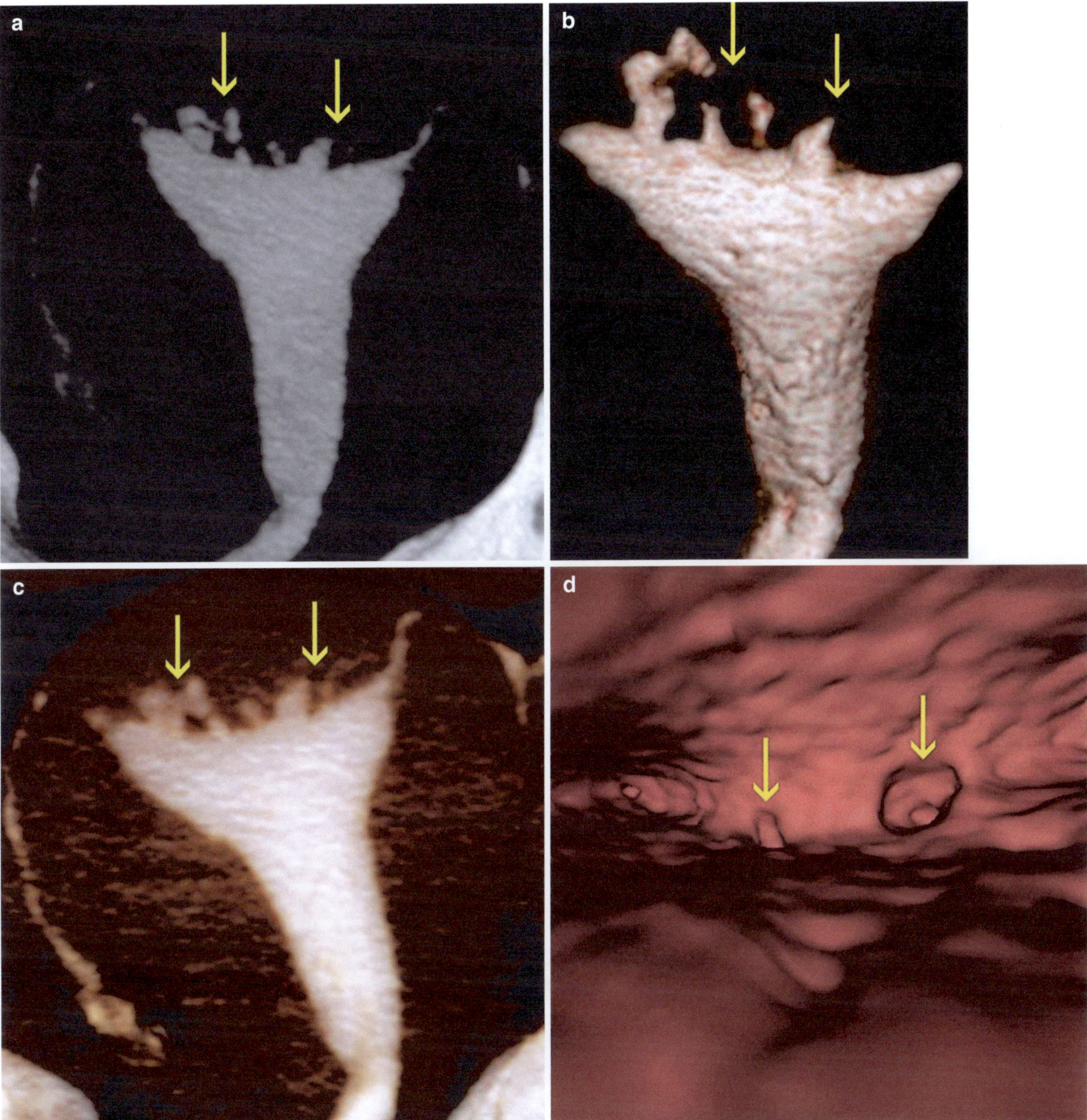

Fig. 7.27 Typical findings of diffuse adenomyosis at the level of the uterine fundus on VHSG study. Multiple lineal and saccular projections into the myometrium beyond the normal outline of the endometrial cavity are appreciated with the injected contrast material (*arrows*). (**a**) Coronal maximum intensity projection image. (**b**, **c**) Coronal 3D volume rendering images. (**d**) Virtual endoscopy image

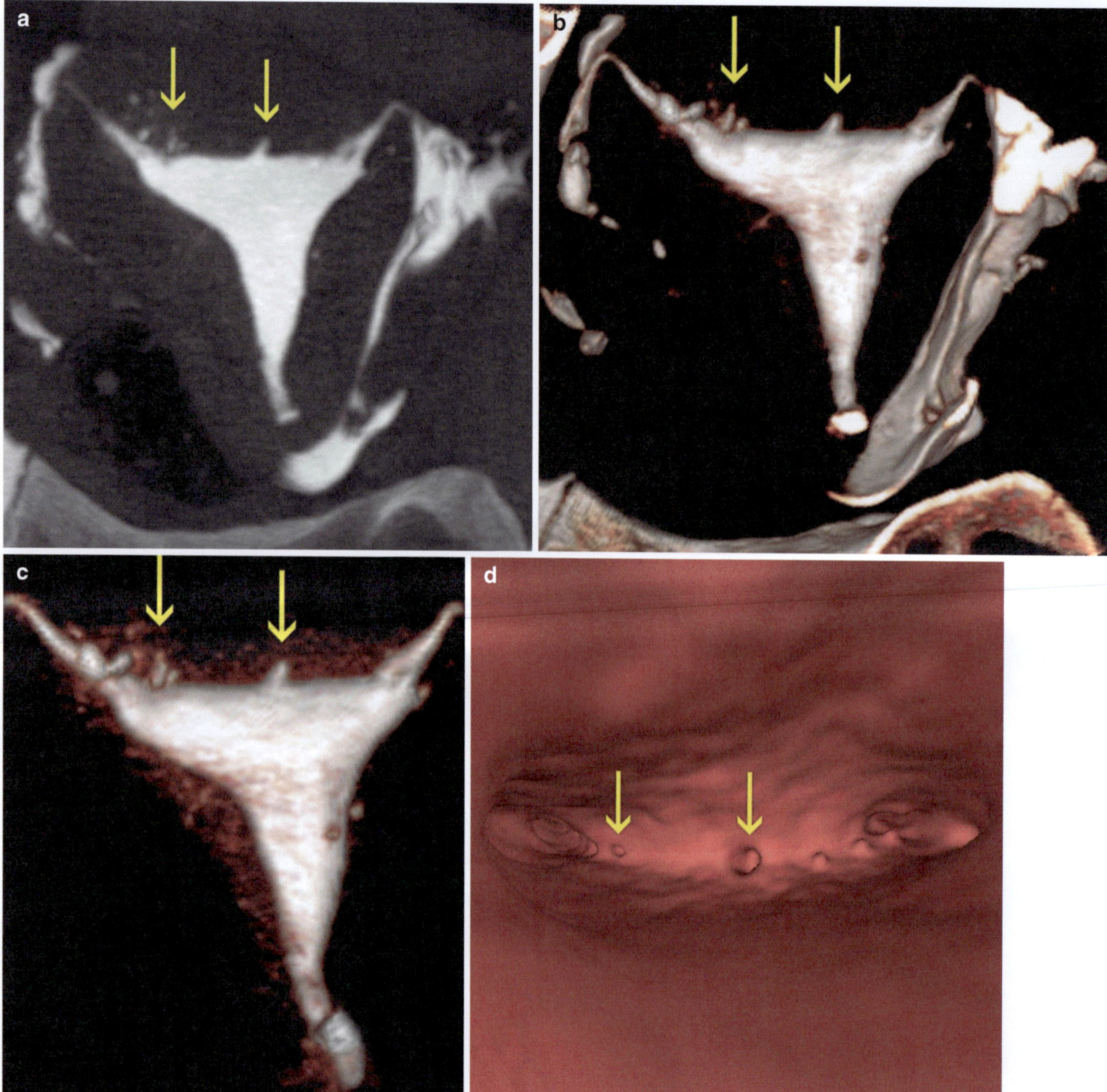

Fig. 7.28 Diffuse adenomyosis findings at the level of the uterine fundus on VHSG study. Multiple lineal and saccular projections into the myometrium beyond the normal outline of the endometrial cavity are appreciated with the injected contrast material (*arrows*). (**a**) Coronal maximum intensity projection image. (**b**, **c**) Coronal 3D volume rendering images. (**d**) Virtual endoscopy image

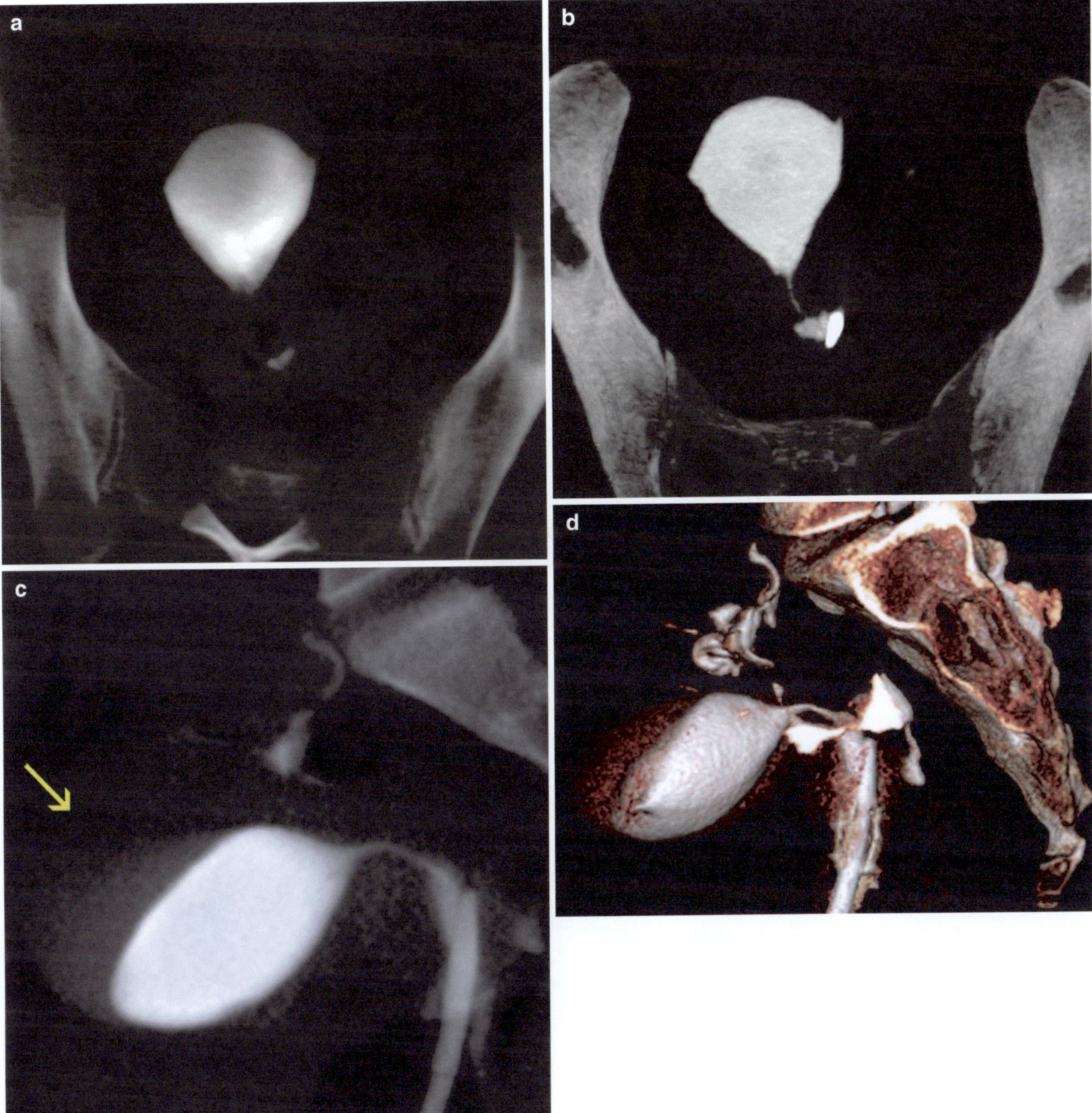

Fig. 7.29 Diffuse adenomyosis at the level of the posterior wall of the uterus on VHSG study. Only a diffuse abnormal thickening of the myometrium (*yellow arrow*) and a larger and deformed uterine cavity are appreciated. (**a**) Coronal multiplanar reconstruction (MPR) image. (**b**) Coronal maximum intensity projection image. (**c**) Sagittal MPR image. (**d**) Sagittal 3D volume rendering image. (**e**) Axial 3D volume rendering image, superior view. (**f**) Virtual endoscopy image. The deformity generated on the endometrial cavity (*white arrow*) can be appreciated

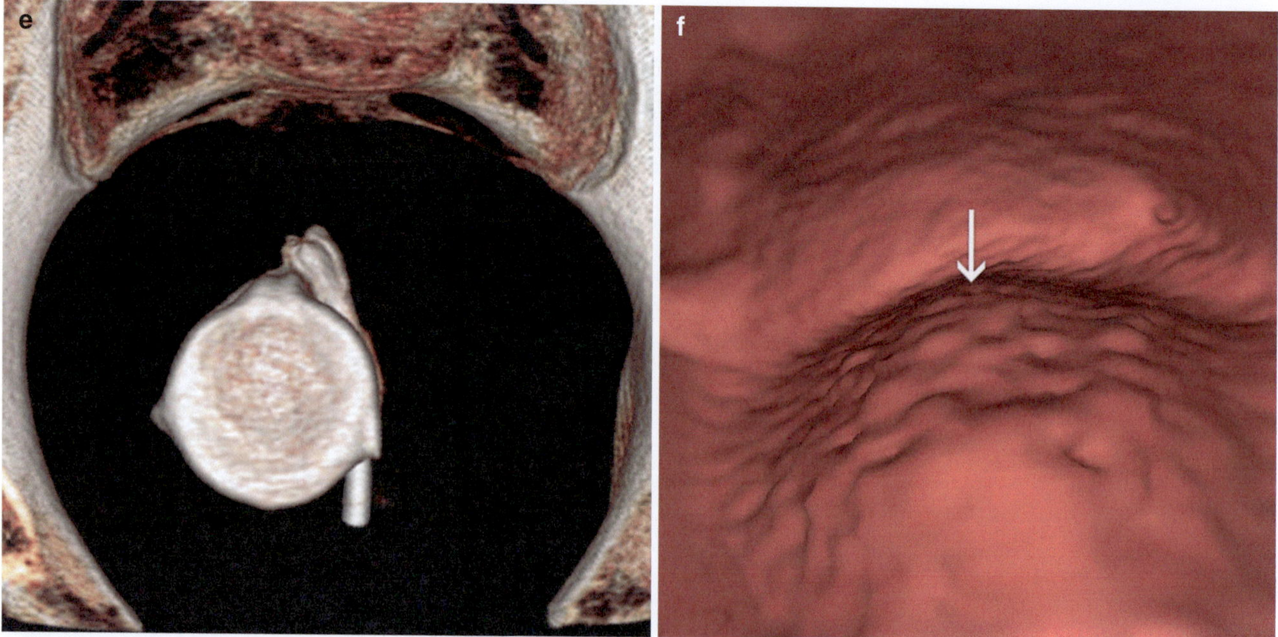

Fig. 7.29 (continued)

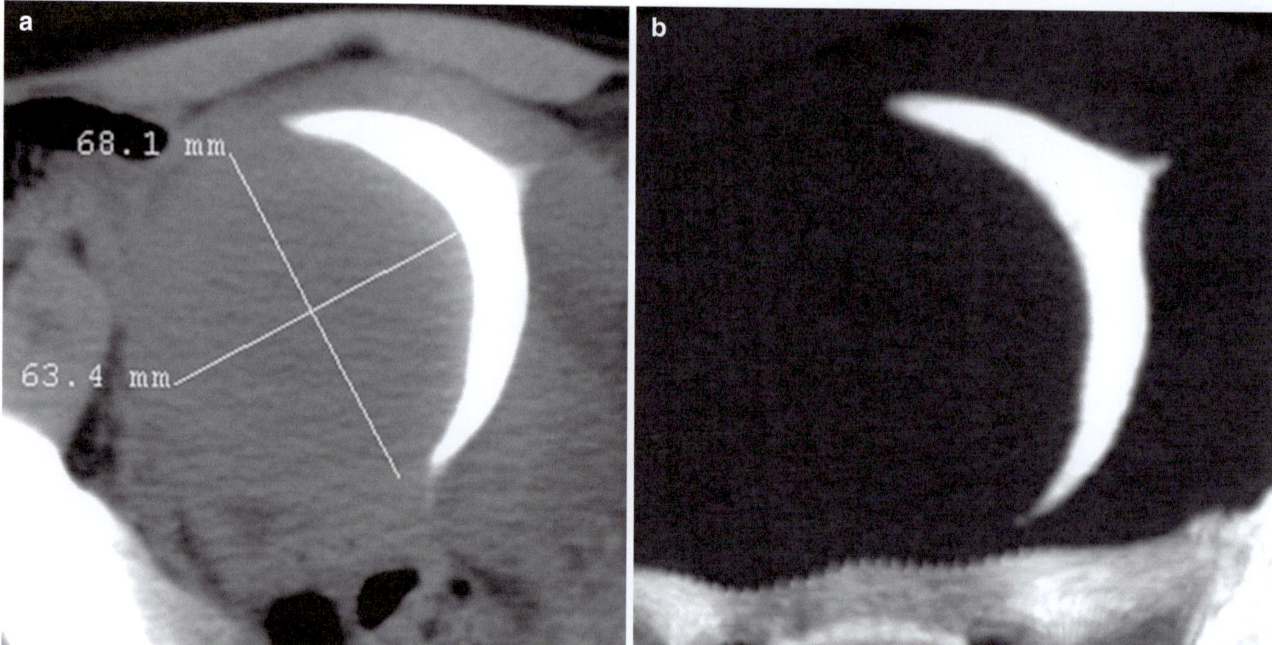

Fig. 7.30 Diffuse adenomyosis at the level of the right lateral wall of the uterus on VHSG study. Only a diffuse abnormal thickening of the myometrium and a larger and deformed uterine cavity are appreciated. (**a**) Coronal multiplanar reconstruction image with soft tissue window. (**b**) Coronal maximum intensity projection image. (**c**) Coronal 3D volume rendering image. (**d**) Virtual endoscopy image

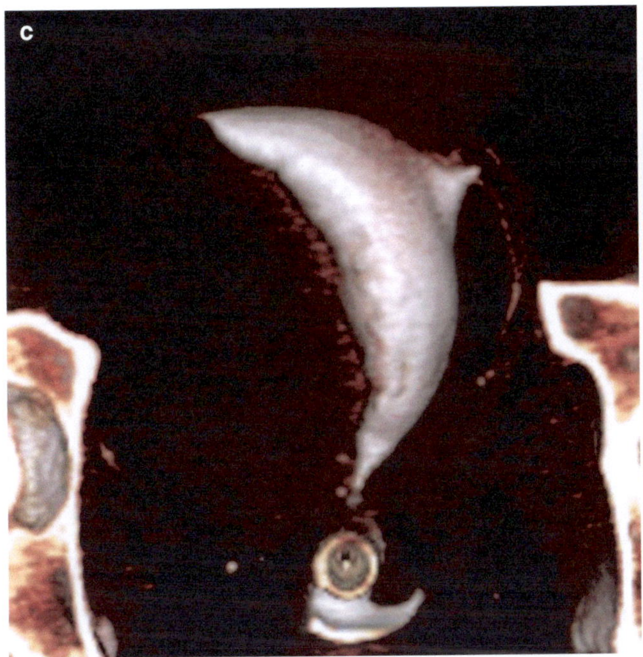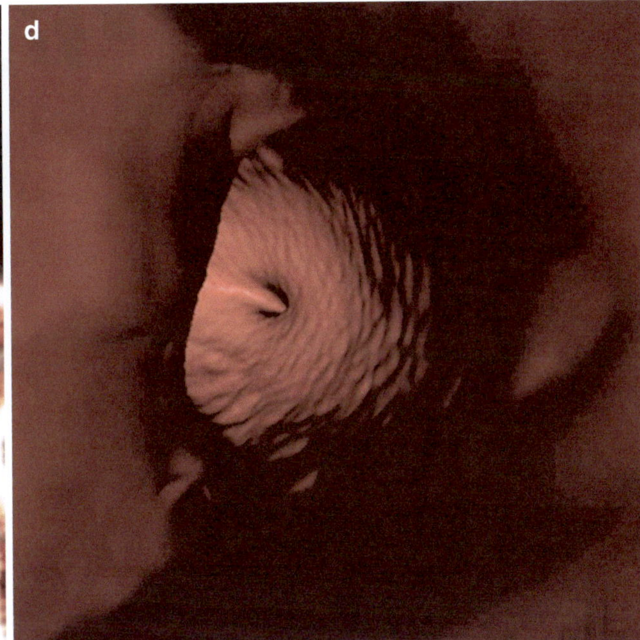

Fig. 7.30 (continued)

Conclusion

The pathological processes that involve the myometrium can be partially visualized and characterized by the VHSG study.

While the diagnostic capacity of the study is superior to that of the conventional radiologic one, the ultrasound and MR, with their different variants, allow a better evaluation of the myometrium and of the different pathologies that affect it.

References

1. Taylor A. ABC of subfertility: extent of the problem. BMJ. 2003;327:434–6.
2. Donnez J, Jadoul P. What are the implications of myomas on fertility? A need for a debate? Hum Reprod. 2002;17:1424–30.
3. Hunt JE, Wallach EE. Uterine factors in infertility – an overview. Clin Obstet Gynecol. 1974;17:44–64.
4. Buttram Jr VC, Reiter RC. Uterine leiomyomata: etiology, symptomatology, and management. Fertil Steril. 1981;36:433–45.
5. Baird D, Dunson D, Hill M, et al. High cumulative incidence of uterine leiomyoma in black and white women: ultrasound evidence. Am J Obstet Gynecol. 2003;188:100–7.
6. Heinemann K, Thiel C, Mohner S, et al. Benign gynecologic tumors: estimated incidence results of the German Cohort Study on Women's Health. Eur J Obstet Gynecol Reprod Biol. 2003;107:78–80.
7. Marino JL, Eskenazi B, Warner M, et al. Uterine leiomyoma and menstrual cycle characteristics in population based cohort study. Hum Reprod. 2004;19:2350–5.
8. Borgfeldt C, Andolf E. Transvaginal ultrasonographic findings in the uterus and endometrium: low prevalence of leiomyoma in a random sample of women age 25–40 years. Acta Obstet Gynecol Scand. 2000;79:202–7.
9. Mendoza Aguilar M, Herrera Flores I, Viramontes Trejo G, et al. Incidencia de patología de útero y anexos diagnosticada por histerosalpingografía en el Hospital General de México. An Radiol Méx. 2009;3:201–9.
10. Rumack CM, Wilson SR, Charboneau JW, Levine D. Diagnostic ultrasound. 4th ed. Elsevier: Mosby; 2010.
11. Wamsterker K, Emanuel MH, de Kruif JH. Transcervical hysteroscopic resection of submucous fibroids for abnormal uterine bleeding: results regarding the degree of intramural extension. Obstet Gynecol. 1993;82:736–40.
12. Dexeus S, Labastida R, Marqués L. Hysteroscopy in daily gynaecologic practice. Acta Eur Fertil. 1986;17:423–5.
13. Wolf DM, Spataro RF. The current state of hysterosalpingography. Radiographics. 1988;8:1041–58.
14. Nalaboff K, Pellerito J, Ben-Levi E. Imaging the endometrium: disease and normal variants. Radiographics. 2001;21:1409–24.
15. Davis P, O'Neill M, Yoder I, et al. Sonohysterographic findings of endometrial and subendometrial conditions. Radiographics. 2002;22:803–16.
16. Capuñay C, Baronio M, Carrascosa P, et al. CT virtual hysterosalpingography in the evaluation of uterine myomas. Fertil Steril. 2010;94(Supplement):S211.
17. Bazot M, Salem C, Frey I, et al. Imaging of myomas: is preoperative MRI useful? Gynecol Obstet Fertil. 2002;30:711–6.
18. Simpson WL, Beitia LG, Mester J. Histerosalpingography: a reemerging study. Radiographics. 2006;26:419–31.
19. Yoder IC, Hall DA. Hysterosalpingography in the 1990s. AJR Am J Roentgenol. 1991;157:675–83.
20. Matalliotakis IM, Katsikis IK, Panidis DK. Adenomyosis: what is the impact on fertility? Curr Opin Obstet Gynecol. 2005;17:261–4.
21. Kunz G, Beil D, Huppert P, et al. Adenomyosis in endometriosis-prevalence and impact on fertility. Evidence from magnetic resonance imaging. Hum Reprod. 2005;20:2309–16.
22. Togashi K, Ozasa H, Konishi I, et al. Enlarged uterus: differentiation between adenomyosis and leiomyoma with MR imaging. Radiology. 1989;171:531–4.

23. Tamai K, Togashi K, Ito T, et al. MR imaging findings of adenomyosis: correlation with histopathologic features and diagnostic pitfalls. Radiographics. 2005;25:21–40.
24. Bohlman ME, Ensor RE, Sanders RC. Sonographic findings in adenomyosis of the uterus. AJR Am J Roentgenol. 1987;148:756–66.
25. Reinhold C, Tafazoli F, Mehio A, et al. Uterine adenomyosis: endovaginal US and MR imaging features with histopathologic correlation. Radiographics. 1999;19:S147–60.
26. Atri M, Reinhold C, Mehio AR, et al. Adenomyosis: US features with histologic correlation in an in vitro study. Radiology. 2000;215:783–90.
27. Carrascosa P, Capuñay C, Mariano B, et al. Virtual hysteroscopy by multidetector computed tomography. Abdom Imaging. 2008;33(4):381–7.
28. Carrascosa P, Capuñay C, Vallejos J, et al. Virtual Hysterosalpingography: a new multidetector CT technique for evaluating the female reproductive system. Radiographics. 2010;30:643–61.

The uterine anomalies are generated by a defect in the fusion or reabsorption of the Müller conducts, in whatever stage of the embryonary development.

The müllerian anomalies cause infertility and, for this reason, its correct identification is fundamental to determine the best treatment to follow. Due to the fact that normal pregnancies can exist in women with congenital anomalies, uterine malformations are usually only detected in patients with fertility complications; hence the prevalence of reported congenital anomalies in the general population is probably underestimated.

The prevalence of utero-vaginal anomalies is of approximately 1–3 % [1–7] in the general population. Women with anomalies can have difficulty getting pregnant; nevertheless the risk of loss of pregnancy is greater, reaching 3 % [3, 4, 8–13]. Some anomalies can be corrected by hysteroscopy and others by laparoscopic surgery.

The uterine malformations are made clinically evident in different stages depending on the specific characteristics or association with other disorders. In a newborn, it can present itself as a palpable pelvic or abdominal mass due to a vaginal or uterine obstruction associated to intramural fluid.

In a teenager with a menarche lateness or primary amenorrhea, with or without liquid retention in the uterus (hematometra) or in the vagina (hematocolpos), can present itself as a painful intra-abdominal tumor. Some patients suffer from cyclic pains. The anomalies can show various infertility problems, like repeated spontaneous abortions, premature deliveries and intrauterine fetal retardment [14–16].

Once one understands the defect in the embryological development, it is possible to comprehend the potential of associated congenital malformations of other organs [17–20].

Renal malformations which may occur are agenesia or renal ectopia [21]. Less frequent are the osseous –anomalies like abnormal scapula, supernumerary or fused ribs and fusion of the spine (Klippel-Feil syndrome).

Associated cardiac malformations have also been described. The morbidity is increased in certain types in which müllerian obstructions are associated with hemato-salpinx (blood retention in the fallopian tubes) or hematocolpos (blood retention in the vagina).

Once the presence of a congenital anomaly is suspected, it is necessary to carry out diagnostic methods for its confirmation as well as for the determination of the adequate therapeutic procedure.

Twenty-five percent of patients with anomalies have fertility complications [11, 13, 22]. Clinically, primary amenorrhea, premature and repeated spontaneous abortions, and complications in the delivery can be produced [23, 24].

Other malformations of the genitalia, urological (25 %) or rectal can be associated. The renal agenesia is the most frequent of these anomalies, as well as the renal ectopy, the renal cystic dysplasia and the duplication of the collector system.

There exist extra uterine and intrauterine factors like the exposition to the ionizing radiation, intrauterine infections and use of drugs with teratogenic effect such as the thalidomide or the synthetic estrogen utilized in the 70s which is related to defects in the genital development.

The recognition of said anomalies is important to distinguish them from other types of processes, to detect if complications have occurred and plan the adequate therapeutic procedure for the patients suffering from sterility. The uterine malformations must be suspected according to the clinical history and the physical exam.

Embryology

The knowledge of the embryology of the female urogenital tract is fundamental to understand the pathogenia of the different types of anomalies.

The female reproductive system is developed from two Müller conducts (paramesonpheric conducts) that begin in the mesoderm lateral to each Wolf conduct (mesonpheric conduct). The pair of Müller conducts develops in a medial and caudal direction. The cranial section remains not fused and forms the Fallopian tubes. The caudal part fuses and forms the uterus and two-thirds of the top of the vagina.

P. Carrascosa et al., *CT Virtual Hysterosalpingography*,
DOI 10.1007/978-3-319-07560-0_8, © Springer International Publishing Switzerland 2014

Table 8.1 Classification of congenital anomalies

I. Müllerian ducts agenesis
II. Unicornuate uterus
(a) With rudimentary horn
(b) Without rudimentary horn
III. Uterus didelphys
IV. Bicornuate uterus
V. Septate uterus
VI. DES exposure uterus

American Fertility Society – 1988 [26]

This is known as lateral fusion. Another known process is the vertical fusion where the medial septum and both conducts regress. The caudal part of the vagina comes from the sino-vaginal bulb and fuses with the inferior Müller ducts.

The ovaries originate from the gonad bridge, a tissue completely different from the mesoderm that gives rise to the genital and urinary systems. For this reason, congenital gynecological and renal anomalies can be associated.

The uterine anomalies are classified in agenesia and hypoplasia, vertical and lateral fusion defects [25, 26]. In 1979, Buttram and Gibbons proposed a classification of anomalies of the müllerian ducts based on the degree of failure of the normal development, and they separated them in classes according to their similar clinical manifestation, treatment and prognosis [27]. This classification was modified by the American Fertility Society and nowadays is universally accepted (Table 8.1).

Diagnostic Methods

Frequently, after the diagnostic suspicion of a malformation, an evaluation is necessary, with the aim of determining the exact diagnosis of the pathology, for which case exists a variety of different imaging methods such as hysterosalpingography (HSG), ultrasound, magnetic resonance (MR) and a recently new method known as Virtual Hysterosalpingography (VHSG).

HSG is a diagnostic modality which allows the evaluation of congenital anomalies. However, it has several limitations. In certain anomalies, knowledge of the morphology is required, not only of the uterine cavity, but also of the myometrial wall. This technique does not offer information on the uterine wall, reason why in certain cases it relies on measurements to estimate, with certain precision, what malformation it could be. These measurements are not always accurate [28].

Ultrasound is a method that permits the transvaginal or pelvic evaluation of congenital anomalies. However, to assess with more precision the morphology of the myometrial

wall, the tridimensional technique is the one which offers better information [29, 30].

MR has been considered the reference method for the evaluation of uterine anomalies due to its great capacity in tissular resolution and in optimally detecting the external margins of the uterine wall [31–33]. Due to its high contrast resolution and use of multiple sagittal planes, coronal and axial in T1, T2 sequences with or without fat saturation, it is able to identify diverse uterine anomalies. The slice width that the MR uses does not allow the exact detection of associated intramural pathologies or the assessment of the tubal morphology and permeability. MR characterizes the uterine anomaly but, to discard other associated factors possibly related to infertility, other complementary methods are required.

There is now a new and very useful method to assess the gynecological apparatus as a whole, the Virtual Histerosalpingography study. It offers information on the cervical and uterine regions, of the tubes and the anexial region with only 1.5 s in the acquisition of the images, using an extremely low dose of radiation (0.3 mSv) and with a reduced rate of complications due to its non invasiveness [34–41].

Agenesia of the Müllerian Conducts

This anomaly consists of segmental agenesia and variable degrees of uterovaginal hypoplasia.

VHSG permits the evaluation of this type of alteration, offering integral 2D and 3D information. In Fig. 8.1, a hypoplastic uterus is shown, characterized for being of small size.

Unicornuate Uterus

In this anomaly, a failure of one müllerian conduct exists, while the other develops normally, resulting in a unicornuate uterus. It presents itself in 20 % of uterine malformation cases; being able to be only one or to present a rudimentary horn with no association to the endometrium in 33 % of the cases.

A rudimentary horn can be communicative if there is communication of the endometrium with the contra-lateral horn (10 %), or not communicative if no such communication exists (22 %) (Fig. 8.2).

Clinical manifestations appear only in cases of non communicative rudimentary horns with symptoms such as dysmenorrhea with hematometra at the time of the menarche. There also is a risk of endometriosis in unicornuate uterus with non communicative rudimentary horns. In 41–62 % of

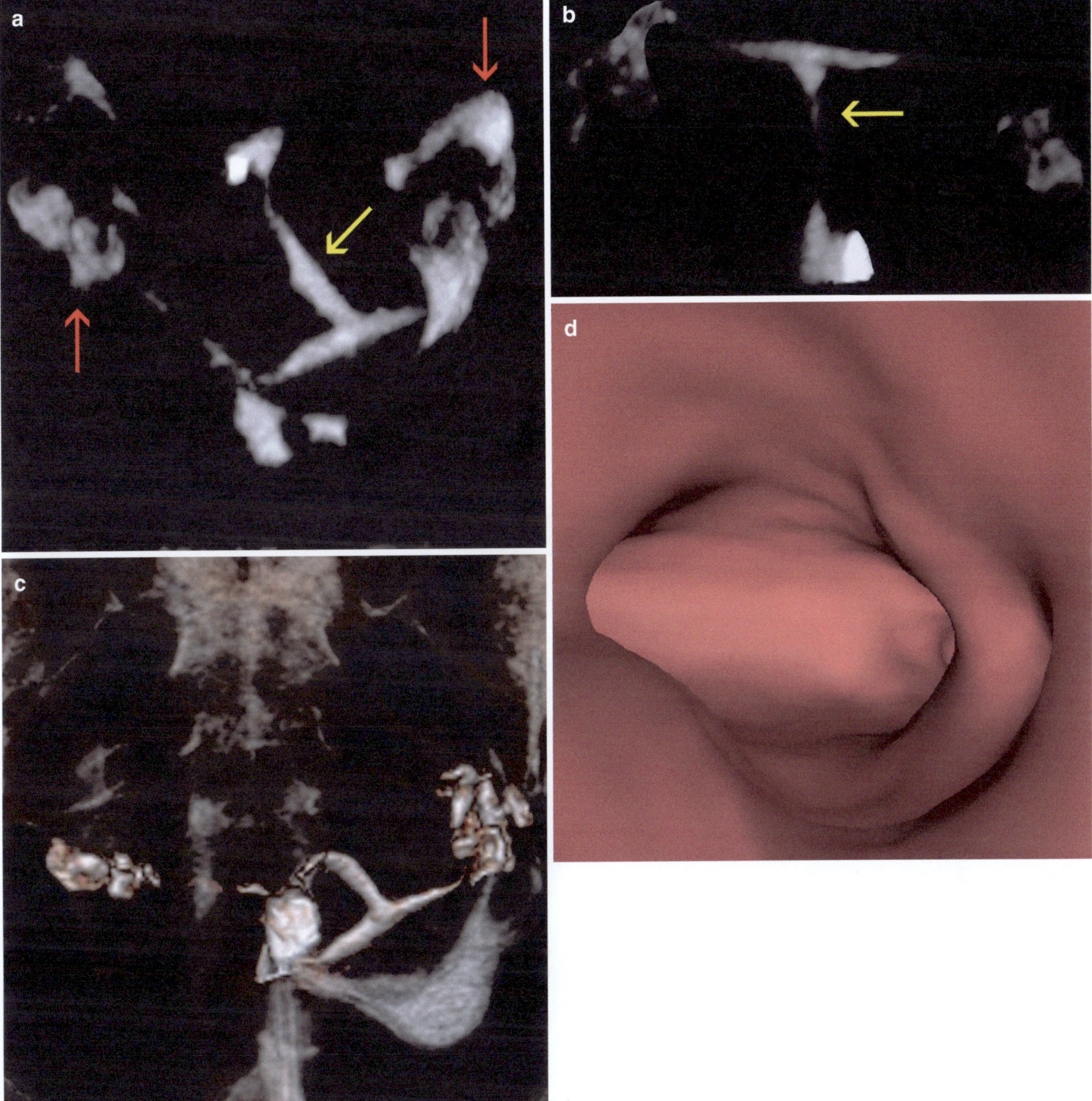

Fig. 8.1 Hypoplastic uterus seen through VHSG. (**a**) Axial CT image with soft tissue window which shows a hypoplastic retroverted uterus lateralized to the left (*yellow arrow*). Both permeable tubes are observed (*red arrows*). (**b**) Axial maximum intensity projection image which exhibits a small uterus (*arrow*) with tubes of normal morphology. (**c**) Coronal 3D volume rendering image illustrates similar findings. (**d**) Virtual endoscopy image shows a small uterine cavity

cases, spontaneous abortions are observed and premature deliveries between 10 and 20 %.

HSG, MR and VHSG show with simplicity this anomaly. The uterus appears curved and elongated with the shape of a banana. The uterine volume reduced. In Figs. 8.3 and 8.4 comparative examples of a unicornuate uterus are observed.

Previously, the limitations of MR in the visualization of associated intramural pathologies were mentioned. In Fig. 8.5 a case of a unicornuate uterus with cervical and uterine polyps identified by VHSG and not seen by MR is shown.

The treatment of this anomaly consists in the resection of the non communicative rudimentary horn to avoid the

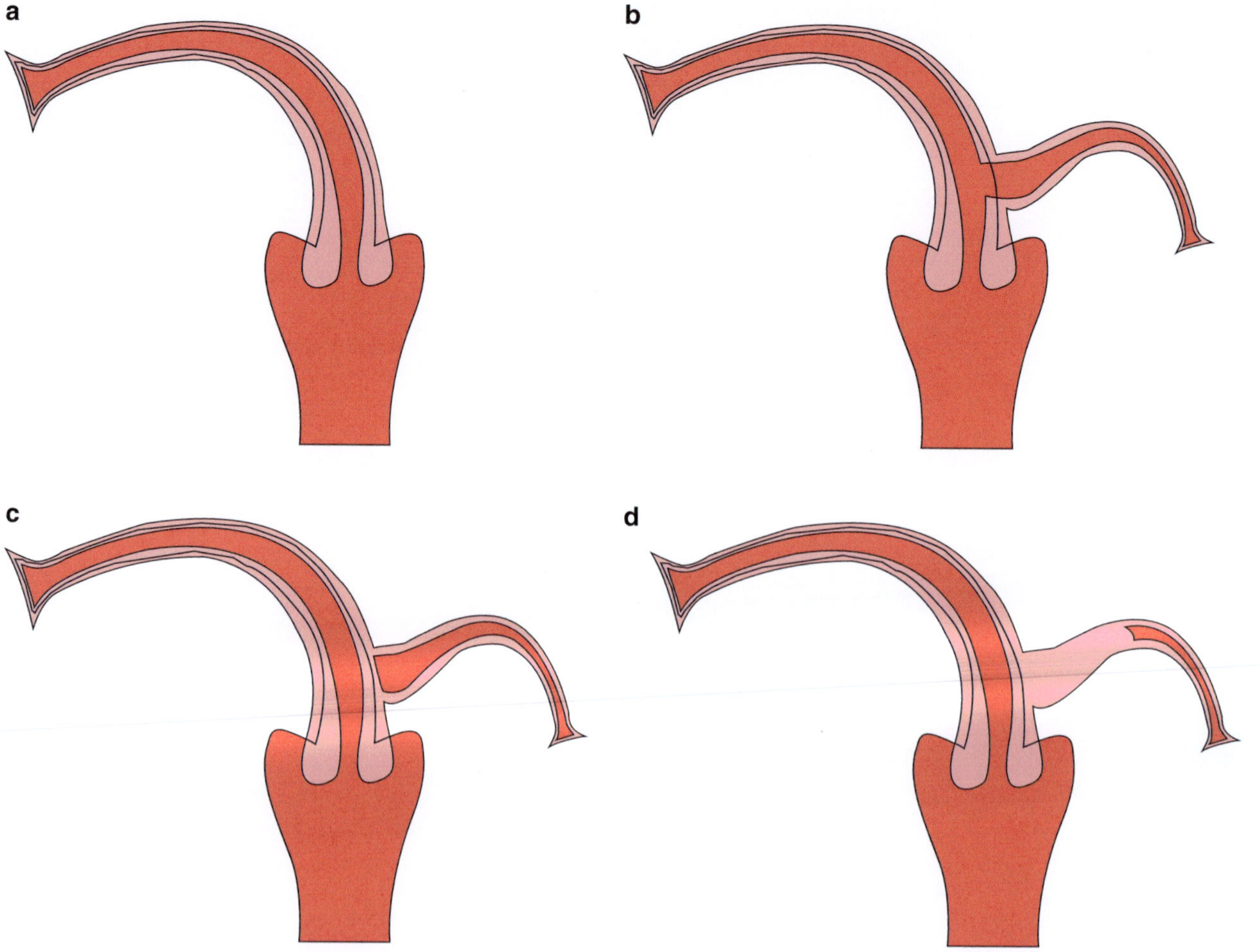

Fig. 8.2 Types of unicornuate uterus. (**a**) Unicornuate uterus without rudimentary horn. (**b**) Unicornuate uterus with rudimentary communicative horn. (**c**) Unicornuate uterus with rudimentary non-communicative horn. (**d**) Unicornuate uterus with rudimentary non-communicative horn without cavity

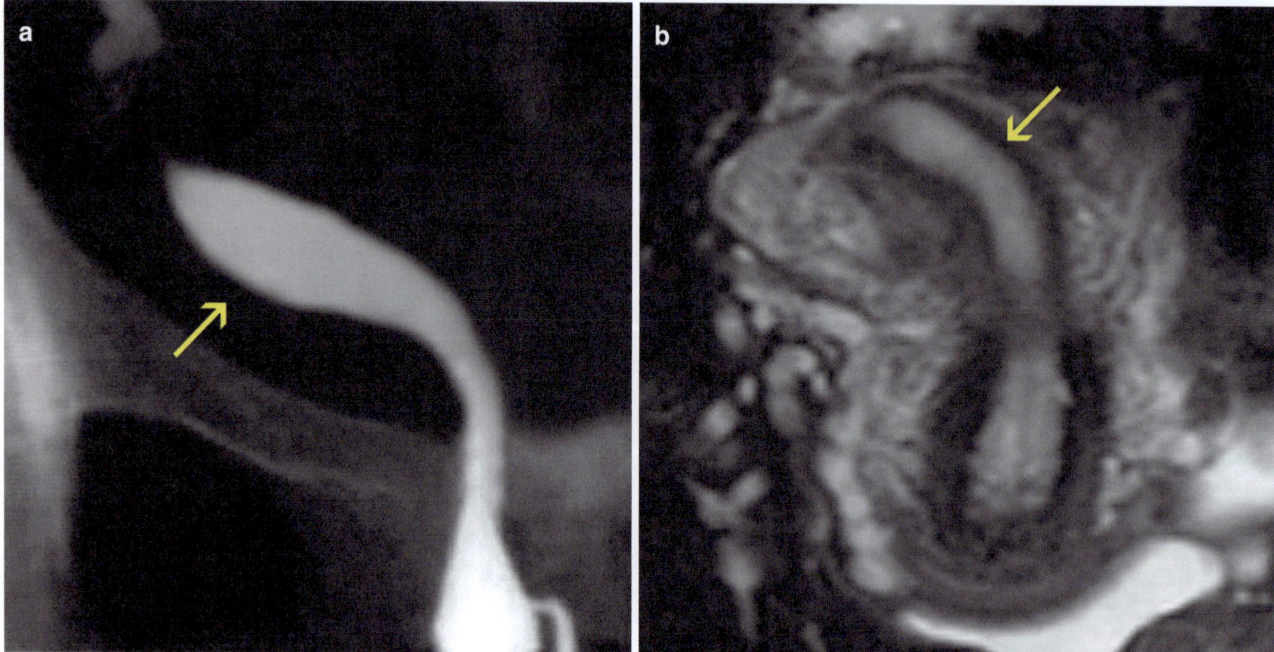

Fig. 8.3 Unicornuate uterus. Comparison of different imaging modalities. (**a**) HSG image, which shows a unicornuate uterus located to the left (*arrow*). The tube is of normal shape and size. (**b**) Axial T2 weighted MRI image with fat suppression which exhibits a unicornuate uterus (*arrow*). (**c–e**) Maximum intensity projection and coronal 3D volume rendering VHSG images that identify similar findings. F. Virtual endoscopy image

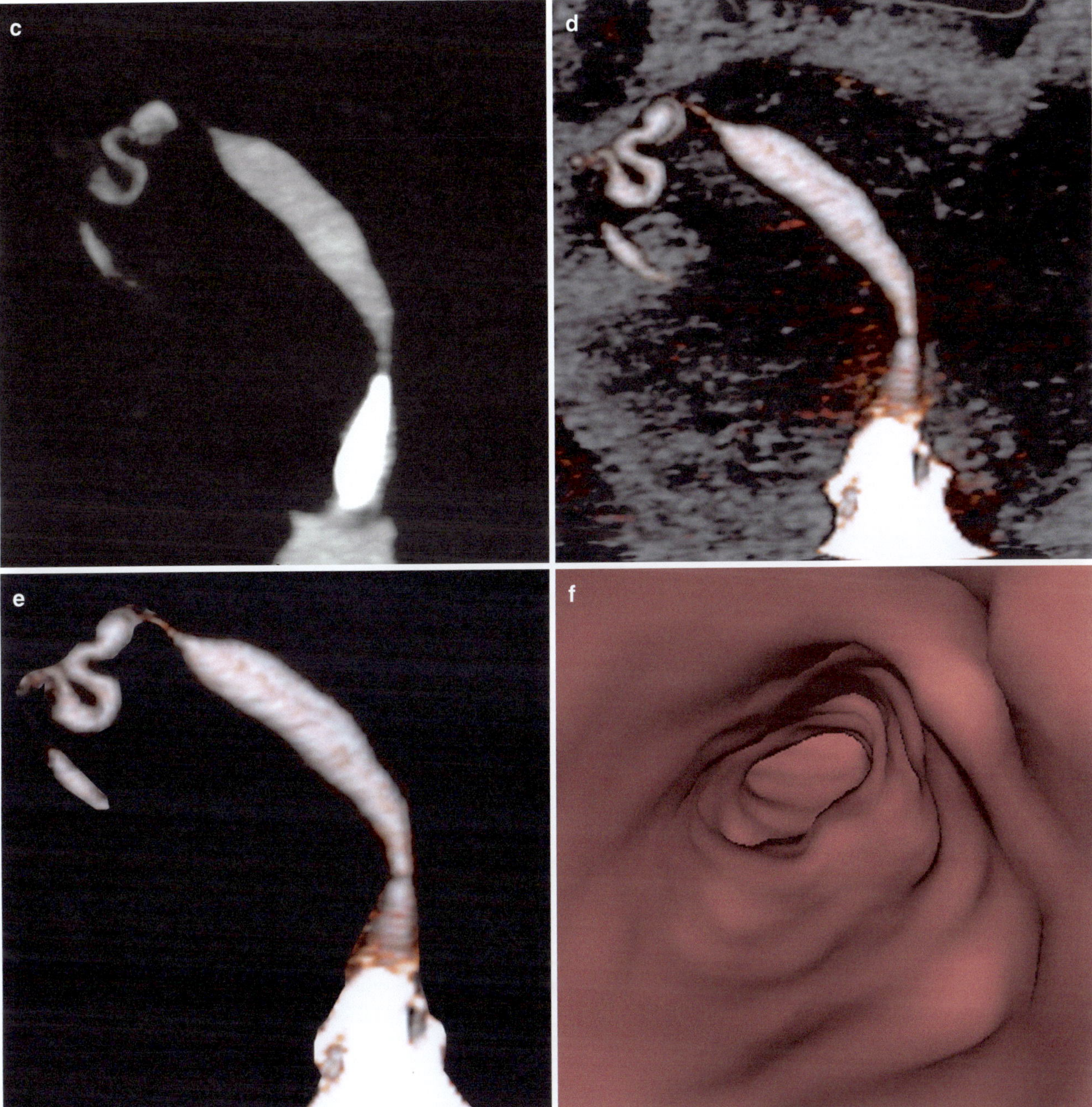

Fig. 8.3 (continued)

possibility of ectopic pregnancies. Associated renal anomalies are observed frequently in 40 % of these patients. This alteration is usually ipsilateral to the rudimentary horn.

Uterus Didelphys

Results from the incomplete fusion of the müllerian ducts and accounts for 5 % of the anomalies. An almost complete fusion failure exists between the endometrial cavities with a lack of communication between both horns (Fig. 8.6).

As each müllerian duct develops its own hemiuterus and cervix, no communication exists between the endometrial cavities. In 75 % of the cases an associated vaginal septum is observed that, at the same time, can complicate itself with a hematometrocolpos.

The non obstructive uterus didelphys is usually asymptomatic, while the ones that present unilateral vaginal obstruction manifest dysmenorrhea. This anomaly is associated with a percentage of spontaneous abortions that oscillates between 32 and 52 % and with premature deliveries in between 20 and 48 %.

As diagnostic methods, HSG, MR and VHSG allow its evaluation, showing the typical findings mentioned of this anomaly.

In Fig. 8.7, a comparative case of the three modalities is shown. It is possible to observe the advantages of

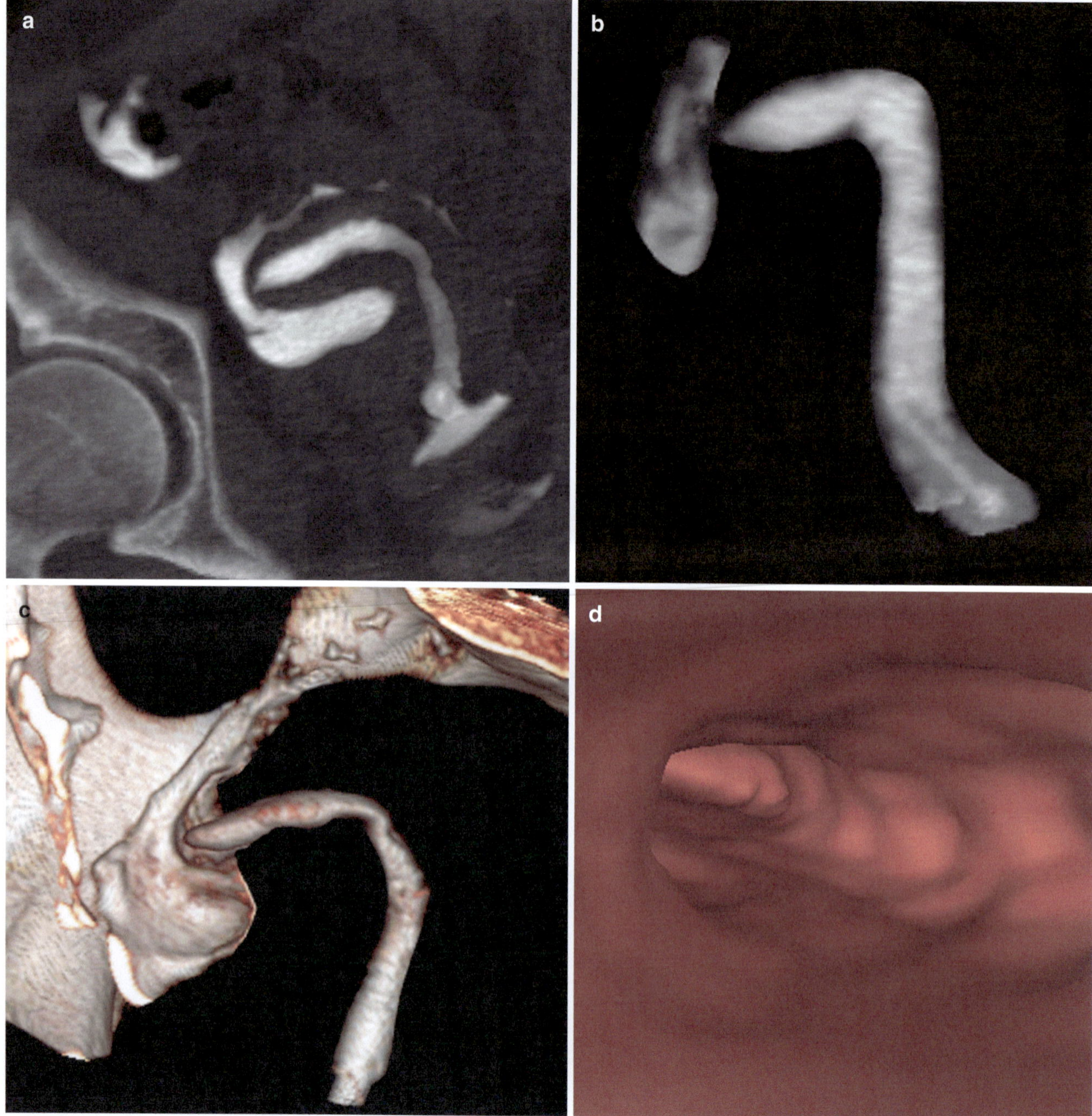

Fig. 8.4 Unicornuate uterus. Comparison between VHSG and MRI. (**a**) Maximum intensity projection (MIP) image which illustrates the morphology of the unicornuate uterus towards the right. (**b**) MIP image showing only the typical morphology of a unicornuate uterus. (**c**) 3D volume rendering image exhibiting similar findings. (**d**) Virtual endoscopy view illustrating a unique horn. (**e**, **f**) Axial T2 weighted MRI image with and without fat suppression displaying the shape of a unicornuate uterus

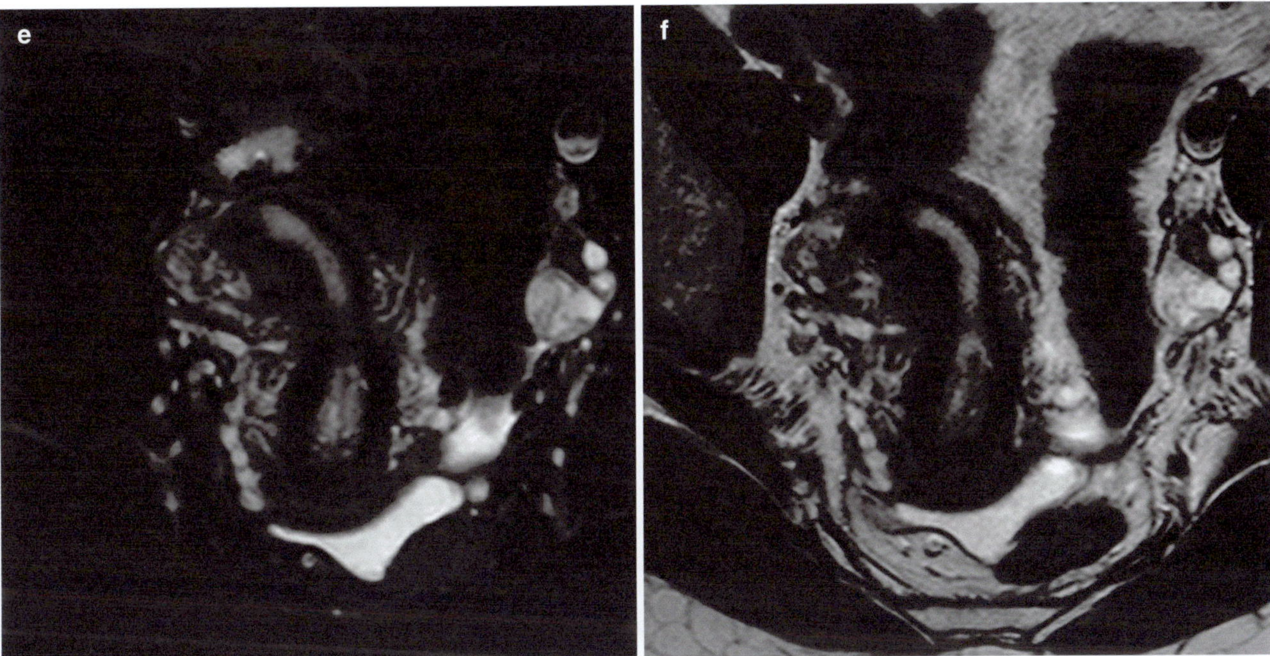

Fig. 8.4 (continued)

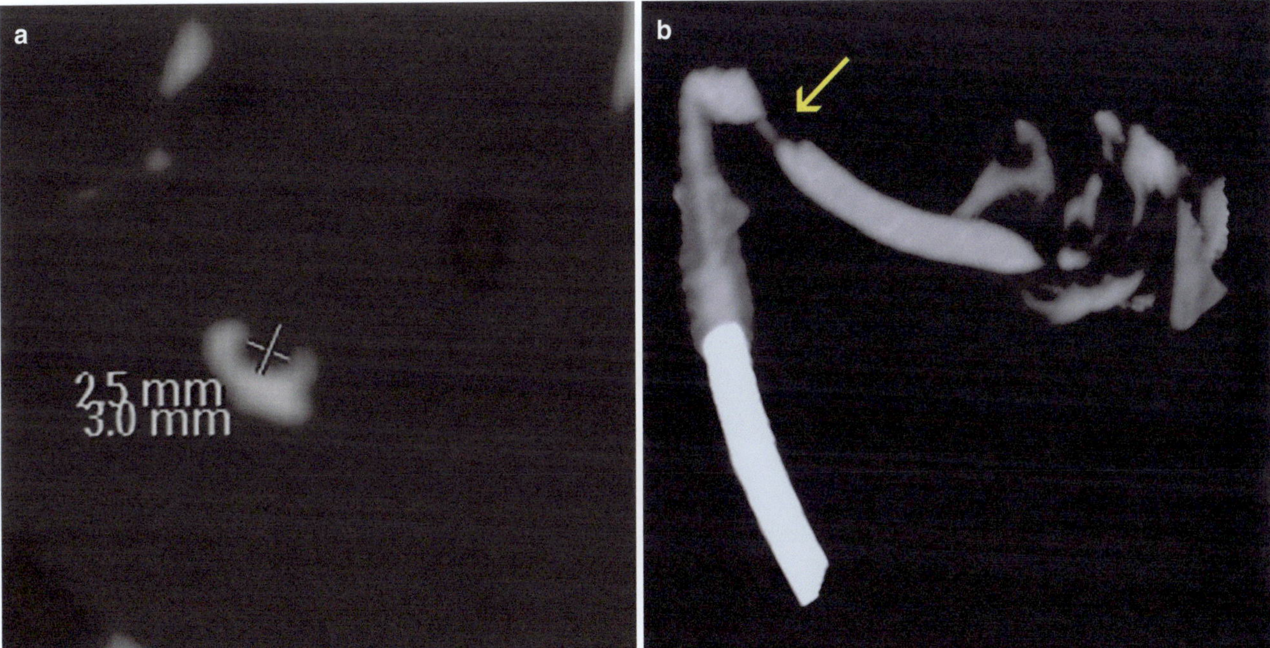

Fig. 8.5 Unicornuate uterus with cervical polyp. (**a**) Axial CT image with soft tissue window showing an elevated endocervical lesion of 2.5×3.0 mm compatible with a polyp. (**b**) Oblique coronal maximum intensity projection image of a unicornuate uterus. A small filling defect is observed in the cervical canal (*arrow*). (**c**) Virtual endoscopy image which exhibits the polyp (*arrow*). (**d**) Magnified virtual endoscopy view. (**e**) Coronal 3D volume rendering image. (**f**) Axial T2 weighted MRI image with fat suppression showing a unicornuate uterus. The polyp was not able to be identified

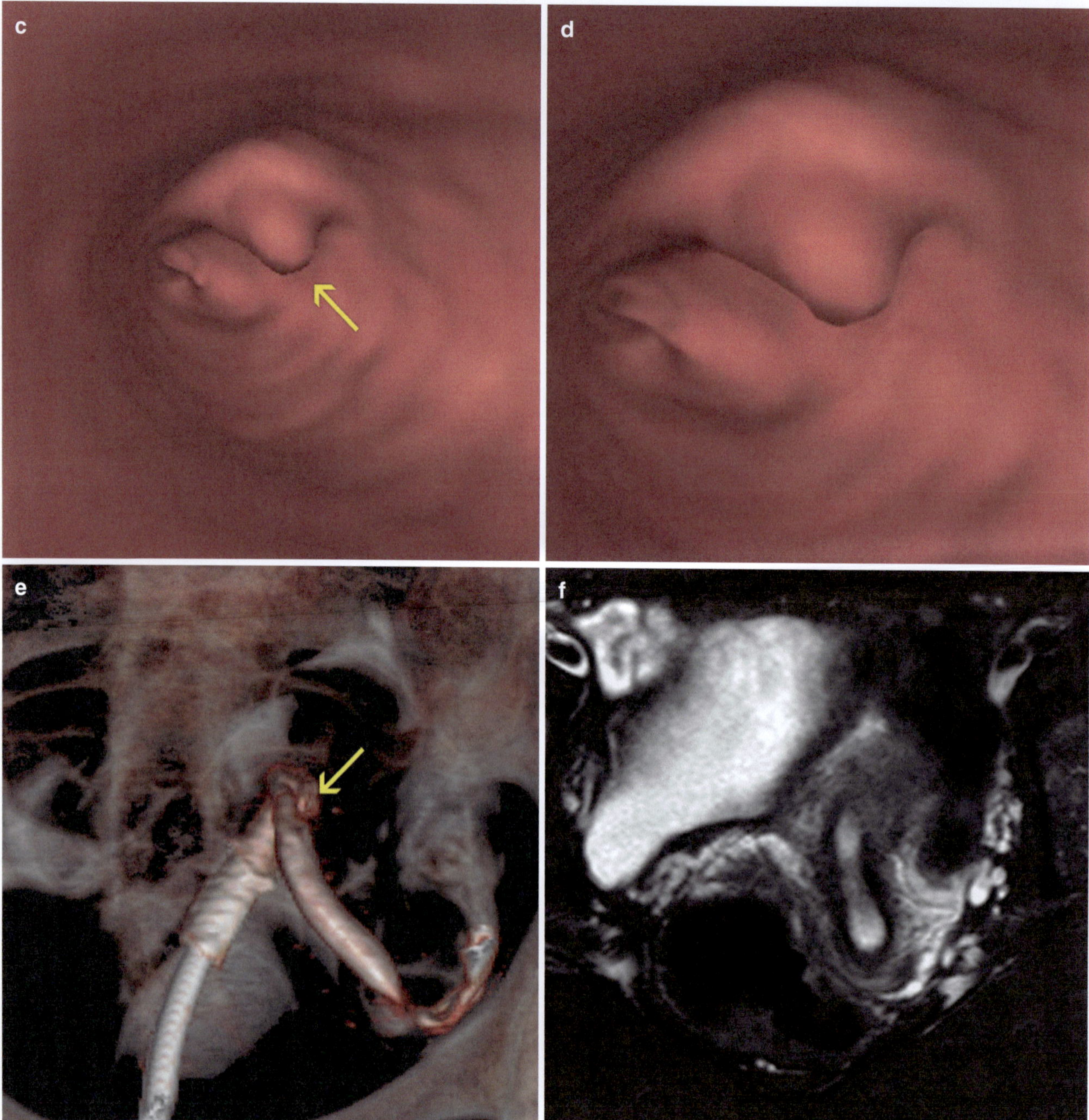

Fig. 8.5 (continued)

VHSG thanks to multiple post-processing techniques such as bidimensional, tridimensional and endoscopic reprocessing.

In Fig. 8.8 didelfos uterus with associated polypoid pathology and normal MR is shown.

Bicornuate Uterus

This anomaly consists of two independent uterine horns that caudally join with communication of the endometrial cavities, frequently at the isthmic-cervical level.

In this anomaly, an incomplete fusion of the upper segments of the utero-vaginal canal is observed. This case constitutes 10 % of the anomalies.

The bicornuate uterus can be of different types: partial, complete or arcuate (Fig. 8.9).

The bicornuate uterus can be unicollis when it extends up to the internal cervical orifice or bicollis when it has a duplicated cervix. It associates in 28–35 % of cases with spontaneous abortions and in 14–23 % with premature deliveries.

Diagnostic methods that offer information are ultrasound, HSG, MR and VHSG.

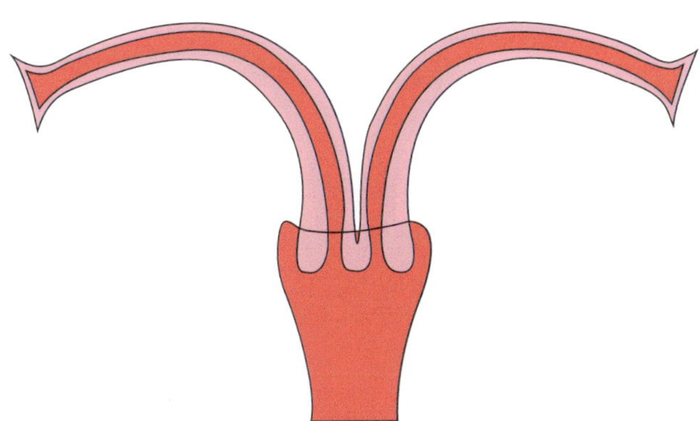

Fig. 8.6 Picture of a uterus didelphys

Ultrasound: two divergent endometrial cavities are observed. In the conventional method, in some cases, results complex to evaluate the uterus fundus, while the tridimensional modality provides a more precise information (Fig. 8.10).

HSG: The uterine horns are well separated with an intercornual angle equal or more than 105° (Fig. 8.11). Each horn is fusiform and ends in each one's respective Fallopian tube (Fig. 8.12).

This method has difficulty in exactly defining the bicornuate uterus and differentiates it of the septate one due to the fact that it does not evaluate the myometrial wall.

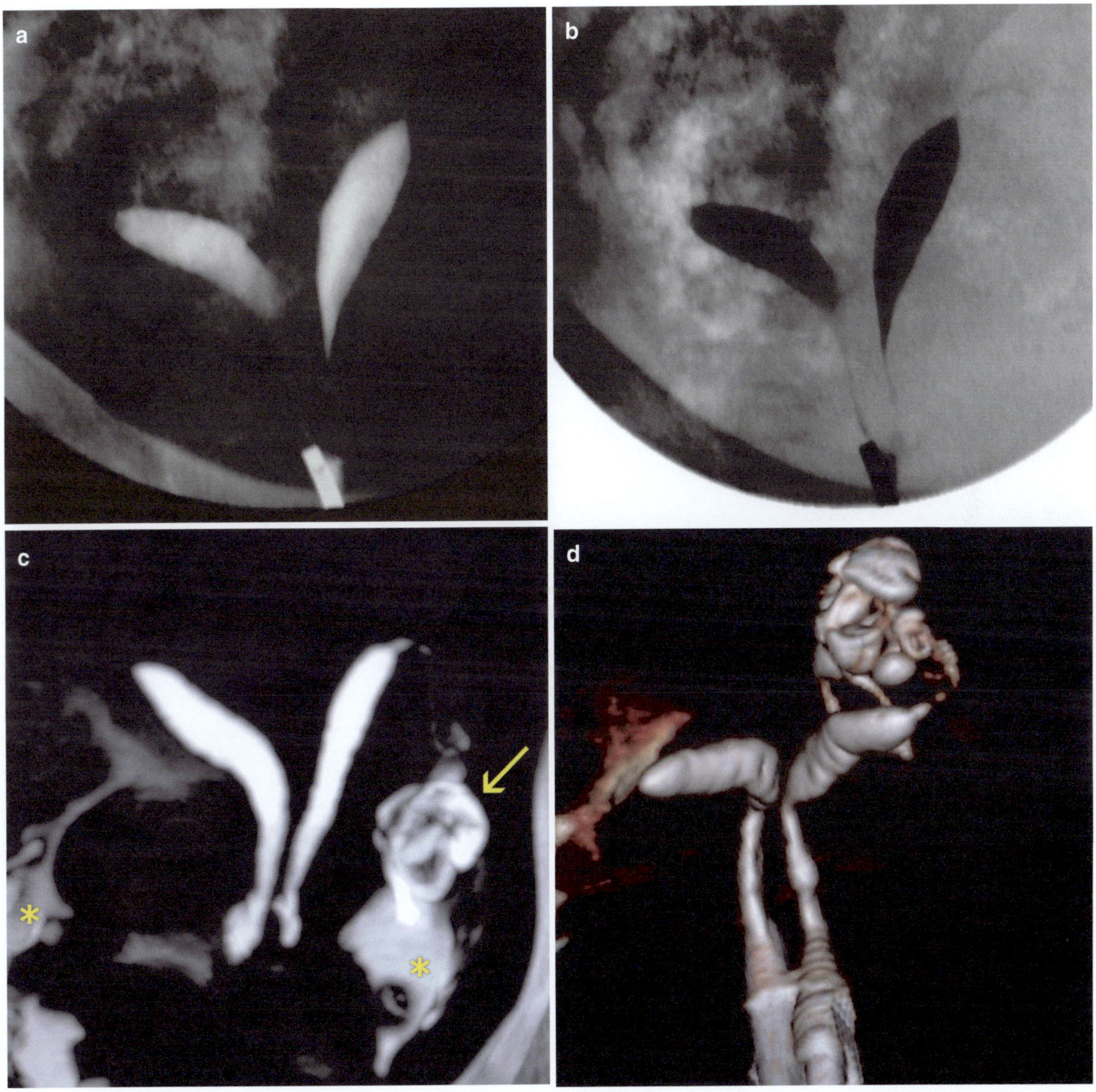

Fig. 8.7 Uterus didelphys. Comparison between HSG, MRI and VHSG. (**a**, **b**) HSG showing a uterus didelphys. Two independent uterine cavities with no communication between them can be observed. (**c**) VHSG: axial maximum intensity projection image of a uterus didelphys. Two non-connected uterine hemicavities can be observed. Each one possesses a normal Fallopian tube (*arrow*) with passage of contrast to the peritoneal cavity (*asterisk*). (**d**) VHSG: Coronal 3D volume rendering image illustrating the morphology of a uterus didelphys. (**e**, **f**) Coronal T2 weighted MRI images showing two uterine hemicavities extending from the cervical region to the uterine body

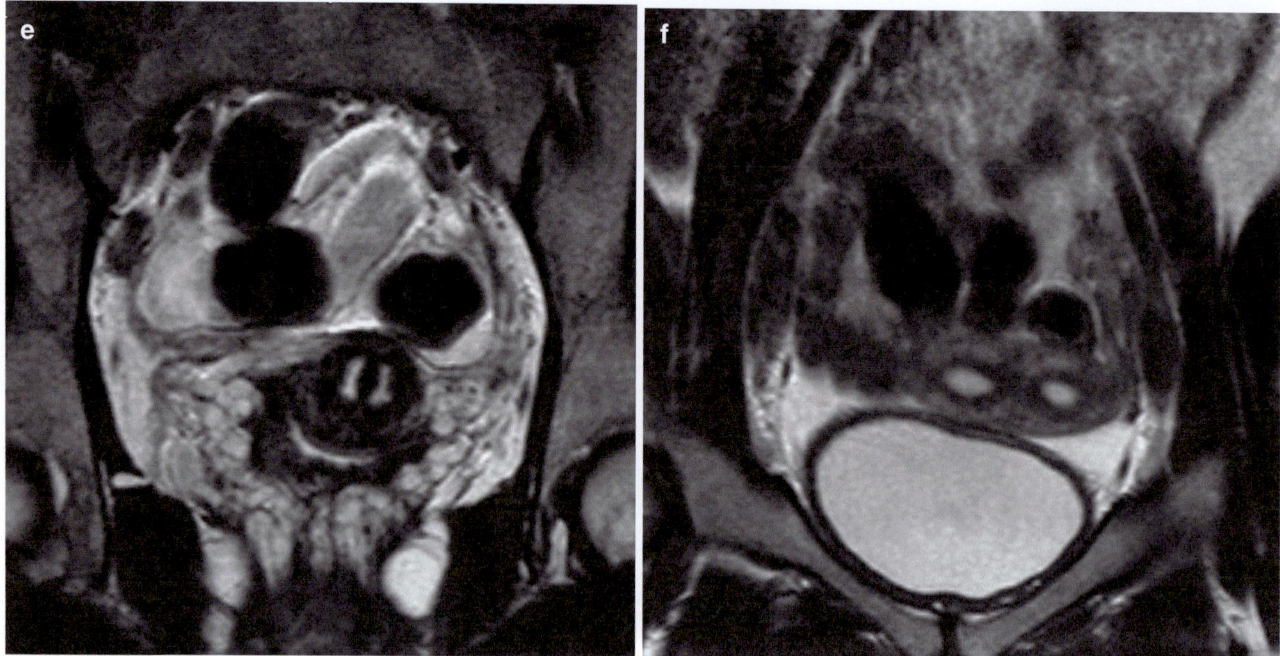

Fig. 8.7 (continued)

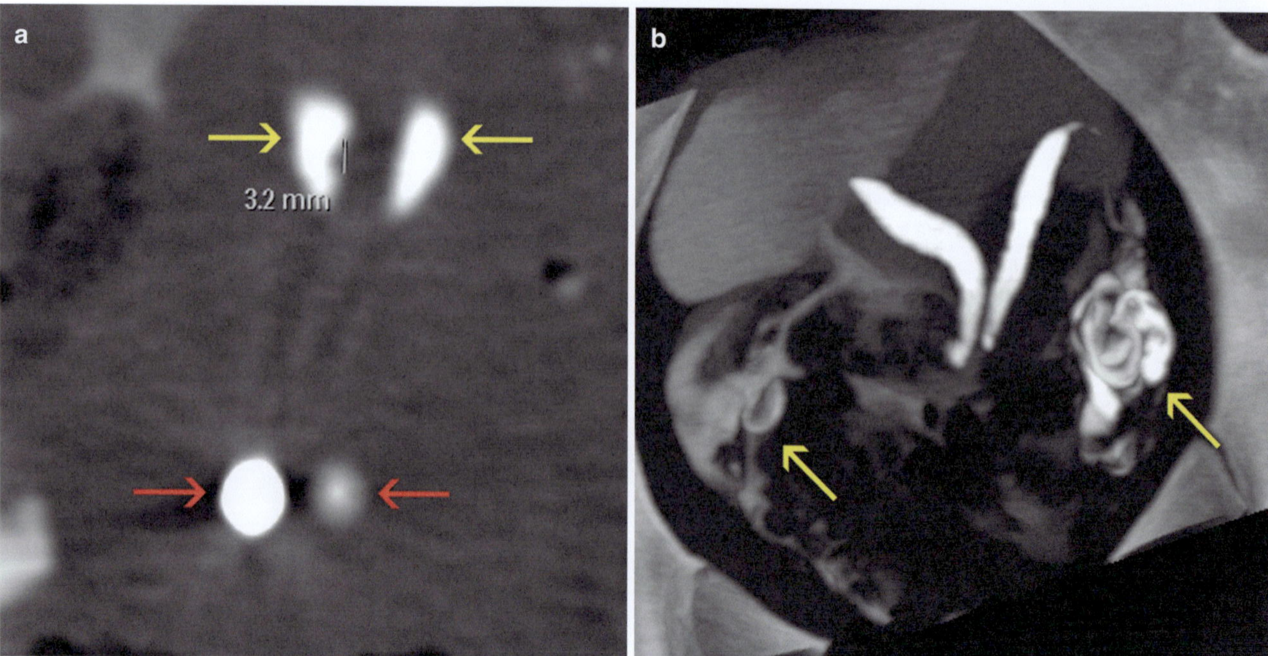

Fig. 8.8 Uterus didelphys with endometrial polyps. VHSG. (**a**) Axial CT image with soft tissue window showing two cervical regions (*red arrows*) and two uterine hemicavities (*yellow arrows*). The right hemicavity presents a polyp of 3.2 mm. (**b**) Axial maximum intensity projection image. Two non-communicated uterine hemicavities. Both tubes are permeable (*arrows*). (**c**) Coronal 3D volume rendering image. Two filling defects can be observed in the right horn compatible with endometrial polyps (*arrows*). (**d, e**) Axial T2 weighted MRI images with and without fat suppression exhibiting the uterus didelphys. However the polyps observed through VHSG cannot be found due to the reduced space resolution of the MRI. (**f**) Coronal T2 weighted MRI image showing two non-communicated uterine hemicavities (*arrows*)

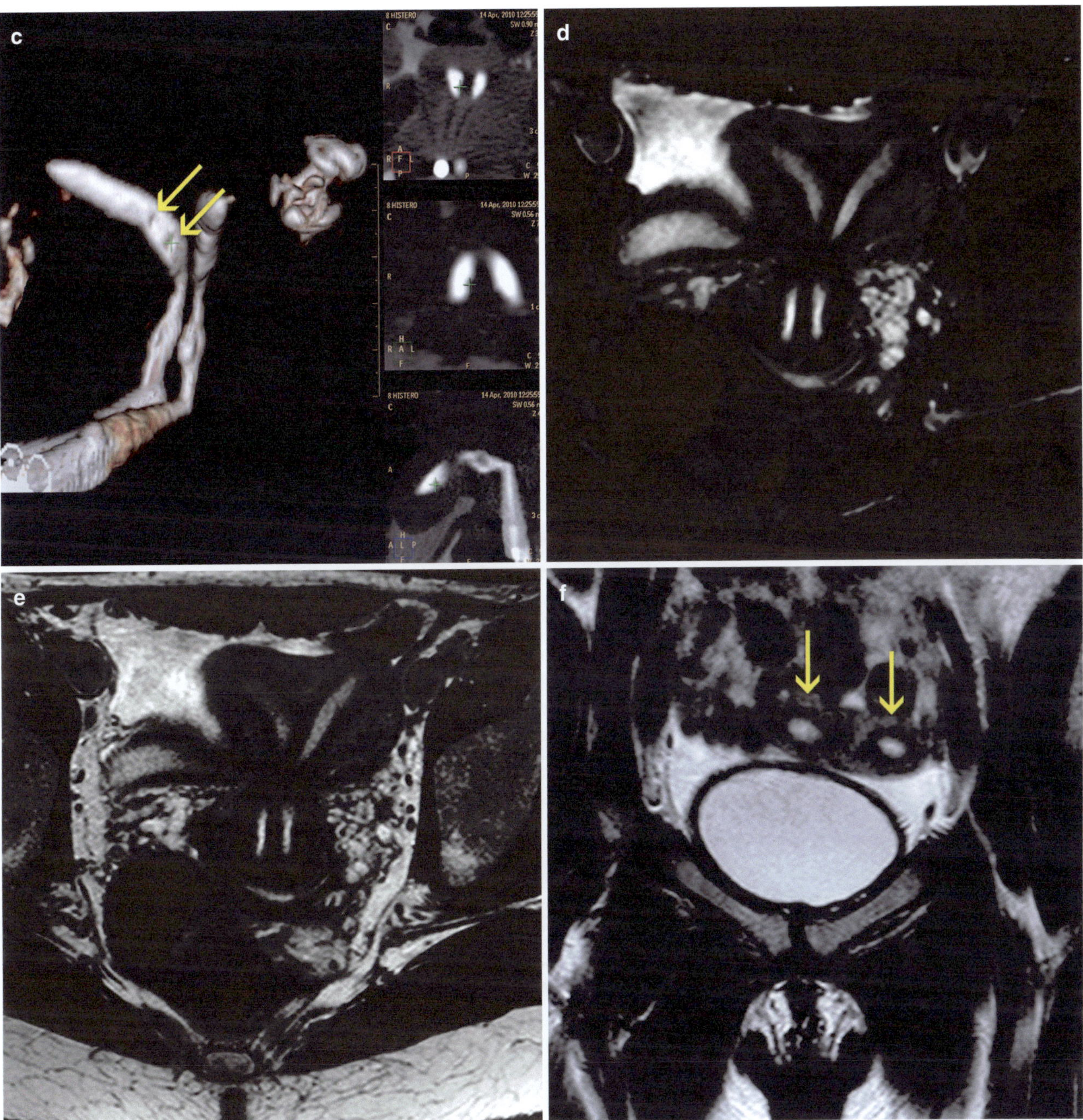

Fig. 8.8 (continued)

MR: provides information of the external myometrial wall, showing the typical morphology with indentation of the fundus larger than 1 cm (Fig. 8.13).

VHSG: This new diagnostic modality is extremely useful in the study of uterine anomalies; this is because it evaluates the uterus lumen as well as uterus wall (Figs. 8.14 and 8.15). In this way is possible to, characterize the uterine anomaly with high diagnostic precision and also evaluate the presence of endoluminal pathologies that may be associated (Figs. 8.16 and 8.17).

VHSG utilizes different forms of bidimensional, tridimensional and endoscopic reconstructions for the diagnosis and classification of uterine malformations.

Bidimensional reconstructions with a soft tissue window show the endometrial cavities in diverse coronary and sagittal planes as well as the myometrial wall, providing similar findings to those in MR, with the indented uterine myometrium fundus

In this type of reconstruction the presence of associated intraluminal pathologies in the cervix, uterus or tubes

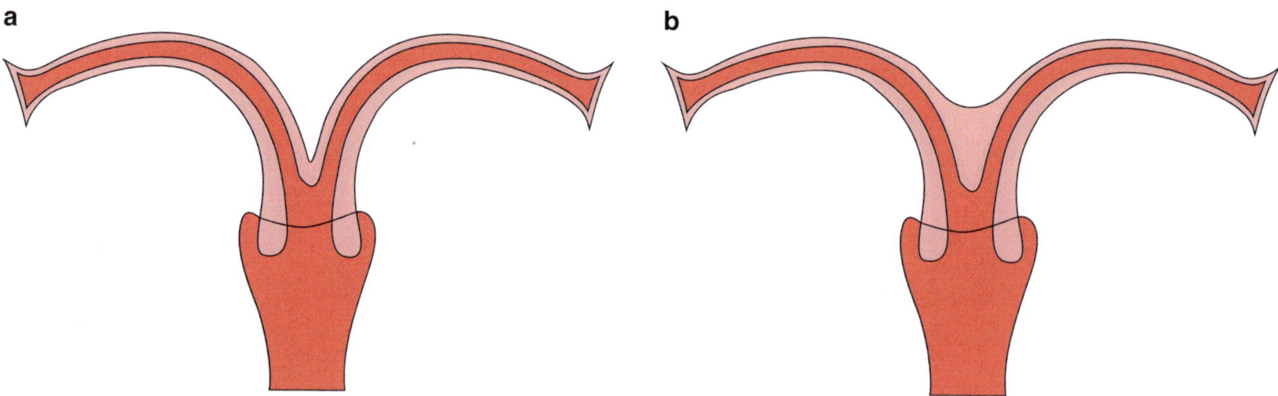

Fig. 8.9 Picture of bicornuate uterus. (**a**) Complete bicornuate uterus. (**b**) Partial bicornuate uterus

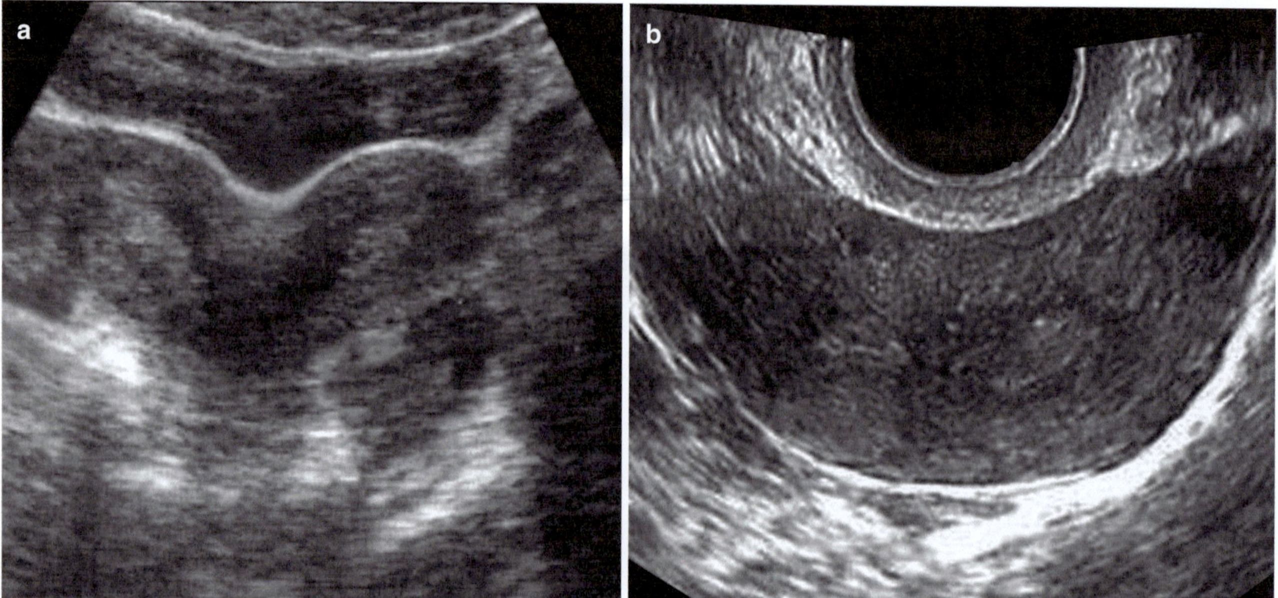

Fig. 8.10 Ultrasound of bicornuate uterus. (**a**) Image showing the typical indentation at the level of the uterine fundus. (**b**) Transverse image showing both endometrial cavities

can be evaluated, like polyps and synechiae among others (Fig. 8.18).

The great space resolution allows the identification of millimetric lesions, offering their exact location.

There exist two different types of tridimensional reconstructions; maximum intensity of projection reconstructions (MIP) and volume rendering reconstructions (VR) (Fig. 8.19).

MIP reconstructions show the uterine morphology, offering similar information to that provided by the HSG but in a tridimensional format. This reconstruction is the one that provides least information.

VR reconstruction is a tridimensional reconstruction that handles windows of opacities and transparencies and allows the reconstruction of the uterus showing the cavity as well as the adjacent myometrial wall. This reconstruction is highly valuable because it exactly defines the type of malformation. Besides, if it identifies associated intraluminal pathology

Virtual endoscopic images show the endocervical and endouterine lumen (Fig. 8.20). There is an alteration in the normal morphology of the uterine fundus However, due to this type of reprocessing, the differentiation between a septate and a bicornuate uterus is not possible. Virtual views also put on evidence the associated intraluminal pathology.

In Fig. 8.21, examples are shown of bicornuate uteruses with associated pathologies visualized through VHSG but not through MR. In Fig. 8.22, and example of a bicornuate uterus is observed through HSG, MR and VHSG.

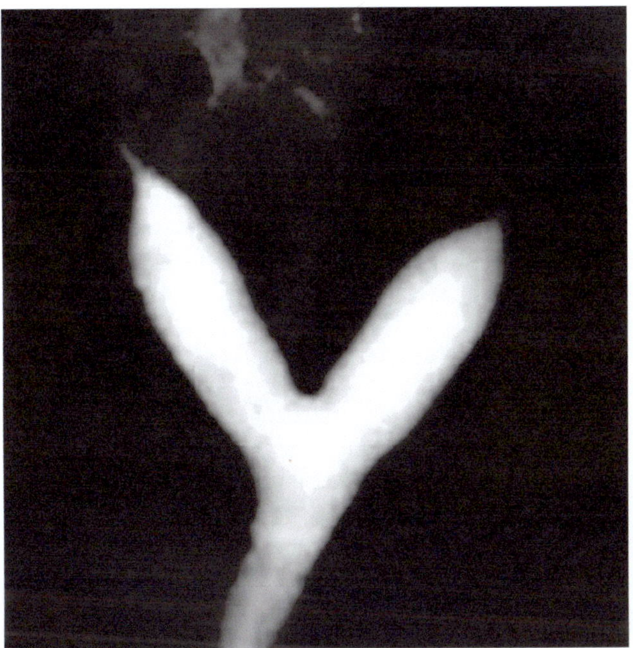

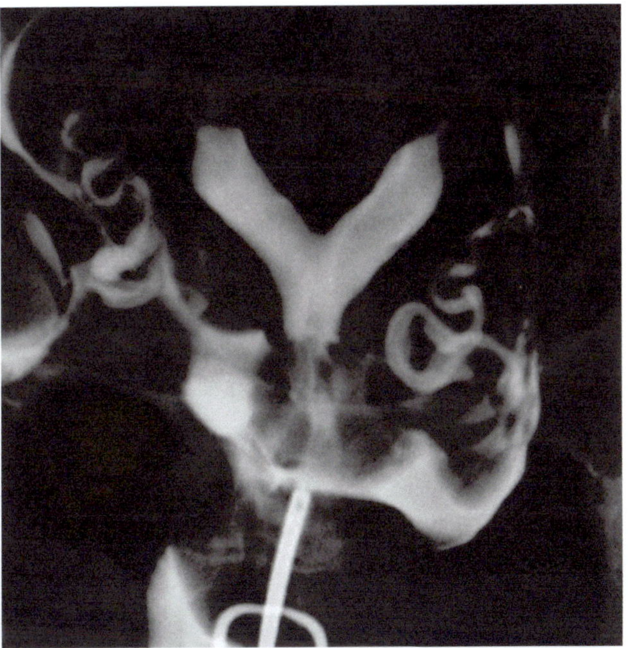

Fig. 8.11 HSG of bicornuate uterus. The separation of both uterine horns is > 105°, typical of this uterine anomaly

Fig. 8.12 HSG of bicornuate uterus. The typical separation of both uterine horns and the two Fallopian tubes are illustrated

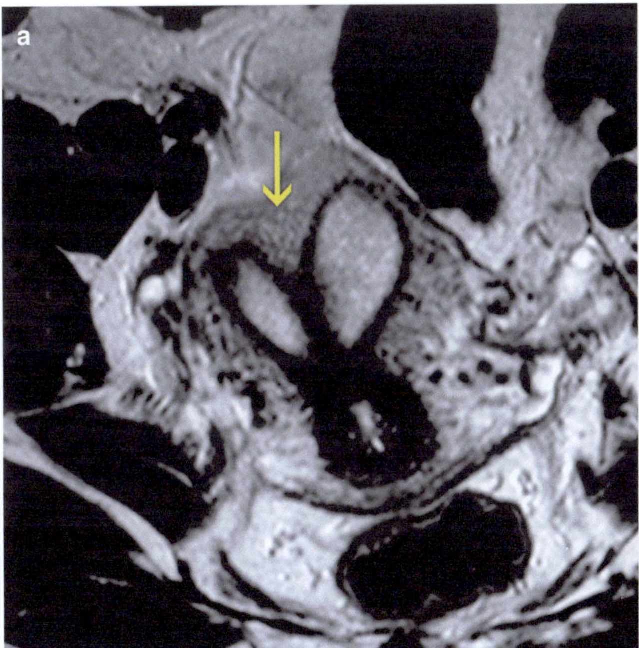

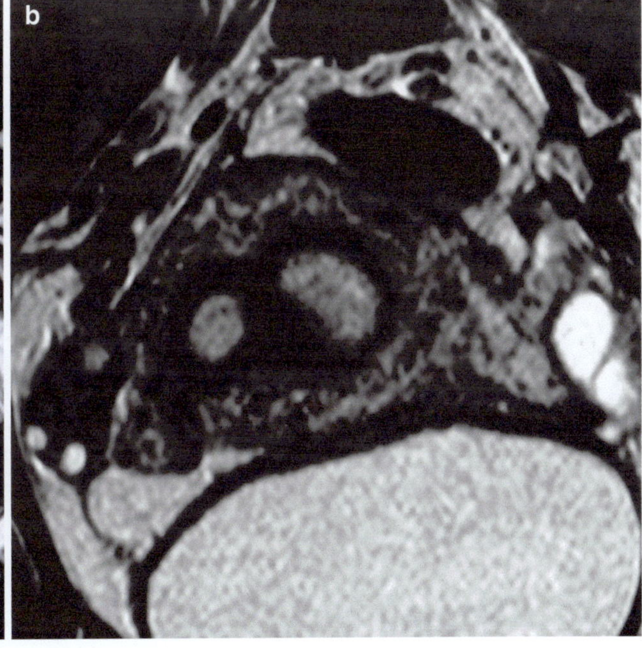

Fig. 8.13 MRI of bicornuate uterus. (**a**) Axial T2 weighted MRI image showing a bicornuate uterus. The depression of the myometrial wall with the typical indentation can be observed at the uterine fundus (*arrow*). (**b**) Coronal T2 weighted MRI image. Both uterine horns with asymmetric sizes are illustrated

Arcuate Uterus

An arcuate uterus is characterized by a mild indentation at the level of the medial sector of the endometrium in the area of the uterine fundus.

In the original classification of Buttram and Gibbons it was considered as a subclassification of the bicornuate uterus in a slight variant. In the arcuate uterus a relation of more than 10 % must exist between the height of the indentation of the depth with the distance between the two apices of the uterine horns (Fig. 8.23).

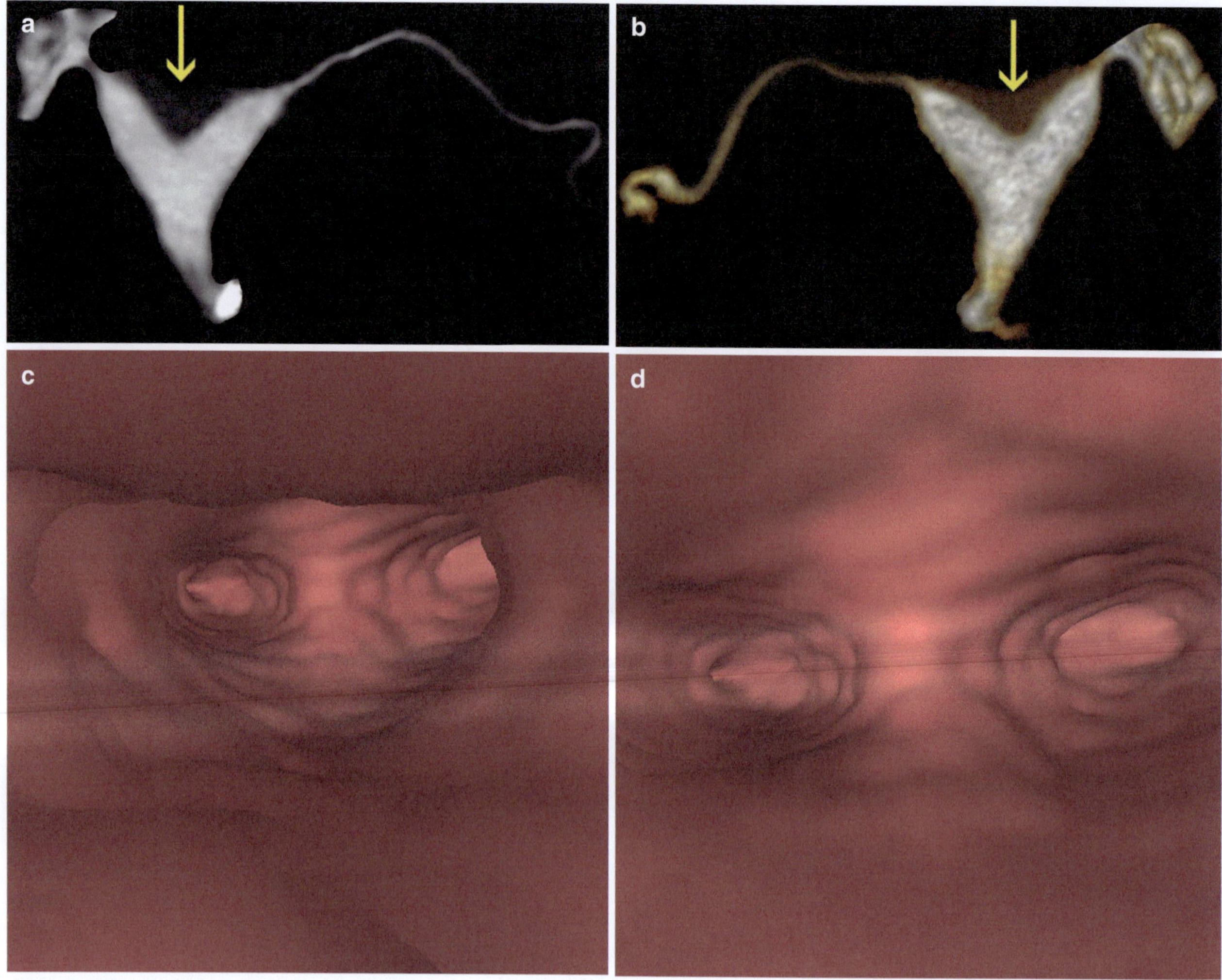

Fig. 8.14 VHSG of bicornuate uterus. (**a, b**) Coronal maximum intensity projection and 3D volume rendering images showing the uterine morphology, with an indentation at the uterine fundus (*arrows*). (**c, d**) Virtual endoscopic views

Diagnostic methods like HSG, MR and VHSG allow a correct evaluation of this type of uterus:

HSG: shows a uterus with normal morphology with an indented fundus (Fig. 8.24).

MR: shows a uterine outline slightly indented with an isointense signal to the normal myometrium (Fig. 8.25). No hypointense areas related to fibrous tissue are detected.

VHSG: allows the identification of the normal uterine morphology with the typical indentation of the fundus (Fig. 8.26). At the same time, it detects associated pathology (Fig. 8.27).

Septated Uterus

The septated uterus is the most frequent anomaly (55 %) and corresponds to the partial or complete non absorption of the utero-vaginal septum (Fig. 8.28).

It associates with poor reproductive chances with a high rate of abortions (26–94 %) and premature deliveries (9–33 %).

The elevated rate of abortions is attributed to the fibrous and vascular composition of the septum. Some theories support that the least bit of connective tissue of the septum could influence in a poor implantation of the embryo, while the rise in muscular tissue could result in an increase in the contractility of the tissue, predisposing the patient to spontaneous abortions. To this is added a smaller size of the uterine cavity at the expense of the septum. The vascularization of the septum is also abnormal.

The septated uterus can be complete when the septum begins in the fundus on the middle line and reaches the external cervical orifice. In 25 % of cases it can extend to the upper margin of the vagina. In partially septated uterus the septum has variable length.

The external morphology of the uterus can be convex, straight or slightly concave (<1.0 cm). The external

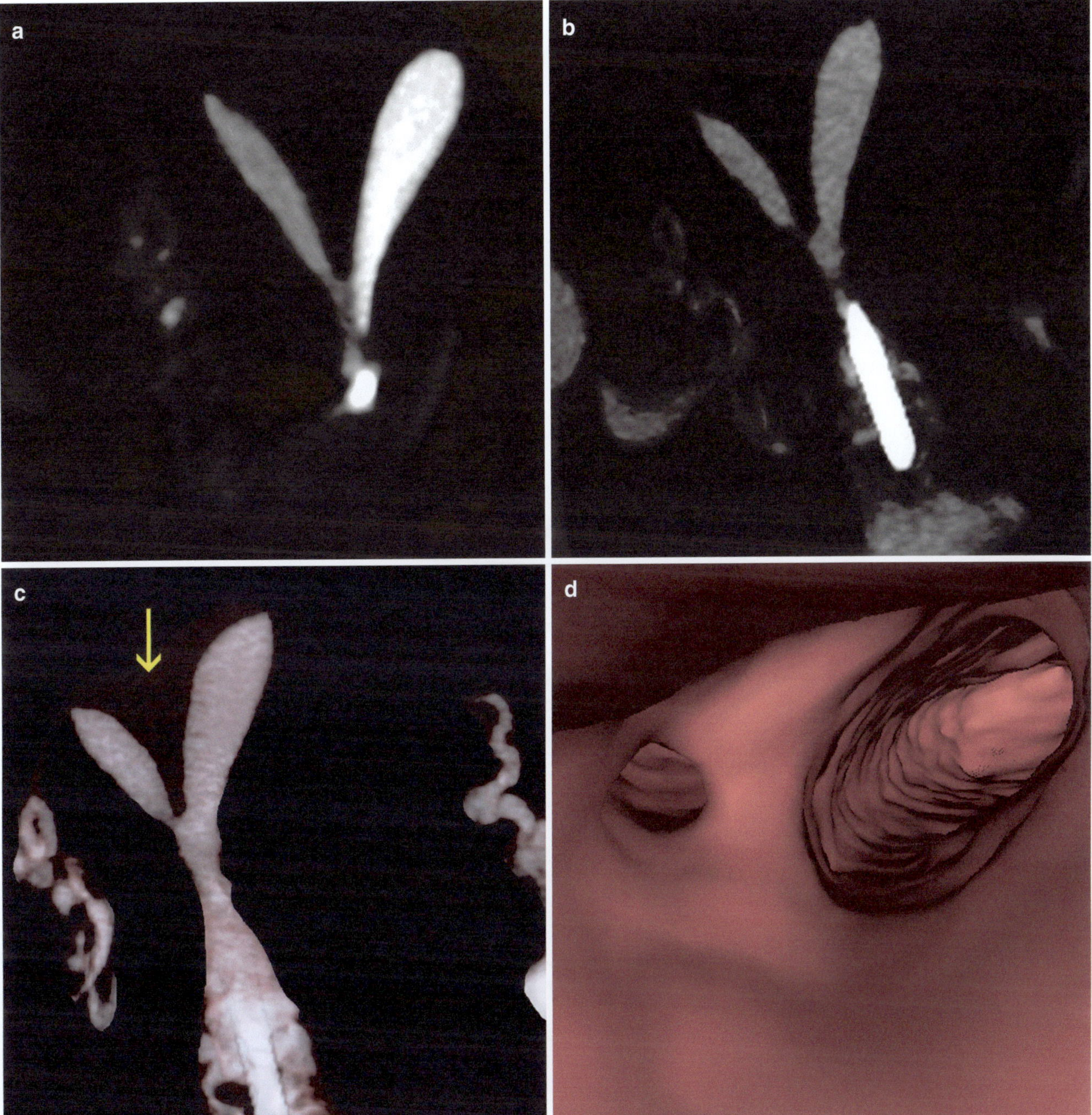

Fig. 8.15 VHSG of bicornuate uterus and its correlation with HSG. (**a**) Thick-slab coronal multiplanar reconstruction image showing the morphology of a uterine cavity with two horns. (**b**) Coronal maximum intensity projection image illustrating similar findings. (**c**) Coronal 3D volume rendering image exhibiting the morphology of the myometrial wall with the typical indentation (*arrow*). (**d**) Virtual endoscopic view illustrating the uterine horns, which have an asymmetric lumen. (**e, f**) HSG images exhibiting exclusively the morphology of the uterine cavity

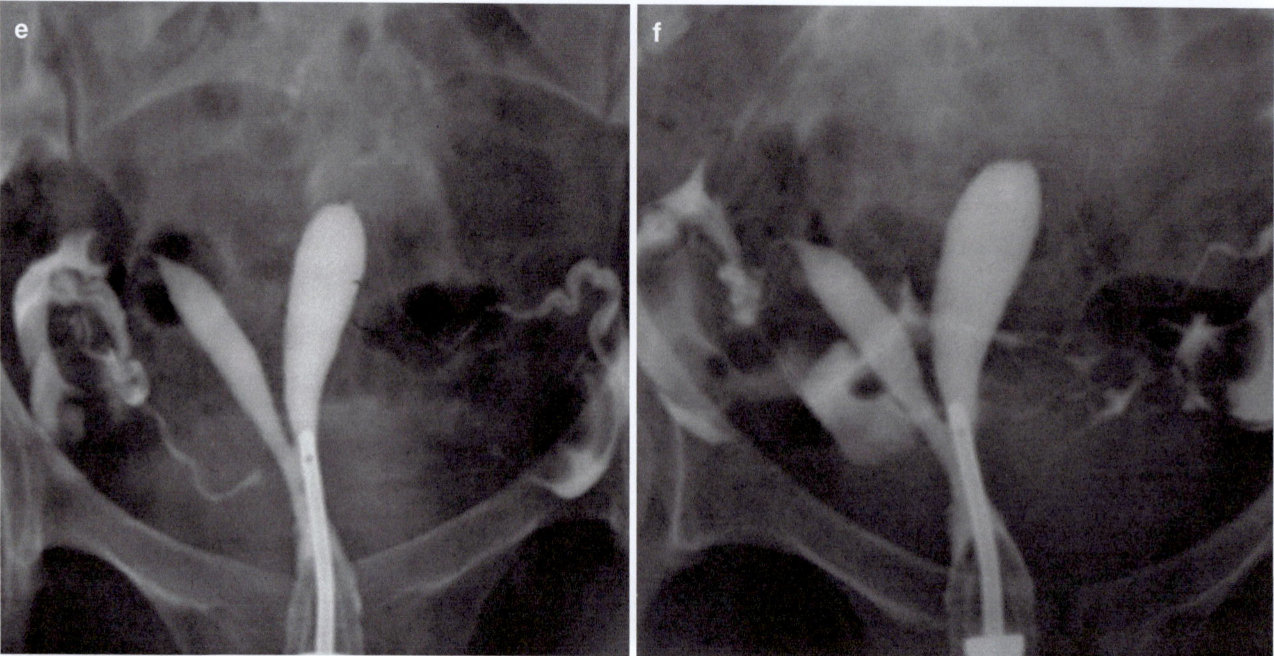

Fig. 8.15 (continued)

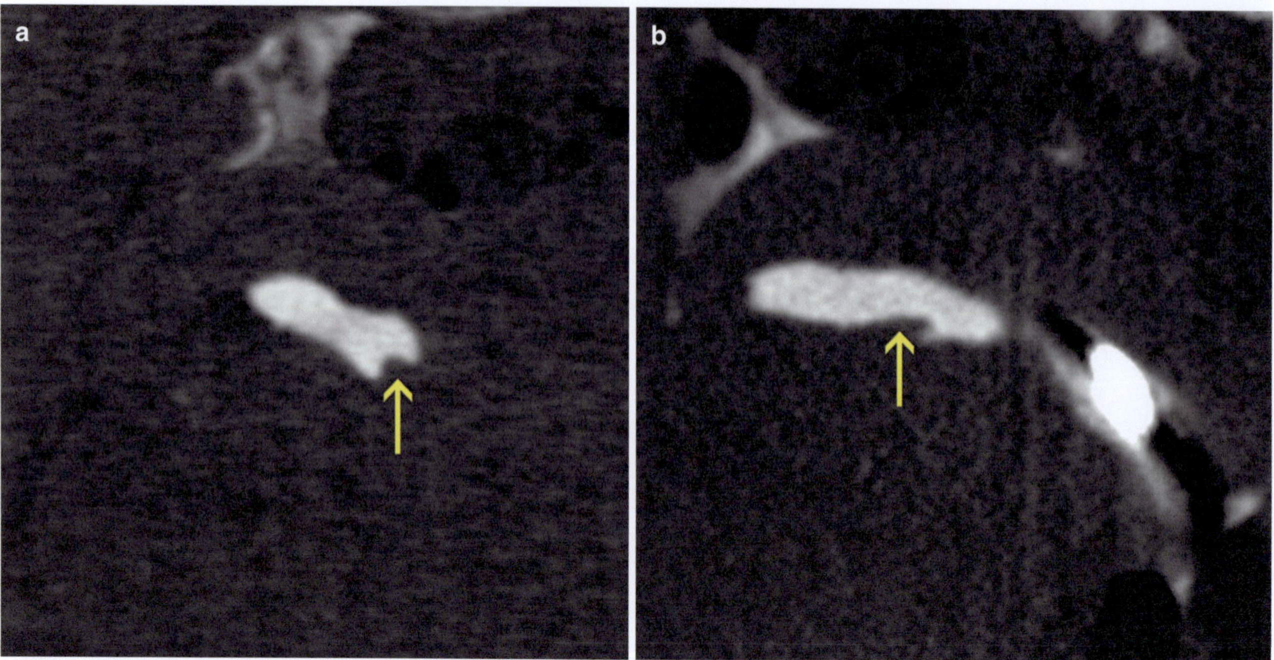

Fig. 8.16 VHSG of bicornuate uterus with the presence of endometrial polyp. (**a**, **b**) Coronal and sagittal multiplanar reconstruction images with soft tissue window showing endometrial polyps (*arrows*). (**c**) Coronal maximum intensity projection image illustrating a bicornuate uterus. (**d**) Thick-slab (5 mm) coronal multiplanar reconstruction image showing the morphology of the uterine cavity with its two uterine horns. (**e**) Coronal 3D volume rendering image additionally showing a filling defect in the left horn compatible with a polyp (*arrow*). (**f**) Virtual endoscopic image

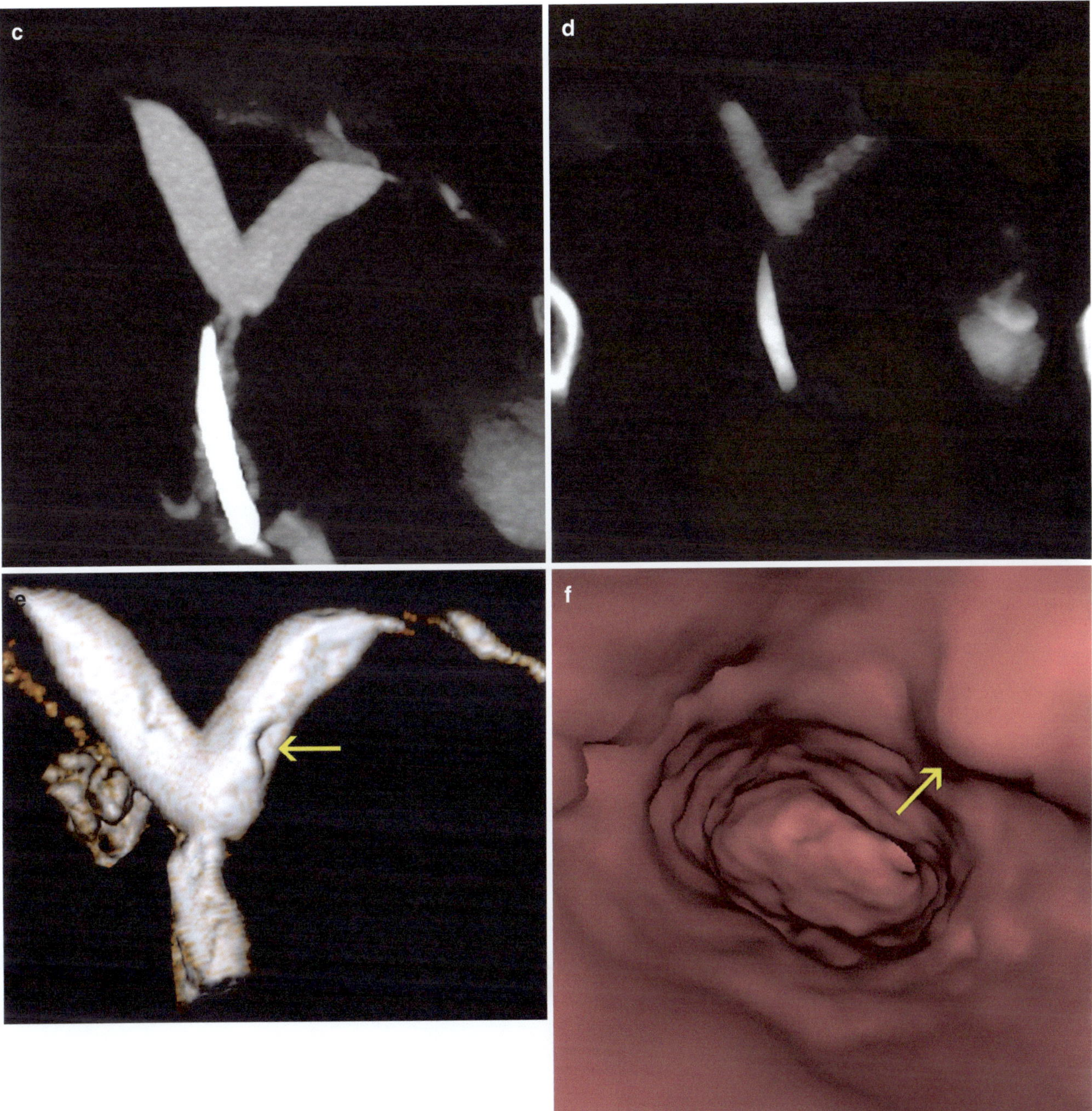

Fig. 8.16 (continued)

configuration of the uterine margin is crucial to differentiate it from the bicornuate uterus.

Diverse diagnostic methods (US, HSG, MR, VHSG) offer specific information.

Ultrasound: In this method the separation of the endometrial cavities by a myometrial tissue with intermediate echogenicity is observed.

In uteruses with complete septum, the inferior segment presents hypoechogenicity due to the fibrous component.

The external myometrial morphology must show a convex, straight or slightly convex shape. This sometimes results difficult to diagnose with this modality.

A line must be drawn that passes through both uterine horns as well as a myometrial indentation in the fundus >5 mm must exist below the interostial line.

HSG: permits the evaluation of the size and extension of the septum.

The diagnostic precision to differentiate between a septated and bicornuate uterus is of 55 %.

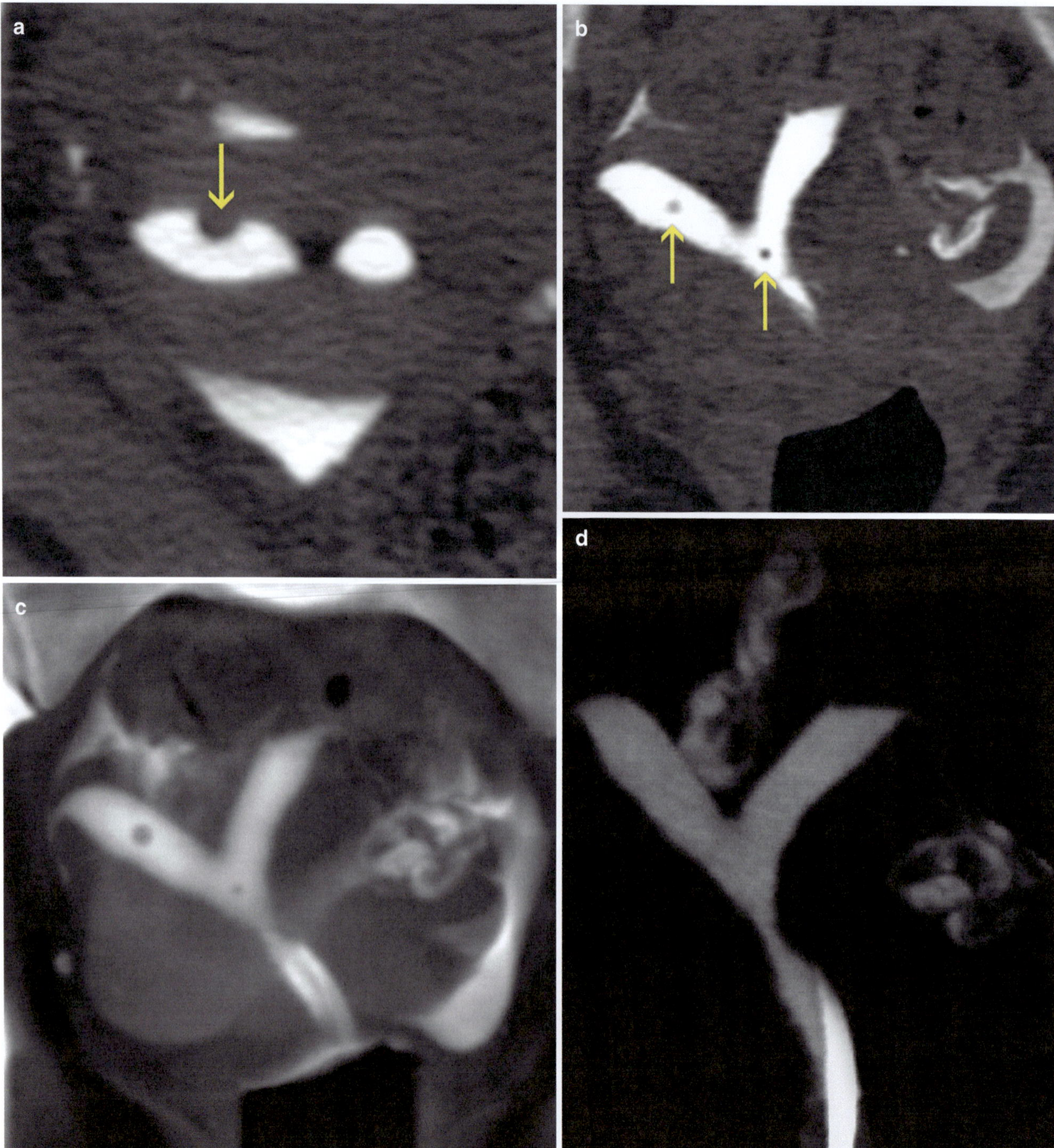

Fig. 8.17 VHSG of bicornuate uterus with multiple polyps. (**a**) Axial CT image with soft tissue window showing a polyp in the right uterine horn (*arrow*). (**b**) Coronal multiplanar reconstruction (MPR) image with soft tissue window illustrating two elevated lesions in the right horn (*arrows*). (**c**) Coronal MPR image of 5 mm exhibiting similar findings. (**d**) Coronal maximum intensity projection image. This type of reconstruction has difficulty in identifying the endoluminal lesions. However it clearly shows the uterine morphology. (**e**, **f**) 3D volume rendering images showing three-dimensionally the uterus with two filling defects compatible with polyps (*arrows*)

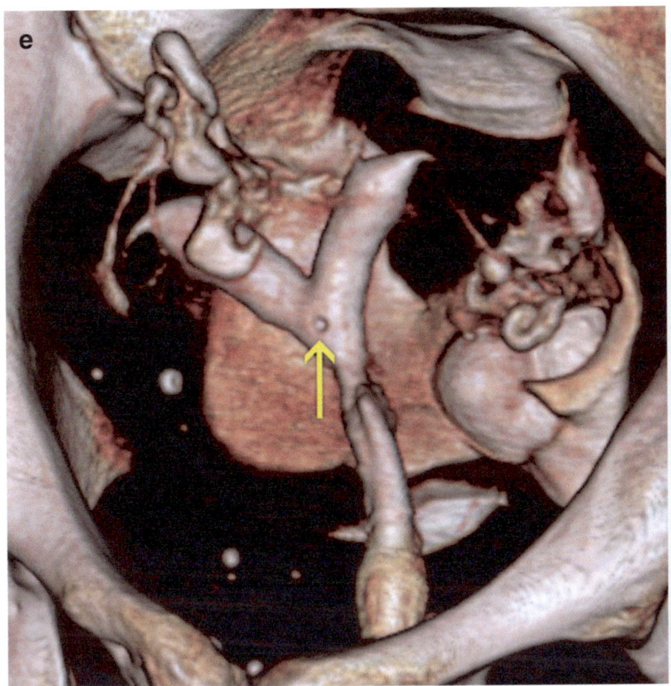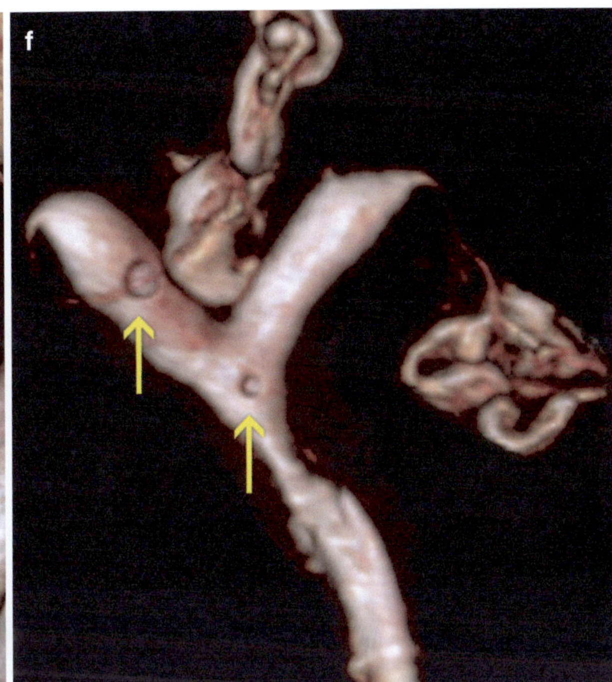

Fig. 8.17 (continued)

An angle <75° between both horns suggests a septated uterus (Fig. 8.29). While if that angle is >105°, it most probably is a bicornuate uterus. However, these measurements can be superposing each other in both pathologies. An intercornual distance <4 cm suggests a septated uterus.

With regards to the treatment, a resection of the septum through hysteroscopy is indicated. This increases the rates of births and reduces the number of abortions.

MR: In this method the uterus is seen with a normal size. However each endometrial cavity appears smaller.

The signal of the septum is isointense with respect to the fundus and lateral walls.

The MR allows the proper visualization of the uterine fundus (Fig. 8.30).

VHSG: This new diagnostic modality is extremely useful in the evaluation of the uterine anomalies due to the fact that it permits intraluminal observation as well as the wall (Figs. 8.31 and 8.32). In this way VHSG can characterize the uterine anomaly with a high diagnostic precision at the same time that it evaluates for the existence of associated endoluminal pathologies (Fig. 8.33).

VHSG utilizes different forms of bidimensional, tridimensional and endoscopic reconstructions for the diagnosis and classification of uterine malformations.

Bidimensional reconstruction with window of soft parts permits the visualization of the endometrial cavities in diverse coronary and sagittary planes. At the same time it provides exact information of the myometrial wall showing,

in the case of a septated uterus, a concave uterine contour (Fig. 8.34).

In this type of reconstruction the presence of associated intraluminal pathologies is also evaluated at the level of the cervix, uterus or tubes Polyps and synechiae are examples among others.

The great space resolution of this new modality permits the identification of millimetric lesions providing their exact location.

Tridimensional reconstructions complement the diagnosis, although VR reconstructions are more useful as they offer information on the lumen and the wall (Fig. 8.35).

Virtual endoscopic images show the endocervical and endouterine lumen. An alteration of the normal morphology of the uterine fundus is observed, it is not possible to differentiate a septated uterus from a bicornuate one (Fig. 8.36). The virtual views also emphasize the associated intraluminal pathologies.

A Diethylstilbestrol (DES) Exposition Sequel

A Diethylstilbestrol (DES) exposition sequels occurs in patients that were exposed to synthetic estrogens which can induce myometrial hypertrophy of the fetal uterus with a T shape. An increased risk exists of developing a carcinoma of the vagina. They constitute complex uterine anomalies.

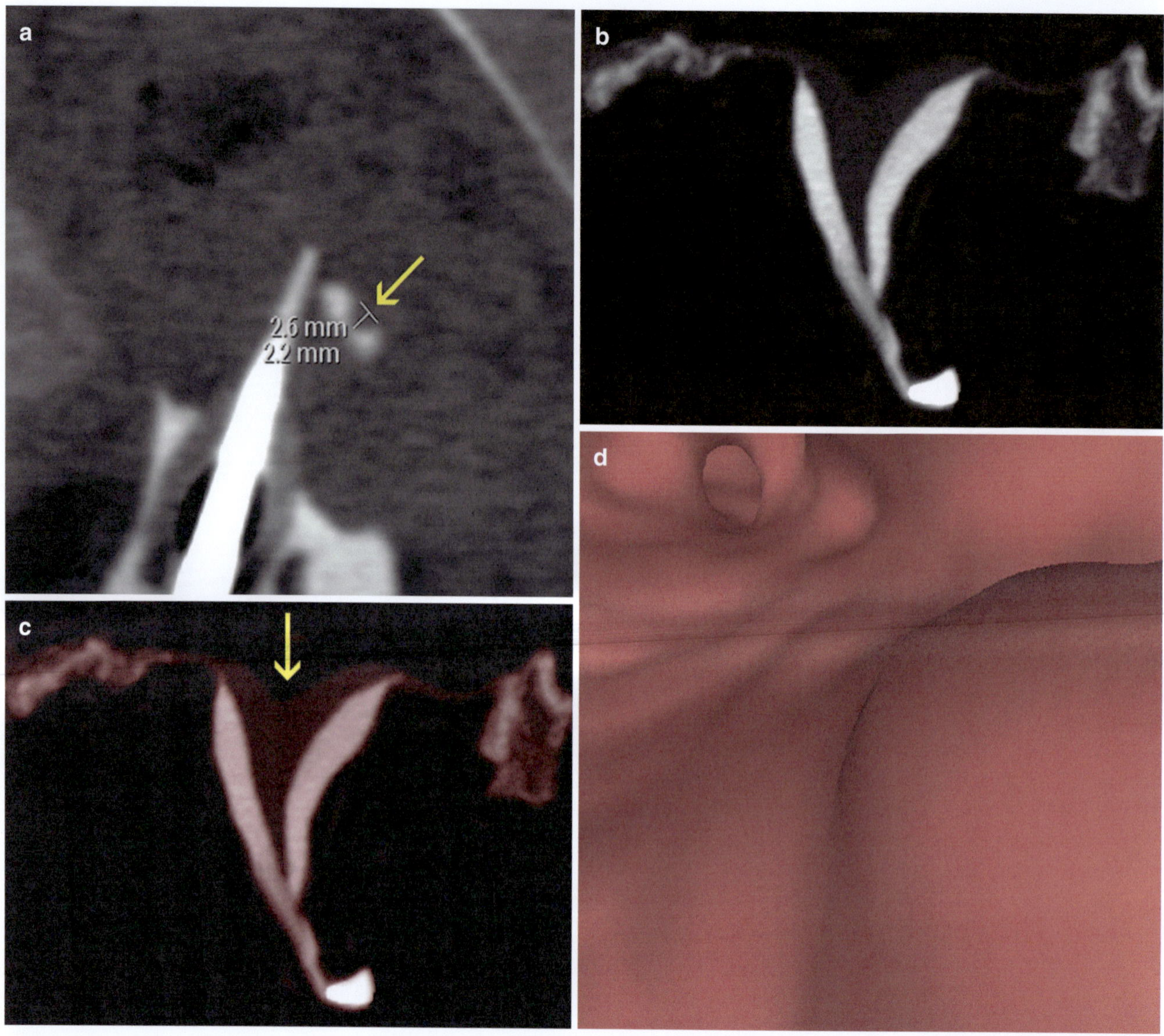

Fig. 8.18 (**a**) Sagittal multiplanar reconstruction image with soft tissue window. A small polyp in the distal cervical canal is observed (*arrow*). (**b**, **c**) Maximum intensity projection and 3D volume rendering images of bicornuate uterus. (**d**) Virtual endoscopic image

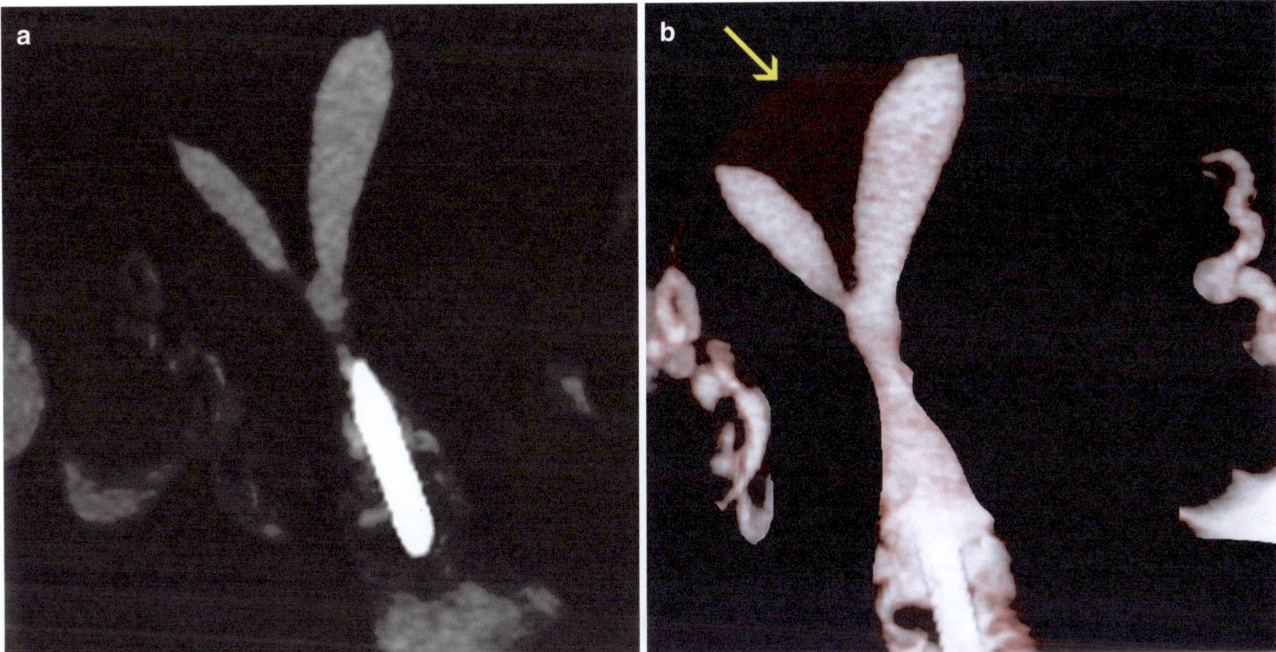

Fig. 8.19 (**a**) Coronal maximum intensity projection image showing a complete bicornuate uterus. (**b**) Coronal 3D volume rendering image also exhibits the myometrial wall (*arrow*)

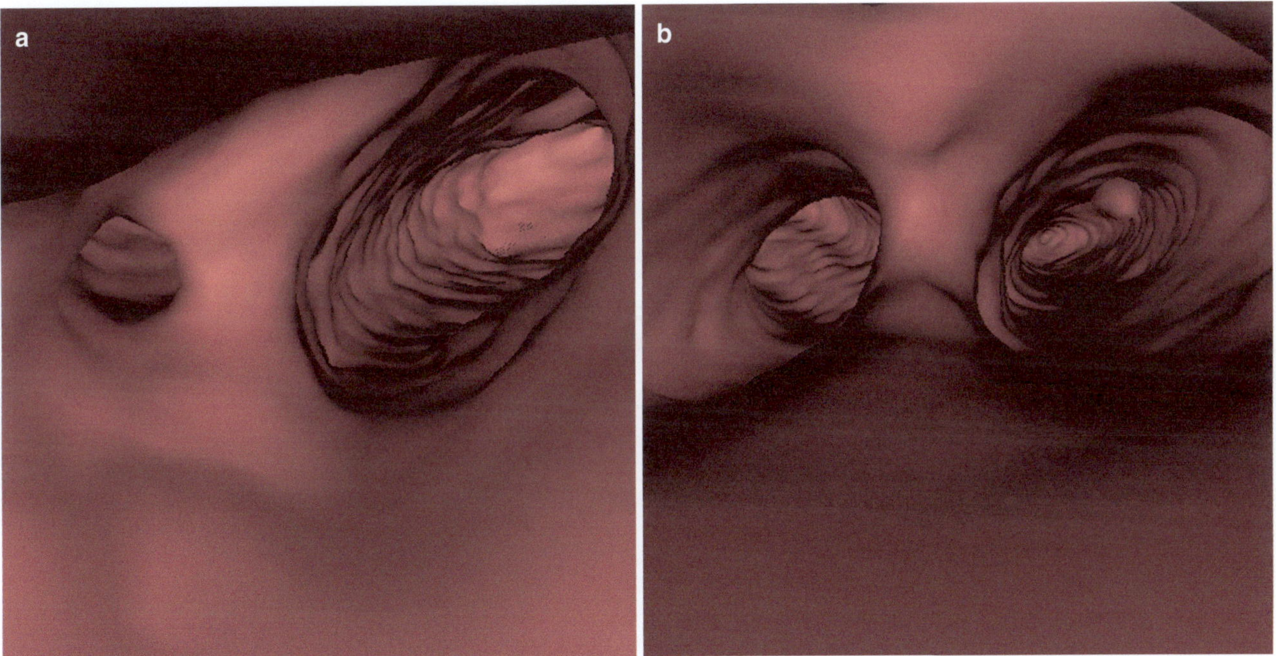

Fig. 8.20 Virtual endoscopic views of bicornuate uterus. (**a**) In this patient, the lumen in both horns is asymmetrical. (**b**) In this case, the lumen in both horns is similar

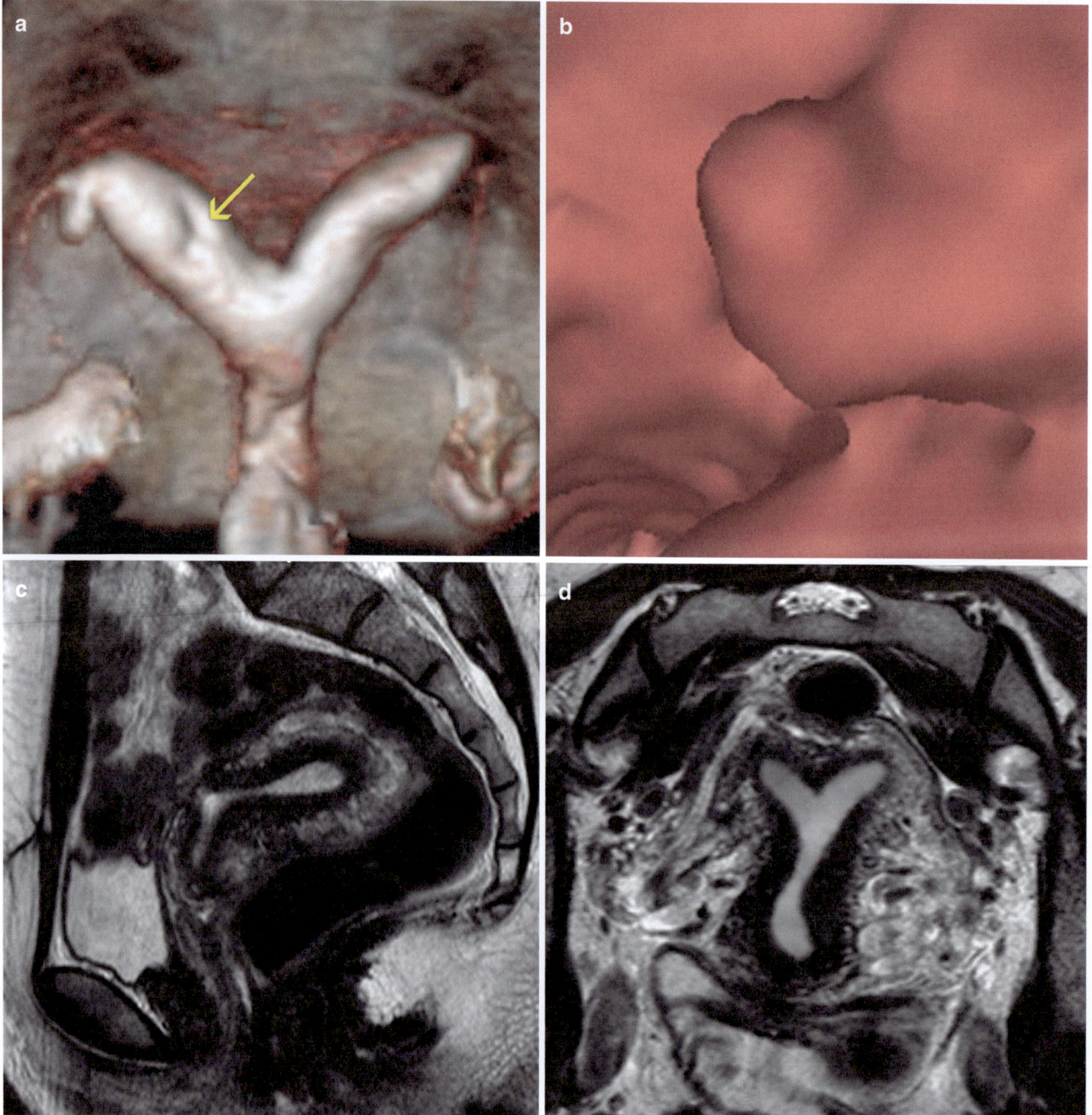

Fig. 8.21 Comparison of bicornuate uterus between VHSG and MRI. (**a**) Coronal 3D volume rendering image with filling defect compatible with a polyp in the right horn (*arrow*). (**b**) Virtual endoscopic image showing the polyp. (**c**) Sagittal T2 weighted MRI image showing a retroverted uterus. (**d**) Axial T2 weighted MRI image which exhibits the morphology of the bicornuate uterus. No polyp is identified

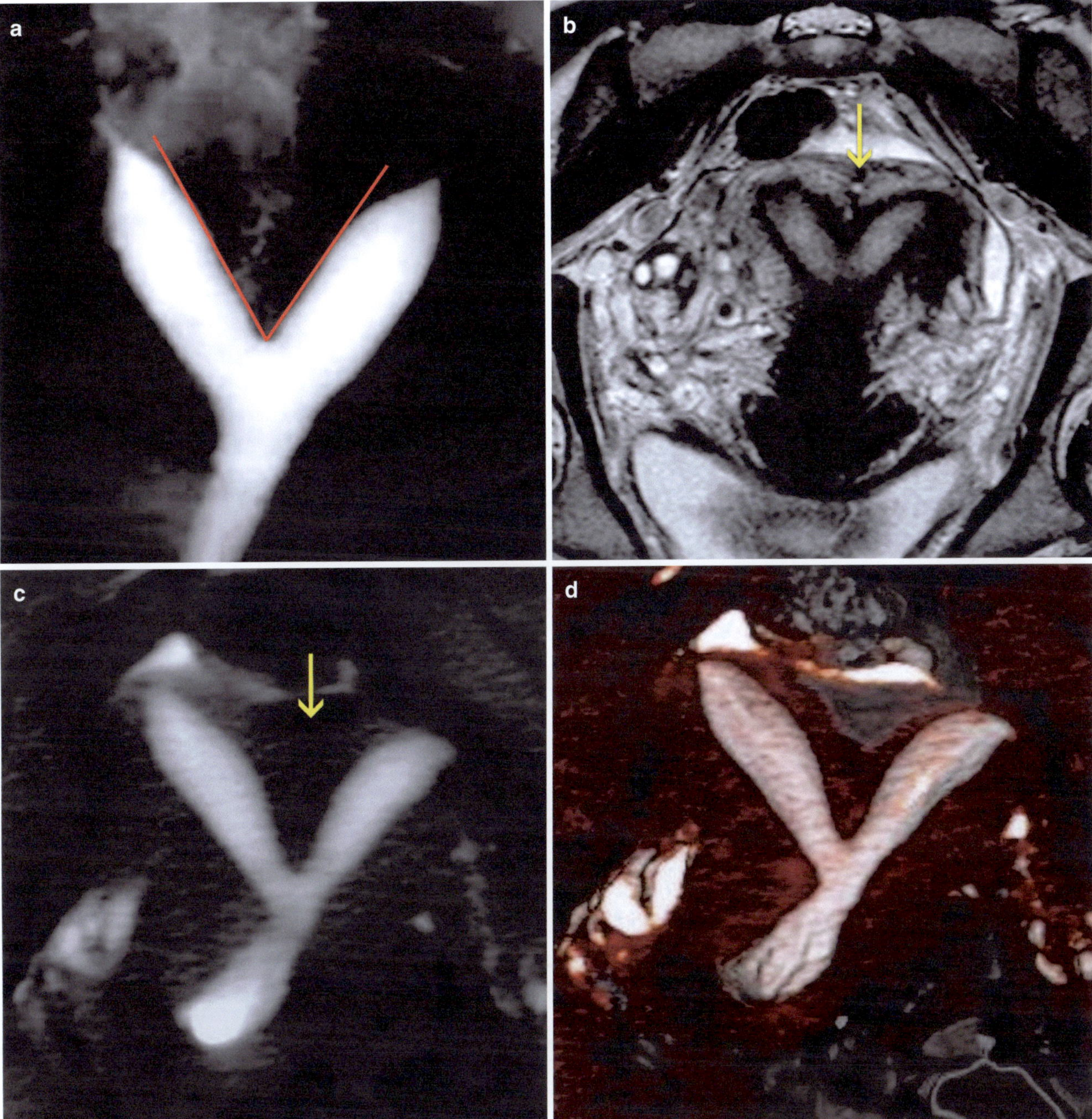

Fig. 8.22 Comparison of bicornuate uterus between HSG, MRI and VHSG. (**a**) HSG. Both uterine horns with an intercornual angle that suggests a bicornuate uterus is observed. (**b**) Axial T2 weighted MRI image. Both uterine horns and the myometrial wall can be observed, which presents a slight indentation in its external margin (*arrow*). (**c**) Thick-slab (5 mm) coronal multiplanar reconstruction image. Similar to MRI, the VHSG permits the evaluation of the miometrium. Slight indentation at the uterine fundus is detected (*arrow*). (**d**) Coronal 3D volume rendering image showing similar findings

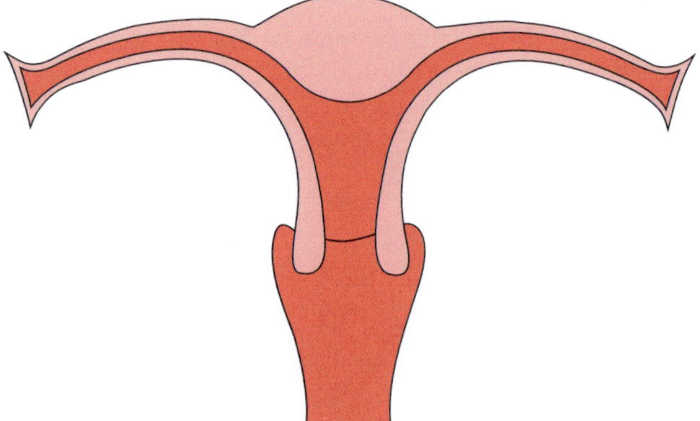

Fig. 8.23 Picture of an arcuate uterus

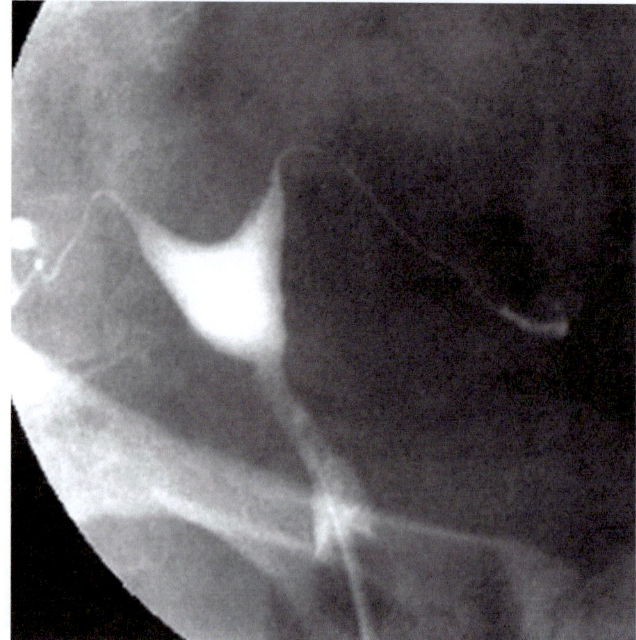

Fig. 8.24 HSG of arcuate uterus

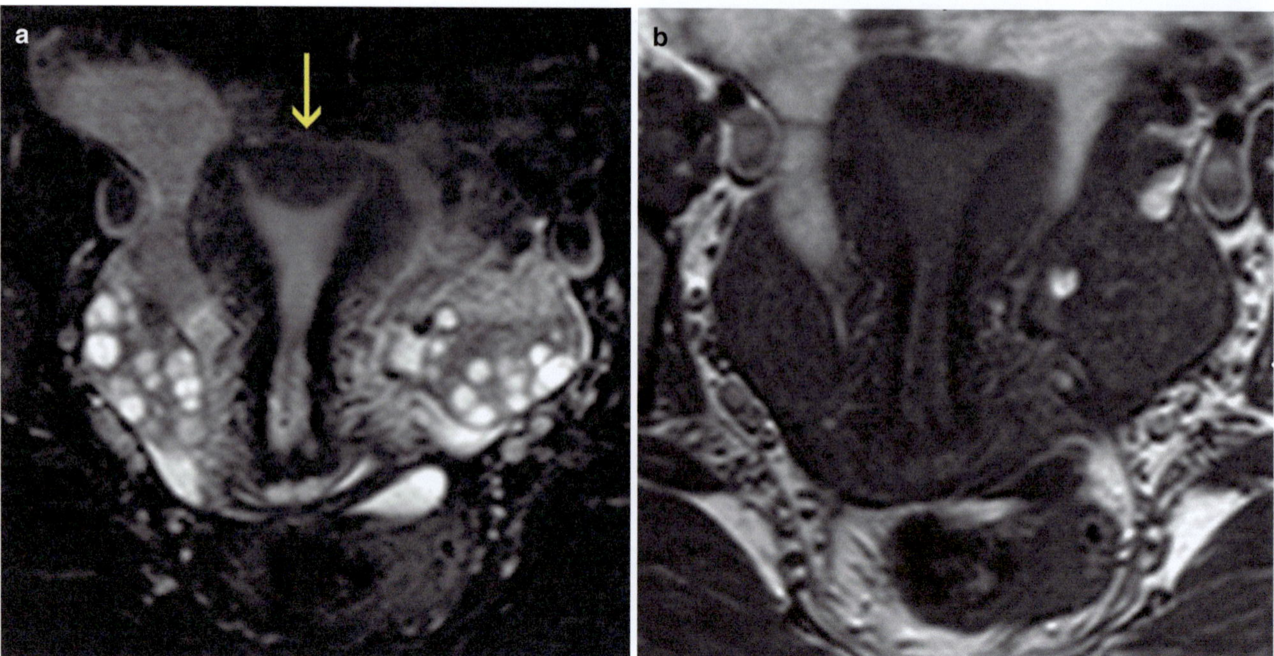

Fig. 8.25 MRI of arcuate uterus. (**a**) Axial T2 weighted MRI image with fat suppression. The endometrial cavity shows a concave shape at the uterine fundus (*arrow*). (**b**) Axial T1 weighted MRI image illustrating similar findings

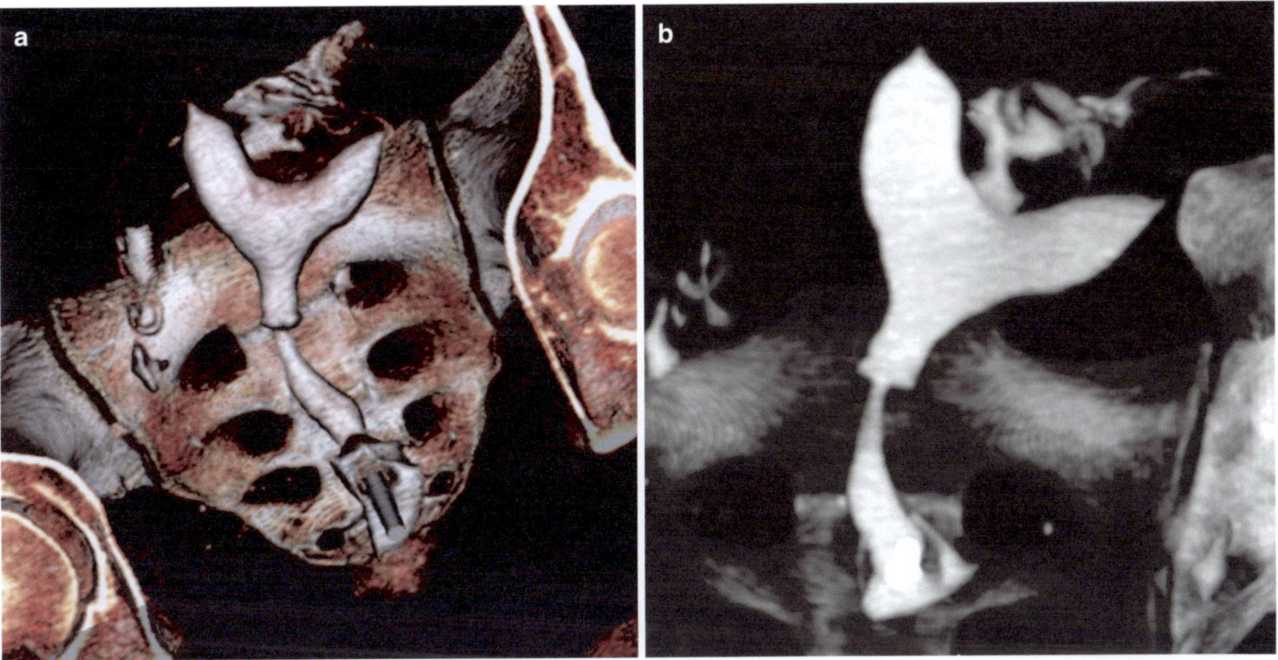

Fig. 8.26 VHSG of a typical arcuate uterus. (**a**) Coronal 3D volume rendering image. (**b**) Coronal maximum intensity projection image illustrating similar findings

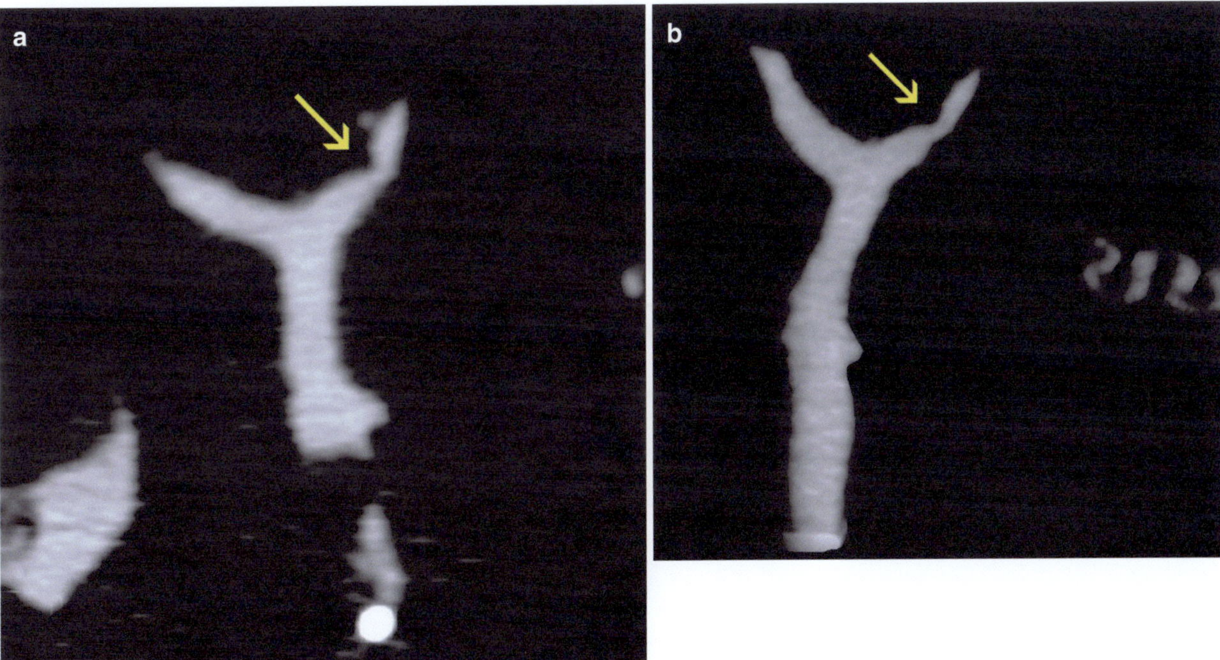

Fig. 8.27 VHSG and MRI of an arcuate uterus. (**a**) VHSG. Axial CT image with soft tissue window showing an arcuate uterus with an endometrial polyp in fundus near the left horn (*arrow*). (**b**) VHSG. Coronal maximum intensity projection image illustrating a focal filling defect in the site of the polyp (*arrow*). (**c**) VHSG. Coronal 3D volume rendering image which exhibits similar findings (*arrow*). (**d, e**) Axial T2 weighted MRI images with and without fat suppression showing the arcuate uterus. The endometrial polyp cannot be identified. (**f**) Axial T1 weighted MRI image. This sequence is useful in the evaluation of the uterine contours

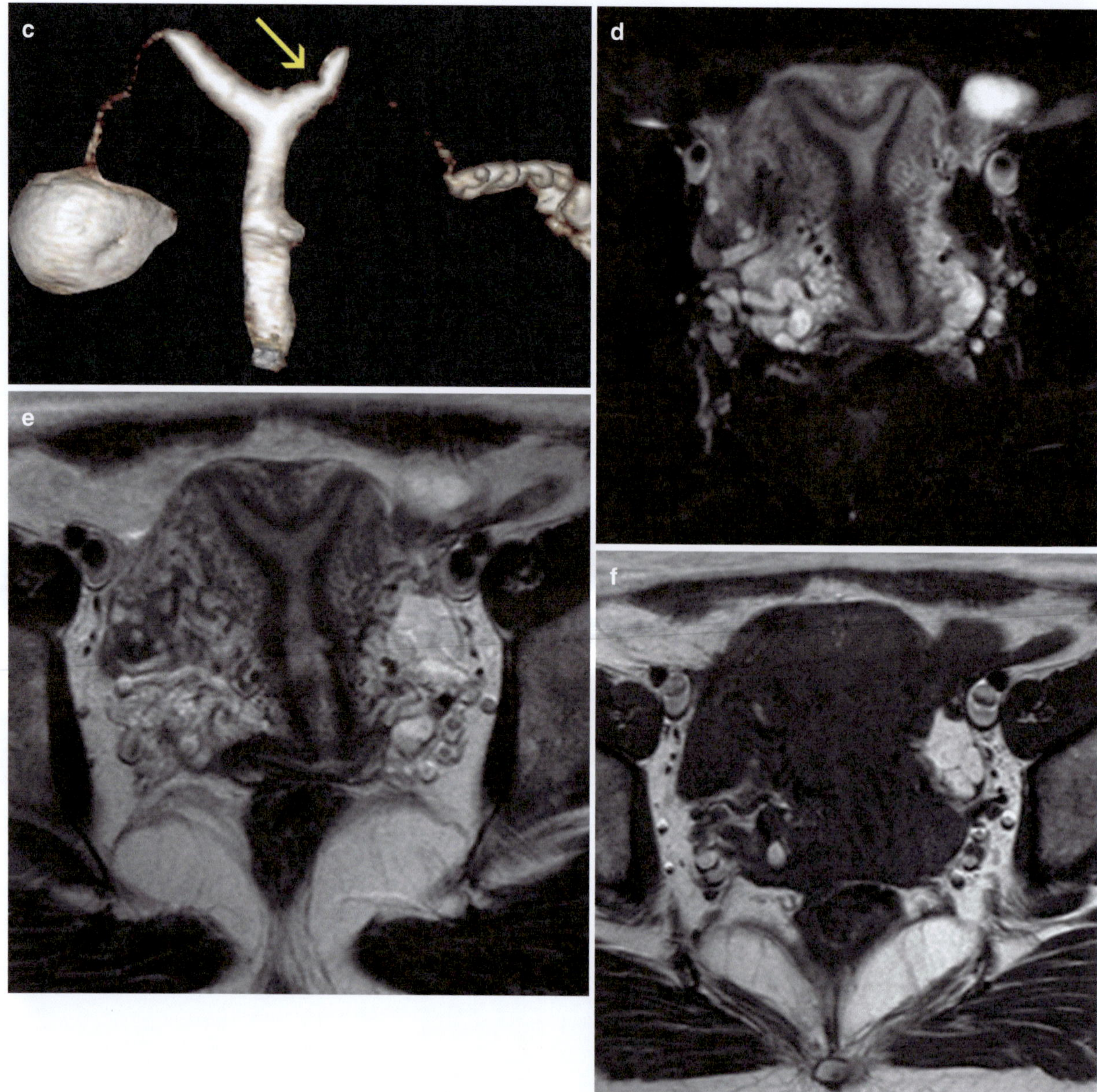

Fig. 8.27 (continued)

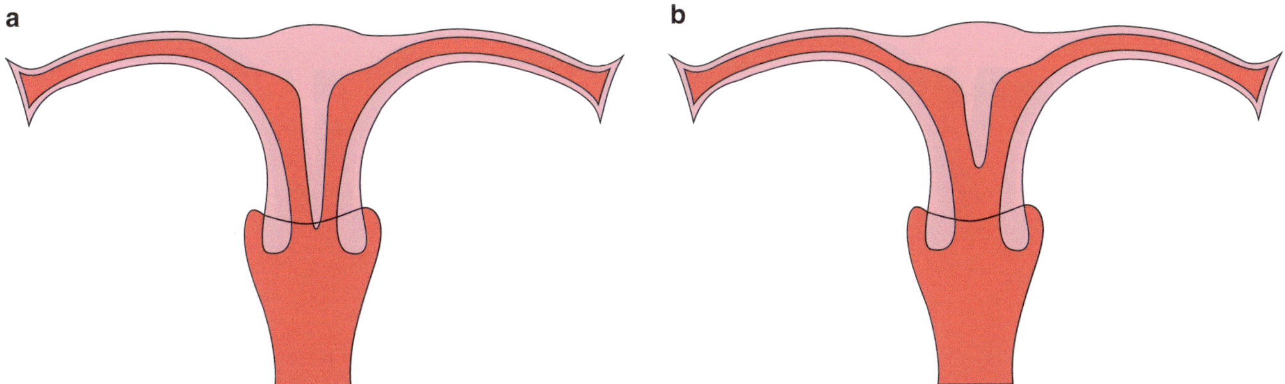

Fig. 8.28 Pictures of septate uterus. (**a**) In a complete septate uterus, a septum extends from the uterine neck to the uterine fundus. (**b**) In a incomplete septate uterus, a septum extends from the medial portion of the endometrial cavity to the uterine fundus

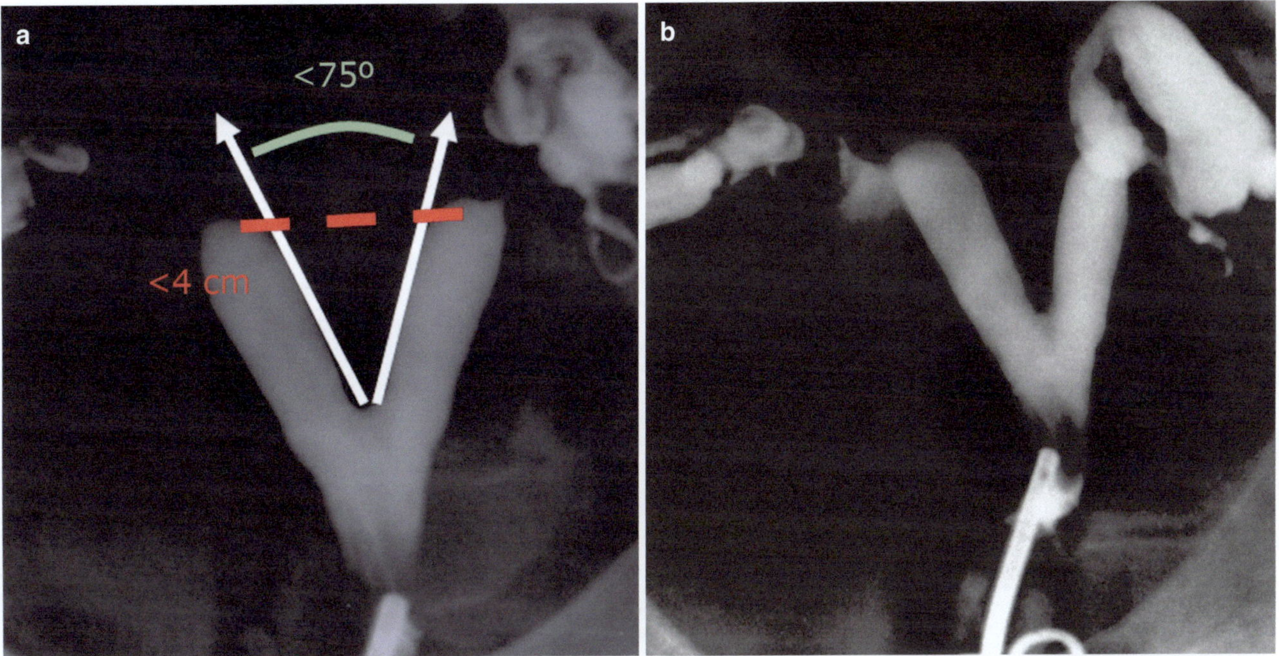

Fig. 8.29 HSG of septate uterus. (**a**) Measurements to diagnose a septate uterus. The intercornual angle must be <75° and the intercornual distance <4 cm. (**b**) Oblique coronal view

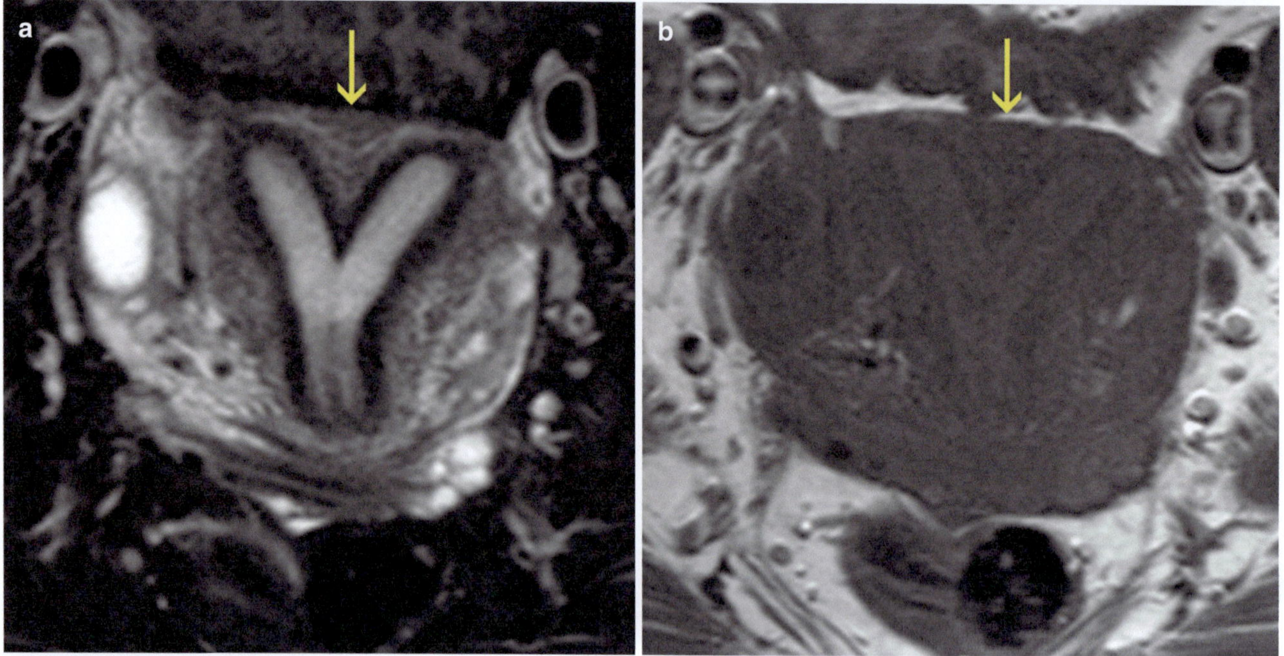

Fig. 8.30 MRI of septate uterus. (**a**) Axial T2 weighted MRI image show two uterine horns and a normal, convex myometrial wall at the uterine fundus (*arrow*). (**b**) Axial T1 weighted MRI image. This sequence is useful to evaluate the morphology of the myometrial wall. The fundal convexity of the uterus is clearly seen (*arrow*)

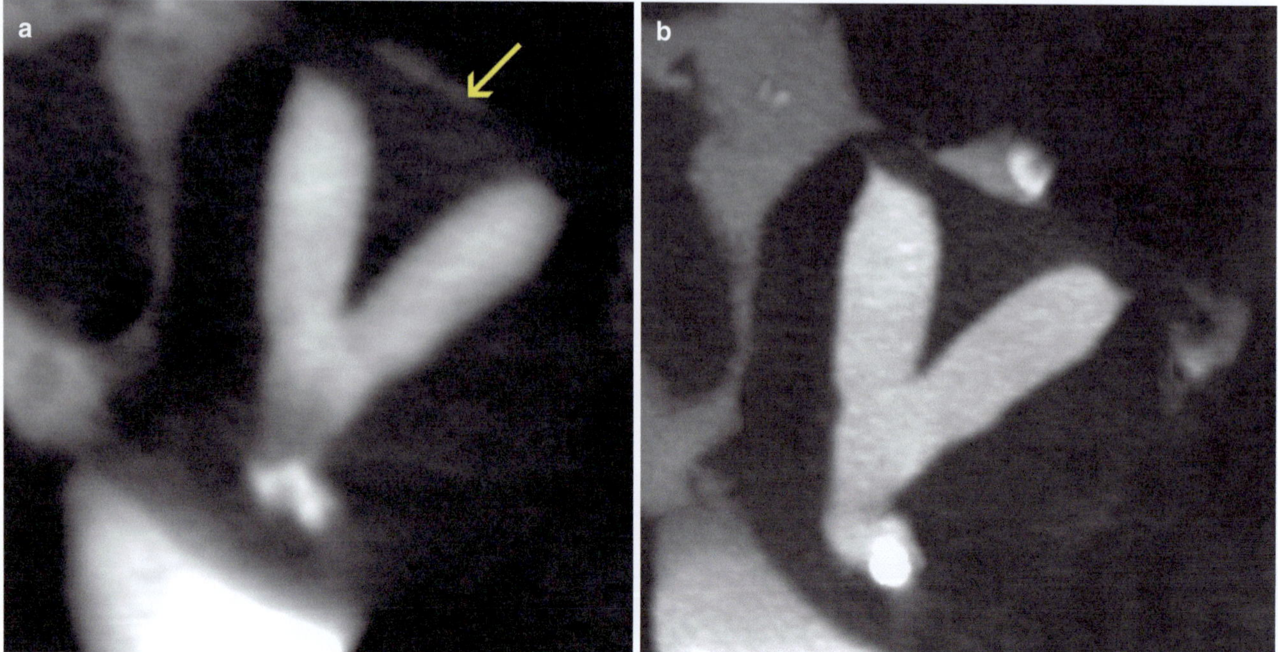

Fig. 8.31 VHSG of septate uterus. (**a**) 10-mm axial CT image with soft tissue window showing the fundal convexity of the uterus (*arrow*). (**b, c**) Coronal maximum intensity projection and 3D volume rendering images showing similar findings. (**d**) Virtual endoscopy image. The septum which divides the endometrial cavity and both uterine horns can be observed

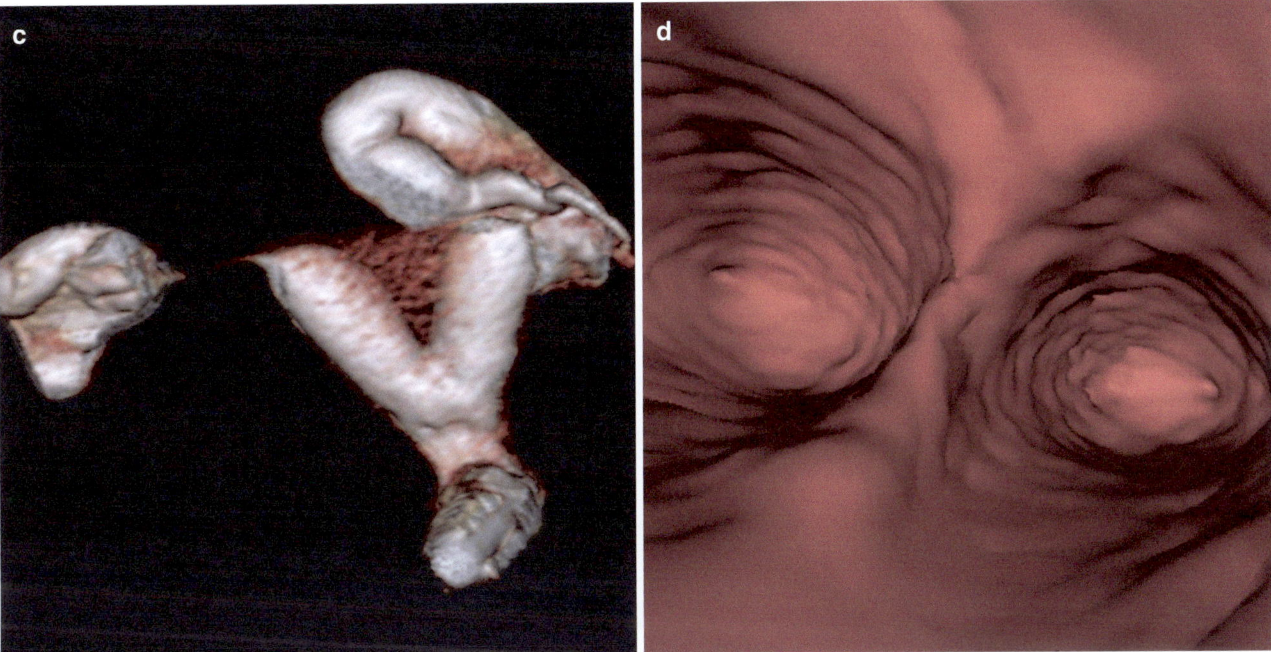

Fig. 8.31 (continued)

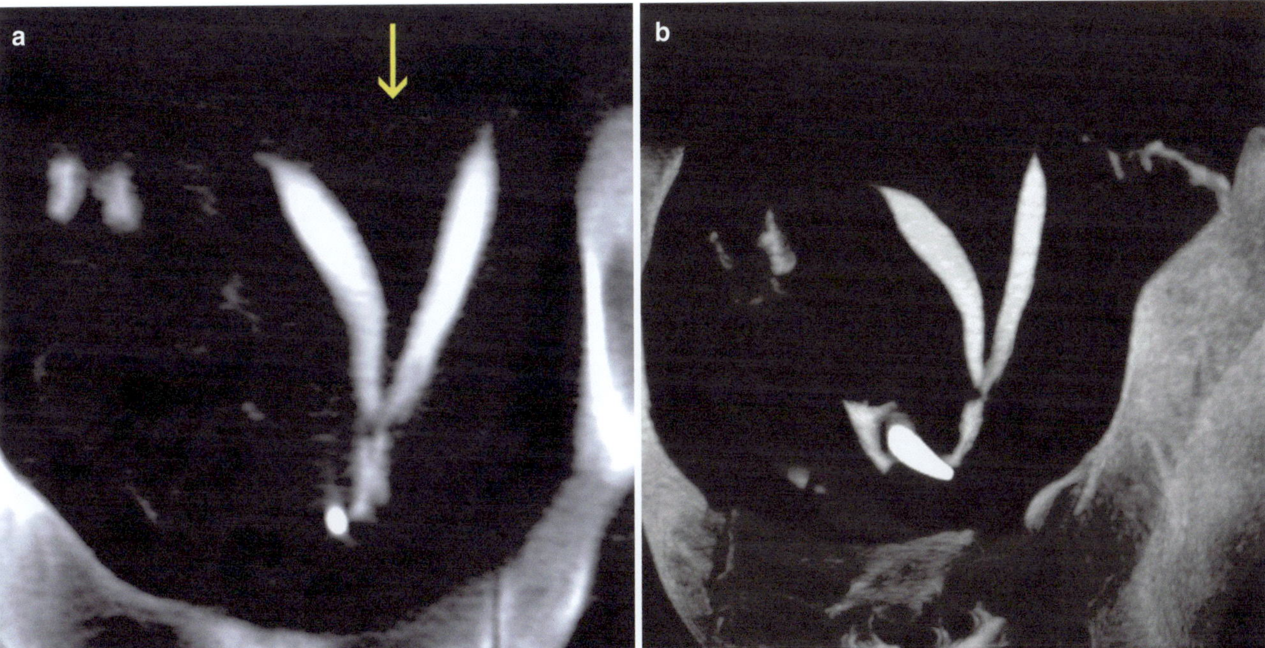

Fig. 8.32 VHSG of septate uterus. (**a**) 10-mm axial CT image with soft tissue window showing the fundal convexity of the uterus (*arrow*). (**b, c**) Oblique coronal maximum intensity projection and 3D volume rendering images showing similar findings. (**d**) Virtual endoscopy image. The septum which divides the endometrial cavity and both uterine horns can be observed

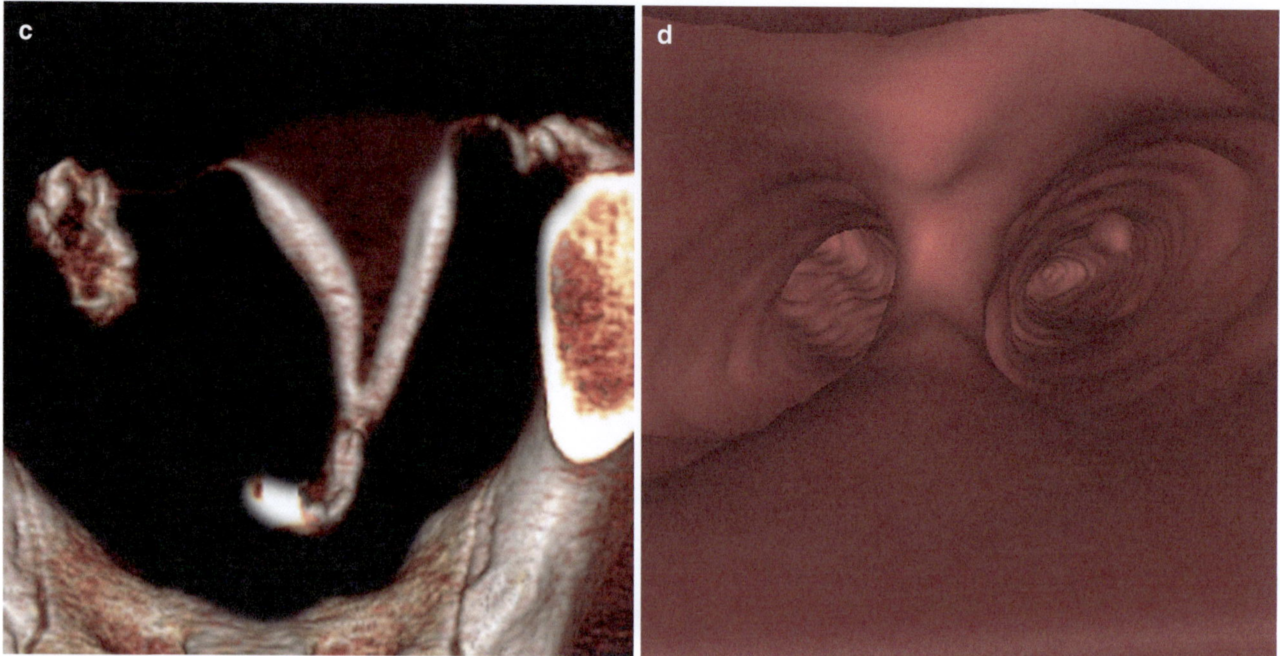

Fig. 8.32 (continued)

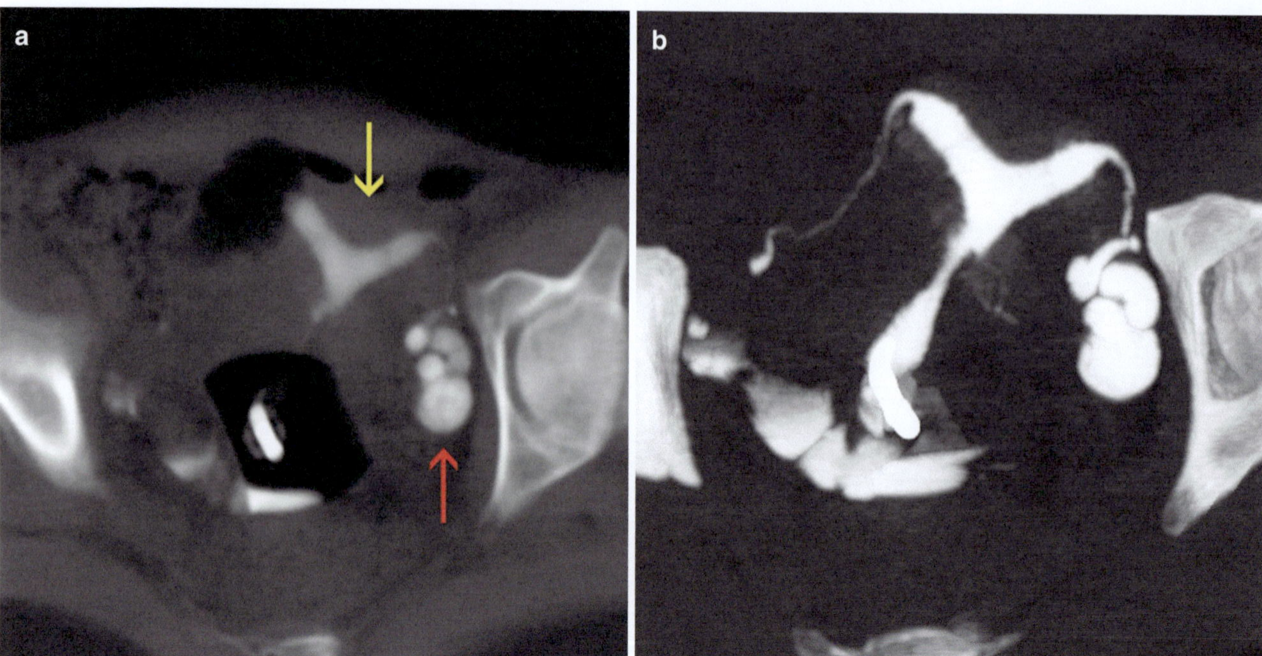

Fig. 8.33 VHSG and MRI of septate uterus. (**a**) 10-mm axial CT image with soft tissue window showing the fundal convexity of the uterus (*yellow arrow*). A left hydrosalpinx is also observed (*red arrow*). (**b**, **c**) Oblique coronal maximum intensity projection and 3D volume rendering images showing similar findings. (**d**) Virtual endoscopy image. The septum which divides the endometrial cavity and both uterine horns can be observed. (**e**, **f**) Axial T2 weighted MRI images with and without fat suppression which show the morphology of the uterus but cannot analyze the Fallopian tubes

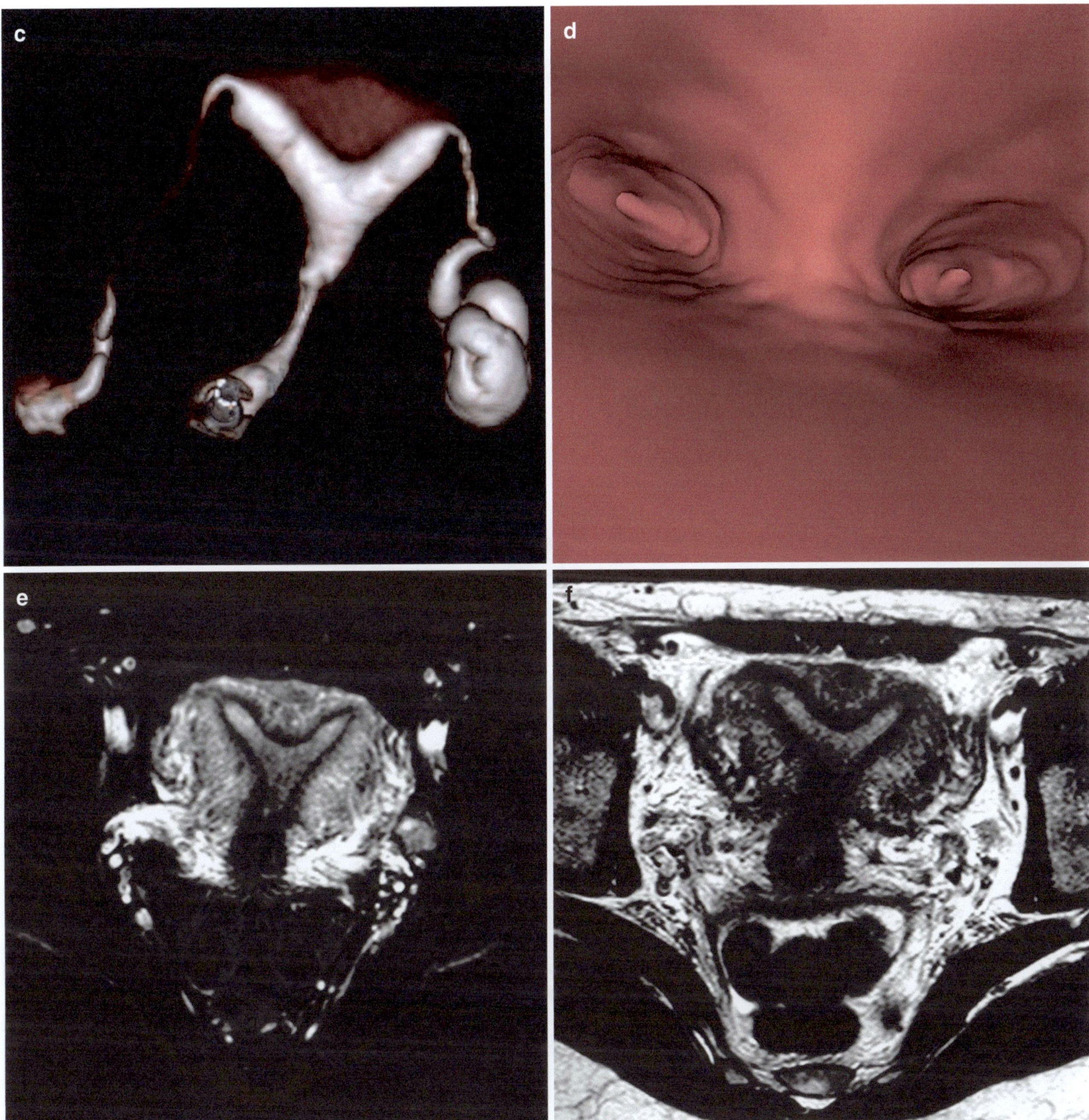

Fig. 8.33 (continued)

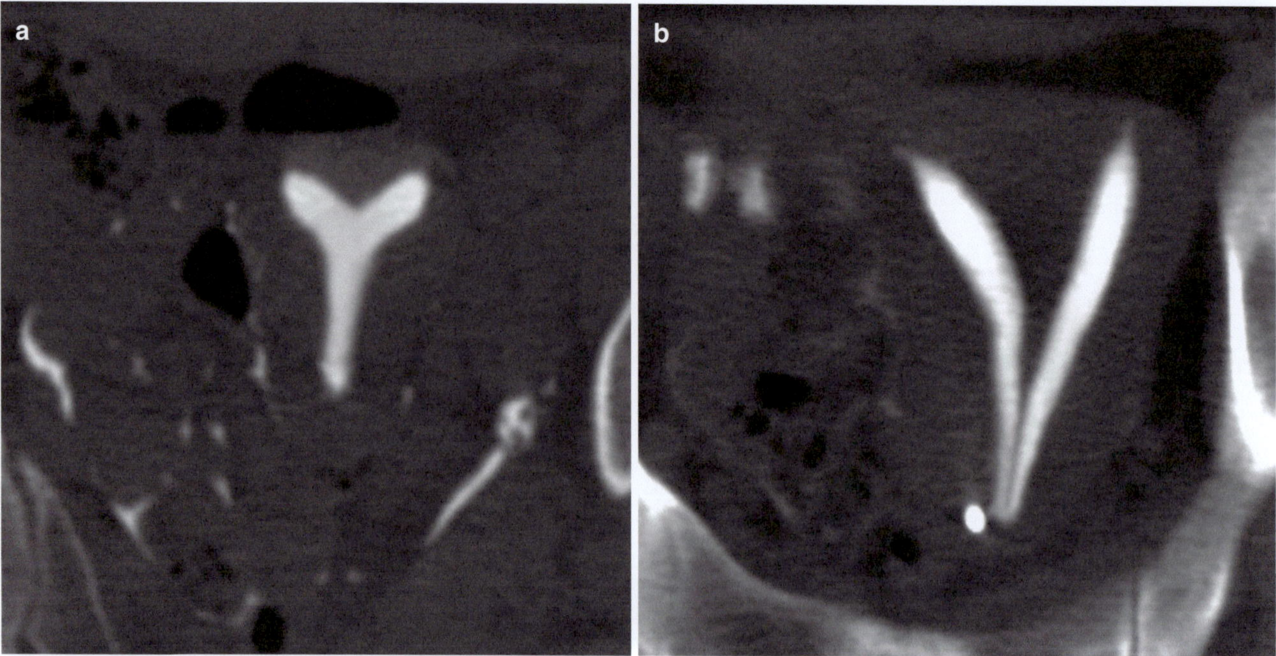

Fig. 8.34 Coronal multiplanar reconstruction images. (**a**) Partial septate uterus. (**b**) Complete septate uterus

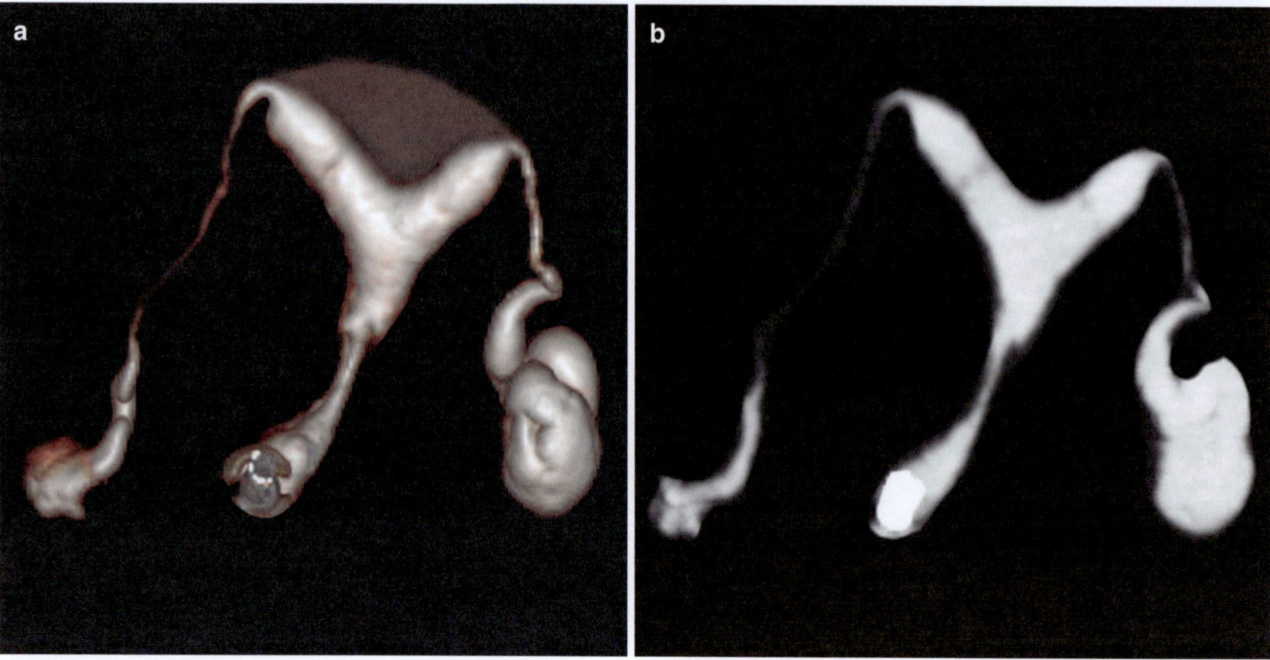

Fig. 8.35 (**a**) 3D volume rendering image illustrating the myometrial wall and the fundal convexity of the uterus. (**b**) Maximum intensity projection image does not allow the evaluation of the miometrium. Only the endometrial cavity can be depicted

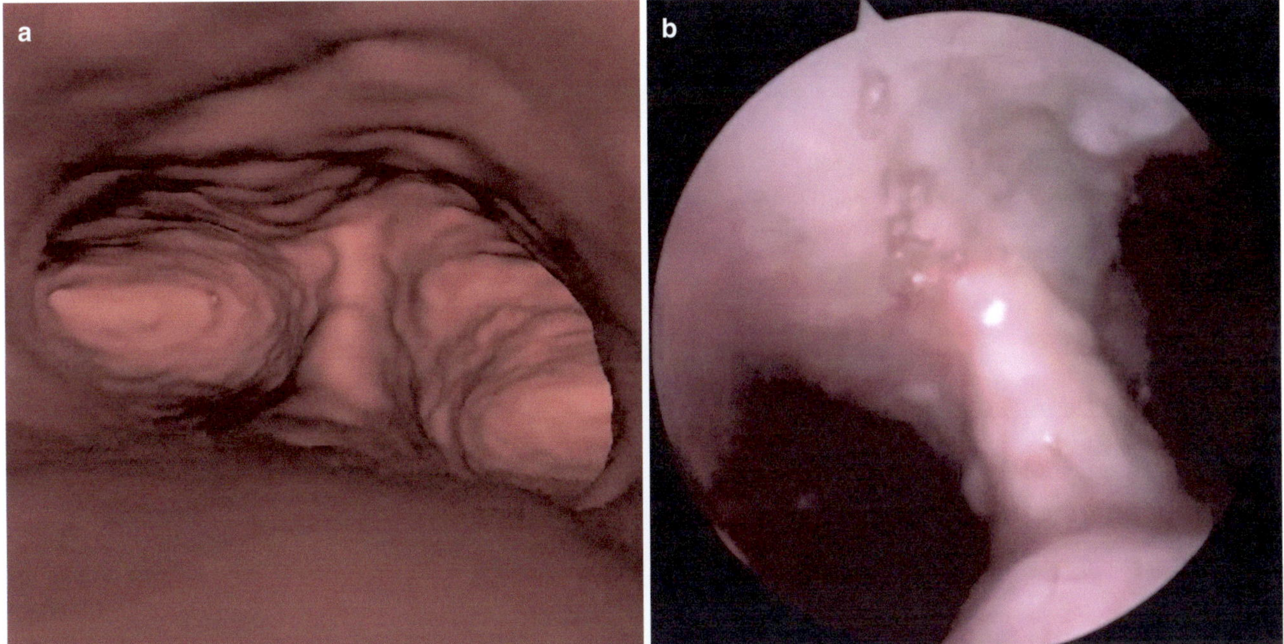

Fig. 8.36 Endoscopic views of septate uterus. (**a**) Virtual endoscopy image where the septum is observed in the middle of the uterine cavity. (**b**) The conventional hysteroscopy illustrates similar findings

Conclusion

The congenital anomalies are a frequent cause of infertility. Those anomalies can be studied via diverse imaging methods. Up until now MR was the gold standard method for their evaluation and characterization. However, said method possesses limitations with regards to the detection of associated intraluminal pathologies as well as the tubarian evaluation. These associated pathologies can also be the cause of infertility, hence the MR requires other diagnostic methods to evaluate patients completely.

VHSG is a new diagnostic method, minimally invasive that utilizes only 0.3 mSV total radiation. The necessary information for a diagnosis is obtained with only one study, through bidimensional, tridimensional and endoscopic reconstructions. In this way it allows to reduce times and enhance the patients' comfort.

References

1. Acien P. Incidence of Mullerian defects in fertile and infertile women. Hum Reprod. 1997;12:1372–6.
2. Ashton D, Amin HK, Richart RM, et al. The incidence of symptomatic uterine anomalies in women undergoing transcervical tubal sterilization. Obstet Gynecol. 1988;72:28–30.
3. Homer HA, Li TC, Cooke ID. The septate uterus: a review of management and reproductive outcome. Fertil Steril. 2000;73:1–14.
4. Raga F, Bauset C, Remohi J, et al. Reproductive impact of congenital Mullerian anomalies. Hum Reprod. 1997;12:2277–81.
5. Saleem SN. MR imaging diagnosis of uterovaginal anomalies: current state of the art. Radiographics. 2003;23:e13.
6. Simon C, Martinez L, Pardo F, et al. Mullerian defects in women with normal reproductive outcome. Fertil Steril. 1991;56:1192–3.
7. Troiano RN, McCarthy SM. Mullerian duct anomalies: imaging and clinical issues. Radiology. 2004;233:19–34.
8. Clifford K, Rai R, Watson H, et al. An informative protocol for the investigation of recurrent miscarriage: preliminary experience of 500 consecutive cases. Hum Reprod. 1994;9:1328–32.
9. Nahum GG. Uterine anomalies. How common are they, and what is their distribution among subtypes? J Reprod Med. 1998;43:877–87.
10. Raziel A, Arieli S, Bukovsky I, et al. Investigation of the uterine cavity in recurrent aborters. Fertil Steril. 1994;62:1080–2.
11. Hassan MA, Lavery SA, Trew GH. Congenital uterine anomalies and their impact on fertility. Womens Health (Lond Engl). 2010;6(3):443–61.
12. Zhang Y, Zhao YY, Qiao J. Obstetric outcome of women with uterine anomalies in China. Chin Med J (Engl). 2010;123(4):418–22.
13. Saravelos SH, Cocksedge KA, Li TC. Prevalence and diagnosis of congenital uterine anomalies in women with reproductive failure: a critical appraisal. Hum Reprod Update. 2008;14(5):415–29.
14. Oystragh P. Pregnancy in uterus didelphys. Med J Aust. 1968;2(9):400–2.
15. Lewis BV, Brant HA. Obstetric and gynecologic complications associated with müllerian duct abnormalities. Obstet Gynecol. 1966;28(3):315–22.
16. Lewis AD, Levine D. Pregnancy complications in women with uterine duplication abnormalities. Ultrasound Q. 2010;26(4):193–200.
17. Guadagno L, Pardini C, Floriddia G, et al. On a case of bilateral total gonado-mullerian agenesis associated with left renal agenesis and ectopy and dysmorphism of the right kidney. Riv Crit Clin Med. 1968;68(4):387–403.
18. Ceci GP, Scapicchi G. Unilateral Wolff-Mullerian agenesis associated with homolateral gonadal agenesis. Atti Accad Fisiocrit Siena Med Fis. 1967;16(1):648–56.
19. Talebian Yazdi A, De Smet K, Ernst C, et al. Uterus didelphys with obstructed hemivagina and renal agenesis: MRI findings. JBR-BTR. 2011;94(1):16–8.

20. Takagi H, Matsunami K, Imai A. Uterovaginal duplication with blind hemivagina and ipsilateral renal agenesis: review of unusual presentation. J Obstet Gynaecol. 2010;30(4):350–3. Review.
21. Acién P, Acién M. Unilateral renal agenesis and female genital tract pathologies. Acta Obstet Gynecol Scand. 2010;89(11):1424–31.
22. Chan YY, Jayaprakasan K, Zamora J, et al. The prevalence of congenital uterine anomalies in unselected and high-risk populations: a systematic review. Hum Reprod Update. 2011;17(6):761–71.
23. Sugiura-Ogasawara M, Ozaki Y, Katano K, et al. Uterine anomaly and recurrent pregnancy loss. Semin Reprod Med. 2011;29(6):514–21.
24. Rock JA, Schlaff WD. The obstetric consequences of uterovaginal anomalies. Fertil Steril. 1985;43:681–92.
25. Chosson J. Attempt at embryologic classification of malformations of Mullerian origin of the female genital system. Rev Fr Gynecol Obstet. 1967;62(12):695–702.
26. The American Fertility Society. The American Fertility Society classifications of adnexal adhesions, distal tubal occlusion, tubal occlusion secondary to tubal ligation, tubal pregnancies, mullerian anomalies and intrauterine adhesions. Fertil Steril. 1988;49:944–55.
27. Buttram Jr VC, Gibbons WE. Mullerian anomalies: a proposed classification. (An analysis of 144 cases). Fertil Steril. 1979;32:40–6.
28. Ubeda B, Paraira M, Alert E, et al. Hysterosalpingography: spectrum of normal variants and nonpathological findings. AJR Am J Roentgenol. 2001;177(1):131–5.
29. Byrne J, Nussbaum-Blask A, Taylor WS, et al. Prevalence of müllerian duct anomalies detected at ultrasound. Am J Med Genet. 2000;94:9–12.
30. Benjaminov O, Atri M. Sonography of the abnormal fallopian tube. AJR Am J Roentgenol. 2004;183(3):737–42.
31. Bermejo C, Ten Martínez P, Cantarero R, et al. Three-dimensional ultrasound in the diagnosis of Müllerian duct anomalies and concordance with magnetic resonance imaging. Ultrasound Obstet Gynecol. 2010;35(5):593–601.
32. Marcal L, Nothaft MA, Coelho F, et al. Mullerian duct anomalies: MR imaging. Abdom Imaging. 2011;36(6):756–64.
33. Winter L, Glücker T, Steimann S, et al. Feasibility of dynamic MR-hysterosalpingography for the diagnostic work-up of infertile women. Acta Radiol. 2010;51(6):693–701.
34. Carrascosa P, Sangster G, Capuñay C, et al. Histerosalpingografía virtual, experiencia inicial. 21st International Congress of Radiology 2000. Abstract.
35. Carrascosa P, Capuñay C, Mariano B, et al. Virtual hysteroscopy by multidetector computed tomography. Abdom Imaging. 2008;33(4):381–7.
36. Carrascosa P, Capuñay C, Baronio M, et al. 64- Row multidetector CT virtual hysterosalpingography. Abdom Imaging. 2009;34:121–33.
37. Carrascosa P, Capuñay C, Vallejos J, et al. Virtual hysterosalpingography: a new multidetector CT technique for evaluating the female reproductive system. Radiographics. 2010;30:643–61.
38. Carrascosa P, Capuñay C, Vallejos J, et al. Virtual hysterosalpingography: experience with over 1000 consecutive patients. Abdom Imaging. 2011;36(1):1–14.
39. Baronio M, Carrascosa P, Capuñay C, et al. Diagnostic performance of CT virtual hysteroscopy in 69 consecutive patients. Fertil Steril. 2010;94(Supplement S77). Abstract.
40. Capuñay C, Baronio M, Carrascosa P, et al. CT virtual hysterosalpingography in the evaluation of uterine myomas. Fertil Steril. 2010;94(Supplement S211). Abstract.
41. Carrascosa P, Baronio JM, Borghi M, et al. Histerosalpingoscopía virtual. Una técnica novedosa y no invasiva para diagnosticar patología intrauterina. Reproducción. 2006;21:19–26.

Tubal factor is one of leading causes associated to infertility in women. There exist diverse pathological conditions that affect the Fallopian tubes and, henceforth, interfere with normal transport of the ovule through them. The most frequent process is pelvic inflammatory disease, which represents a wide spectrum that includes salpingitis, piosalpinx and the tube-ovary abscess. Other frequent entities, and some more rare, can compromise the Fallopian tubes. The differential diagnosis with other pelvic entities is of the utmost importance for treating the patients. There exist diverse diagnostic methods that are utilized in the study of uterine tubes. Hysterosalpingography is the modality which has traditionally been used to investigate the tuboperitoneal factor. Ultrasound and Magnetic Resonance Imaging (MRI) present limitations to the direct visualization of tubes. In the last years enhancements in these methods have been developed, like the sono-hysterosalpingography and the MR-hysterosalpingography, but they still have not reached an adequate resolution for the diagnosis of the tubal pathology. Laparoscopy is the method of reference and is reserved for the confirmation of the radiologic findings and for therapeutic procedures.

Virtual hysterosalpingography (VHSG) is a new diagnostic modality that utilizes a similar procedure as the conventional study based on computed tomography studies. Volumetric images of high spatial resolution are obtained through the opacification of the uterine cavity and Fallopian tubes, which allows achieving high quality images and virtual endoscopic navigation [1].

The increasing use of diagnostic imaging forces the familiarization with an extensive pathological process that affects uterine tubes. The knowledge of the diseases of uterine tubes and their appearance in images of normal and abnormal conditions is crucial for optimal diagnosis and treatment. In this chapter the anatomical fundaments will be presented, as well as the spectrum of typical and pathological findings in the uterine tubes and in VHSG studies.

Uterine Tubes Study

Hysterosalpingography is the study which has been utilized for the initial evaluation of patients with infertility. Besides offering a morphological assessment of uterine cavity, hysterosalpingography provides important information about the anatomy of the Fallopian tubes and tubal patency (Fig. 9.1). The distribution of contrast material into pelvic cavity can be documented and a possible peritoneal factor inferred indirectly. Nevertheless, the results for the diagnosis of the tubal occlusion (sensibility of 65 % and specificity of 83 %) are limited when compared with laparoscopy [2]. For this reason, other techniques were, and are, being constantly tested for the evaluation of the tubal patency. In routine ultrasound, Fallopian tubes cannot be visualized unless they are dilated or when a sufficient amount of fluid exists in the pelvic cavity that allows individualization within the wide ligament [3]. Another technique consists in carrying out a sonographic evaluation after an injection of saline solution into the pelvic cavity. In these cases, the tubal patency is not evaluated, but only tubal diameters. A modified technique is denominated sonohysterosalpingography, in which saline solution is injected through the cervical canal and distention of uterine cavity is under control by ultrasound [4, 5]. This technique does not allow the evaluation of the tubal anatomy. Nuclear medicine was also used in the assessment of tubal patency with radionuclide detection in the peritoneal cavity that had previously been placed at the end of the vagina. This technique is denominated nuclear hysterogram, which has limitations in the morphologic evaluation of the tubes and in the detection of unilateral tubal obstructions [6]. Recently, different experiences in the evaluation of uterine tubes with MRI were published [7–9]. Although the results are promising, limitations exist with regards to spatial resolution and, henceforth, in the complete visualization of tubes and intratubal anatomy. Definite diagnosis and treatment of tubal disease is carried out with surgical intervention either with a laparoscopy or a

P. Carrascosa et al., *CT Virtual Hysterosalpingography*,
DOI 10.1007/978-3-319-07560-0_9, © Springer International Publishing Switzerland 2014

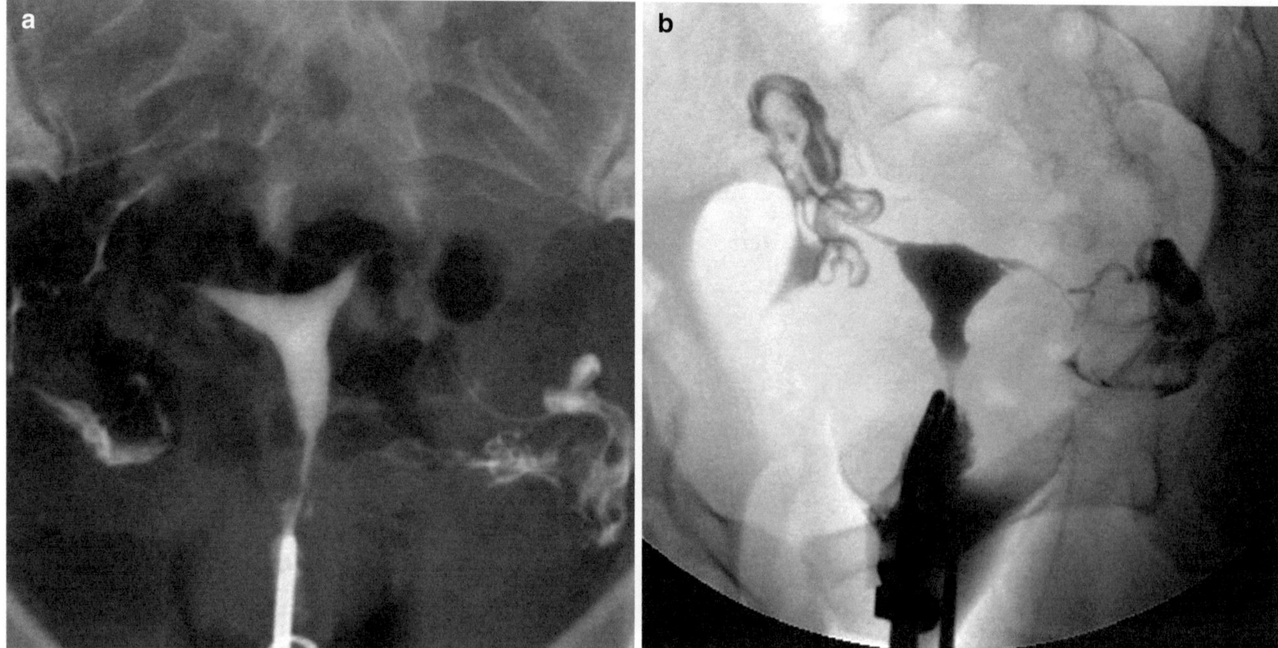

Fig. 9.1 (**a**) HSG showing the normal anatomy of the uterine tubes and the bilateral spillage of contrast into peritoneum. (**b**) HSG with inverted window, where the normal tubal morphology and patency are appreciated

laparatomy. When combining the direct visualization of the tubes with the blue methylene injection via hysteroscopy, the patency is proven. The internal evaluation of tubes can be achieved by introduction of the laparoscope through a tiny incision done by the surgeon. In this way the fold and mucus pattern can be visualized, especially in the ampullar or dilated region of the tubes. This technique is called falloscopy. A complete internal visualization can also be accessed through the canulization of a microhysteroscope, known as a salpingography. In recent years, the selective salpingography guided by fluoroscopy was developed, an interventionist procedure for patients with proximal tubal occlusion [10]. The success rates of repermeabilization and visualization of the distal anatomy of the tube were of 76–95 %. However, reocclusion was observed in 15–30 % of the cases and there was a prevalence of 10 % of ectopic pregnancies after the procedure. All novel techniques described still require an adequate evaluation with large controlled and randomized studies in search of high levels of scientific evidence [11].

Radiological Approach

Tubal pathology is classified from the radiological point of view in those that affect tubal visualization, caliber, filling defects and their morphology. Partial or absent tubal visualization may be due to a variety of technical factors or pathologic processes. Hence, this finding is nonspecific and can be related to an insufficient amount of contrast, cornual spasms or mucous plugs [12]. During the VHSG study, these circumstances are avoided with an adequate preparation of the patient and a protocol procedure [13]. The administration of oral antispasmodics an hour before the exam prevents cornual spasms and the presence of mucosal plugging within the tubes [14]. While employing a controlled administration of the contrast medium with an injector pump, the exact moment of the image acquisition is calculated, verifying a volume of contrast that is enough for the complete opacification of the uterine cavity and of the tubes. An excessive quantity would be non productive for the tubal visualization due to the fact that the contrast material poured into the peritoneal cavity could hide the tubes. Hence, the calculation of the moment of the image acquisition becomes of vital importance for the success of the study; it avoids rescan which means an increase in the radiation dose. Pathological obstructions can occur at any level. Inflammatory obstruction typically affects the ampullary portion (Fig. 9.2). On the other hand, when the occlusion is post-surgery (salpingectomy or tubal ligation), in general the visualization is partial and the obstruction is at the level os the isthmus (Fig. 9.3).

The tubal dilatations are due usually to inflammatory pelvic diseases or endometriosis (Fig. 9.4). Dilatation may be associated with complete obstruction (hydrosalpinx) or with some peritoneal spillage (Fig. 9.5).

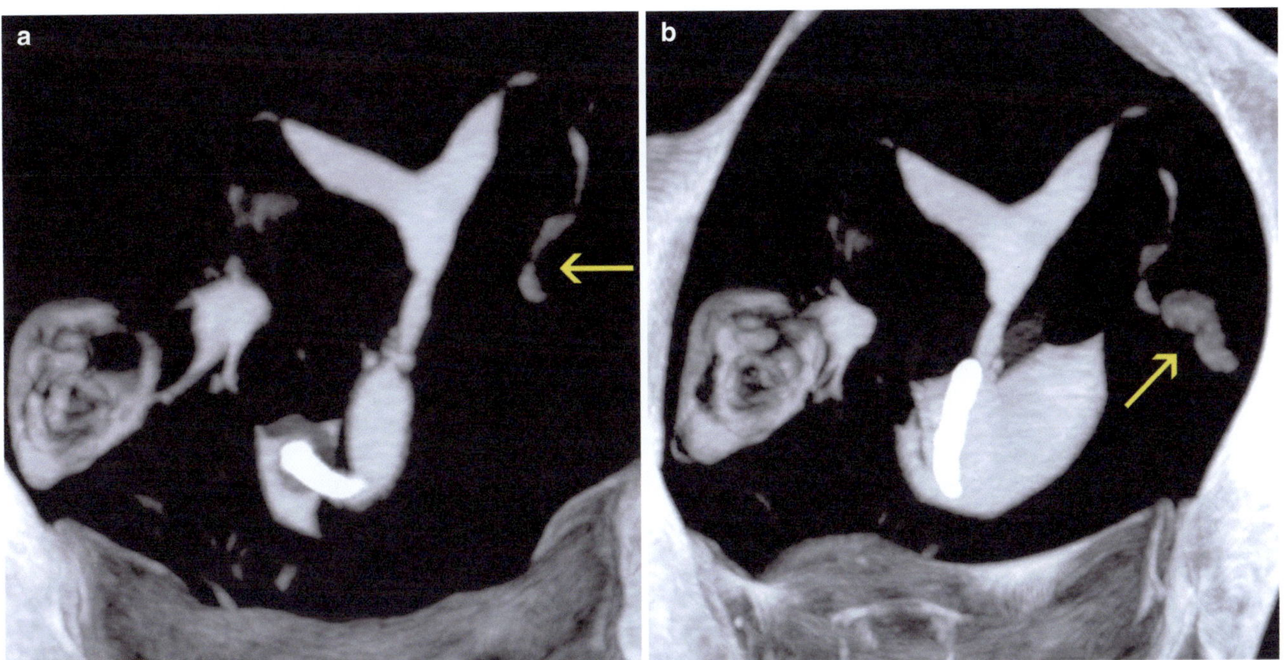

Fig. 9.2 Distal tubal obstruction. (**a**, **b**) Coronal oblique maximum intensity projection images showing absence of the contrast spillage into the peritoneal cavity through the left tube, which is opacified up to its distal portion (*arrows*)

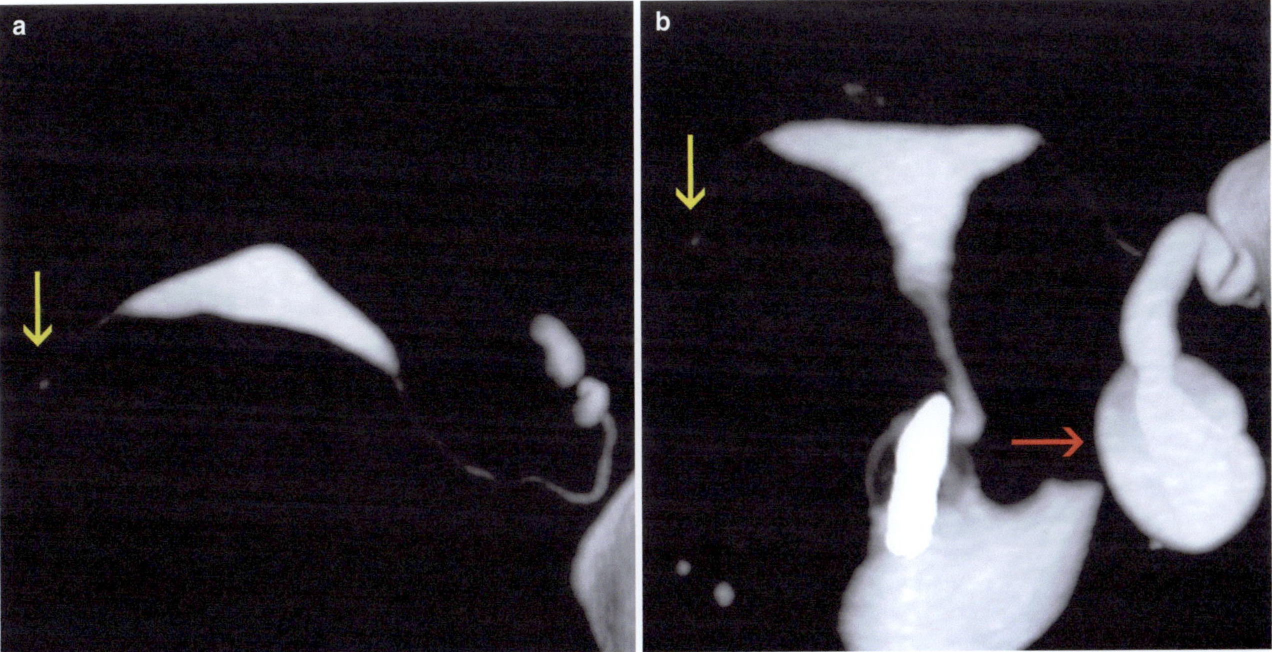

Fig. 9.3 Post-surgery tubal obstruction. (**a**, **b**) Axial and coronal maximum intensity projection images showing opacification of proximal portion of right uterine tube (*yellow arrow*), in a patient with a history of ectopic pregnancy and right salpingectomy. Note that the left tube is dilated (*red arrow*)

The filling defects within the tubes are rare and can be visualized as elevated endoluminal lesions in the virtual endoscopic images. The presence of air bubbles introduced during the procedure of the study is easily identified due to its density, and should not be considered pathological (Fig. 9.6). The tubal polyps are the most frequently observed

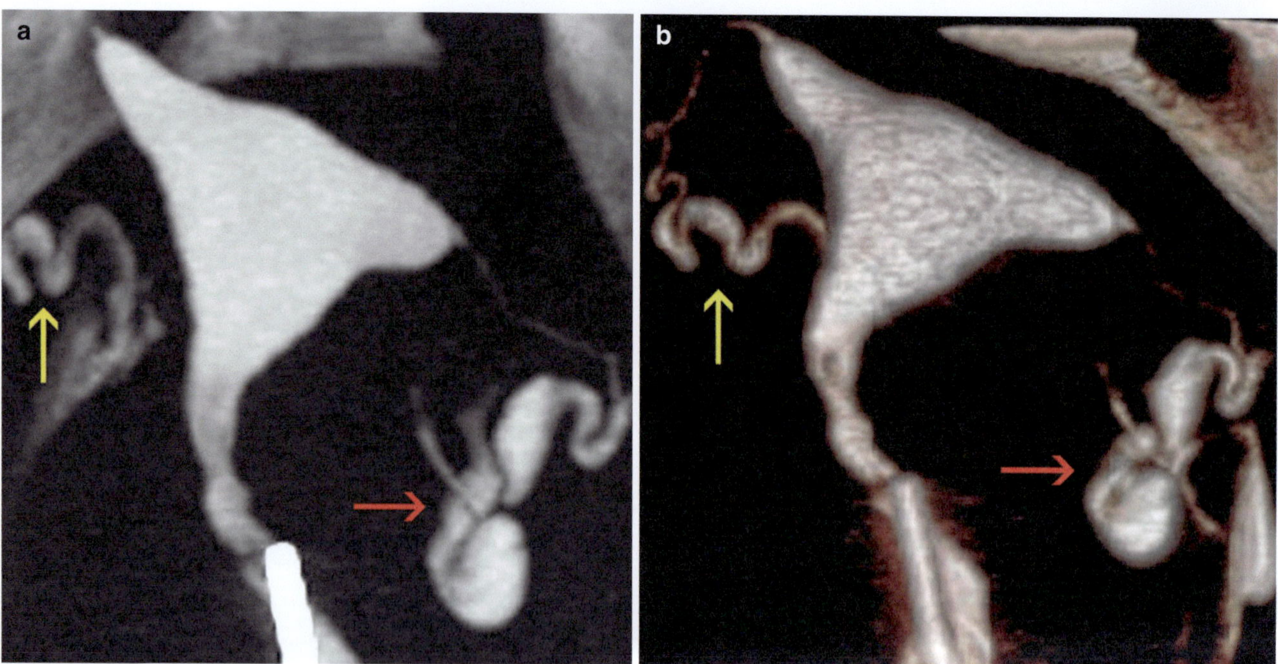

Fig. 9.4 Tubal dilatation. Mild ampullary dilatation of the left uterine tube, with scarce passage of contrast into the peritoneal cavity (*red arrow*). The right tube is normal in caliber (*yellow arrow*). (**a**) Maximum intensity projection image. (**b**) 3D volume rendering image

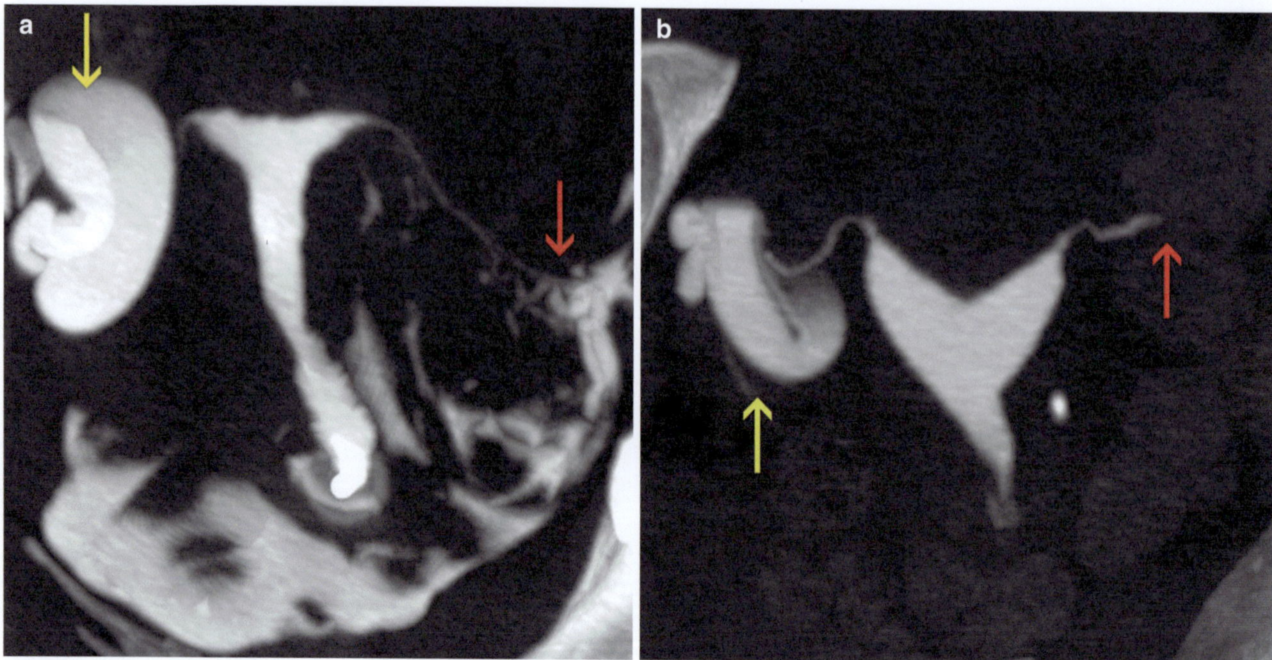

Fig. 9.5 Hydrosalpinx. (**a**) Maximum intensity projection image showing a severe dilatation of the right uterine tube (*yellow arrow*), without passage of contrast to the peritoneal cavity. On the other hand, the left tube is visualized with normal caliber and ample passage of contrast to the peritoneal cavity (*red arrow*). (**b**) Another case of right unilateral hydrosalpinx (*yellow arrow*). The left tube shows only opacification of the interstitial portion due to salpingectomy (*red arrow*)

in the proximal region to the tubes (Fig. 9.7). On the other hand, in the ampullar region, linear and irregular filling defects that correspond to intratubal synechiae are observed more frequently, in general related to inflammatory processes (Fig. 9.8).

The alterations of the tubal morphology manifest themselves as irregularities of their edges or with a beaded pattern that alternates stenosis and segmental dilatations. The salpingitis isthmica nodosa is presented as multiple and small pseudodiverticula dilatations of the tubes that generally compromise the isthmic portion (Fig. 9.9). Other inflammatory processes and postsurgical changes can alter the tubal outline and simulate a salpingitis isthmica nodosa, although the most usual presentation form is the beaded pattern (Figs. 9.10 and 9.11) [15].

Most Frequent Tubal Pathologies

The alterations of the uterine tubes are frequent causes of infertility. Diverse pathological conditions are usually observed in daily clinical practice, but the inflammatory pelvic disease and endometriosis are the most common.

Congenital Anomalies

The congenital anomalies that exclusively compromise the Fallopian tubes are rare and are comprised by aplasia, hypoplasia, accessory ostium, and congenital diverticula. The agenesis of the tubal segment of the müllerian ducts can simulate an acquired tubal obstruction. Typically the occlusion is observed in the isthmic-ampullar junction of the tube. Tubal anomalies associated to uterine malformations are observed most frequently, like in the bicornuate uterus, where the tube of the affected side can be absent or with a rudimentary development.

Inflammatory Pelvic Disease

The inflammatory processes of the pelvic cavity usually affect the uterine tubes leading to tubal dysfunction and obstruction, frequent causes of infertility. The most common dissemination route is by ascendant infection from the distal uterine tract. When initial compromise of the vagina or

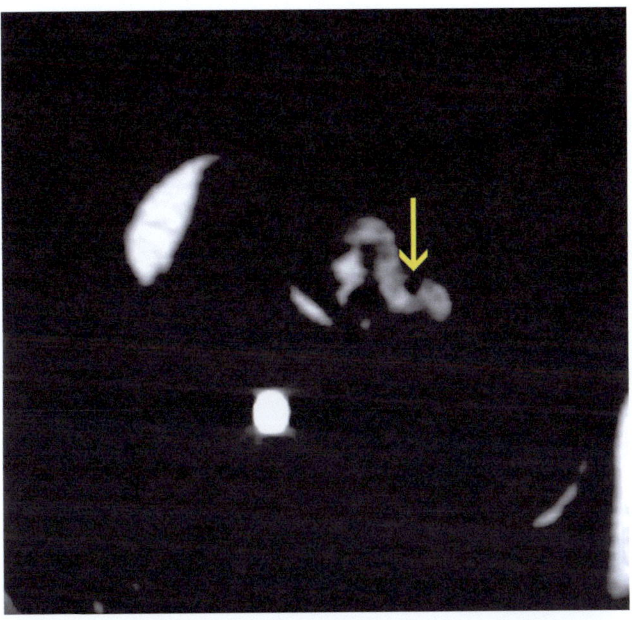

Fig. 9.6 Air bubble. Axial CT image showing a focal filling defect of low density in the ampullary region of the left tube (*arrow*) corresponding to an air bubble

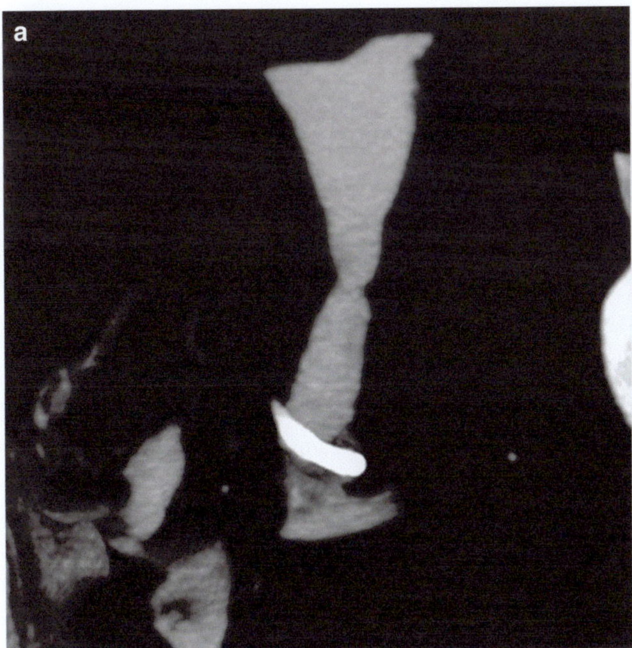

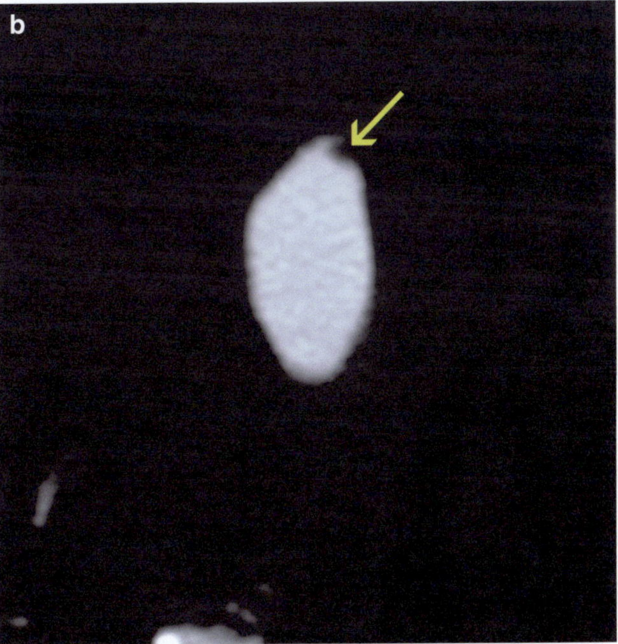

Fig. 9.7 Tubal polyp. (**a**) Maximum intensity projection image where absence of opacification of the left uterine tube is evidenced. (**b**) Amplified axial CT image of the left cornual region showing an elevated 3-mm lesion projecting into the intramural portion of the left uterine tube (*arrow*), causing the tubal obstruction

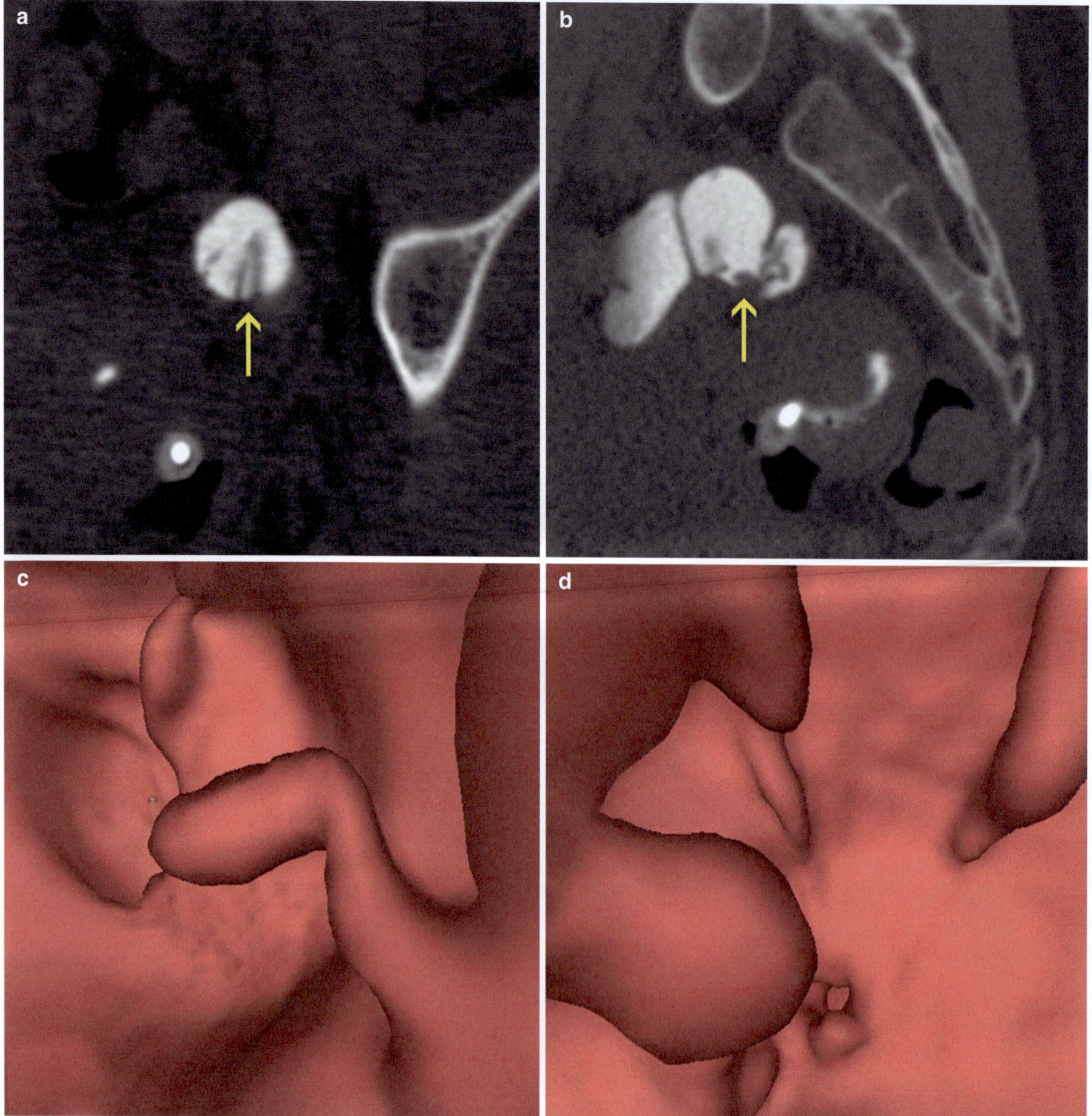

Fig. 9.8 Intra-tubal synechiae. (**a**, **b**) Axial and sagittal CT images at the level of the left uterine tube, which is dilated and has lineal and irregular filling defect in its interior (*arrows*). (**c**, **d**) Virtual endoscopy images confirming the presence of intra-tubal synechiae

cervix exists, or before the presence of an intrauterine gadget, the infection extends to the uterine cavity causing endometritis, and if it progresses it leads to salpingitis and pelvic infection. Other causes of tubal infection are the invasive or instrumental procedures like curettage, hysteroscopies, etc. or in the puerperium. The most frequent ethiological agents are bacterial, including gram-negative, gram-positive, anaerobe and gonococcus germs. The trachomatis Chlamydia is the most frequent anaerobia bacteria. In the infections associated to intrauterine gadgets, species of Actinomyces are usually found, and the tubal affection is usually characteristically unilateral. Currently, tuberculosis causes salpingitis in rare occasions. As the affliction is chronic, there exist irregularities in the outline of the ampullar region of the tube and is usually associated to calcifications.

In the context of an acute tubal infectious process, the germs infiltrate the mucosa's cells causing stromal edema. The folds then turn prominent and adherent. Next, the inflammation extends towards the depths of the wall affecting the muscular and serosa layer, and consequently produces peritonitis. A hypersecretion exists at the level of the mucosa, and the tubal lightfills with serous or purulent fluid, resulting in hydrosalpinx or piosalpinx, respectively. When

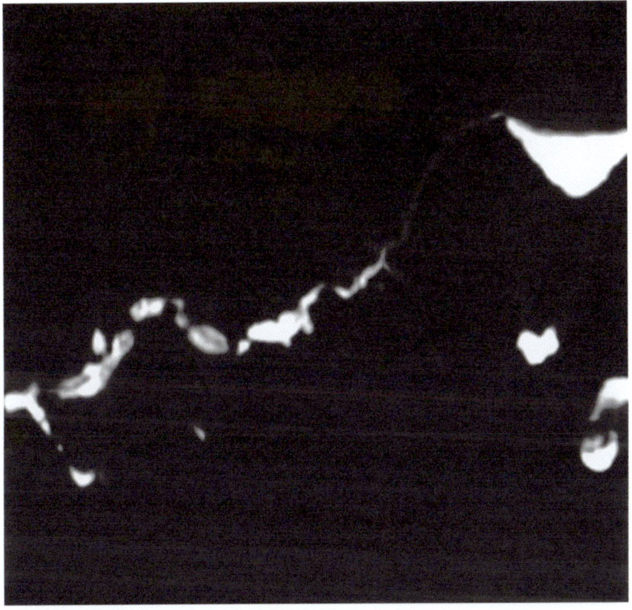

Fig. 9.9 Maximum intensity projection image showing irregularity in the right tubal outline with the presence of multiple nodular diverticular spaces, characteristic findings of salpingitis isthmica nodosa

the tubal infection is resolved, intratubal synechiae and perifimbrial adherences are formed, which contribute to the obstruction of the affected tube [16].

It is worth stating that the hysterosalpingography study is counter indicated when an acute infectious process exists. Ultrasound as well as magnetic resonance can show the presence of piosalpinx, tubo-ovaric abscesses and fluid in the pelvic cavity. In VHSG studies, scars of tubal infections can be observed. The findings depend on the severity and location of the infection. The study is normal if the sequels are limited to scarce peritubal adhesions. In these cases, the contrast poured into the peritoneum does not flow freely and remains loculated adjacent to the infundibulum (Fig. 9.12). On occasions the adherences cause deformation in the ampullar region. Other findings of larger gravity are dilatations, hydroosalpinx (Fig. 9.13) and intratubarian synechiae, which imply a tubal dysfunction and, hence, signs of bad chances of achieving a pregnancy after a surgical reconstruction of the affected tube.

Salpingitis Isthmica Nodosa

Even though the name salpingitis suggests an inflammatory etiology, the origin of this infrequent pathology is unclear. A probable congenital or degenerative cause was also described. The patients tend to possess a history of pelvic infections, infertility, and ectopic pregnancies. In most cases

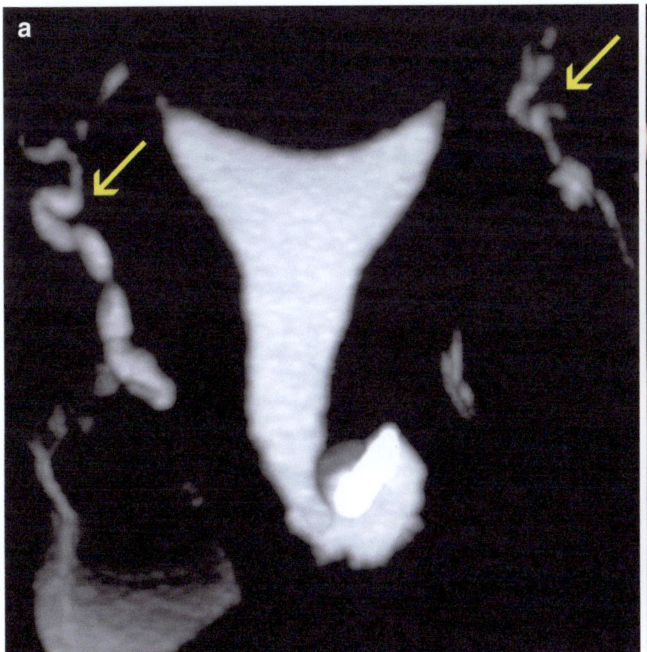

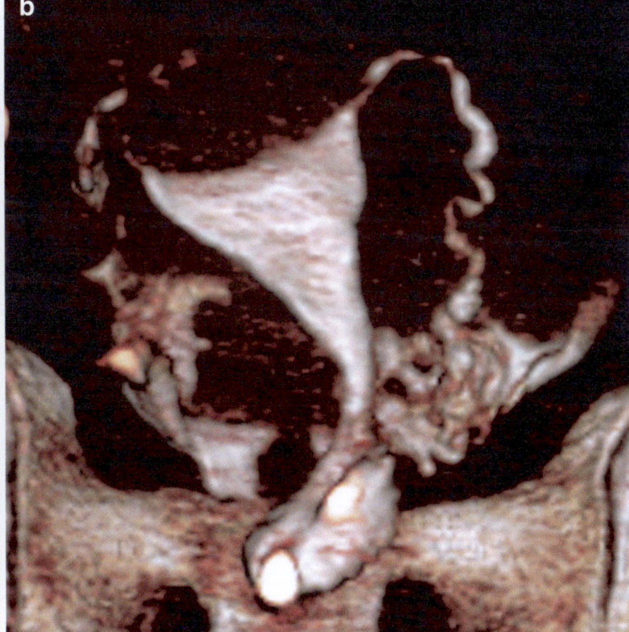

Fig. 9.10 Post-inflammatory tubal morphological changes. (**a**) Maximum intensity projection image shows alteration in the morphology of both tubes manifested by irregularities in their outline, beaded appearance which alternates stenosis and segmental dilations (*arrows*). (**b**) 3D volume rendering image of another patient with tubal morphological changes

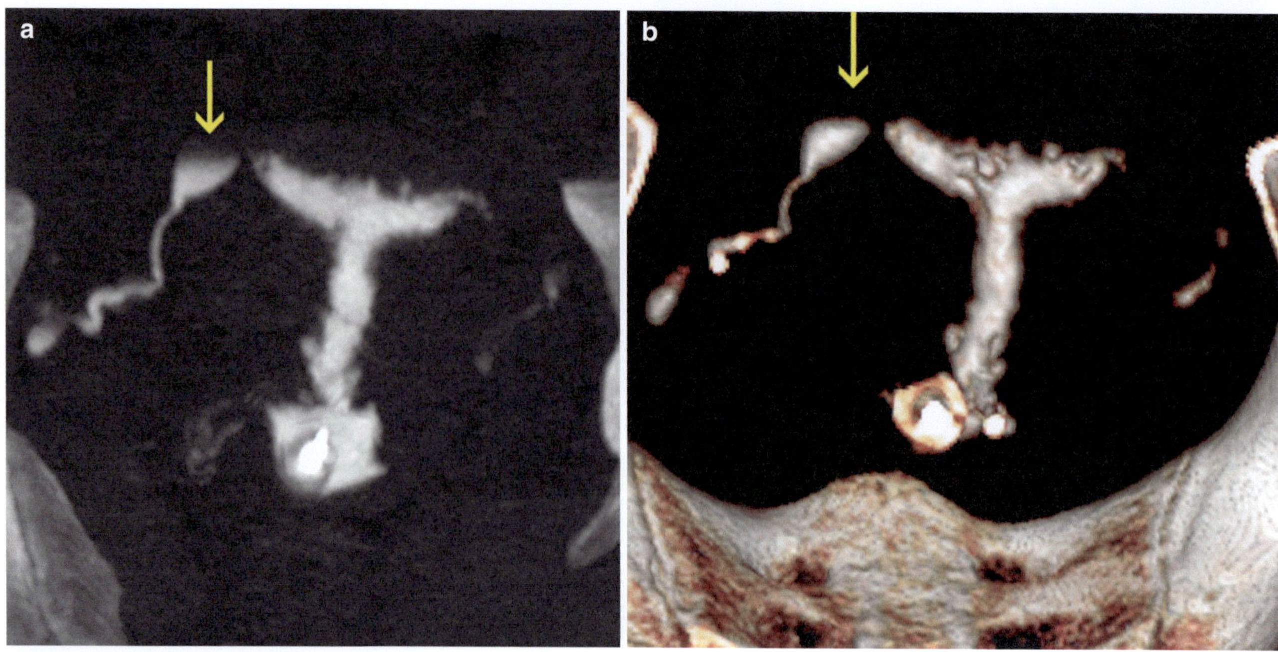

Fig. 9.11 Twenty-eight-year old patient with a history of inflammatory pelvic disease. Post-inflammatory morphological changes such as irregularity in the outline of the uterine cavity and segmental dilation of the proximal portion of the right uterine tube (*arrows*) are visualized. (**a**) Maximum intensity projection image. (**b**) 3D volume rendering image

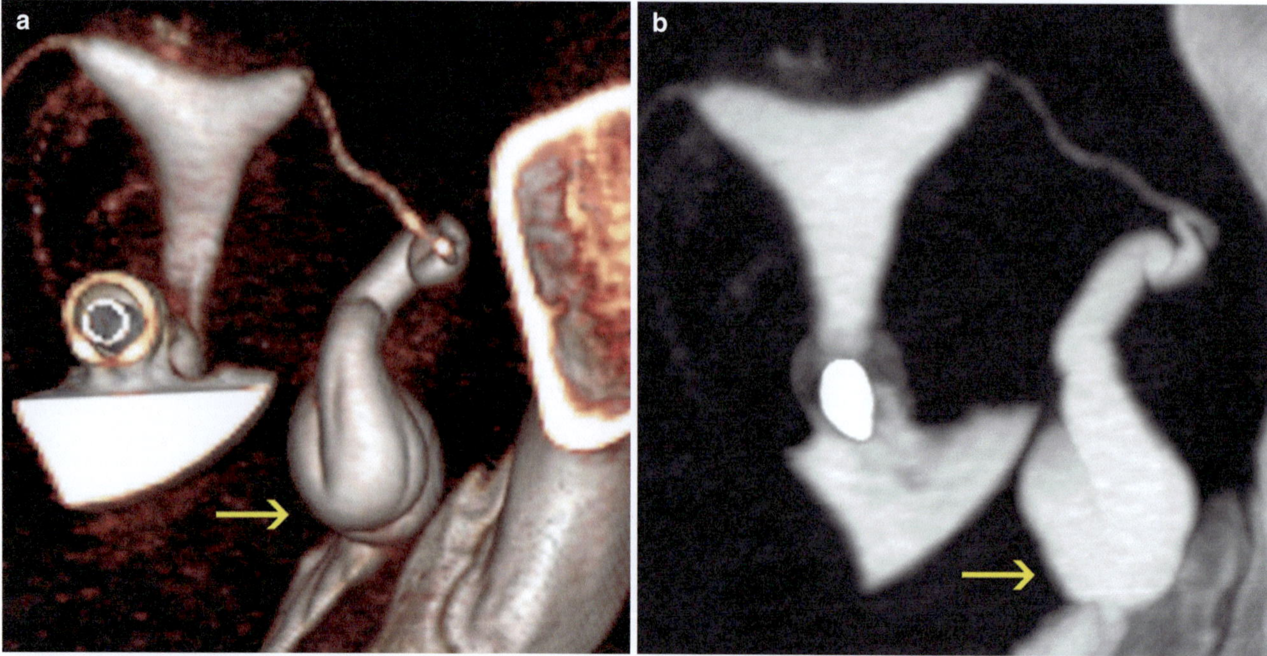

Fig. 9.12 Thirty-three-year old patient with a history of inflammatory pelvic disease. Dilatation of the ampullary region of the left uterine tube can be observed, with scarce passage of contrast, without free dispersion, into the peritoneal cavity, suggesting loculation and blockage by peritoneal adhesions (*arrow*). (**a**) 3D volume rendering image. (**b**) Maximum intensity projection image

it affects the isthmic region of both tubes, and is usually associated to ampullar obstruction and dilatation. Macroscopically, tubal nodularity is observed (hence the nodal denomination). On the other hand, microscopically, a proliferation of the glands of the mucosa and muscular hyperplasia exists. The isolated glands that invade the muscular layer maintain their communication with the tubal light, forming pseudodiverticulae. This entity must not be

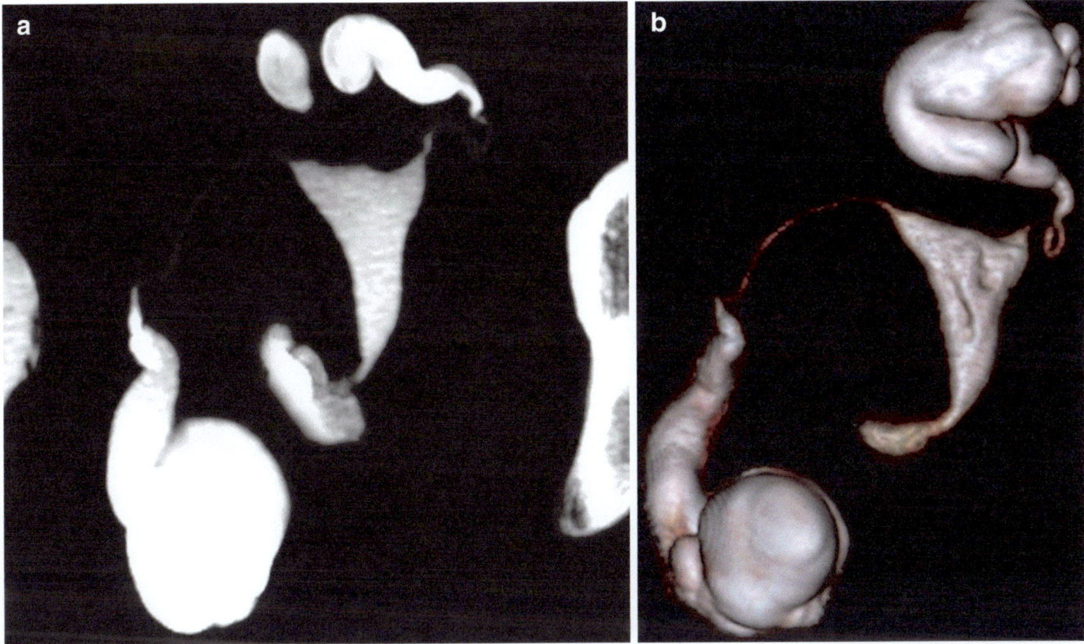

Fig. 9.13 Bilateral hydrosalpinx. Severe dilatation of both uterine tubes, without spillage of contrast into the peritoneal cavity. (**a**) Maximum intensity projection image. (**b**) 3D volume rendering image

confused with tubal adenomyosis where intramural nuclei of endometrial glands exist. In radiologic studies an irregularity in the tubal outline is observed, typically of the isthmic portion.

The characteristic finding is the presence of multiple and small bilateral diverticulae, although depending on the severity of the disease, one can visualize a compromise of a small segment with slight irregularity in moderate cases, up to extensive affectation of all the tubal portions with innumerable and big diverticular dilatations [17].

Endometriosis

The endometriosis is characterized by the presence of endometrial implants in ectopic locations. The site of most affectation is the peritoneal cavity where it can compromise the ovaries, the uterine tubes, intestinal serosa and the parietal peritoneum. The pathogenesis is unknown, but many mechanisms were described such as retrograde menstruation, methaplasia of the celomic epithelium and hematogene or lymphatic dissemination of the endometrium. The tubal endometriosis usually affects the intramural portion, although it can extend to other segments. The nuclei of endometrial implants may cause nodularity and thickening of the tubal wall, or polypoidal excretions and light stretching. In pelvic endometriosis, the affectation can be focal or diffuse with extensive nodularity that compromises various

locations. The nodules usually measure less than 1 cm and vary with the menstrual cycle by bleeding and proliferation. This generates peritoneal irritation, inflammation and fibrosis in chronic stages. Consequently, hemorrhagic cysts (endometriomas), focal scarring and diffuse adhesive disease are formed.

Clinical presentation of the endometriosis is variable. It usually manifests itself in women who menstruate, and regresses in the menopause. Patients can be asymptomatic and the finding occurs incidentally. The symptoms vary depending on the severity of the disease and the affected site. Frequently it causes pelvic pains, dysmenorrhea and dyspareunia. These symptoms worsen during menstruation. Usually it is associated with infertility and the level of severity has prognostic and therapeutic implications. Magnetic resonance is utilized to achieve the diagnosis and determine the extent of the disease non-invasively. But because the endometriosis is a disease surgically resolved, due to the fact that it rarely responds to medical treatment, the laparoscopy is routinely utilized in the stratification and treatment through the removal of the pelvic implants [18].

Both the conventional hysterosalpingography and the virtual one are limited studies in the evaluation of endometriosis due to the impossibility of directly visualizing the endometriosis implants. However, indirect signs can be observed such as dilatation, deformity and tubal obstruction due to periampullar adherences (Fig. 9.14) [19]. The tubal endometriosis can also manifest itself with a

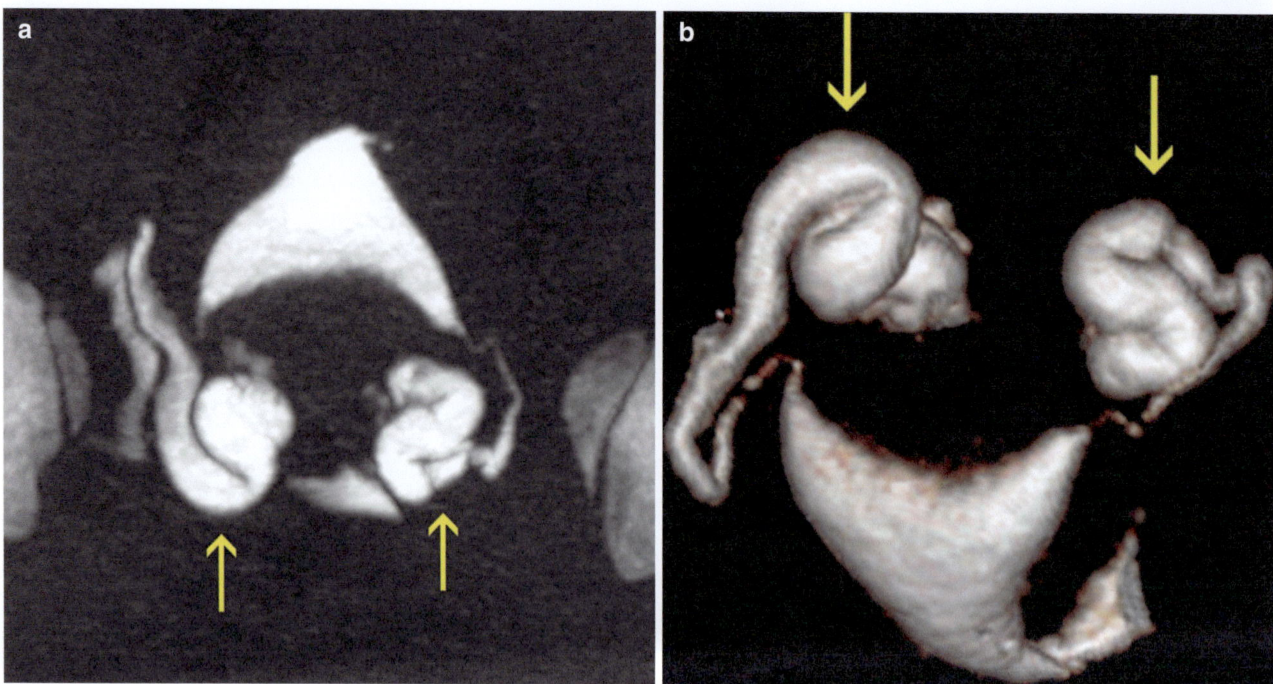

Fig. 9.14 Abnormal upwards and backwards disposition of both uterine tubes, with ampullary dilatation (*arrows*), secondary to retractile adhesion due to chronic endometriosis. (**a**) Maximum intensity projection image. (**b**) 3D volume rendering image

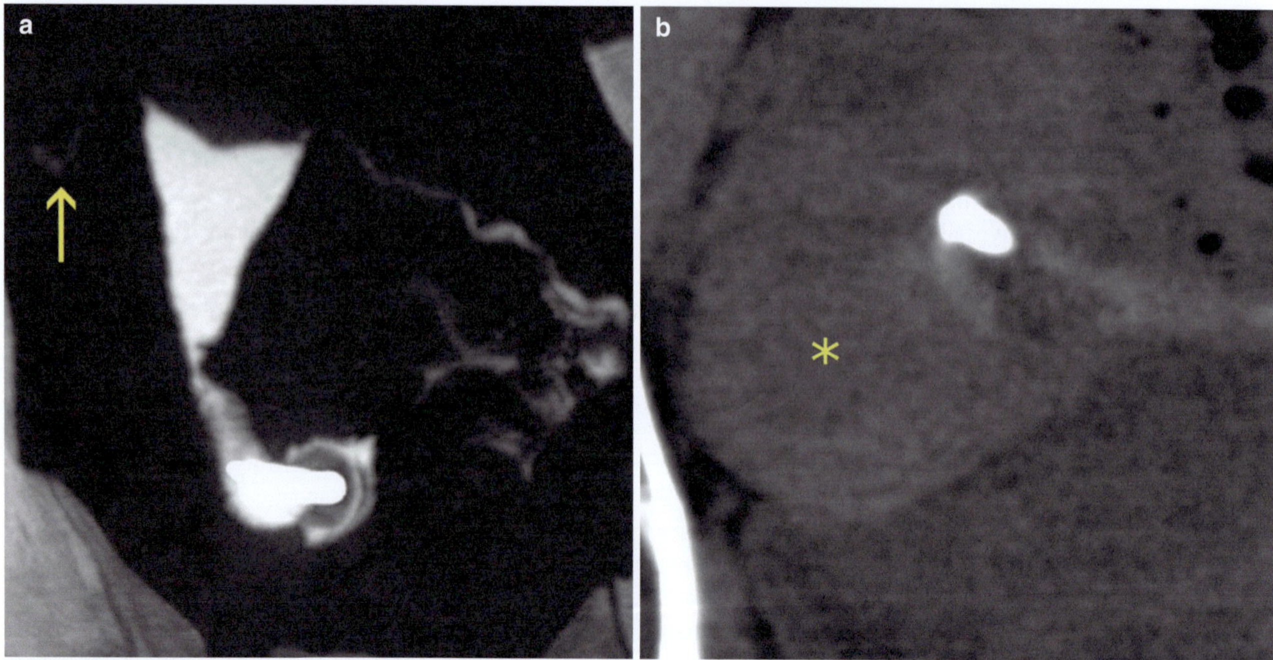

Fig. 9.15 Twenty-nine-year old patient with a history of endometriosis. (**a**) Maximum intensity projection image showing partial and incomplete opacification of the right uterine tube (*arrow*). (**b**) Axial CT image showing a slightly hyperdense rounded image (*asterisk*) in the right adnexal region, suggesting endometrioma

beaded appearance caused by multiple focal stenosis belonging to the endometrial deposits. On occasions, in the VHSG study, the endometriomas can be distinguished as discretely hyperdense collections due to their high protein content (Fig. 9.15).

Polyps and Neoplasias

Polyp lesions are rare and are typically observed in the intramural portion. The non-neoplasic polyps can be mucosal and endometriotic. They are usually observed as round images

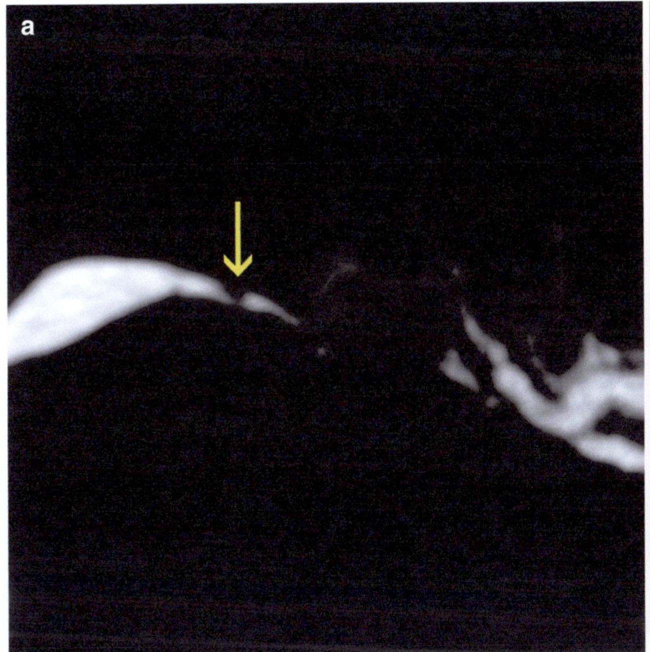

Fig. 9.16 Tubal polyp. (**a**) Maximum intensity projection image of the left tube showing a focal filling defect with a base of implantation in the posterior wall, which partially obstructs the tubal lumen (*arrow*), compatible with a tubal polyp. (**b**) Virtual endoscopy image confirming the tubal polyp (*arrow*)

with focal filling defect or as elevated lesions that protrude in the tubal lumen in virtual endoscopic views, and are associated to obstruction or tube dilatation (Fig. 9.16) [20].

Air bubbles may be introduced in the tube during the procedure of the study, and can simulate or appear as a polyp in the conventional hysterosalpingography. But bubbles are easily distinguished because of their density in the virtual studies. Both the benign and malign tubal neoplasia are not very frequent and present themselves in postmenopausal patients, reasons why they are rarely observed in hysterosalpingography studies [21].

Postsurgical Changes

The knowledge of the available surgical techniques for the treatment of tubal abnormalities is fundamental for the interpretation of the radiological findings in those patients that were subject to these therapies. The sterilization procedures include the bilateral tubal ligation and its variants. The medial isthmic region is the one chosen with most frequency for the blockage. In the VHSG a partial filling of the tubes with an abrupt termination as well as characteristic discrete bulbous dilatation are observed (Fig. 9.17). Segmental resection may be done for the treatment of the ectopic pregnancies, salpingitis isthmica nodosa and other focal abnormalities. In radiologic studies, the intervened tube will appear shorter and with deformities in the site of the operation. Other more conservative techniques imply

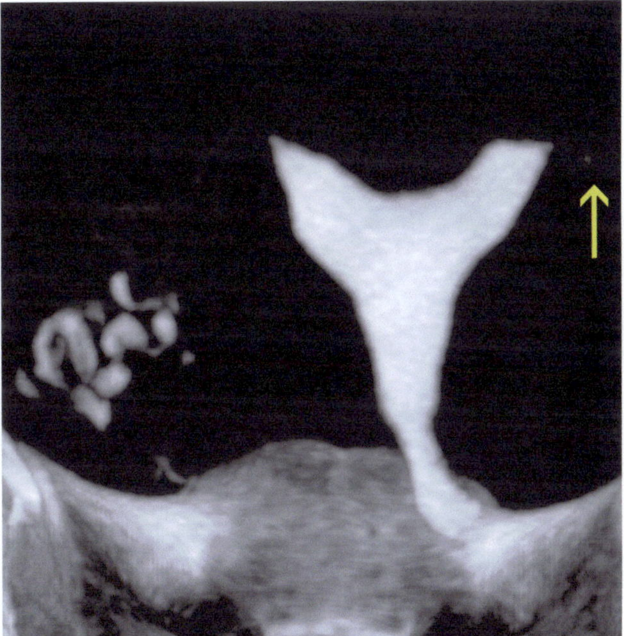

Fig. 9.17 Thirty-two-year old patient with a history of tubal surgery. The maximum intensity projection image shows post-surgery left tubal occlusion (*arrow*)

tubal reconstruction for the correction of the inflammatory and endometriotic sequels with removal of peri and intra-tubal adherences. The surgical changes include the recovery of the permeability and diminishment of the tubal dilatation [22].

Conclusion

The virtual hysterosalpingography is an excellent method in the evaluation of the uterine tubes. The diverse tubal pathologies that cause infertility can be detected by this novel method. The technological advantages that the VHSG study offers allow a detailed assessment of the tubal anatomy and a precise exam with different visualization tools. The radiologist must be familiarized with the normal findings, as well as the signs and presentation of the pathological processes that with high frequency affect the uterine tubes.

References

1. Carrascosa PM, Capuñay C, Vallejos J, et al. Virtual hysterosalpingography: a new multidetector CT technique for evaluating the female reproductive system. Radiographics. 2010;30(3):643–61.
2. Swart P, Mol BW, van der Veen F, et al. The accuracy of hysterosalpingography in the diagnosis of tubal pathology: a meta-analysis. Fertil Steril. 1995;64(3):486–91.
3. Benjaminov O, Atri M. Sonography of the abnormal fallopian tube. AJR Am J Roentgenol. 2004;183(3):737–42.
4. Hamed HO, Shahin AY, Elsamman AM. Hysterosalpingo-contrast sonography versus radiographic hysterosalpingography in the evaluation of tubal patency. Int J Gynaecol Obstet. 2009;105(3): 215–7.
5. Sankpal RS, Confino E, Matzel A, et al. Investigation of the uterine cavity and fallopian tubes using three-dimensional saline sonohysterosalpingography. Int J Gynaecol Obstet. 2001;73(2): 125–9.
6. Lundberg S, Wramsby H, Bremmer S, et al. Radionuclide hysterosalpingography is not predictive in the diagnosis of infertility. Fertil Steril. 1998;69(2):216–20.
7. Unterweger M, De Geyter C, Fröhlich JM, et al. Three-dimensional dynamic MR-hysterosalpingography; a new, low invasive, radiation-free and less painful radiological approach to female infertility. Hum Reprod. 2002;17(12):3138–41.
8. Winter L, Glücker T, Steimann S, et al. Feasibility of dynamic MR-hysterosalpingography for the diagnostic work-up of infertile women. Acta Radiol. 2010;51(6):693–701.
9. Sadowski EA, Ochsner JE, Riherd JM, et al. MR hysterosalpingography with an angiographic time-resolved 3D pulse sequence: assessment of tubal patency. AJR Am J Roentgenol. 2008;191(5):1381–5.
10. Vardhana PA, Silberzweig JE, Guarnaccia M, et al. Hysterosalpingography with selective salpingography. J Reprod Med. 2009;54(3):126–32.
11. Papaioannou S, Bourdrez P, Varma R, et al. Tubal evaluation in the investigation of subfertility: a structured comparison of tests. BJOG. 2004;111(12):1313–21.
12. Chalazonitis A, Tzovara I, Laspas F, et al. Hysterosalpingography: technique and applications. Curr Probl Diagn Radiol. 2009; 38(5):199–205.
13. Carrascosa P, Capuñay C, Vallejos J, et al. Virtual hysterosalpingography: experience with over 1000 consecutive patients. Abdom Imaging. 2011;36(1):1–14.
14. Winfield AC, Pittaway D, Maxson W, et al. Apparent cornual occlusion in hysterosalpingography: reversal by glucagon. AJR Am J Roentgenol. 1982;139(3):525–7.
15. Simpson Jr WL, Beitia LG, Mester J. Hysterosalpingography: a reemerging study. Radiographics. 2006;26(2):419–31.
16. Sam JW, Jacobs JE, Birnbaum BA. Spectrum of CT findings in acute pyogenic pelvic inflammatory disease. Radiographics. 2002;22(6):1327–34.
17. Ott DJ, Fayez JA. Tubal and adnexal abnormalities. In: Ott DJ, Fayez JA, Zagoria RJ, editors. Hysterosalpingography: a text and atlas. 2nd ed. Baltimore: Williams & Wilkins; 1998. p. 90–3.
18. Woodward PJ, Sohaey R, Mezzetti Jr TP. Endometriosis: radiologic-pathologic correlation. Radiographics. 2001;21(1):193–216.
19. Karasick S, Goldfarb AF. Peritubal adhesions in infertile women: diagnosis with hysterosalpingography. AJR Am J Roentgenol. 1989;152(4):777–9.
20. Lee A, Ying YK, Novy MJ. Hysteroscopy, hysterosalpingography and tubal ostial polyps in infertility patients. J Reprod Med. 1997;42(6):337–41.
21. Kawakami S, Togashi K, Kimura I, et al. Primary malignant tumor of the fallopian tube: appearance at CT and MR imaging. Radiology. 1993;186(2):503–8.
22. Letterie GS, Haggerty MF, Fellows DW. Sensitivity of hysterosalpingography after tubal surgery. Arch Gynecol Obstet. 1992;251(4):175–80.

Part III

Miscellaneous

The uterine silhouette is a settling place for different malformations and pathological processes, some of which can require surgical treatment, may it be via the abdomen (laparotomy, laparoscopy) or the vagina (hysteroscopy, laparoscopy) [1–3]. In certain opportunities one can also turn to endovascular treatment, as is the case of the chemoembolization of uterine myomas [4–6].

These procedures on the uterus can generate morphological changes that are visible in virtual hysterosalpingography (VHSG) studies. Different are the motives to carry out these therapeutic measures, among them is found the resection of myomas, the reparation of uterine anomalies, the removal of synechiae and the cesarean section [7, 8].

In this chapter the cases related to diverse therapeutic procedures their sequels and/or complications will be shown.

Myomas

The uterine myomatosis is a frequent entity in women older than 30 [9, 10]. The myomas can be intramural, submucosal and subserous. Their relation with fertility is controversial, with different opinions on when and in what level do the myomas influence in the success of the pregnancy [11–15].

Different are also the therapeutic strategies, depending on the number, size, maternity wishes and age of the patient. Submucosal myomas can be dried with hysteroscopy; subserosal or intramural myomas removed through laparotomy or preferably through laparoscopic surgery [1, 2, 16, 17]. The surgical drying of these tumors can generate significant changes in the morphology of the uterus according to the size, location and number of removed myomas. In the case of small intramural or subserous fibroids, the uterine cavity does not generally present any changes. However, the removal of submucosal or intramural myomas of larger size can deform the cavity after the myomectomy [7, 8].

Currently, another therapeutic option that has earned a place amid the different variants of available treatments is the chemoembolization [4–6]. This procedure provides also

changes at the level of the uterus and/or of the cavity that can be appreciated in imaging studies.

Case 1

A 34-year old patient, G0P0, with primary infertility. The VHSG shows the presence of a subserous myoma on the left lateral and anterior wall of $5 \times 5.5 \times 8$ cm that deforms the uterine silhouette, and a uterine cavity of normal morphology and regular outlines (Fig. 10.1). Its surgical removal is decided prior the start of the infertility treatment. The control VHSG carried out 2 months after the surgery shows a uterus of conservative size and normal morphology (Fig. 10.2).

Case 2

A 29-year old patient, G1P1, with secondary infertility of 18 months. The VHSG exam shows a deformity in the uterine cavity at the level of the fundus, on the right horn, secondary to the presence of a posterior submucosal myoma of medium size (Fig. 10.3). Given these characteristics, and its potential influence in the success of the conception, it is proceeded with its removal via hysteroscopy (Fig. 10.4). The control VHSG after 3 months shows a uterine cavity of normal morphology with regular outlines, with no evidence of postsurgical sequels (Fig. 10.5).

Case 3

A 36-year old patient, G0P0, with primary infertility and multiple symptomatic uterine myomatosis of 7 years of evolution. The presence of an intramural myoma on the right lateral uterine wall of $44 \times 42 \times 41$ mm stands out, with an approximate volume of 39 cm³ (Fig. 10.6). The patient carried out medical treatment with agonists of the GnRh for 6 months, previous to the uterine embolization treatment, taking part of an immediate post-procedure without complications. A year later she returns for a reevaluation for her primary infertility. A control transvaginal ecography is done, identifying iso-hipoecogenic areas on the right myometrial wall in the location of the treated myoma, with thickening and endometrial liquid. Upon the 10th day, a conventional

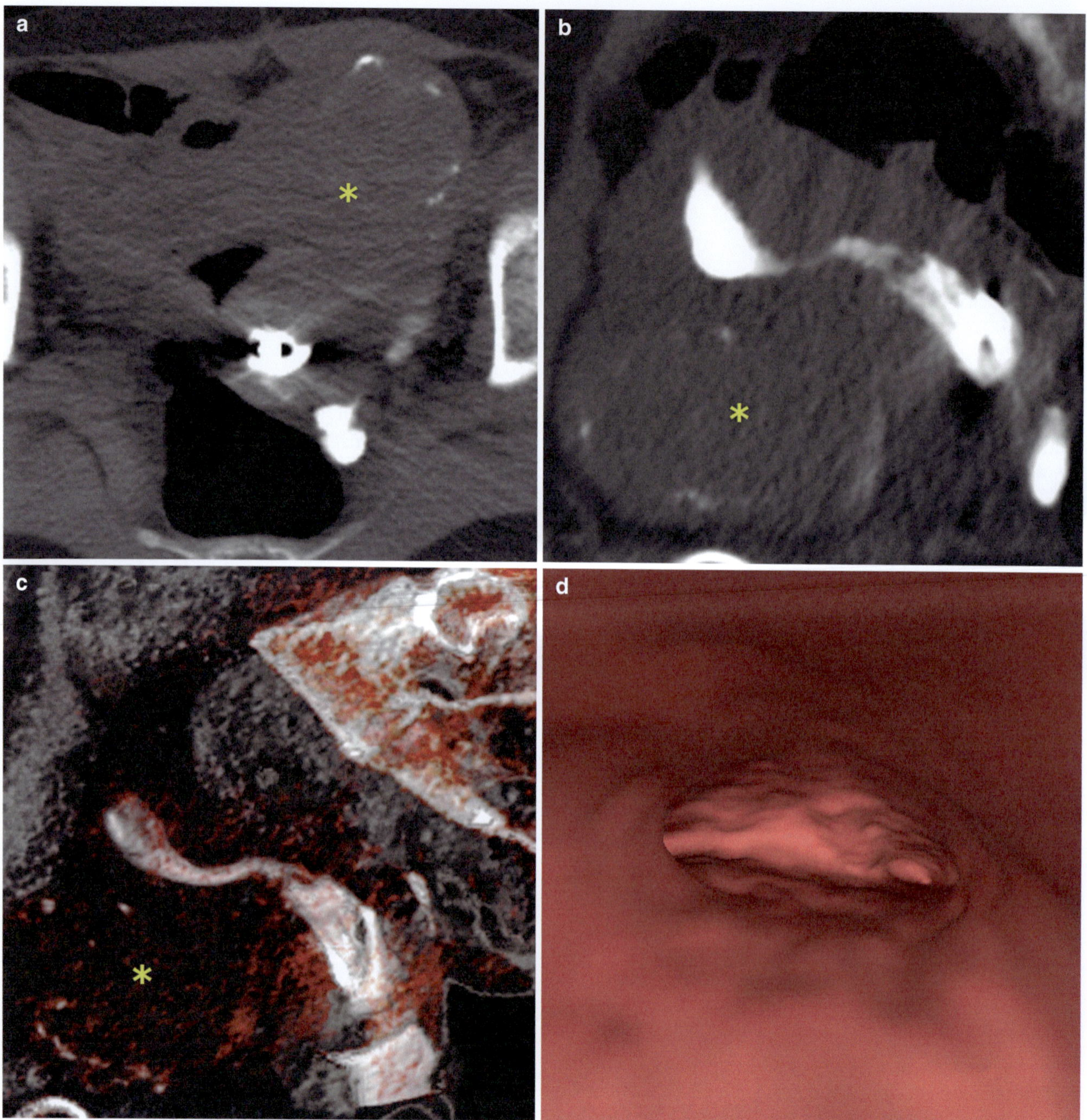

Fig. 10.1 VHSG study showing an anteverted uterus increased in size with the presence of an anterior subserosal myoma, with fine peripheral calcifications (*asterisk*). (**a**) Axial maximum intensity projection (MIP) image. (**b**) Sagittal MIP image. (**c**) Sagittal 3D volume rendering image. (**d**) Virtual endoscopy image showing a normal endometrial cavity

X-ray hysterosalpingography is done that shows passage of the instilled contrast through the external cervical os towards a pseudocavity located on the right uterine wall (Fig. 10.7). The exam is completed with the realization of a VHSG to value with higher precision the state of the endometrial cavity and plan the next procedure of assisted fertilization. The study shows the presence of fistula between the endometrial cavity and the residual post-embolization cavity, allowing the clear visualization of the diameter and length of the fistula trajectory, the parietal thickness of the residual pseudocavity and the absence of perforation towards the peritoneal cavity (Fig. 10.8).

Uterine Malformations

The plastic and reconstructive uterus operations in patients with uterine anomalies, whether it is a septated or bicornuate uterus, are an alternative for those women who want to achieve a successful pregnancy [3, 13]. In patients with a septated uterus,

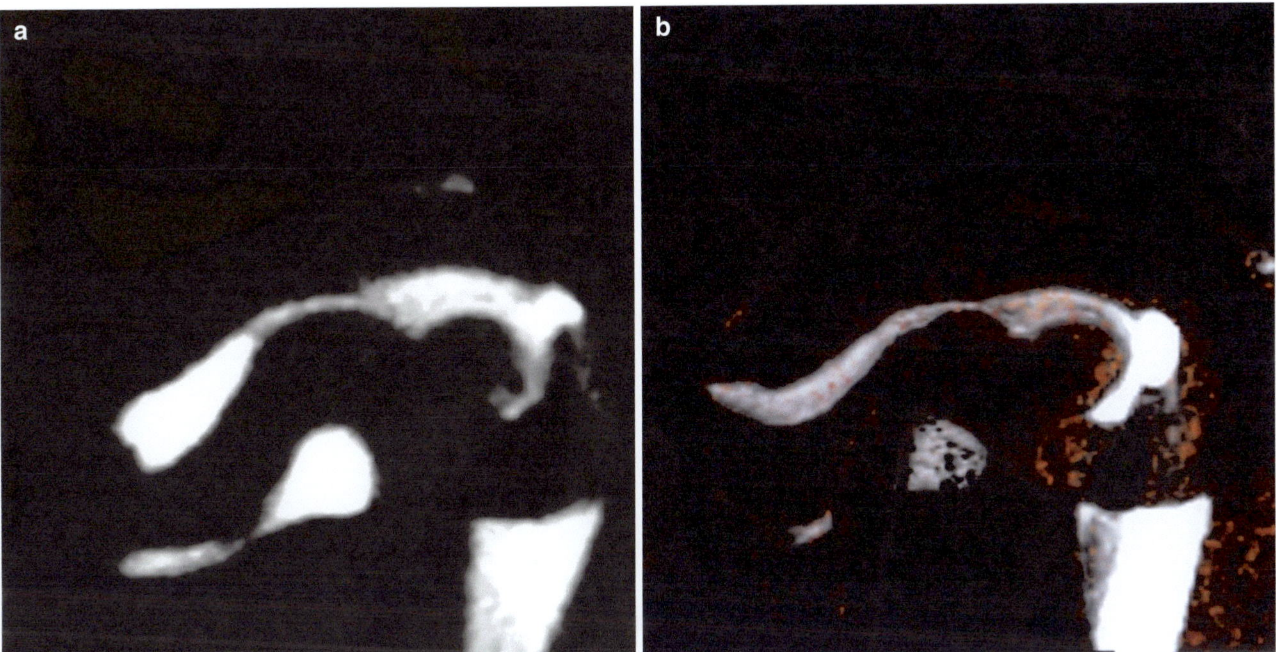

Fig. 10.2 Post-surgery VHSG study showing an anteverted uterus of normal size. (**a**) Sagittal maximum intensity projection image. (**b**) Sagittal 3D volume rendering image

the removal of the uterine septum via hysteroscopy is a surgical technique of growing application in the treatment of this uterine anomaly. Among the complications of this technique, an incomplete removal of the uterine septum and the formation of adherences or intrauterine synechiae are included [18, 19].

Case 4

A 24-year old patient, G3P0A3, with a history of spontaneous abortions during the first trimester. A diagnosis of a partial septated uterus is done (Fig. 10.9). As a therapeutic strategy, the removal via hysteroscopy of the uterine septum is decided. The VHSG study post-treatment shows a more ample uterine cavity, with a small indentation at the level of the fundus corresponding to the normal postsurgical remnant (Fig. 10.10).

Case 5

A 25-year old patient, G2P0A2, with diagnosis of bicornuate uterus (Fig. 10.11). The patient is subject to a Strassman surgery as the reparation technique. In the post-treatment VHSG study carried out on the third month, a larger endometrial cavity could be appreciated, with a slight deformity at the level of the fundus, of regular margins and with no filling defects (Fig. 10.12).

Synechiae

The intrauterine adherences represent scars in the uterine cavity result of an infection or trauma. The removal via hysteroscopy is today the most utilized procedure and consid-

ered of reference for the diagnosis and treatment [20, 21]. The most secure, less traumatic and most precise technique consists in the adhesiolisis, through the combination of surgical dissection and electrosurgery, and the postsurgical administration of high doses of estrogens, and/or progestogens and antibiotics, important in the prevention of the recurrence. The use of intrauterine contraceptive devices after the resection of the synechiae is considered useful by some groups, while other propose the use of hyaluronic acid as an alternative [22–24].

Case 6

A 29-year old patient, G2P0A2, with secondary infertility of 3 years of evolution, and a history of abortions with uterine curettage. As part of the diagnostic algorithm, the patient carries out a VHSG that demonstrates the presence of an irregular endometrial cavity, with lineal, irregular and thick filling defects that correspond to synechiae. The presence of a subserous myoma is also appreciated (Fig. 10.13). Treatment consists in the hysteroscopic removal of the synechiae and the laparoscopic resection of the myoma. The VHSG control carried out after 3 months shows the incomplete removal of the adherences, with a residual synechia around the right uterine horn. The subserosal myoma cannot be appreciated (Fig. 10.14).

Case 7

A 34-year old patient, G1P1, with secondary infertility lasting 15 years' duration. The VHSG study showed a permeable cervical canal and an endometrial cavity of normal morphology, with the presence of an endoluminal elevated filling defect on the posterior wall compatible with an endometrial polyp (Fig. 10.15). In the control VHSG study, after the hysteroscopic treatment, a complete removal of the polypoid lesion was appreciated. However, a lineal image is visualized on the cervical canal extending from wall to wall, which is compatible with an endocervical synechia, secondary to the therapeutic treatment (Fig. 10.16).

Cesarean Section

Currently in medicine the births by cesarean section have increased along the years for different reasons (Table 10.1). Cesarean constitutes a regular surgical practice that involves the uterine silhouette, and in obstetrics being the most frequent surgery. Its incidence has grown significantly, in some countries reaching a rate between 17 and 25 % [25]. The cesarean section implies an incision done above the lower

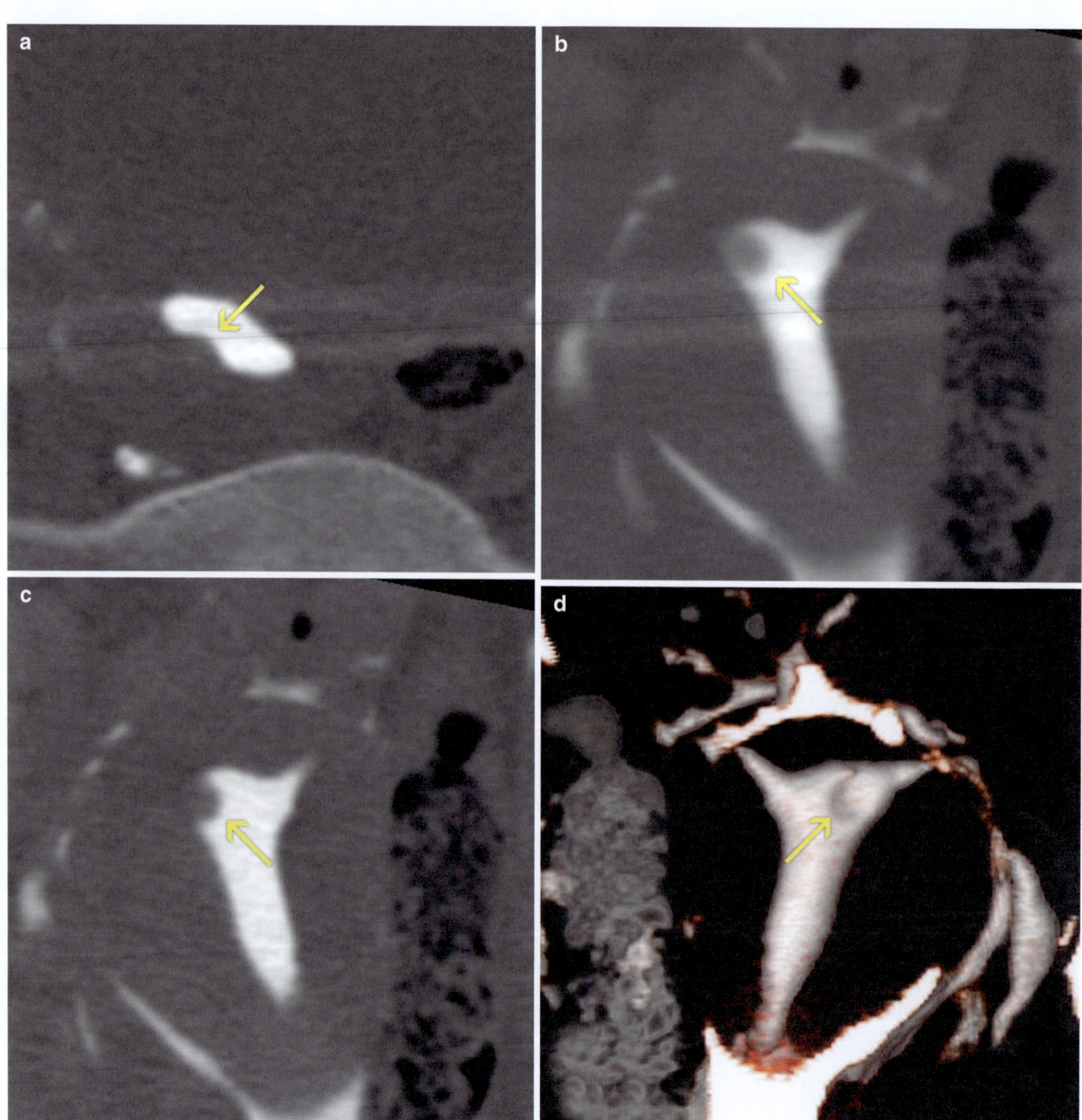

Fig. 10.3 VHSG study which shows an elevated image on the posterior wall of the uterus that protrudes into the endometrial cavity compatible with a submucosal myoma (*arrows*). (**a**) Axial maximum intensity projection (MIP) image. (**b**) 5-mm coronal multiplanar reconstruction image. (**c**) Coronal MIP image. (**d**) Coronal 3D volume rendering image, posterior view. (**e, f**) Virtual endoscopy images

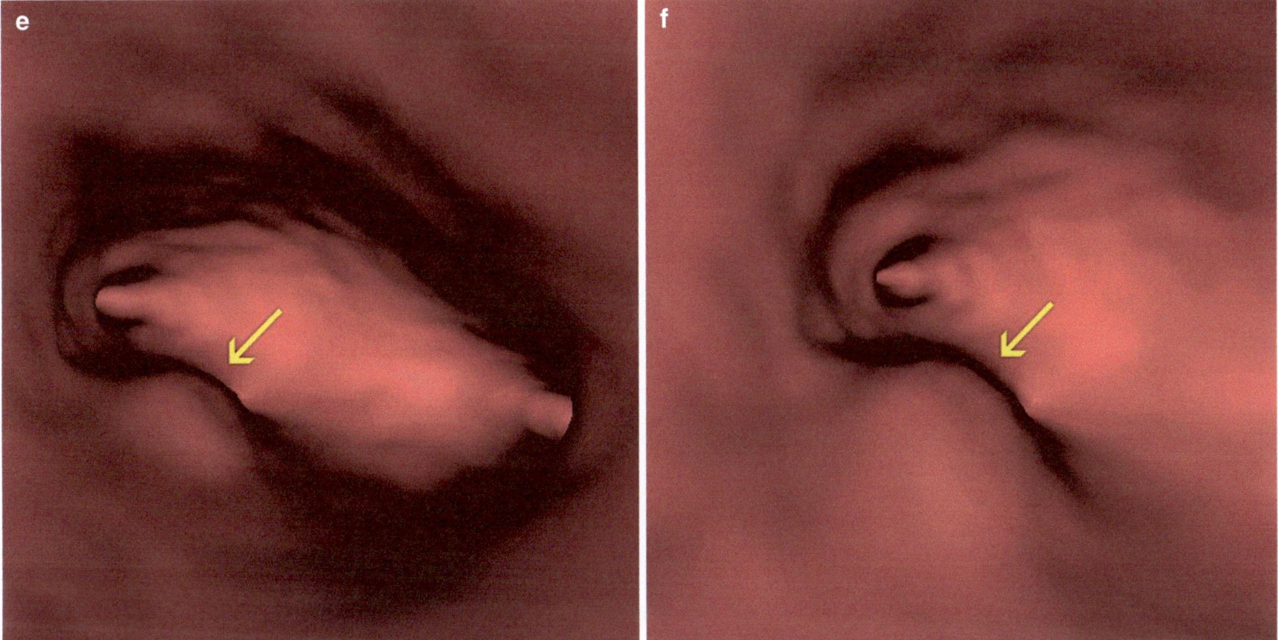

Fig. 10.3 (continued)

section of the uterus. The surgical techniques are each time more systematized and the post intervention sequels lower. However, on occasions potential complications can be appreciated. One of the most frequent and with potential influence in future pregnancies is the postsurgical defect associated with the scar. In patients subject to cesarean section, the width of the myometrium wall in the zone of the scar is thinner, and in a number of occasions a residual pseudocavity of diverticular area persists that presents communication with the endometrial cavity and whose size is variable (Figs. 10.17, 10.18, and 10.19). The niche in the scar, as it is also denominated, is defined as a triangular area in the site of the incision, with a depth that varies between 4.2 and 6.2 mm [26–28]. The width of the myometrium in these cases is also thinner with an average width of 6.5 ± 2.7 mm (range 0–10.9 mm) while in operated patient with no presence of a niche, the myometrium measures 8.9 ± 2 mm (6–13.9 mm) [27]. When the niche surpasses 80 % of the depth of the width of the former myometrium is called dehiscence. The VHSG allows the clear visualization of these continuity defects of the myometrial fibers of the isthmic region, their diameters, their depths, and also their volume (Fig. 10.18). It is also possible to measure the width of the myometrial wall in that segment, significantly thinner in comparison with patients with no history of cesarean section. The work presented by Dr. Capuñay and colleagues [29] in the Argentine Congress of Radiology 2011 proved that the width of the myometrial wall in the isthmic region in patients with no history of cesarean is of 11.5 mm, while in those with a history of cesarean is of 5.3 mm, with a statistically significant dif-

ference ($p < 0.001$). The volume of the surgical scar is also variable. Diverse articles have evaluated the relation between the width of the wall at the cesarean scar, valuated with transvaginal ecography, and the risk of dehiscence during pregnancy, showing the real possibility of a rupture. The knowledge of the anatomical information before a pregnancy can be of potential utility; hence it is necessary to show it clinically.

The dehiscence or rupture does not only occur during pregnancy, but can also happen in the absence of one. On occasions there exists a poor scarring process of the surgical incision, following the development of an utero-peritoneal fistula [30].

Case 8

Patient of 35 years of age, G2-P0-C2, with a history of 2 cesareas, the last one 15 months ago. Given the intention of a new pregnancy, a conventional hysterosalpingography study is commended for the assessment of the cesarean scar (Fig. 10.19). A VHSG study, as a complement of the conventional study, corroborates the dehiscence (Fig. 10.20).

Case 9

A 36-year old patient, G2P1C1, with a history of a cesarean section 5 months ago, presents during the last days menstrual bleeding, colic pelvic pain, along with low urinary symptoms, dysuria and polaquiuria. The control transvaginal ecographies carried out in the days where the symptoms of the patient were present did not show significant utero-ovarian

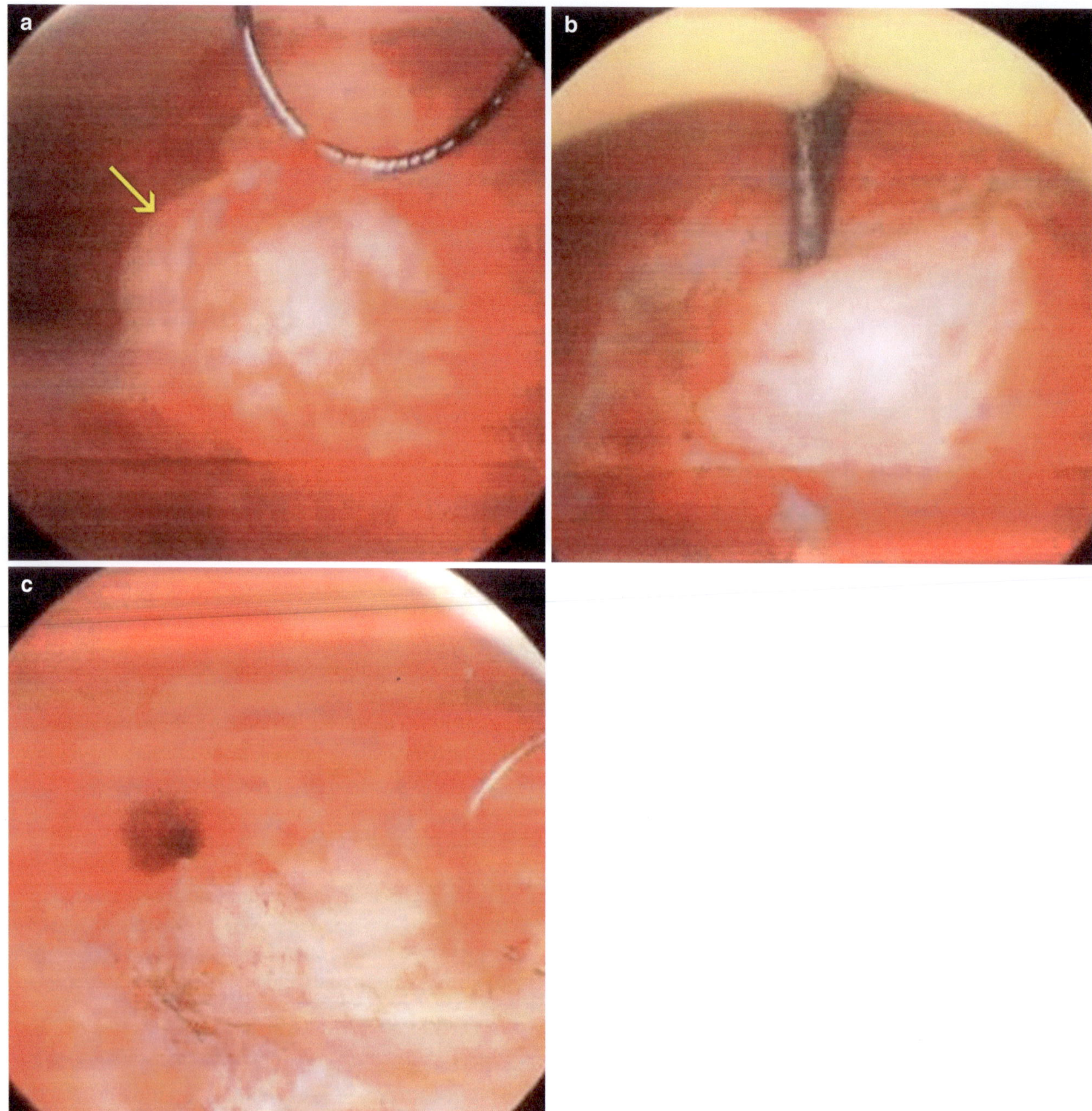

Fig. 10.4 Conventional hysteroscopy images. (**a**) Submucosal myoma on the posterior wall of the uterine cavity (*arrow*). (**b**) Myomectomy. (**c**) Post-surgical sequelae

findings, with a normal quantity of fluid in the peritoneal cavity. It is decided to carry out a VHSG to evaluate the state of the cesarean scar, identifying during the instillation of the contrast the passage of it through the zone of the scar to the peritoneal cavity, proving the presence of a uteroperitoneal fistula (Fig. 10.21). The cesarean scar was wide, of $6.5 \times 7.0 \times 10.2$ mm, with a volume of 5.94 cm^3. The myometrial wall was very thin in the compromised segment (Fig. 10.22).

Fallopian Tubes

The postsurgical modifications at the level of the tubes are related to the total or partial resection in patients with tubo-ovarian ectopic pregnancies, patients with hydrosalpinx, or subject to tubal ligation as part of the birth control strategies [31–35]. Structural changes at the level of the tubes can also be appreciated in patients operated through endometriosis.

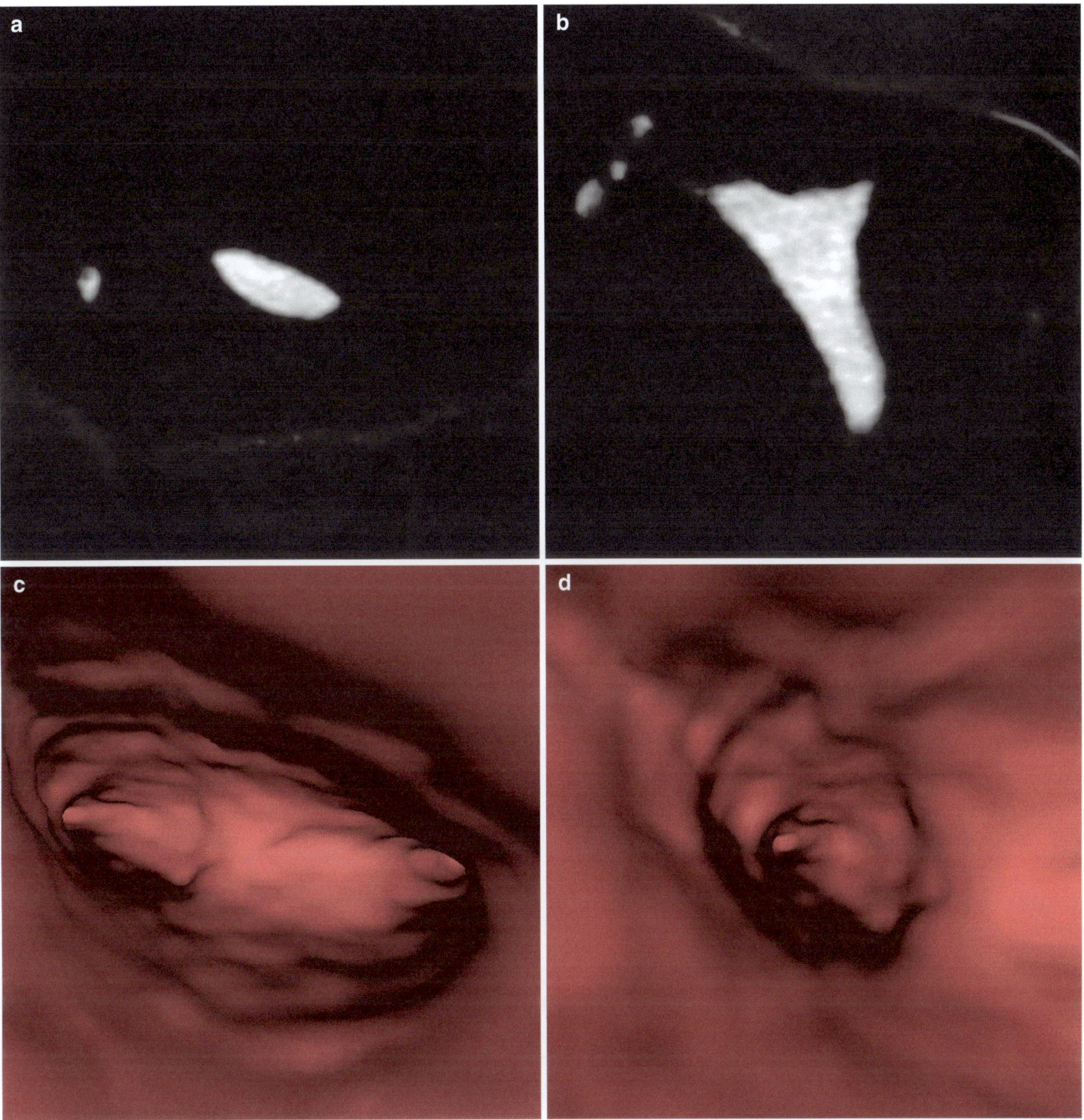

Fig. 10.5 Post-myomectomy VHSG study. An endometrial cavity without endoluminal lesion is observed. (**a**) Axial maximum intensity projection (MIP) image. (**b**) Coronal MIP image. (**c, d**) Virtual endoscopy images

Case 10

A 32-year old patient, G1P0, with a history of uterine tube resection secondary to right tubo-ovarian pregnancy. The VHSG effectuated 2 years after shows the amputation of the right uterine tube 2 cm away from the cornual region, with discrete pseudodiverticular focal dilatation. The left uterine tube is permeable (Fig. 10.23).

Case 11

A 34-year old patient, G1P1, with a history of a surgical resection of both Fallopian tubes as treatment of bilateral hydrosalpinx secondary to endometriosis. The VHSG indicated for the evaluation of the endometrial cavity previous to the start of the assisted fertilization procedure shows the amputation of both uterine tubes, with the identification of only the proximal segment of them, with absence of the passage of contrast to the peritoneum (Fig. 10.24).

Case 12

A-28 year old patient, G2P0A2, with a history of endometriosis and surgical resection of the left uterine tube because of an ectopic pregnancy, in a study for 24 month infertility. The first VHSG carried out showed a cavity free of disease, the amputation of the left tube in accordance to the surgical background and the presence of right hydrosalpinx (Fig. 10.25). The patient is subjected to a laparoscopy surgery to liberate the right tube, with a resection of the endometriosis nuclei. The VHSG control study carried out 2 months after the surgical intervention shows a right uterine tube of normal morphology, with a persistent slight dilatation at the ampulla, and an adequate spillage of contrast to the peritoneal cavity (Fig. 10.26).

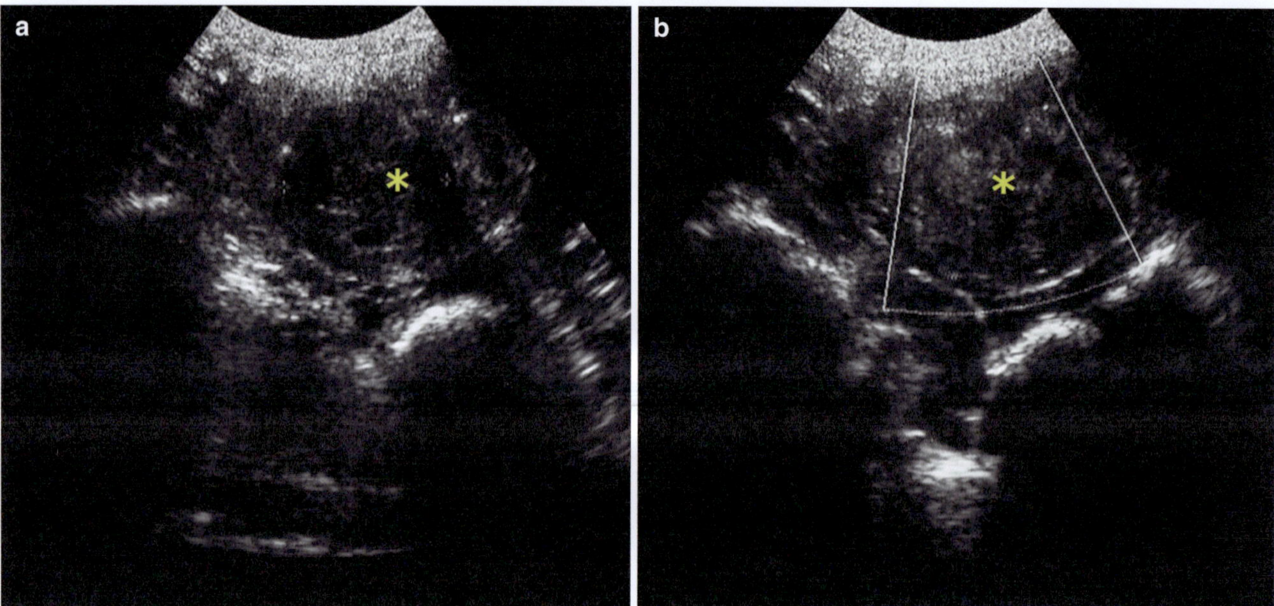

Fig. 10.6 Transvaginal ultrasound. Presence of intramural myoma on the right lateral uterine wall, of 44×42×41 mm in size, with a volume of 39 cm³ (*asterisk*). (**a**) Transverse image (**b**) Transverse image with Doppler

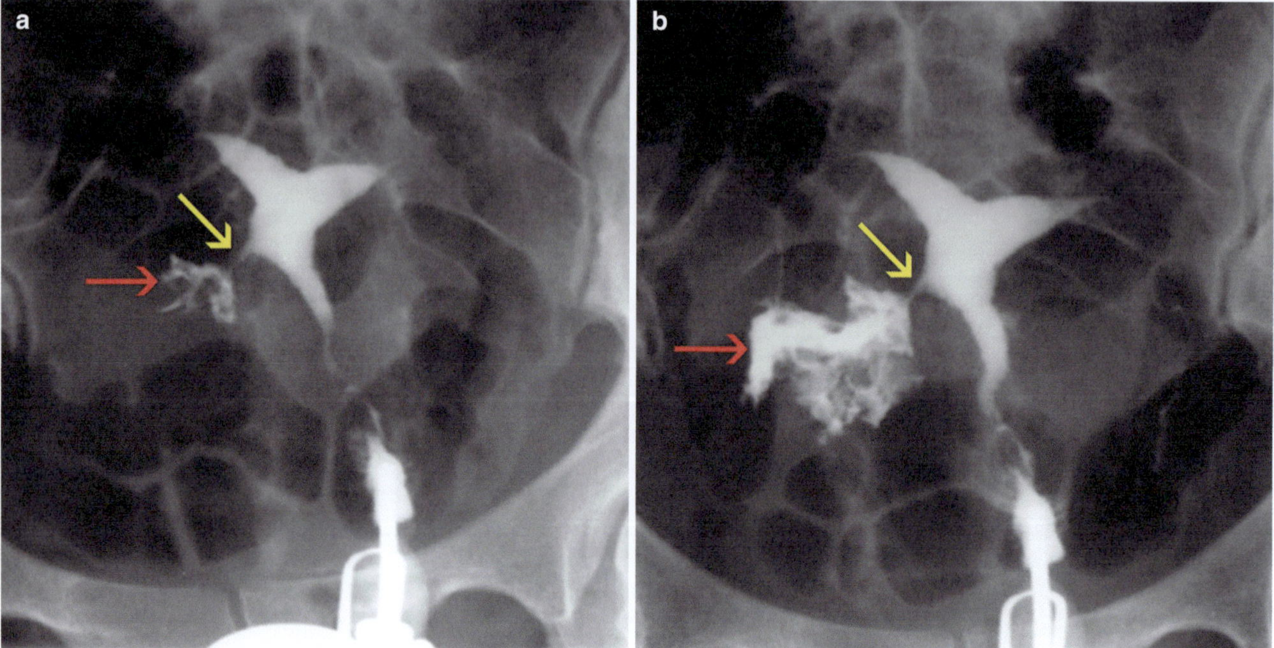

Fig. 10.7 (**a–c**) HSG images post embolization treatment. A progressive filling of an irregular cavity is appreciated on the right uterine wall (*red arrows*). The presence of a fistulous tract (*yellow arrows*) between the endometrial cavity and the uterine wall cavity is demonstrated

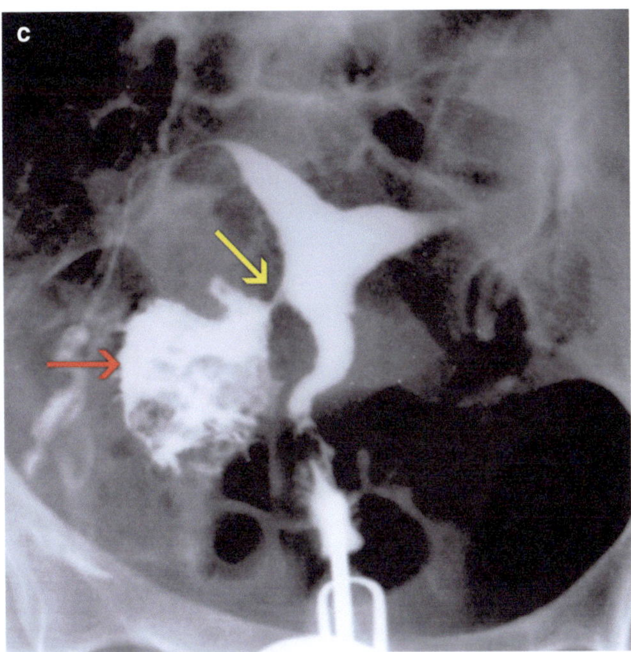

Fig. 10.7 (continued)

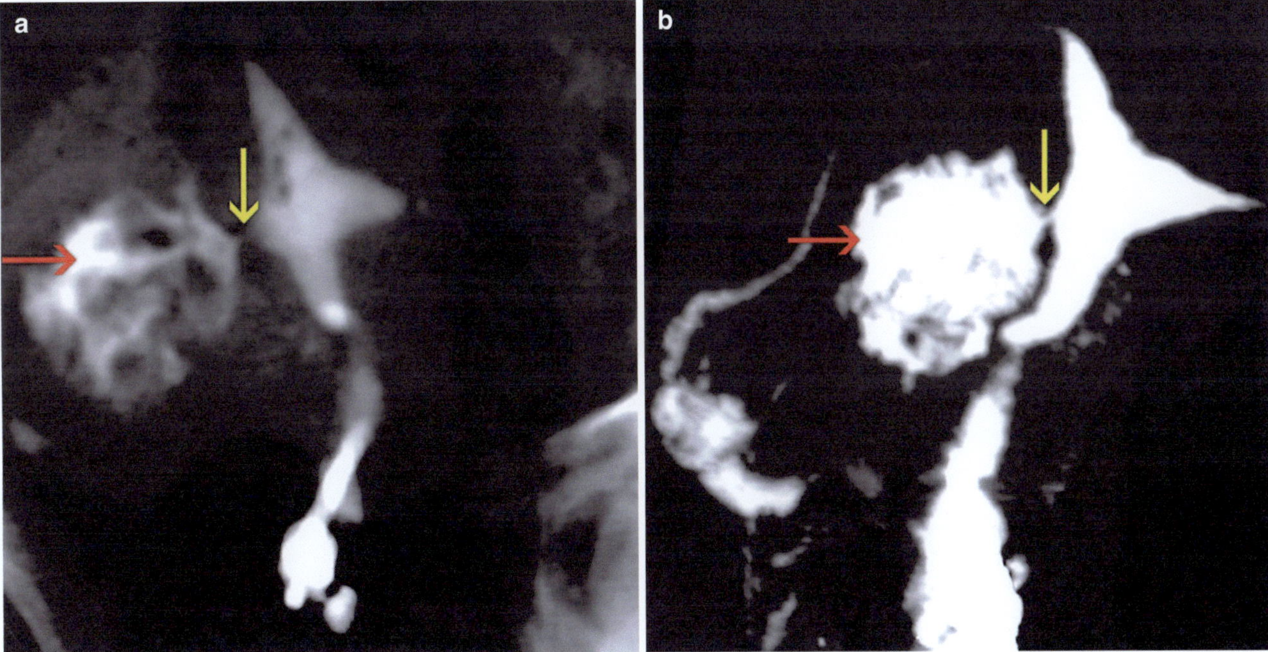

Fig. 10.8 VHSG study post embolization treatment. A progressive filling of an irregular cavity is appreciated on the right uterine wall (*red arrows*), with the presence of a fistulous tract to the endometrial cavity (*yellow arrows*). (**a**) 5-mm coronal multiplanar reconstruction image. (**b**) Coronal maximum intensity projection image. (**c**) Coronal 3D volume rendering image. (**d**) Virtual endoscopy image which shows the orifice of the fistula in the right wall of the endometrial cavity. (**e**) Virtual endoscopy image at the level of the fistulous tract. (**f**) Virtual endoscopy image of the residual post-embolization cavity on the right uterine wall

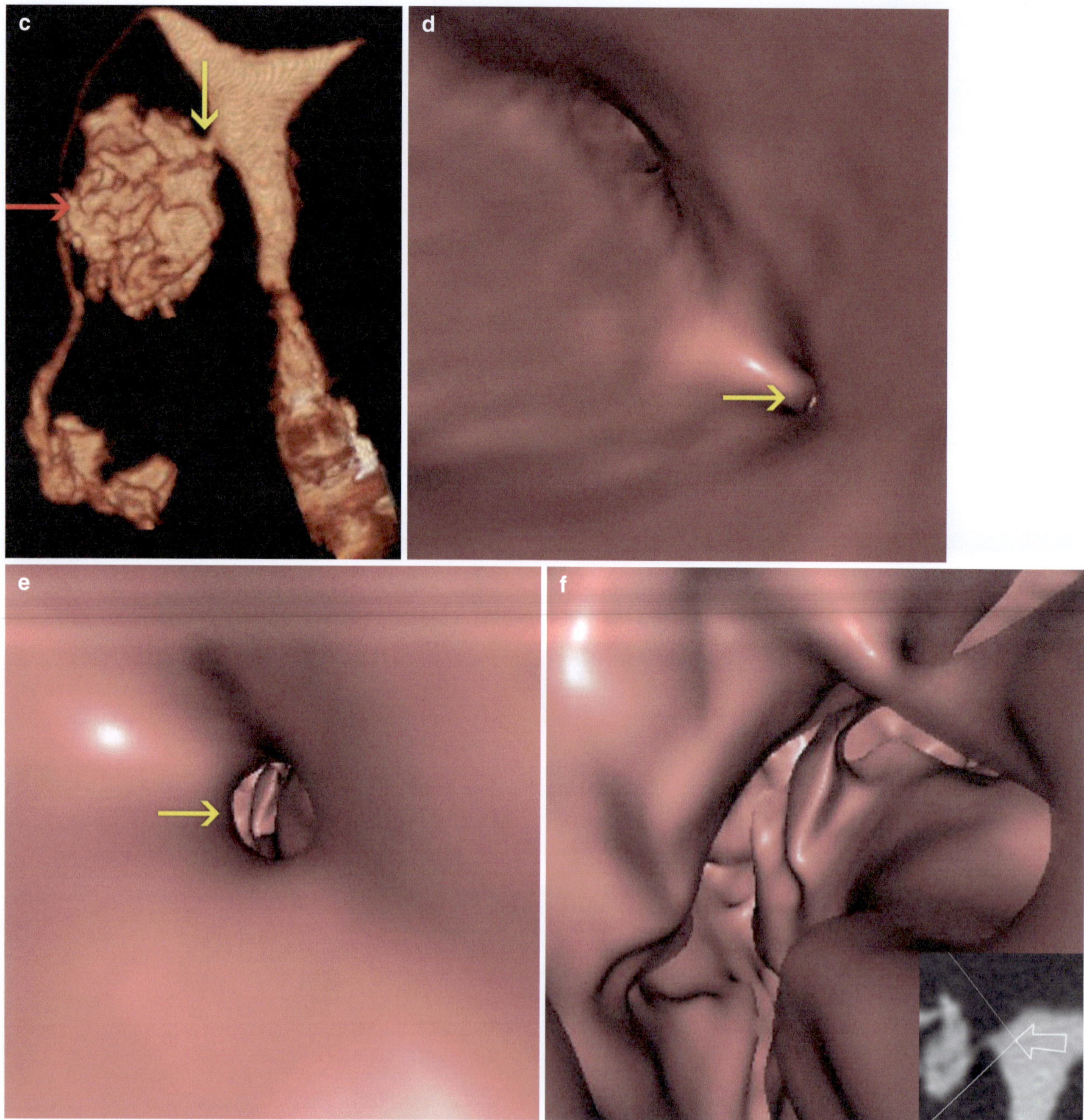

Fig. 10.8 (continued)

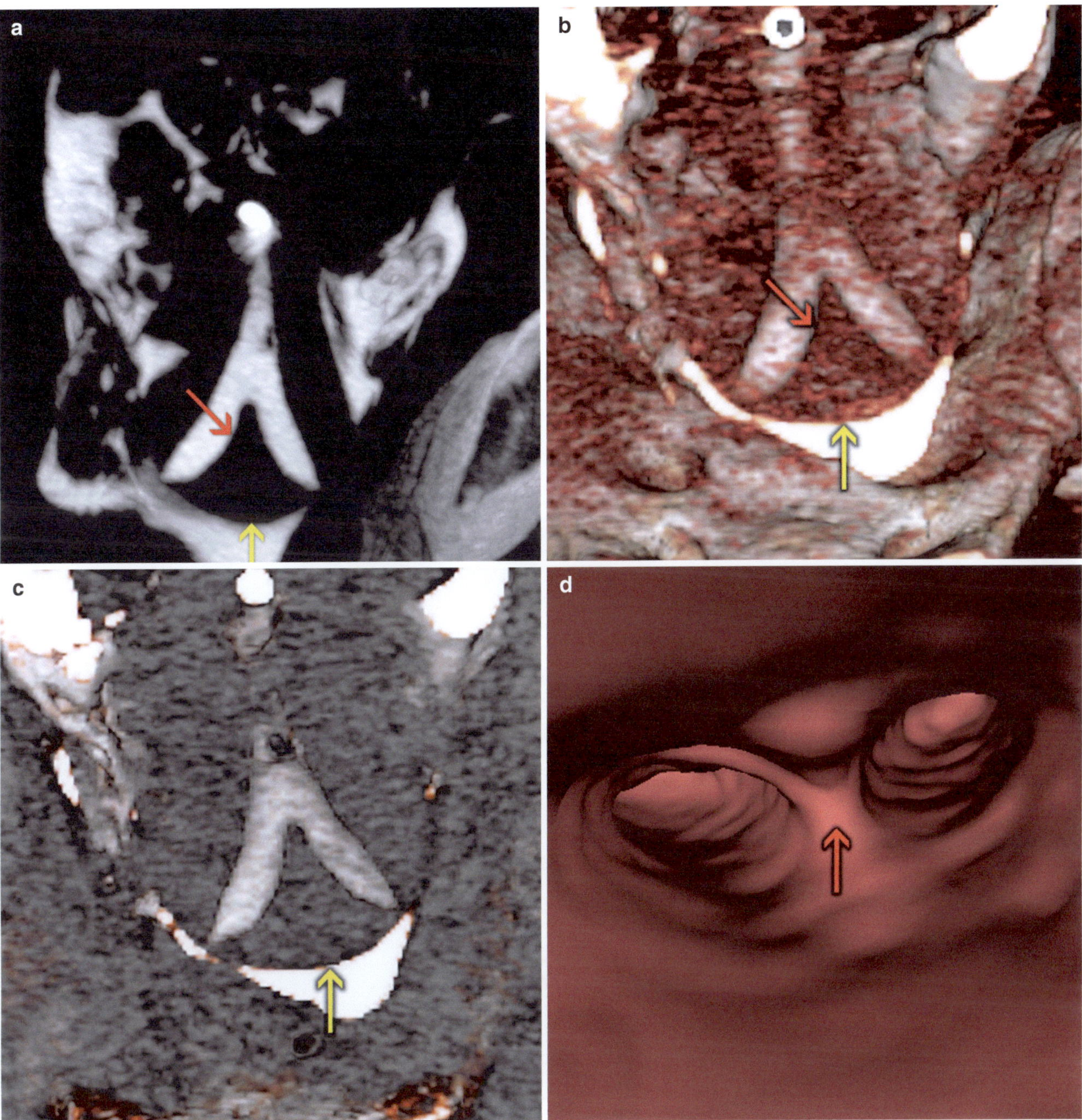

Fig. 10.9 VHSG study showing a partial septate retroverted uterus. A normal external configuration of the uterus is appreciated (*yellow arrows*) as well as the septum which divides the endometrial cavity (*red arrows*). (**a**) Coronal maximum intensity projection image. (**b**, **c**) Coronal 3D volume rendering images. (**d**) Virtual endoscopy image

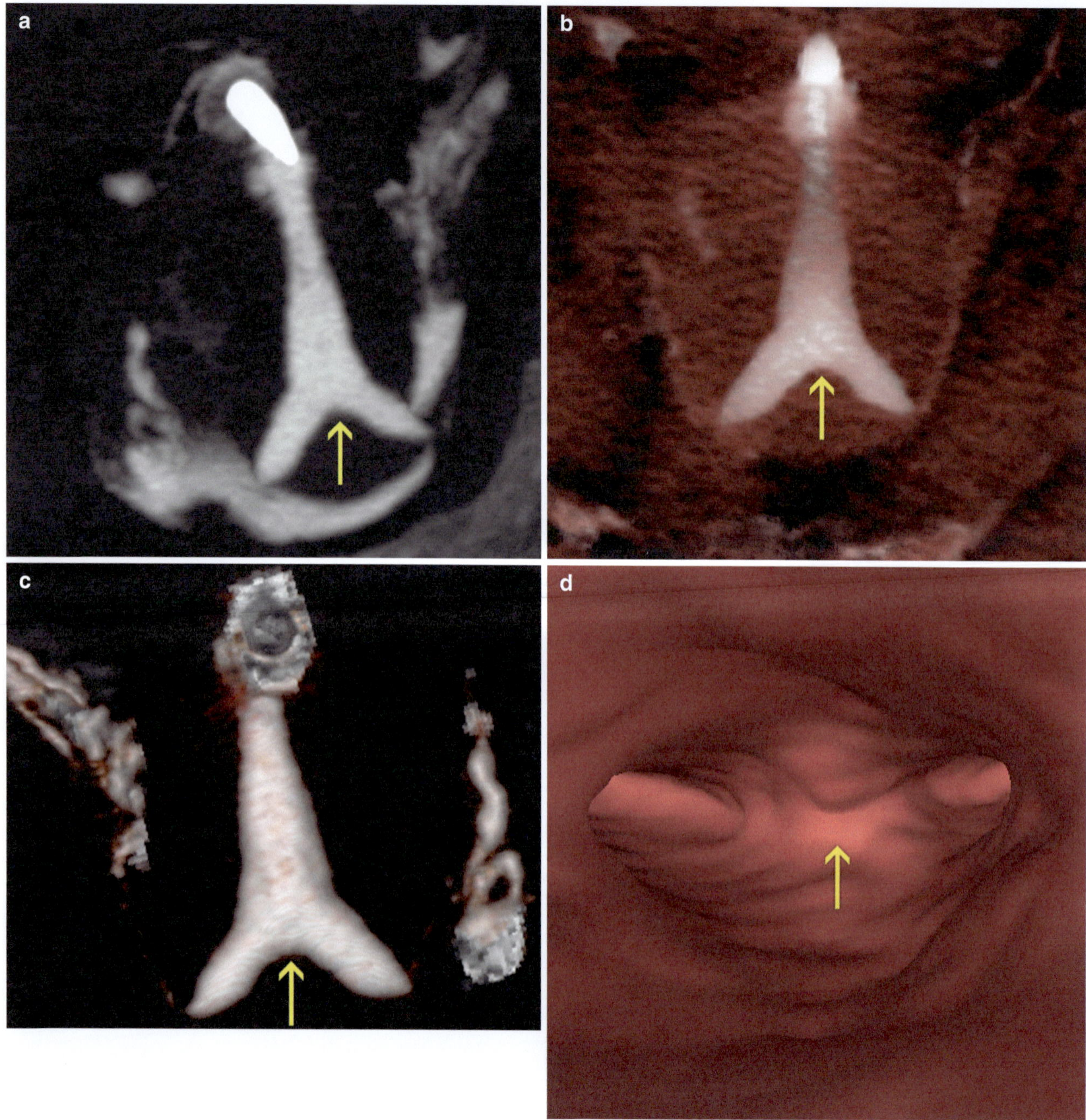

Fig. 10.10 Control VHSG study after the hysteroscopy treatment. The removal of the uterine septum and the presence of a small indentation at the level of the fundus, which corresponds to the normal post-surgical septum remnant can be appreciated (*arrows*). (**a**) Coronal maximum intensity projection image. (**b**, **c**) Coronal 3D volume rendering images. (**d**) Virtual endoscopy image

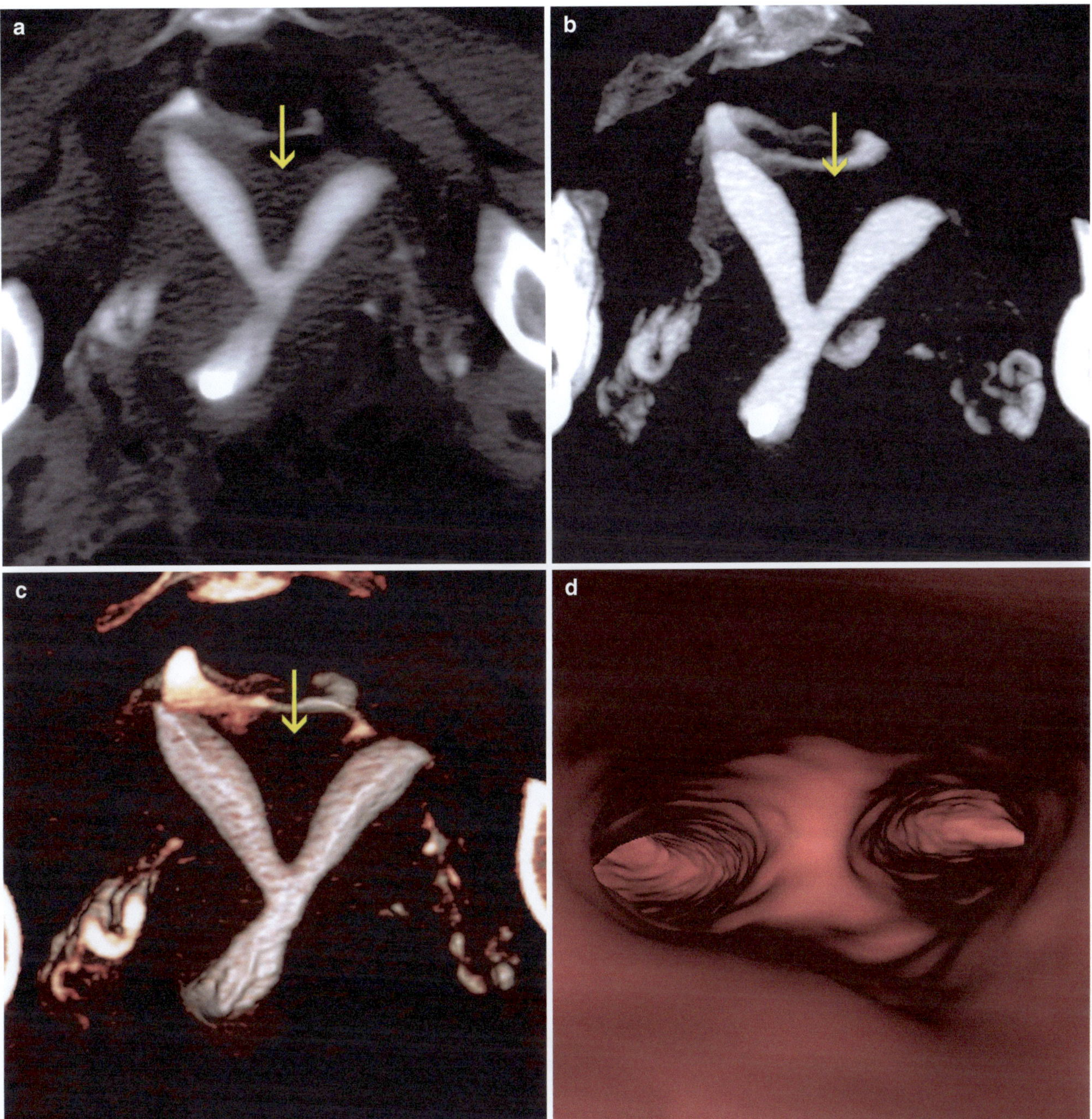

Fig. 10.11 VHSG study showing a retroverted bicornuate uterus. The concave external configuration (*arrows*) and the divergence of the uterine horns can be appreciated. (**a**) 5-mm coronal multiplanar reconstruction image. (**b**) Coronal maximum intensity projection image. (**c**) Coronal 3D volume rendering image. (**d**) Virtual endoscopy image

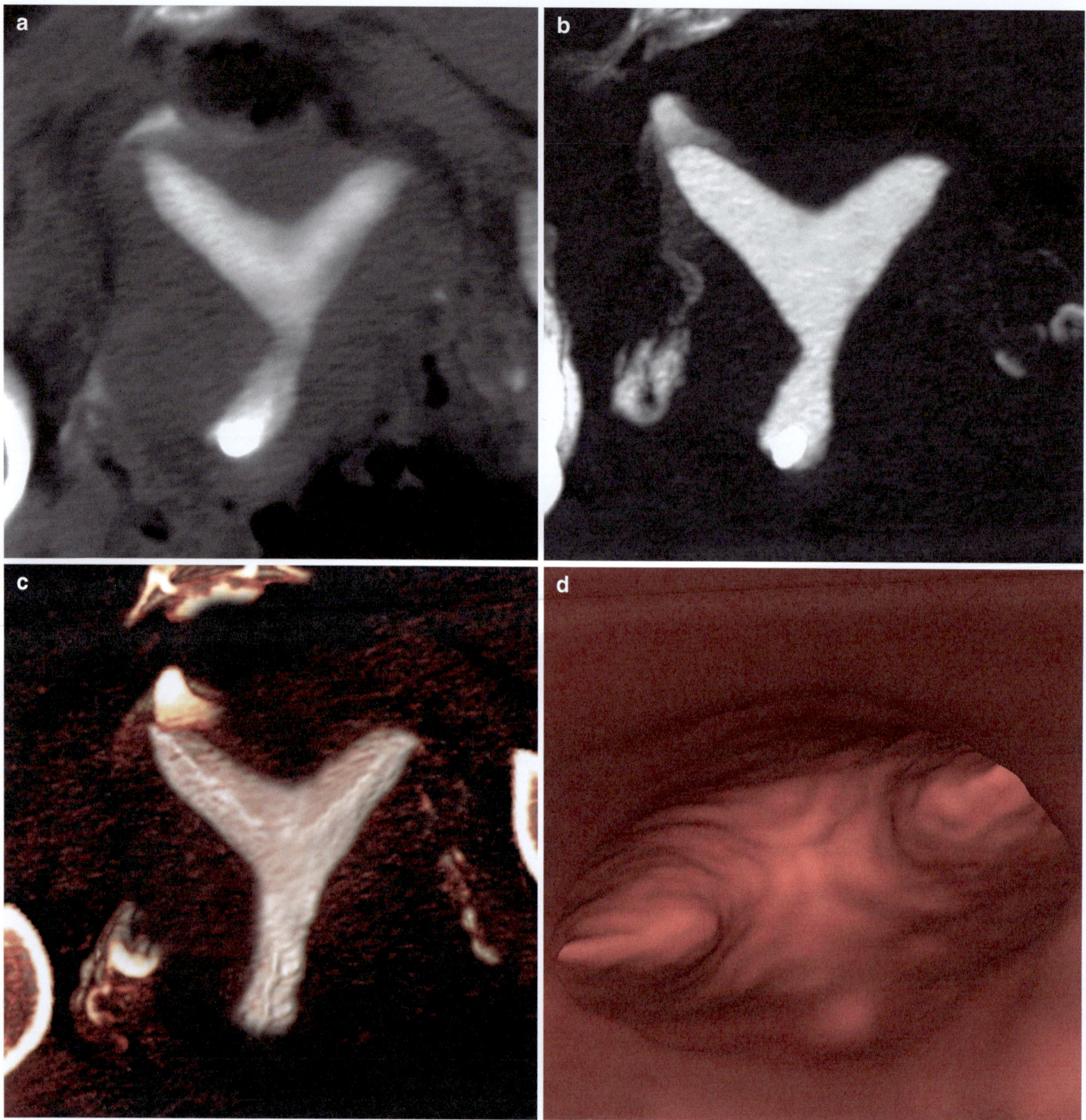

Fig. 10.12 Control VHSG study after uterine repair of a bicornuate uterus. A broader endometrial cavity can be appreciated. (**a**) 5-mm coronal multiplanar reconstruction image. (**b**) Coronal maximum intensity projection image. (**c**) Coronal 3D volume rendering image. (**d**) Virtual endoscopy image

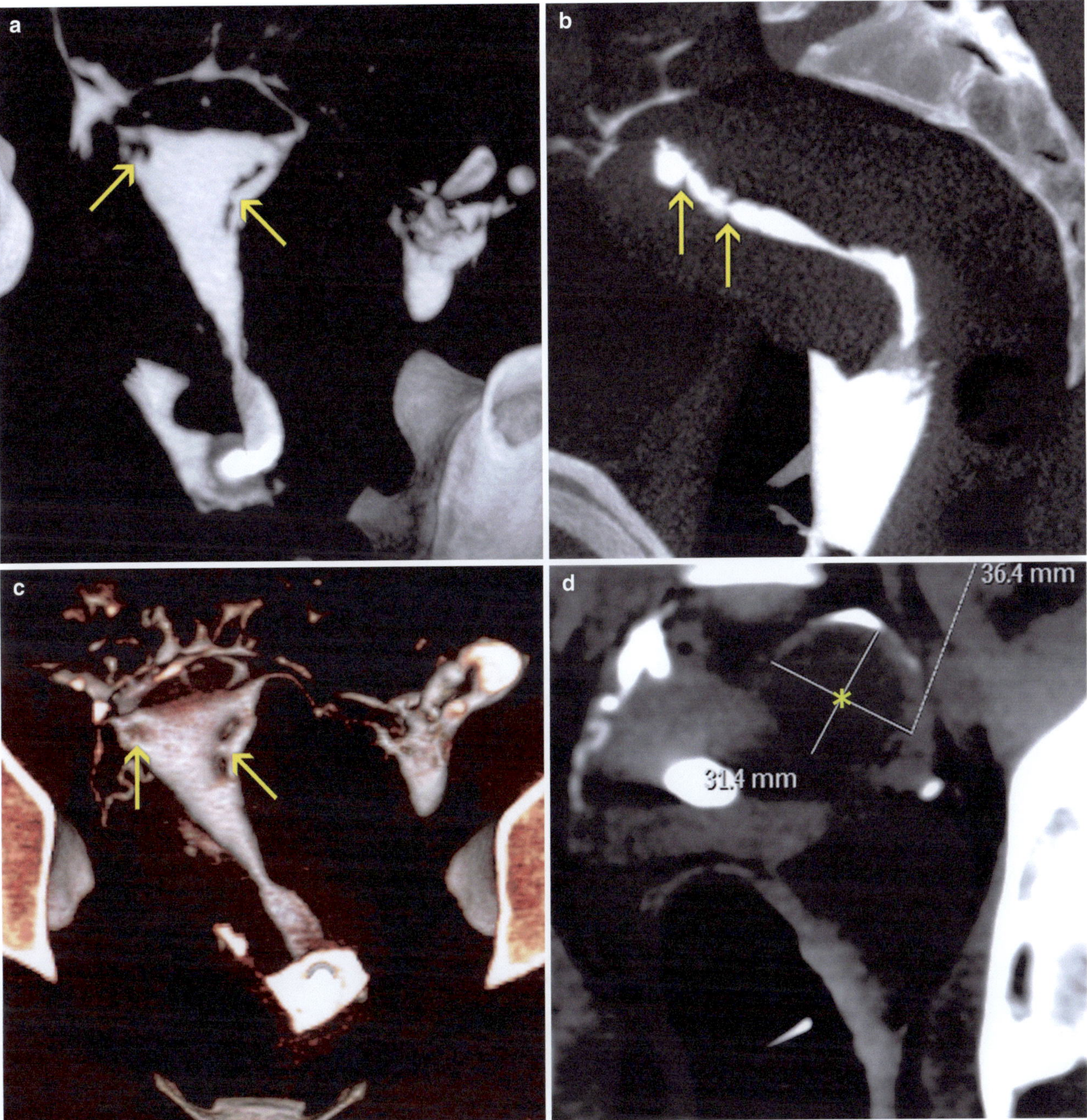

Fig. 10.13 VHSG study showing the presence uterine synechiae (*arrows*). A subserosal myoma on the left lateral wall can also be appreciated (*asterisk*). (**a**) Coronal maximum intensity projection (MIP) image. (**b**) Sagittal MIP image. (**c**) Coronal 3D volume rendering image. (**d**) Axial MIP image. (**e**, **f**) Virtual endoscopy images

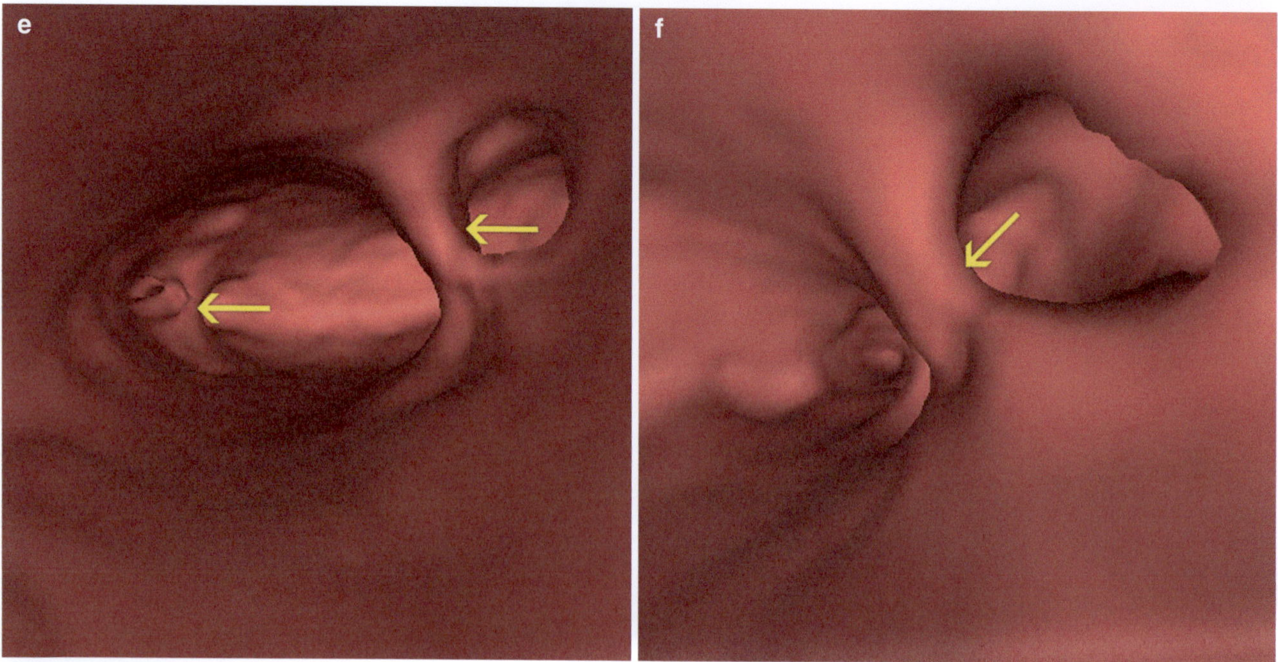

Fig. 10.13 (continued)

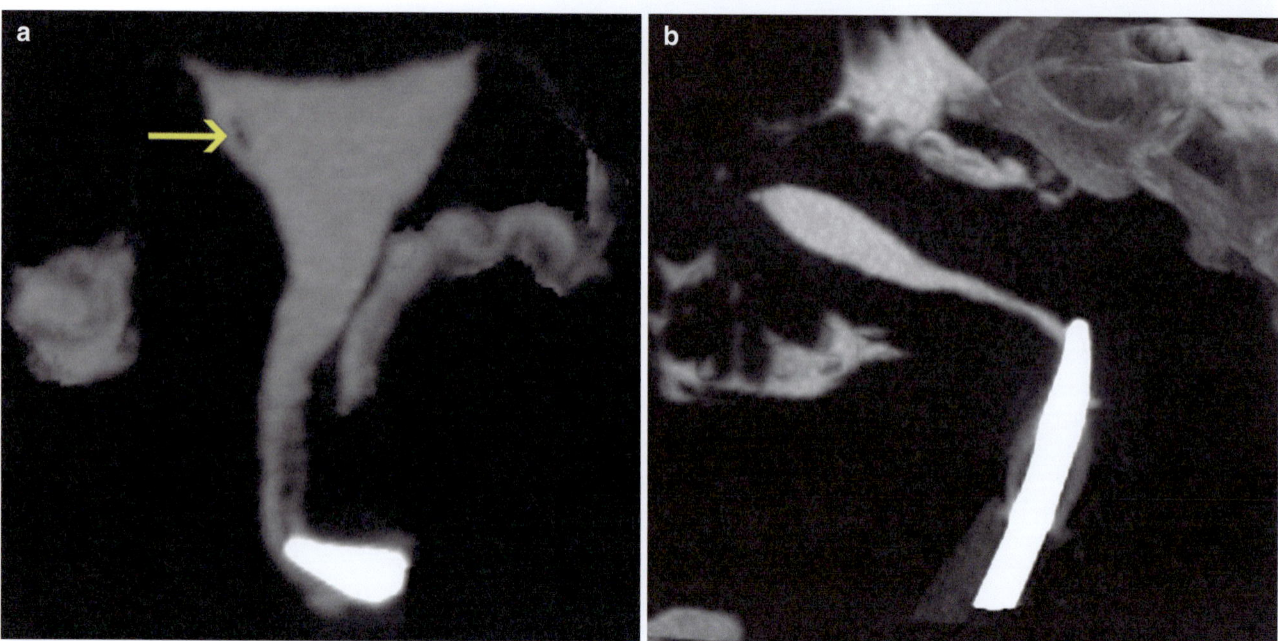

Fig. 10.14 Control VHSG study post-treatment. A small synechiae persists at the level of the uterine cavity on the right horn (*arrows*). The subserosal myoma on the left lateral wall is not visualized. (**a**) Coronal maximum intensity projection (MIP) image. (**b**) Sagittal MIP image. (**c**) Coronal 3D volume rendering image. (**d**) Axial MIP image. (**e**, **f**) Virtual endoscopy images

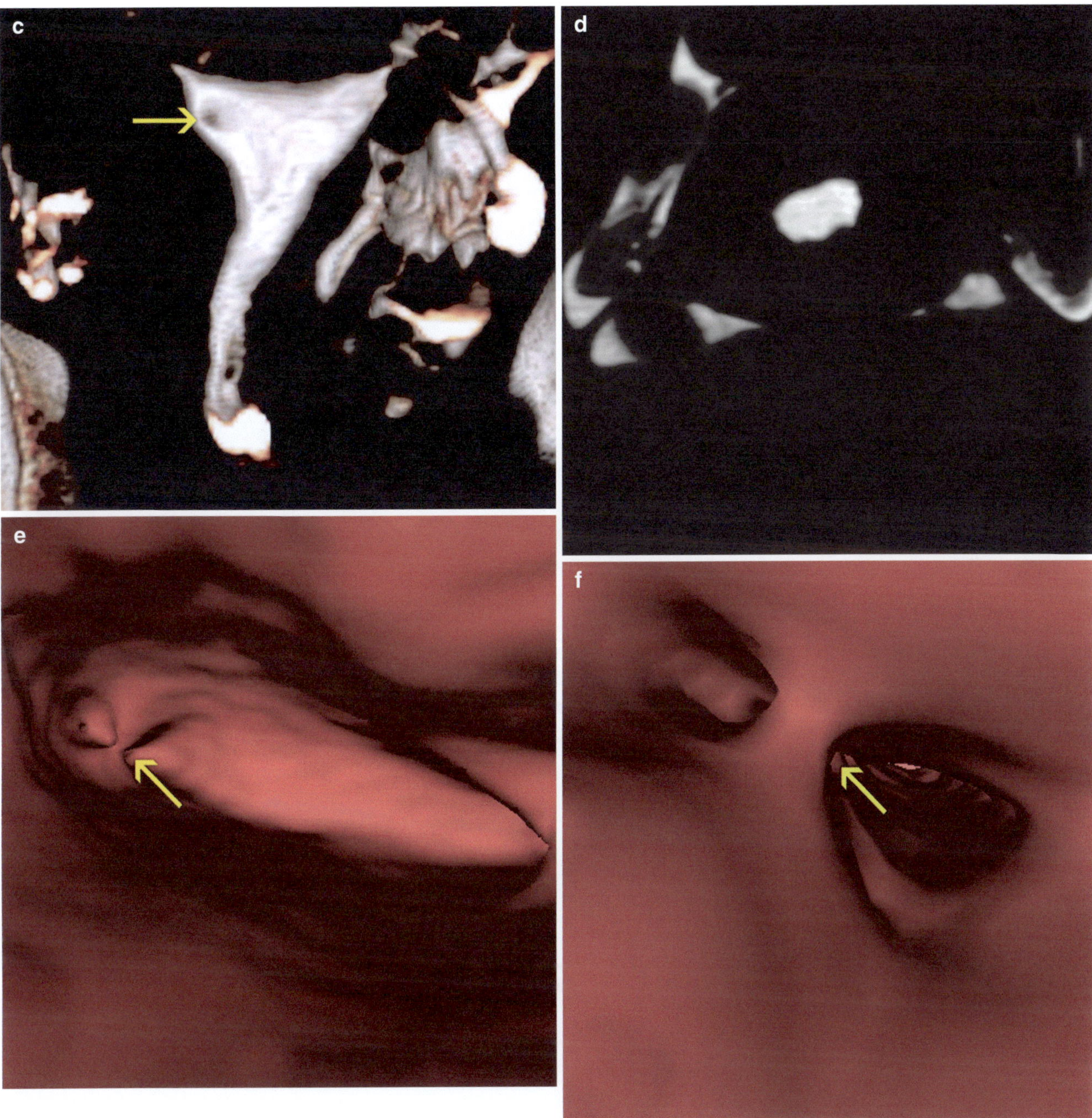

Fig. 10.14 (continued)

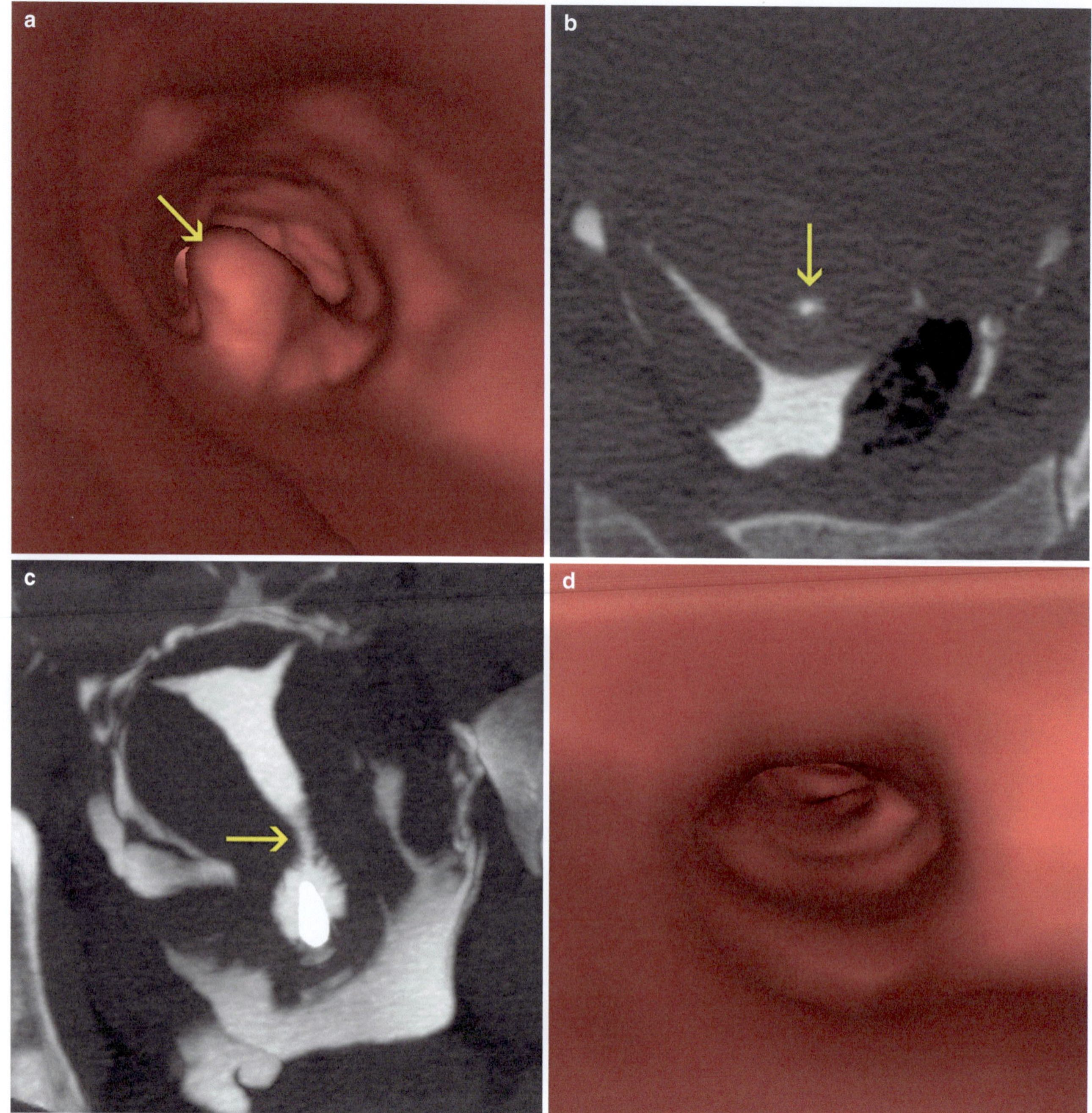

Fig. 10.15 VHSG study. Presence of polyp in endometrial cavity (*arrows*). The cervical canal is normal. (**a**) Virtual endoscopy image. (**b**) Axial CT image of the cervical canal. (**c**) Coronal maximum intensity projection image. (**d**) Virtual endoscopy image

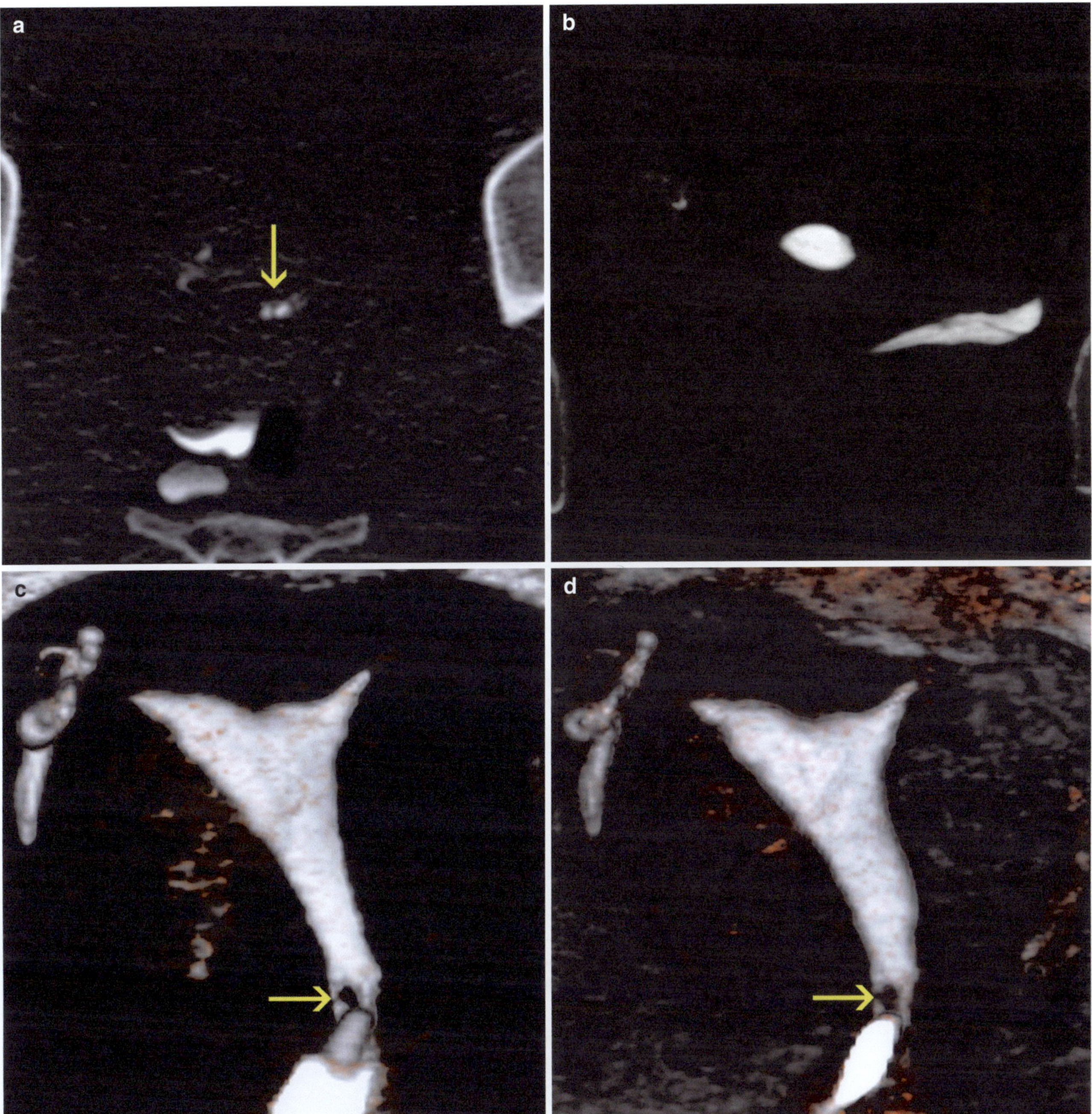

Fig. 10.16 Control VHSG study, after the endometrial polyp resection. An endoluminal lineal image is identified at the level of the cervix compatible with synechiae (*arrows*). The endometrial cavity does not show endoluminal lesions. (**a**) Axial CT image of the cervical canal. (**b**) Axial CT image of the endometrial cavity. (**c**) Coronal maximum intensity projection image. (**d**) Coronal 3D volume rendering image. (**e**) Virtual endoscopy image of the cervical canal. (**f**) Virtual endoscopy image of the endometrial cavity

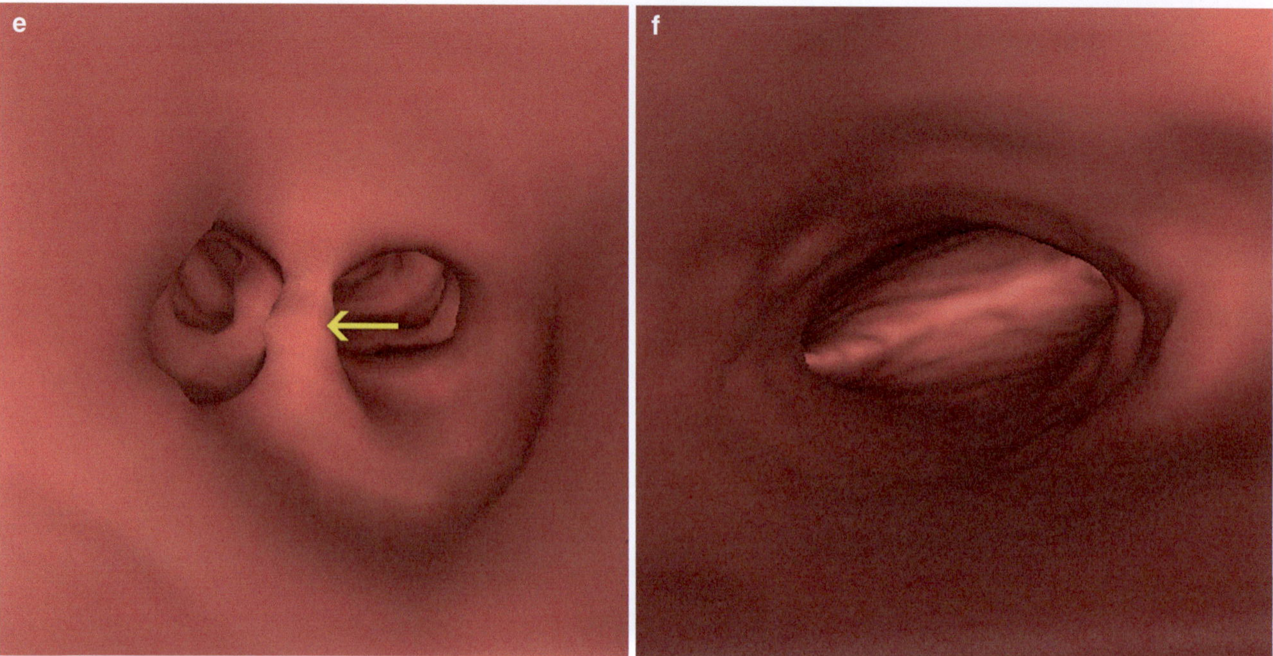

Fig. 10.16 (continued)

Table 10.1 Cesarean indications

Schedule C-section
Baby positions
Breech position
Transverse position
Multiple births
Active genital herpes
Placenta previa
Maternal diseases
Diabetes
Preeclampsia
Repeat cesarean/previous uterine surgeries
Urgent C-section
Placental disorders
Placental abruption
Bleeding placenta previa
Cephalopelvic disproportion
Fetal distress
Umbilical cord prolapsed
Failure to progress in labor

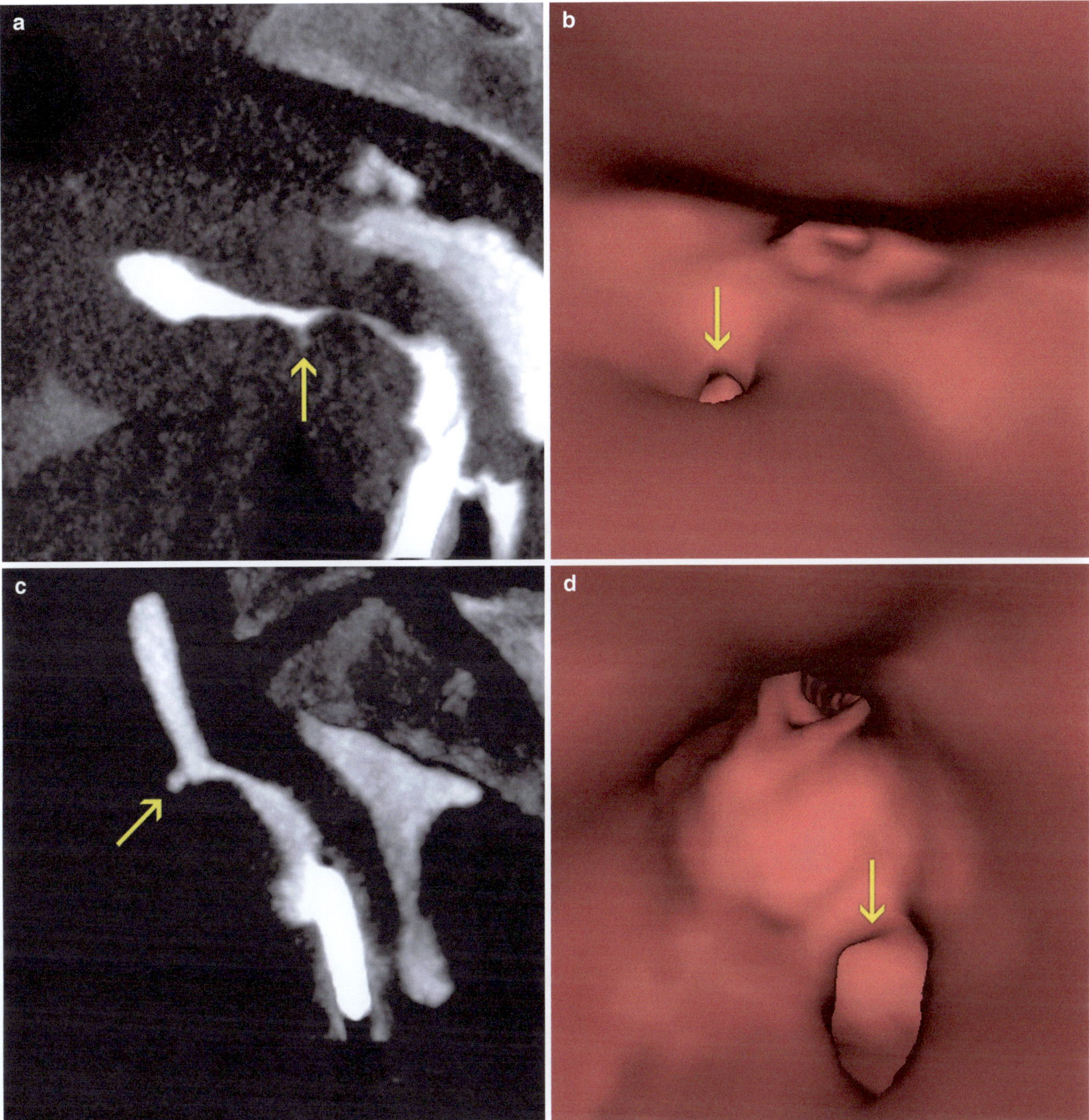

Fig. 10.17 VHSG images in patients with history of cesarean sections. The size of the cesarean scar niche is variable (*arrows*). (**a, b**) Sagittal maximum intensity projection (MIP) image and virtual endoscopy image of a patient with a small scar niche. (**c, d**) Sagittal MIP image and virtual endoscopy image of a patient with a medium sized scar niche. (**e, f**) Sagittal MIP image and virtual endoscopy image of a patient with a large scar niche

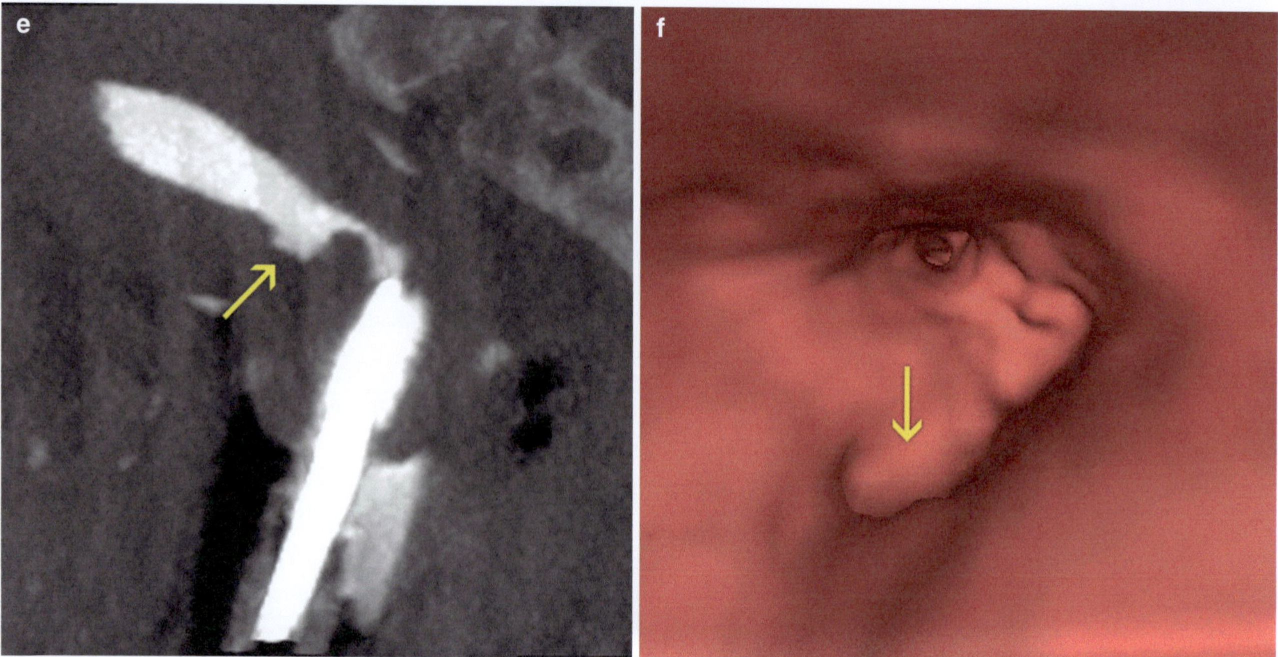

Fig. 10.17 (continued)

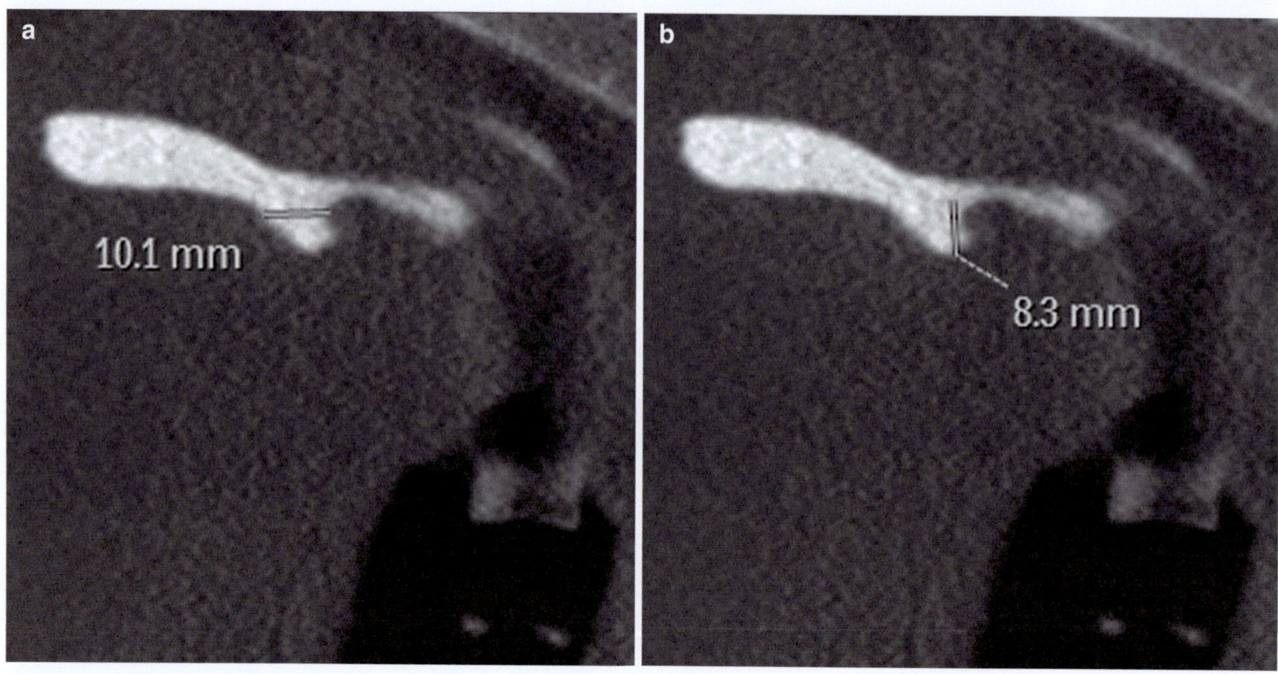

Fig. 10.18 VHSG images that evaluate the cesarean scar niche. (**a–c**) Sagittal maximum intensity projection (MIP) images which measure the diameters and depth of the cesarean scar niche. (**d**) Sagittal 3D volume rendering image. (**e, f**) 3D surface reconstruction images with measurement of the scar niche volume

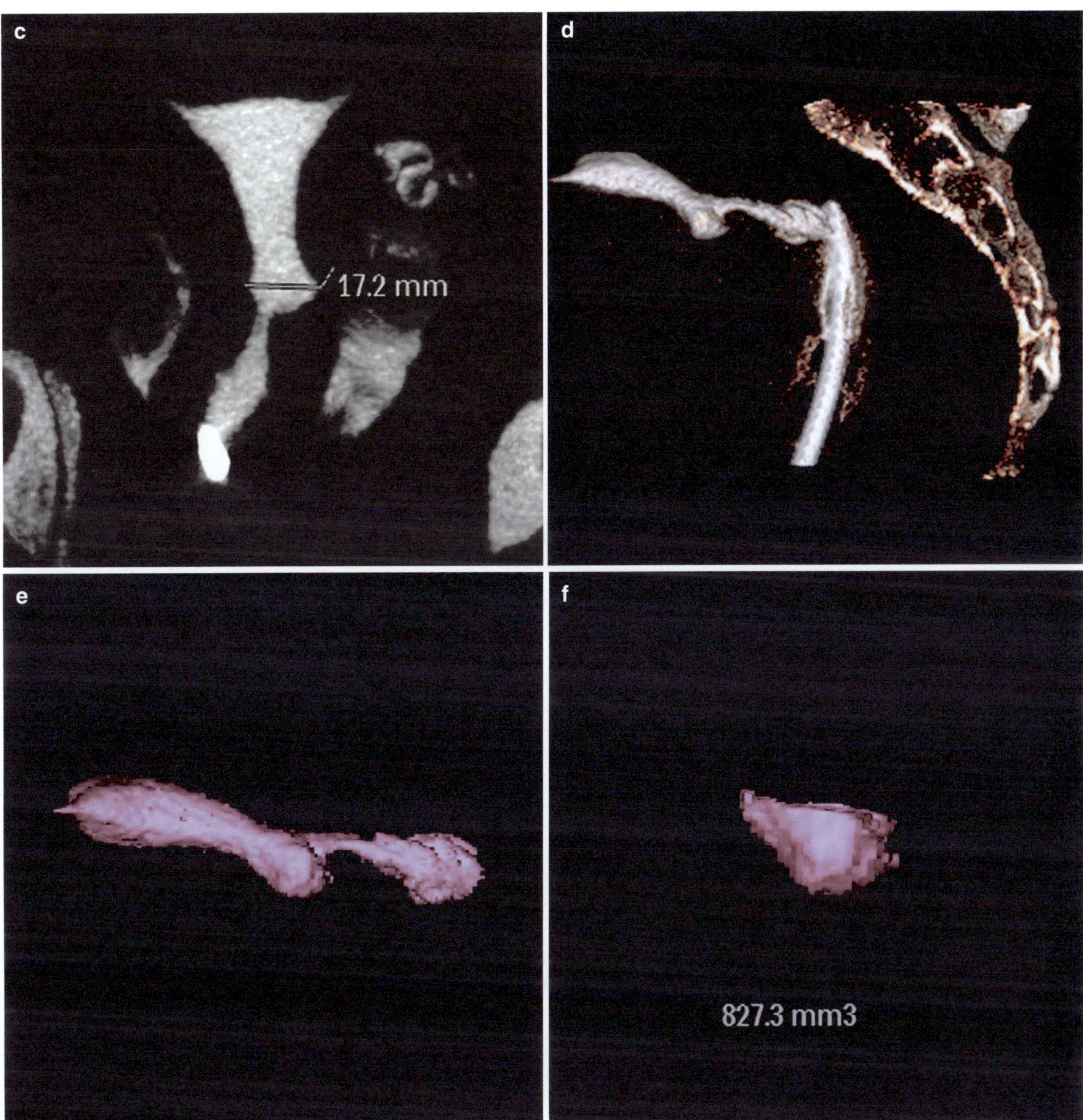

Fig. 10.18 (continued)

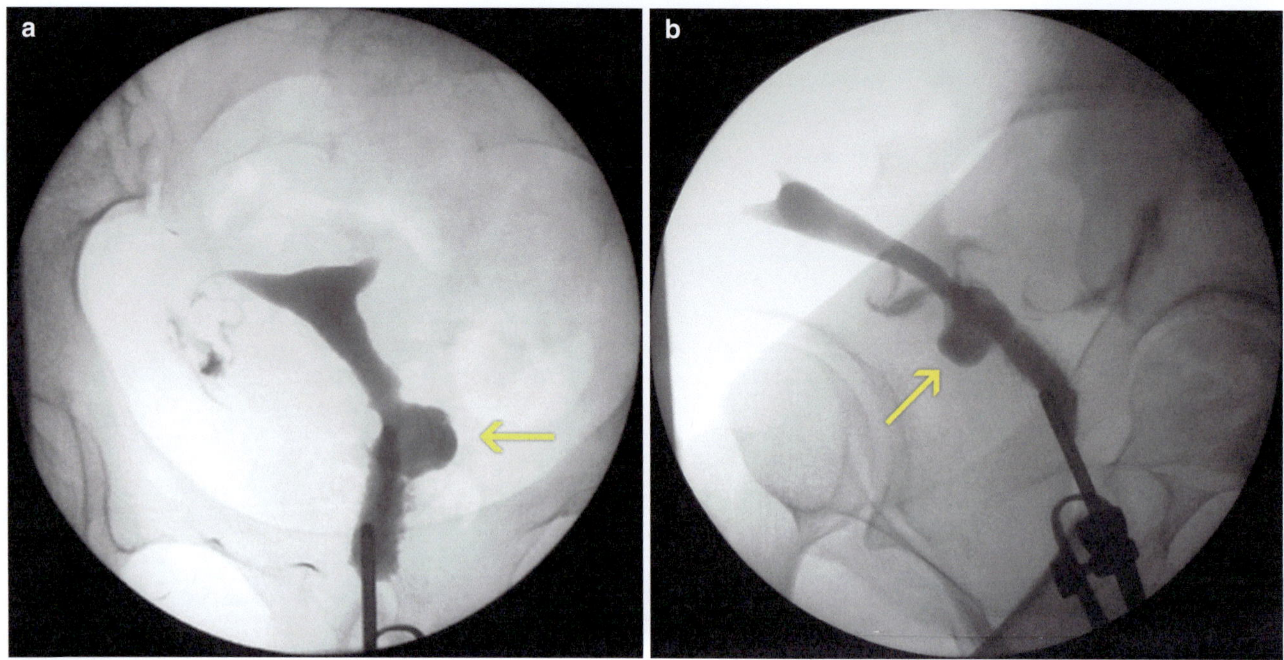

Fig. 10.19   HSG images which show a dehiscence at the level of the cesarean scar (*arrows*). (**a**) Coronal view. (**b**) Lateral view

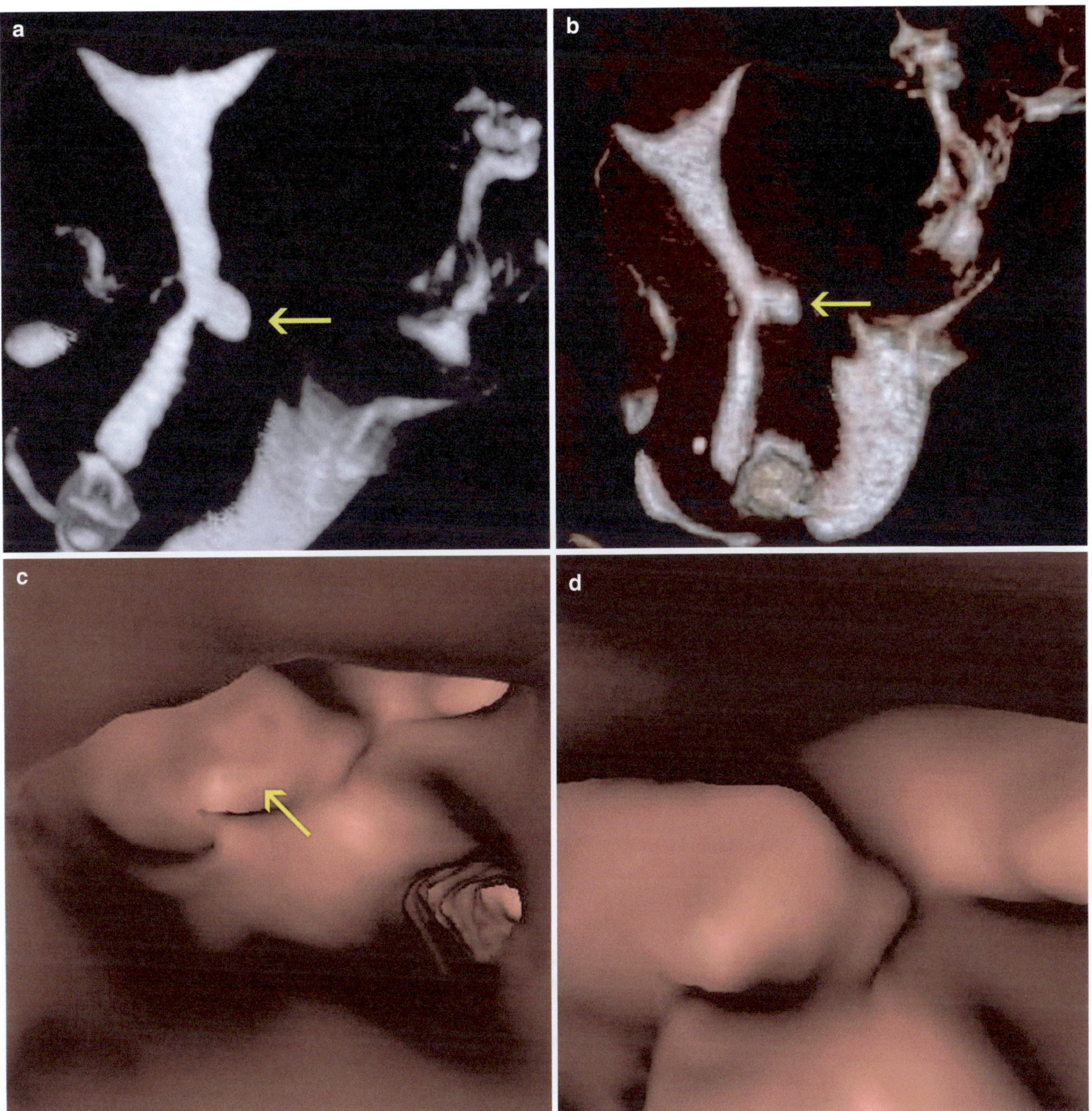

Fig. 10.20 VHSG images showing a dehiscence at the level of the cesarean scar (*arrows*). (**a**) Coronal maximum intensity projection image. (**b**) Coronal 3D volume rendering image. (**c**, **d**) Virtual endoscopy images

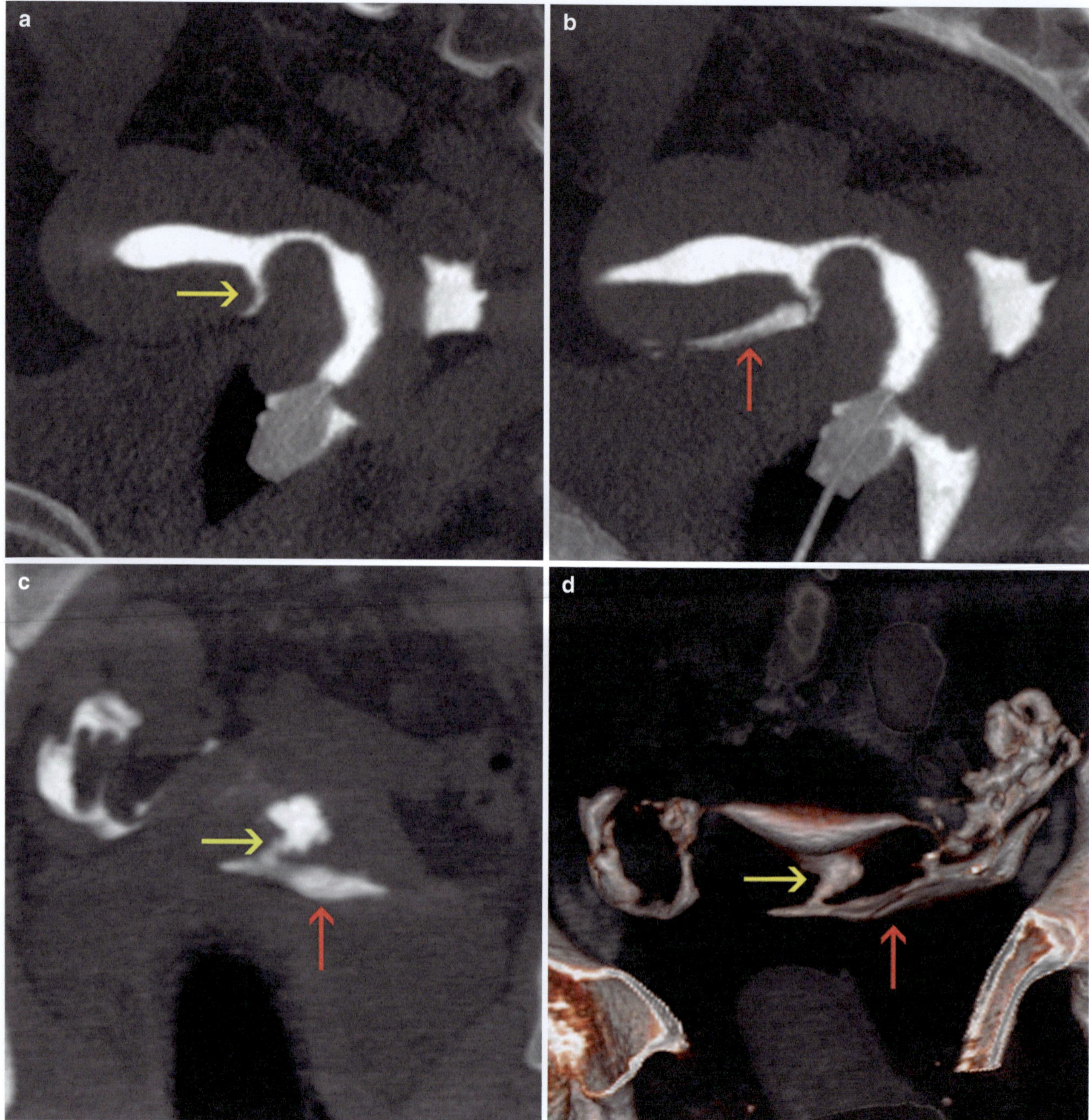

Fig. 10.21 VHSG images showing the cesarean scar niche (*yellow arrows*) and the passage of the instilled contrast to the peritoneal cavity, compatible with utero-peritoneal fistula (*red arrows*). (**a, b**) Sagittal maximum intensity projection (MIP) images. (**c**) Coronal MIP image. (**d**) 3D volume rendering image, anterior view

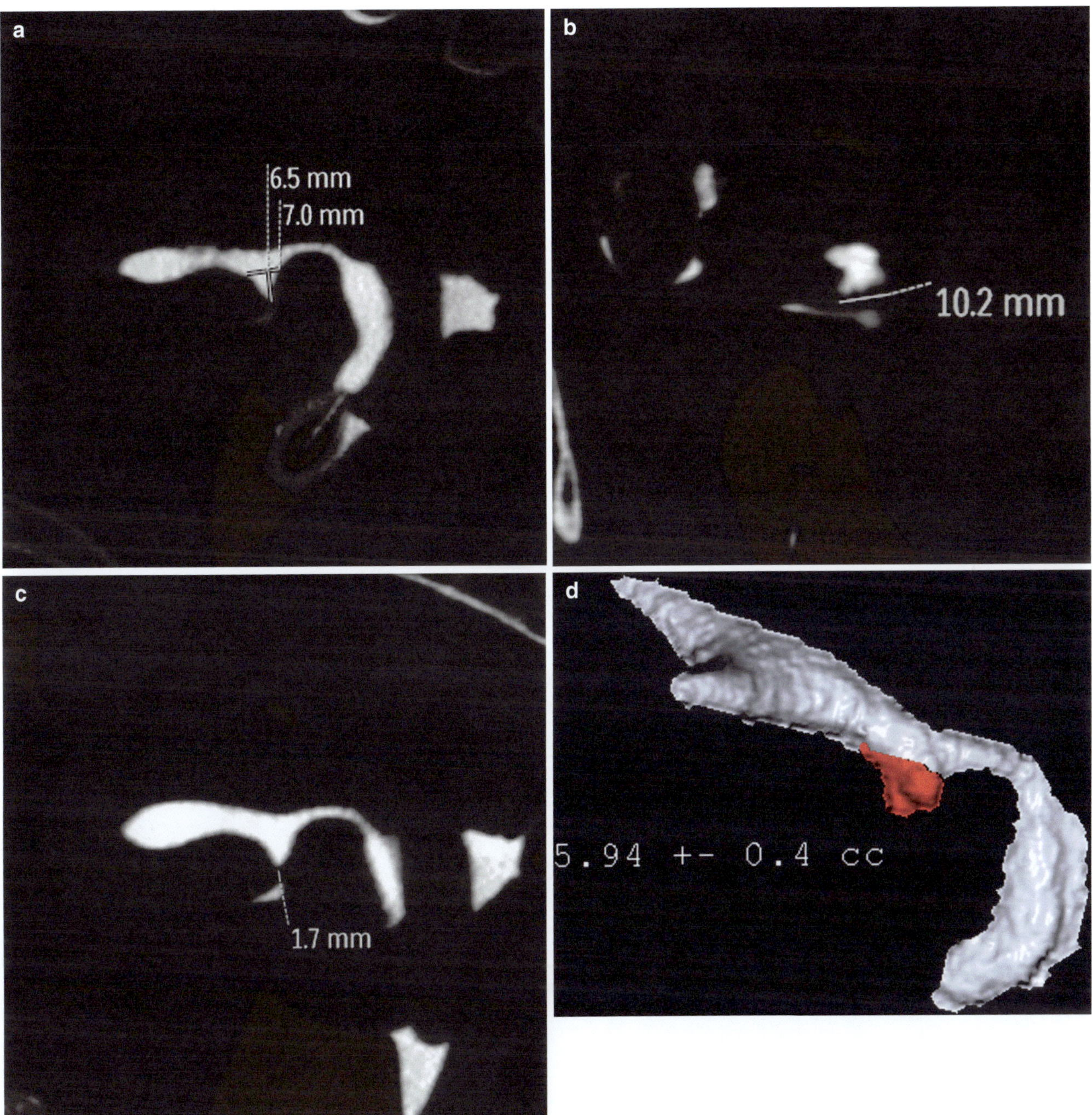

Fig. 10.22 VHSG images showing the size of the cesarean scar niche and the orifice of the utero-peritoneal fistula (*arrow*). (**a**) Sagittal maximum intensity projection (MIP) image. (**b**) Coronal MIP image. (**c**) Sagittal MIP image showing an important thinning of the myometrial wall (1.7 mm). (**d**) 3D surface reconstruction image with measurement of the scar niche volume. (**e**, **f**) Virtual endoscopy images

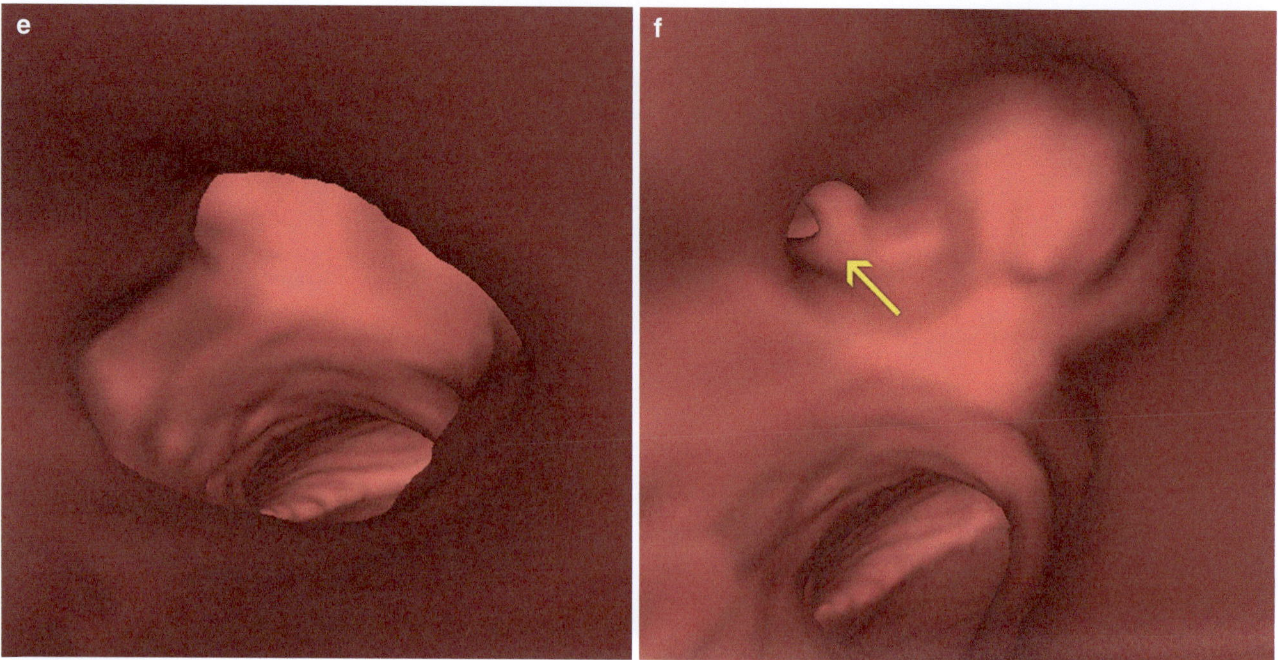

Fig. 10.22 (continued)

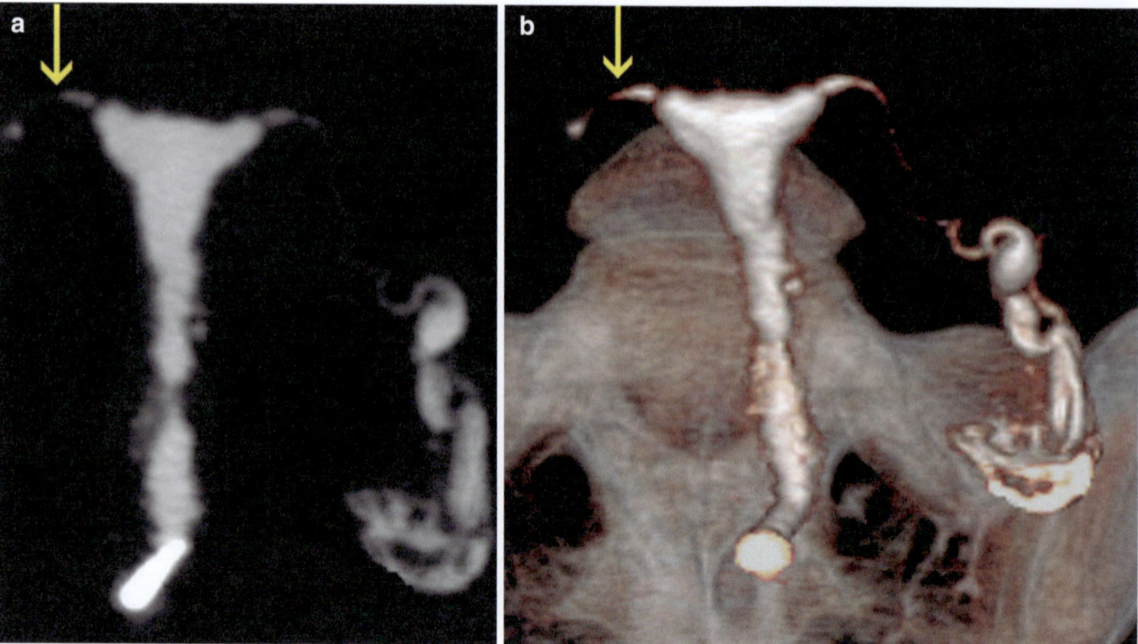

Fig. 10.23 VHSG images showing the amputation of the right uterine tube (*arrows*) in a patient with a history of ectopic pregnancy. (**a**) Coronal maximum intensity projection image. (**b**) Coronal 3D volume rendering image

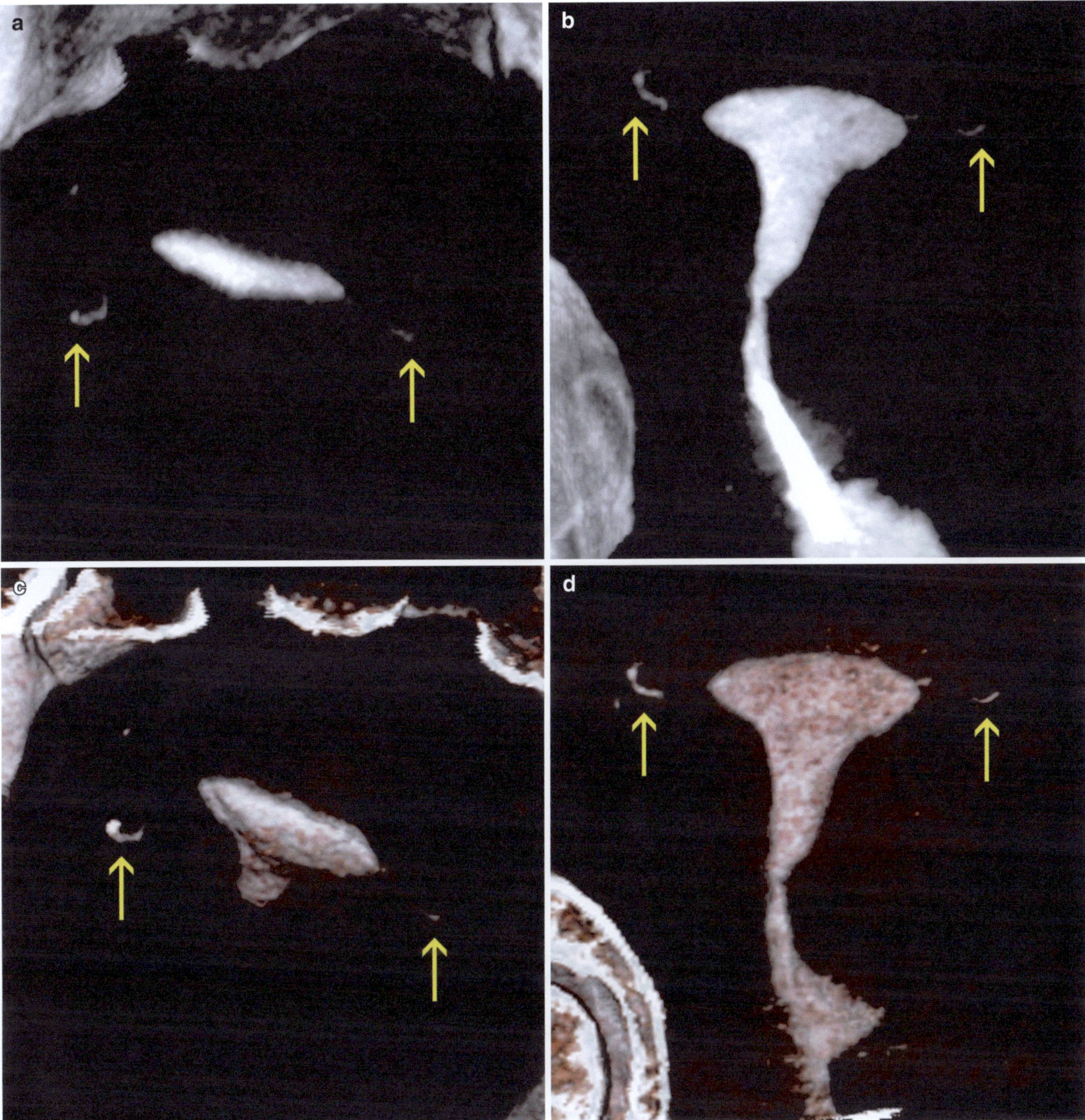

Fig. 10.24 VHSG images showing the amputation of both uterine tubes (*arrows*) due to surgical resection in a patient with bilateral hydrosalpinx and endometriosis. (**a**) Axial maximum intensity projection (MIP) image. (**b**) Coronal MIP image. (**c**) Axial 3D volume rendering image. (**d**) Coronal 3D volume rendering image

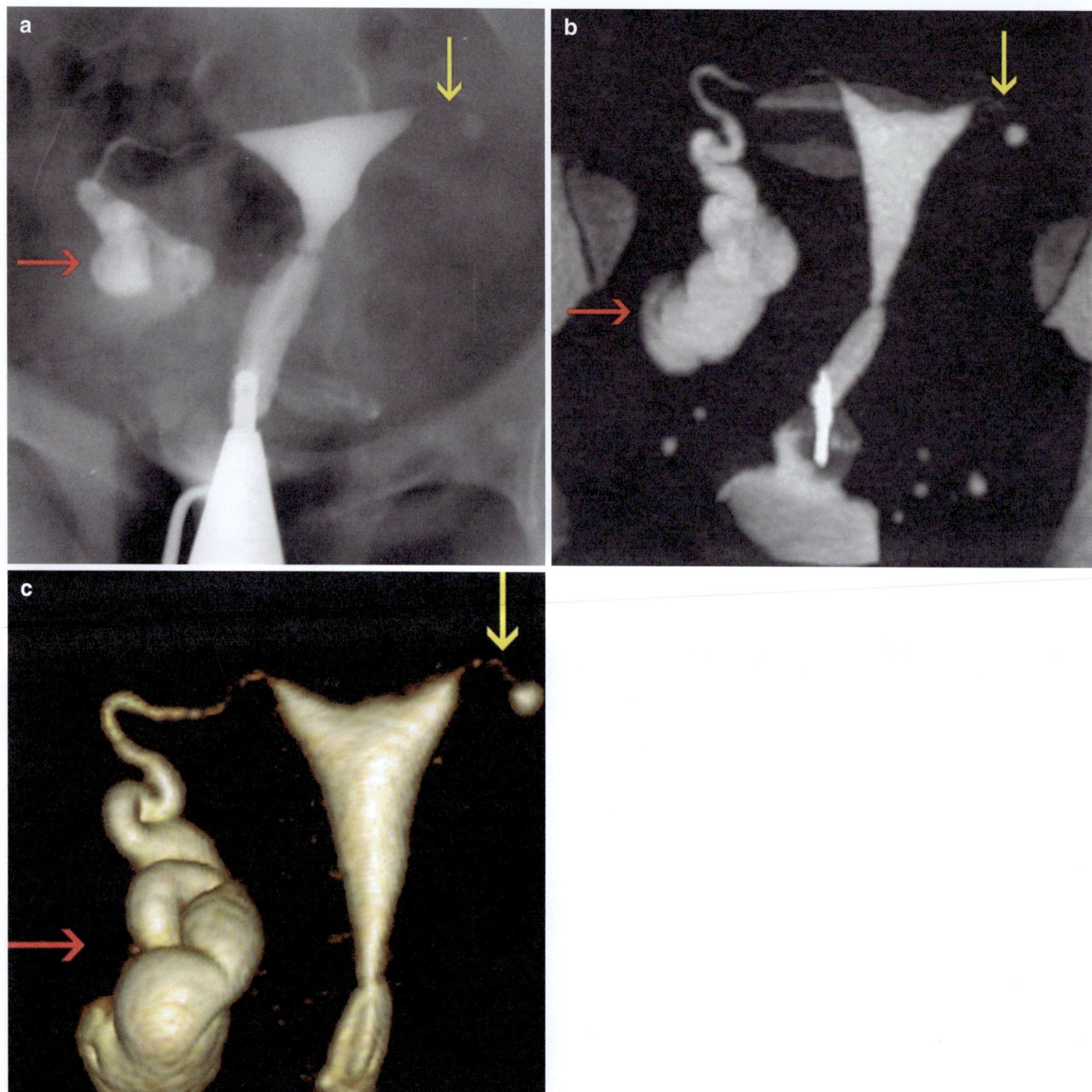

Fig. 10.25 Surgical resection of the left uterine tube due to ectopic pregnancy (*yellow arrows*). Right hydrosalpinx secondary to endometriosis (*red arrows*). (**a**) HSG image. (**b**) Coronal maximum intensity projection VHSG image. (**c**) Coronal 3D volume rendering VHSG image

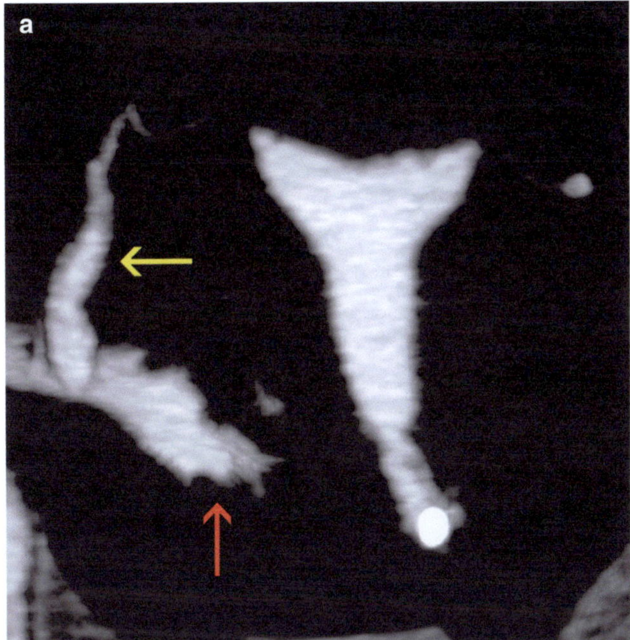

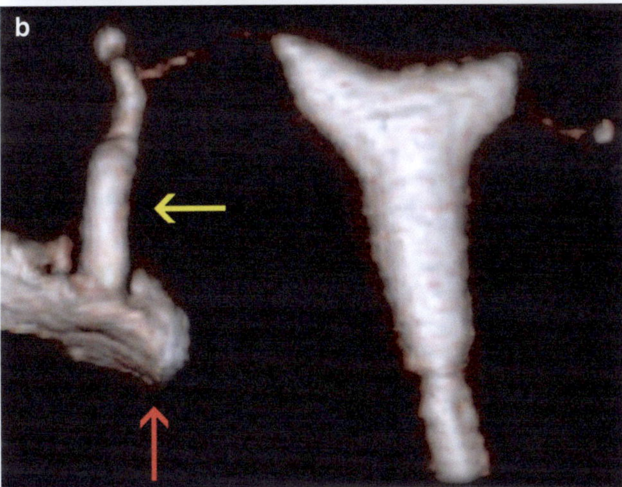

Fig. 10.26 VHSG images post laparoscopic treatment of right hydrosalpinx. The uterine tube shows a slight residual ampullary dilatation (*yellow arrows*), with passage of contrast to the peritoneal cavity (*red arrows*). (**a**) Coronal maximum intensity projection image. (**b**) Coronal 3D volume rendering image

Conclusion

The uterine silhouette and the Fallopian tubes show, on diverse occasions, changes in their morphology and normal anatomy, or suffer complication after the different therapeutic procedures to which they can be subject to in relation to the anatomical or pathological alteration of the base that is present. The VHSG is an integral diagnostic method that allows the precise visualization of said modifications, constituting and excellent diagnostic tool for the monitoring and control of operated patients.

References

1. Macciò A, Madeddu C, Caffiero A, et al. Successful pregnancy following myomectomy of a giant uterine myoma: role of a combined surgical approach. Arch Gynecol Obstet. 2012;285:1577–80.
2. Fernandez H, Kadoch O, Capella-Allouc S, et al. Hysteroscopic resection of submucous myomas: long term results. Ann Chir. 2001;126:58–64.
3. Paradisi R, Barzanti R, Natali F, et al. Metroplasty in a large population of women with septate uterus. J Minim Invasive Gynecol. 2011;18:449–54.
4. Golfieri R, Muzzi C, De Iaco P, et al. The percutaneous treatment of uterine fibromas by means of transcatheter arterial embolization. Radiol Med. 2000;100:48–55.
5. Gupta JK, Sinha A, Lumsden MA, et al. Uterine artery embolization for symptomatic uterine fibroids. Cochrane Database Syst Rev. 2012;(5):CD005073.
6. Kahn V, Fohlen A, Pelage JP. Role of embolization in the management of uterine fibroids. J Gynecol Obstet Biol Reprod (Paris). 2011;40:918–27.
7. Lev-Toaff AS, Karasick S, Toaff ME. Hysterosalpingography before and after myomectomy: clinical value and imaging findings. AJR Am J Roentgenol. 1993;160:803–7.
8. Chen MY, Edwards VH, Ott DJ, et al. Hysterosalpingography after hysteroscopic surgery. Abdom Imaging. 1994;19:477–80.
9. Baird D, Dunson D, Hill M, et al. High cumulative incidence of uterine leiomyoma in black and white women: ultrasound evidence. Am J Obstet Gynecol. 2003;188:100–7.
10. Heinemann K, Thiel C, Mohner S, et al. Benign gynecologic tumors: estimated incidence results of the German Cohort Study on Women's Health. Eur J Obstet Gynecol Reprod Biol. 2003;107:78–80.
11. Donnez J, Jadoul P. What are the implications of myomas on fertility? A need for a debate? Hum Reprod. 2002;17:1424–30.
12. Hunt JE, Wallach EE. Uterine factors in infertility-an overview. Clin Obstet Gynecol. 1974;17:44–64.
13. Dalal RJ, Pai HD, Palshetkar NP, et al. Hysteroscopic metroplasty in women with primary infertility and septate uterus: reproductive performance after surgery. J Reprod Med. 2012;57:13–6.
14. Yoshino O, Nishii O, Osuga Y, et al. Myomectomy decreases abnormal uterine peristalsis and increases pregnancy rate. J Minim Invasive Gynecol. 2012;19:63–7.
15. Suvitie P, Perheentupa A. Myomas and fertility. Duodecim. 2011;127:1848–56.
16. Bourdel N, Bonnefoy C, Jardon K, et al. Hysteroscopic myomectomy: recurrence and satisfaction survey at short- and long-term. J Gynecol Obstet Biol Reprod (Paris). 2011;40:116–22.
17. Hackethal A, Westermann A, Tchartchian G, et al. Laparoscopic myomectomy in patients with uterine myomas associated with infertility. Minim Invasive Ther Allied Technol. 2011;20:338–45.
18. Sentilhes L, Bouet PE, Mezzadri M, et al. Against the routinely hysteroscopic metroplasty for septate uterus. Gynecol Obstet Fertil. 2011;39:394–7.
19. Brucker SY, Rall K, Campo R, et al. Treatment of congenital malformations. Semin Reprod Med. 2011;29:101–12.
20. Pace S, Stentella P, Catania R, et al. Endoscopic treatment of intrauterine adhesions. Clin Exp Obstet Gynecol. 2003;30:26–8.
21. Socolov R, Anton E, Butureanu S, et al. The endoscopic management of uterine synechiae. A clinical study of 78 cases. Chirurgia (Bucur). 2010;105:515–8.
22. Fedele L, Vercellini P, Viezzoli T, et al. Intrauterine adhesions: current diagnostic and therapeutic trends. Acta Eur Fertil. 1986;17:31–7.
23. Kdous M, Hachicha R, Zhiou F, et al. Fertility after hysteroscopic treatment of intra-uterine adhesions. Gynecol Obstet Fertil. 2003;31:422–8.

24. Thomson AJ, Abbott JA, Deans R, et al. The management of intrauterine synechiae. Curr Opin Obstet Gynecol. 2009;21:335–41.

25. Seffah JD. Re-laparotomy after cesarean section. Int J Gynaecol Obstet. 2005;88:253–7.

26. Monteagudo A, Carreno C, Timor-Tritsch IE. Saline infusion sonohysterography in nonpregnant women with previous cesarean delivery: the "niche" in the scar. J Ultrasound Med. 2001;20:1105–15.

27. Regnard C, Nosbusch M, Fellemans C, et al. Cesarean section scar evaluation by saline contrast sonohysterography. Ultrasound Obstet Gynecol. 2004;23:289–92.

28. Donnez O, Jadoul P, Squifflet J, et al. Laparoscopic repair of wide and deep uterine scar dehiscence after cesarean section. Fertil Steril. 2008;89:974–80.

29. Capuñay C, Carrascosa P, Vallejos J, et al. Evaluación de espesor de la pared uterina en el sitio de cicatriz de cesárea anterior en estudios de histerosalpingografía virtual. Congreso Argentino de Radiologia; 2011. http://sar2011.postersenlinea.com/topics.php.

30. Lim PS, Shafiee MN, Ahmad S, et al. Utero-cutaneous fistula after caesarean section secondary to red degeneration of intramural fibroid. Sex Reprod Healthc. 2012;3:95–6.

31. Lang EK, Dunaway Jr HE. Efficacy of salpingography and transcervical recanalization in diagnosis, categorization, and treatment of fallopian tube obstruction. Cardiovasc Intervent Radiol. 2000;23:417–22.

32. Massey JB. Endometriosis and tuboperitoneal fistulas after tubal ligation. Fertil Steril. 1981;36:417–8.

33. Fylstra DL. Uteroperitoneal fistula formation after proximal salpingectomy with harmonic scalpel resulting in a third consecutive fallopian tube ectopic pregnancy: a case report. J Reprod Med. 2009;54:330–2.

34. Stock L, Milad M. Surgical management of ectopic pregnancy. Clin Obstet Gynecol. 2012;55:448–54.

35. Practice Committee of American Society for Reproductive Medicine in collaboration with Society of Reproductive Surgeons. Salpingectomy for hydrosalpinx prior to in vitro fertilization. Fertil Steril. 2008;90:S66–8.

One of the distinct characteristics of the virtual studies is the possibility of obtaining images of the pelvic structures, with sufficient quality so as to be evaluated. Because it is an exam done through computed tomography, it possesses all the diagnostic capacity that derives from this method, allowing the observation of lesions located in other organs and structures. In this way, the extra-uterine findings constitute an unavoidable part of the virtual hysterosalpingography (VHSG).

The implication of the incidental findings was shown in other areas like in virtual colonoscopy [1–3]. In these cases the exam can be utilized as a screening method, allowing the detection of pathologies in a pre-clinical state, leading to an early diagnosis and treatment of some previously unknown conditions in asymptomatic patients. This particular situation is benefited because in the ethereal group of the population in study, in general over 50 years old, the prevalence of chronic pathologies is higher than usual [4, 5]. On the other hand, in patients with fertility problems and 35 year-old in average, the prevalence of extra-uterine pathology is lower.

Besides, one must take into account that the diagnosis of an unexpected finding has a potential impact on different levels. A report with an unexpected finding usually produces a certain level of anxiety, which can be excessive in some patients. The economic impact generated by the complementary exams and treatments that derive from the incidental finding of these lesions must also be taken into account, as well as a possible increase in the morbid-mortality risk if the patient is subjected to invasive procedures [6, 7].

Classification

Similar to the extra colonic findings in virtual colonoscopy studies [8], the incidental diagnosis in VHSG can be classified according to its clinical importance: high, moderate and low.

(i) Findings of high clinical importance:
They are those which require an immediate intervention or the carrying out of other complementary exams. The following have been reported within this group: pelvic limphadenopathies, suspicious ovarian masses, complicated colonic diverticula, pelvic collections, fistulas, and suspicious lytic or blastic bone lesions (Fig. 11.1).

(ii) Findings of moderate clinical importance:
They are generally benign and their re-evaluation can be deferred. Reported in this group are: undetermined adnexal masses, inguinal hernias, non complicated colonic diverticula and undetermined bone lesions (Fig. 11.2).

(iii) Findings of low clinical importance:
They are the ones that do not require another type of analysis or treatment. The most frequent benign lesions are: ovarian cysts and teratomas, vascular calcifications, sacral perirradicular cysts and degenerative bone lesions (Fig. 11.3).

Incidence and Valorization of Extra-Uterine Findings

The report of the unexpected lesions is of great responsibility for the radiologist because the next steps to follow depend on its valuation. On the other hand, the referral physician must know the reaches of the method requested and be ready to face the results comprehensively. It is imperative to consider at this point the importance of the extra time the radiologist puts into the exploration of the rest of the soft and bone pelvis. It is necessary to analyze the acquired axial images in their totality and give them a different treatment than the uterine evaluation.

As mentioned before, the frequency of these incidental lesions is low due to the fact that most of the patients are young, asymptomatic and are in a study for infertility.

P. Carrascosa et al., *CT Virtual Hysterosalpingography*,
DOI 10.1007/978-3-319-07560-0_11, © Springer International Publishing Switzerland 2014

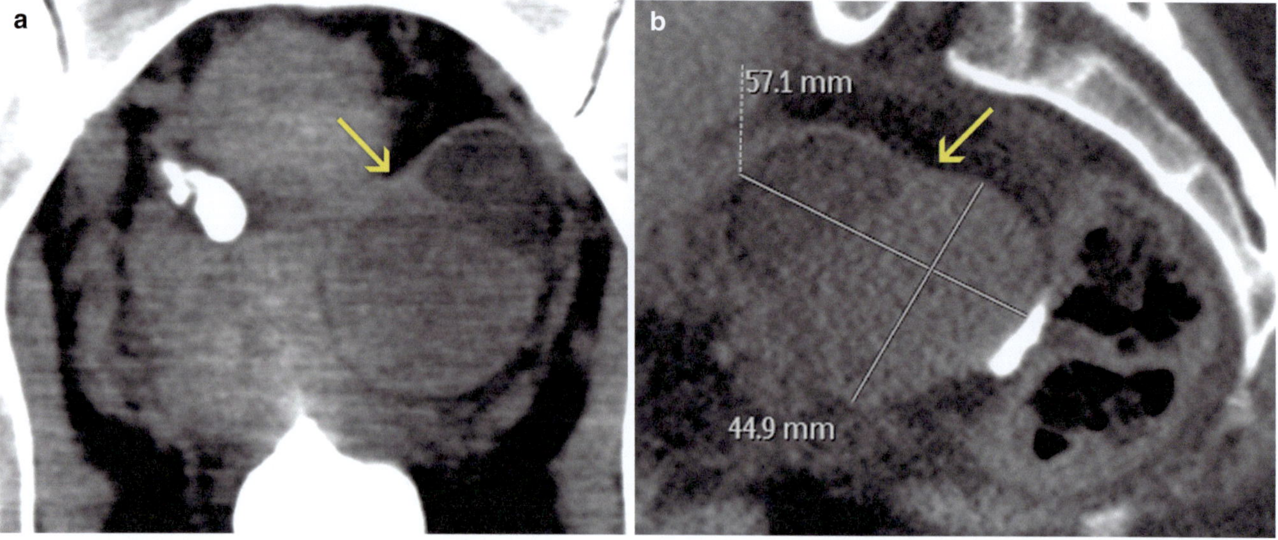

Fig. 11.1 Findings of high clinical importance. (**a**, **b**) Coronal and sagittal VHSG images with soft tissue window. An ovoid lesion can be observed in the left adnexal region (*arrow*) with heterogeneous density and internal septa, suggesting a suspicious malignant ovarian mass. It requires continuing diagnostic algorithm for its classification

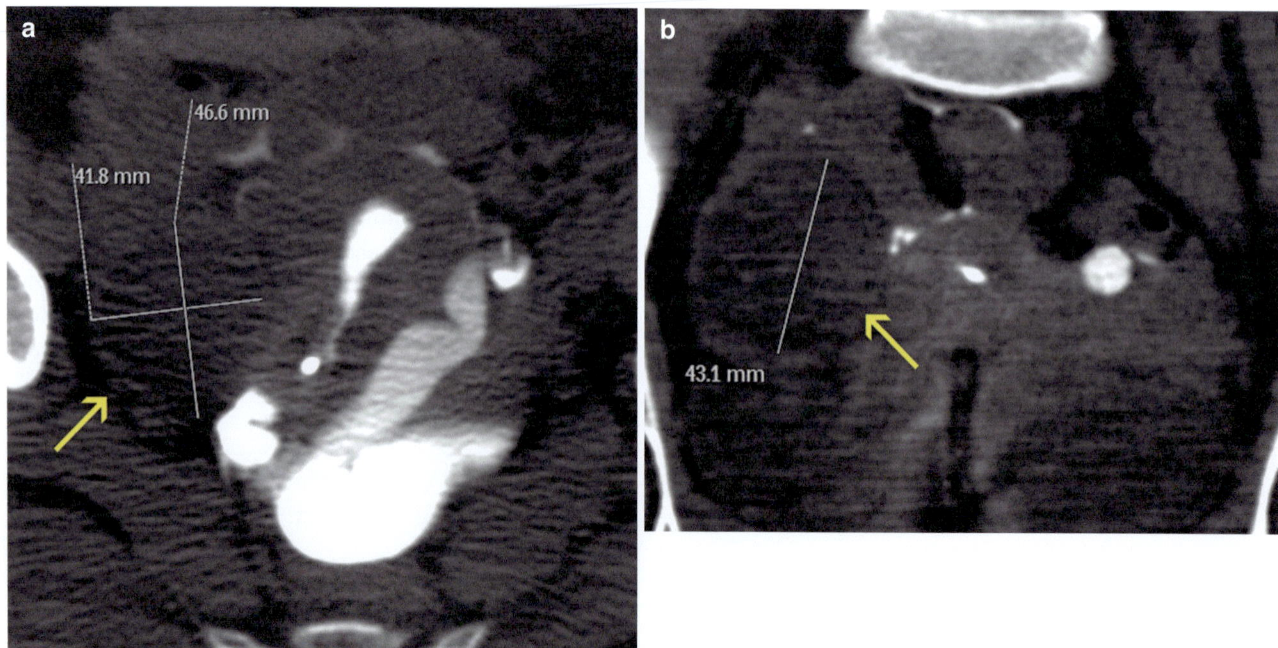

Fig. 11.2 Findings of moderate clinical importance. (**a**, **b**) Axial and coronal VHSG images with soft tissue window. An ovoid lesion larger than 4 cm (*arrows*) can be observed in the right adnexal region, with well defined walls and homogeneous low density. As an undetermined ovarian mass, requires a differed evaluation with a specific method

The unexpected findings of low clinical significance represent a large part of the reports, and generally do not require complementary exams to clarify their diagnosis. The lesions of moderate importance are usually doubtful or undetermined diagnoses, hence the anxiety produced by the uncertainty. In these cases a re-evaluation is vital, and its following depends on each particular case. One example is the unspecific bone lesions, that require new short term imaging studies. The potentially important findings are extremely rare in this group of patients. These are the ones that can affect the health of the patient. Despite their infrequency, one must always be watchful and ready for these findings due to their high impact on morbi-mortality.

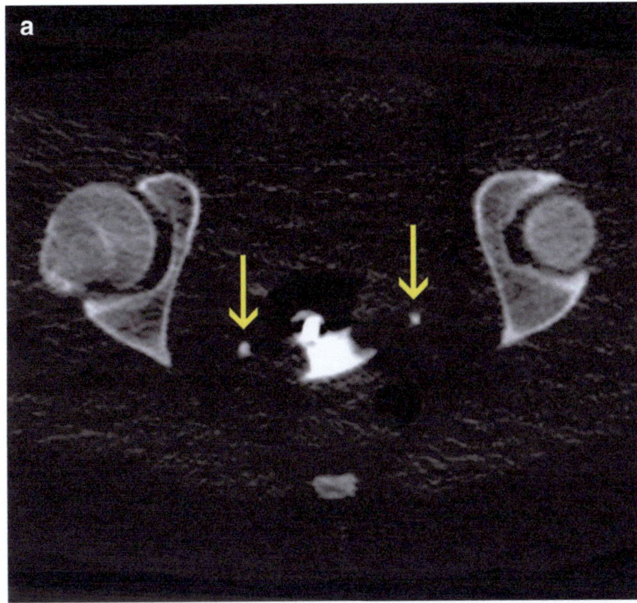
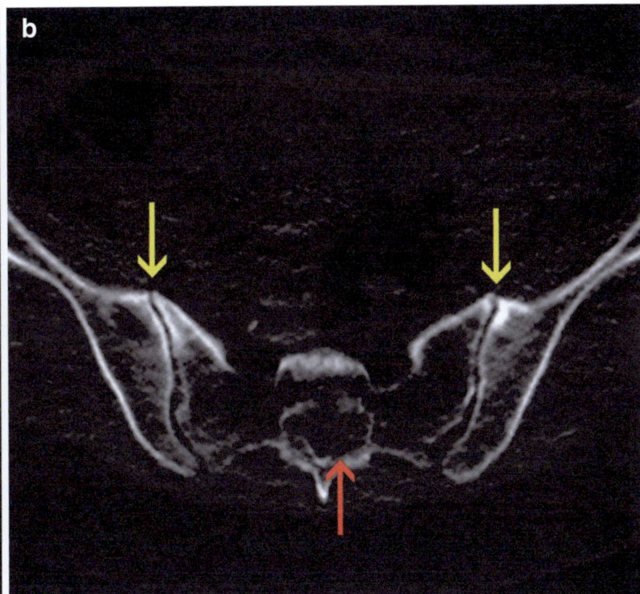

Fig. 11.3 Findings of low clinical importance. (**a**) Axial VHSG image showing two focal images with calcium density (*arrows*) in the lower region of the pelvic cavity, corresponding to vascular calcifications (phleboliths) and should not be confused with urinary stones. (**b**) Axial VHSG image showing deformity in the sacral spinal canal due to the presence of a periradicular cyst (*red arrow*) and degenerative sclerosis in the anterior region of the sacroiliac joints (*yellow arrows*)

Ovarian Pathology

Both functional as well as structural abnormalities affect the ovaries and can be the cause of infertility. For the fecundation to be a success, it is necessary that the ovulation process and follicular development be normal [9]. The study which evaluates these functional parameters, as well as the structural anatomic characteristics, is ultrasound [10]. The conventional hysterosalpingography studies can only infer the existence of an abnormality in the ovary size when displacement and compression is observed in the adjacent uterine tube [11]. Nevertheless, these findings are not specific, because the tubes have a variable position and because other processes can generate a mass effect of the ovaries. On the other hand, in VHSG exams, one can correctly individualize the ovaries, measure their size, and evaluate their density and position in order to characterize pathologic processes (Fig. 11.4). The instilled contrast material which passes to the peritoneal cavity helps delineate the ovaries outline. One disadvantage is associated to the lack of intravenous contrast which is fundamental to detect solid areas and pathologic signs.

The polycystic ovary syndrome is the structural abnormality that most frequently causes infertility [9]. The ovary is enlarged and multiple cysts of different sizes are distinguished in its interior (Fig. 11.5). There exist cases where a complicated cyst can be found, with a high density content that suggests hematologic remains, frequent in endometriosis

cases (Fig. 11.6). Another finding difficult to diagnose are mature cystic ovarian teratomas. They are round or ovoid masses of different dimensions that characteristically present a heterogeneous density, predominantly fat, alternated with solid and calcium areas (Fig. 11.7). When the ovarian masses are not typically benign, a complementary evaluation is required for its improved characterization. The parameters that suggest a malignity are: an ovarian size larger than 4 cm, mixed internal structure (solid-cystic), parietal or septal thickening, and the presence of associated swollen lymph nodes or ascites [12, 13] (Fig. 11.8).

Intestinal Pathology

The sigmoid colon and the rectum are housed in the pelvic cavity, as well as some loops of the distal small intestine. Due to the age range in which the VHSG studies are performed, structural intestinal pathology is infrequent. Only in certain opportunities can diverticula be detected in the sigmoid colon (Fig. 11.9), which is the more frequent site for this disease.

It is also rare to find signs of inflammatory intestinal disease. When it is diagnosed, the adjacent structures must be thoroughly evaluated for complications. The inflammatory pelvic disease and endometriosis favor the presence of adherences in the peritoneal cavity which can, secondly, generate alteration in the normal bowel movements and sub-occlusive

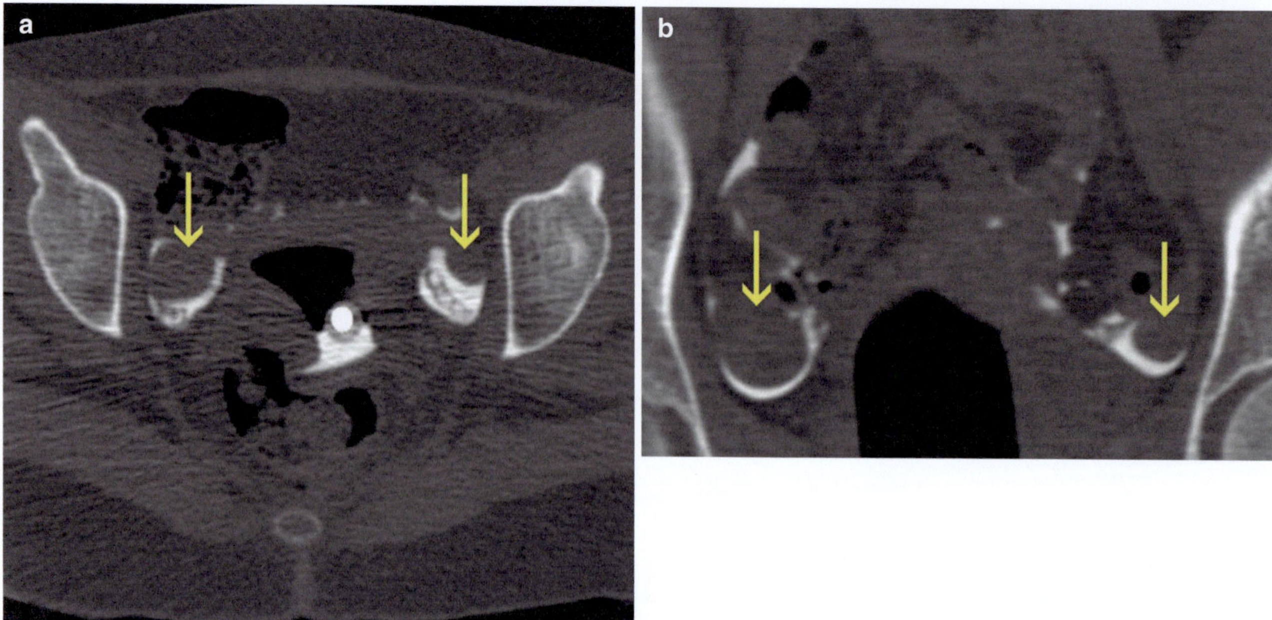

Fig. 11.4 Normal ovaries. (**a**, **b**) Axial and coronal VHSG images where both ovaries of normal size and morphology can be observed (*arrows*) surrounded by contrast material in the peritoneal cavity

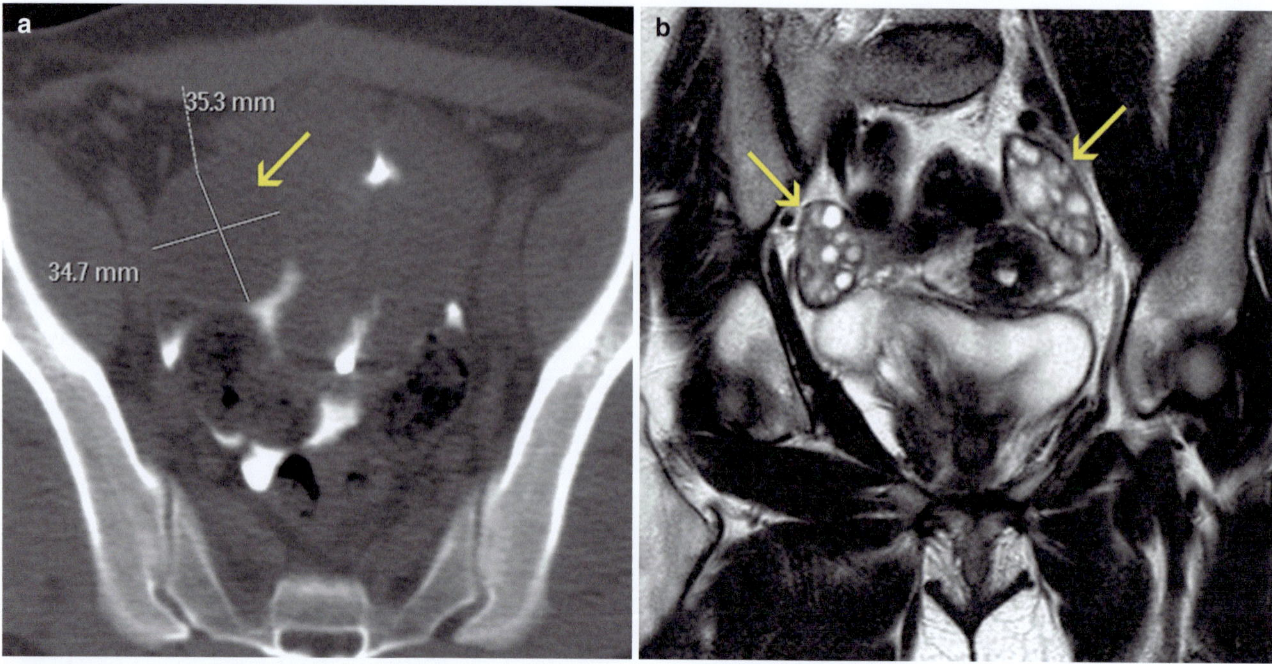

Fig. 11.5 Thirty-four-year old patient with polycystic ovary syndrome. (**a**) Axial VHSG image showing a right enlarged ovary (*arrow*); the internal structure cannot be appreciated. (**b**) Coronal T2 weighted MR image of the same patient showing both enlarged ovaries with multiple small follicles (*arrows*)

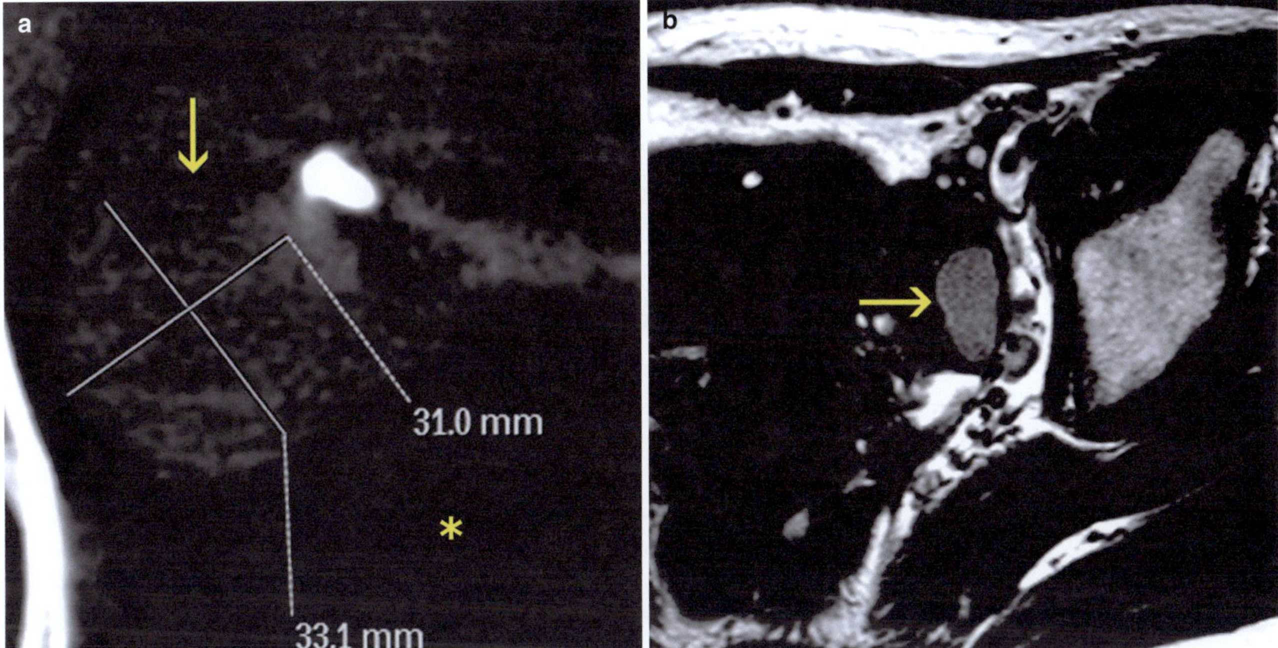

Fig. 11.6 Hemorrhagic cyst. (**a**) Coronal VHSG image with soft tissue window, showing an ovoid lesion in the right adnexal region (*arrow*) which presents higher density than the bladder (*asterisk*), suggesting an hemorrhagic cyst. (**b**) Axial T1 weighted MR image showing an ovoid lesion in the left ovary (*arrow*) which presents a hyperintense signal suggesting hemorrhagic content (endometrioma)

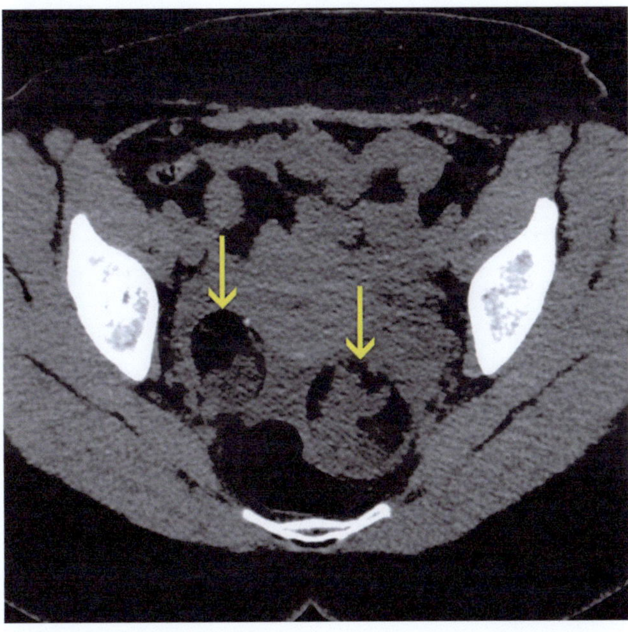

Fig. 11.7 Teratomas. Axial CT image showing two focal heterogeneous lesions (*arrows*) with areas of fat density, alternating with soft tissue and punctiform calcifications, compatible with teratomas

setting. Another lesion which can be detected is the presence of fistulas which communicate the uterine tubes with the digestive tract (Fig. 11.10).

Pelvic Cavity Pathology

It is infrequent to find pathologic processes in the pelvic cavity in VHSG studies. The presence of small quantities of free liquid is considered physiological and is imperceptible in VHSG exams due to the fact that it mixes with the contrast material which free spillage into the cavity through the fallopian tubes. A larger quantity of fluid is catalogued as ascites and is observed in cases of malignant ovarian pathology, among other causes [12]. The inflammatory collections are usually symptomatic; hence the VHSG study would be contraindicated. They are observed as organized fluid collections of thick walls. The herniations of the pelvic content can also be diagnosed through the inguinal, crural, obturatriz and anterior abdominal wall rings (Fig. 11.11). In these cases the hernia content and the signs that suggest complications have to be evaluated.

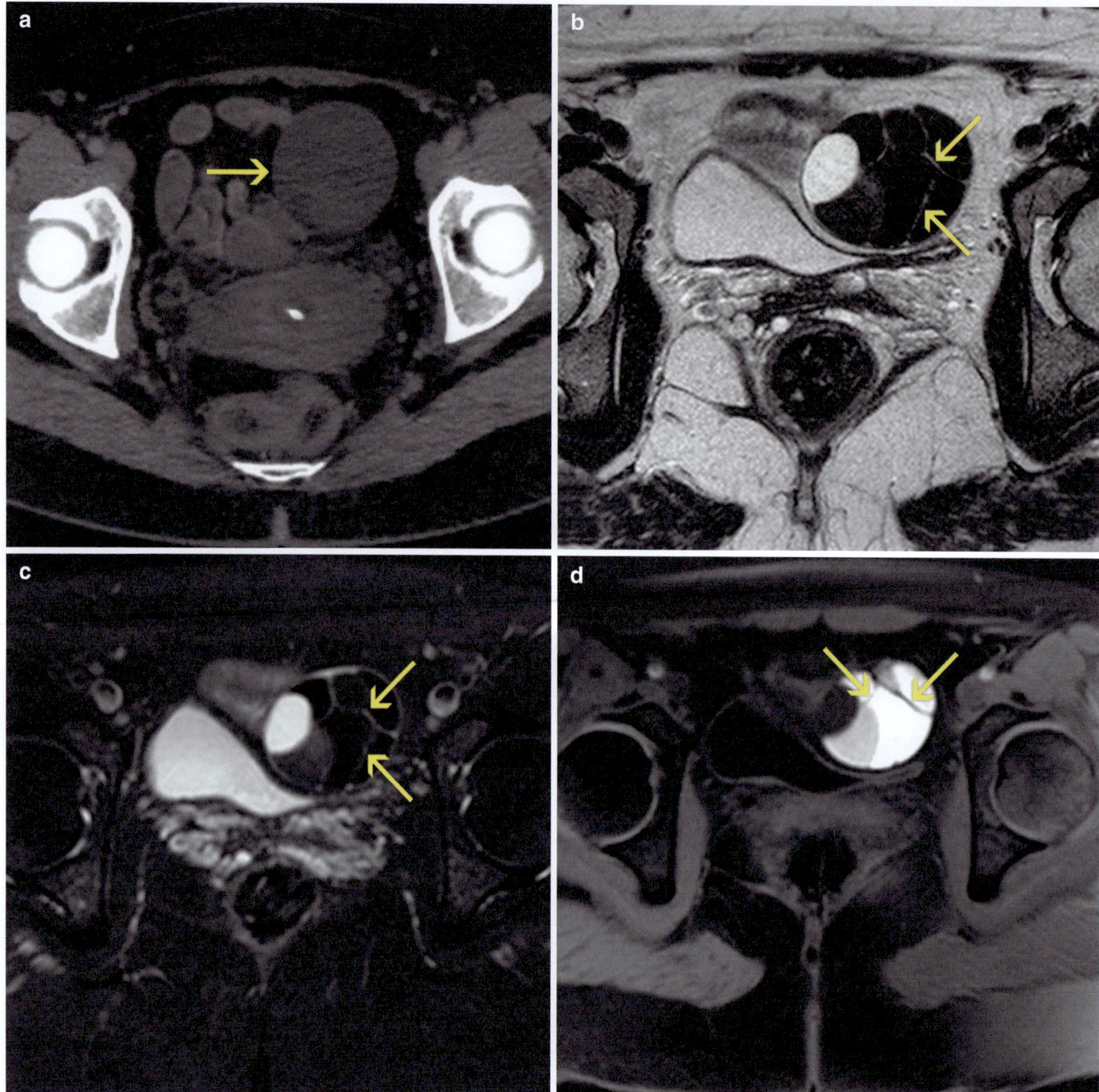

Fig. 11.8 Ovarian carcinoma. (**a**) Axial VHSG image with soft tissue window showing an ovoid mass with heterogeneous density (*arrow*) in the left anterior sector of the pelvic cavity. (**b**) Axial T2 weighted MR image. (**c**) Axial T2 weighted MR image with fat suppression. (**d**) Axial T1 weighted MR image with fat suppression. The mass has heterogeneous signal, predominantly hyperintense on T1 and hypointense on T2 weighted MR images, with multiple internal septa (*arrows*), suggesting an ovarian mucinous cystic tumor

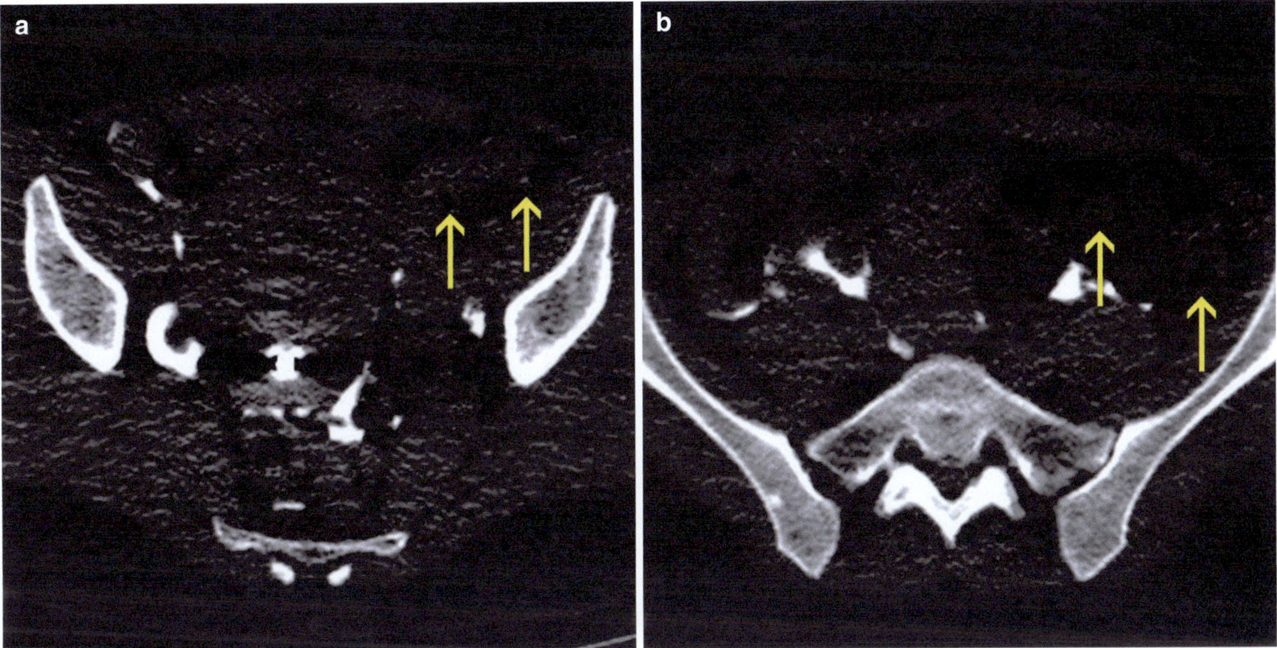

Fig. 11.9 Colon diverticula. (**a**) Axial VHSG image with soft tissue window of a 35-year old patient, showing isolated diverticula in the sigmoid colon (*arrows*), without signs of complications. (**b**) Axial VHSG image in another 41-year old patient who also presented isolated diverticula of larger size in the sigmoid colon (*arrows*), without signs of complications

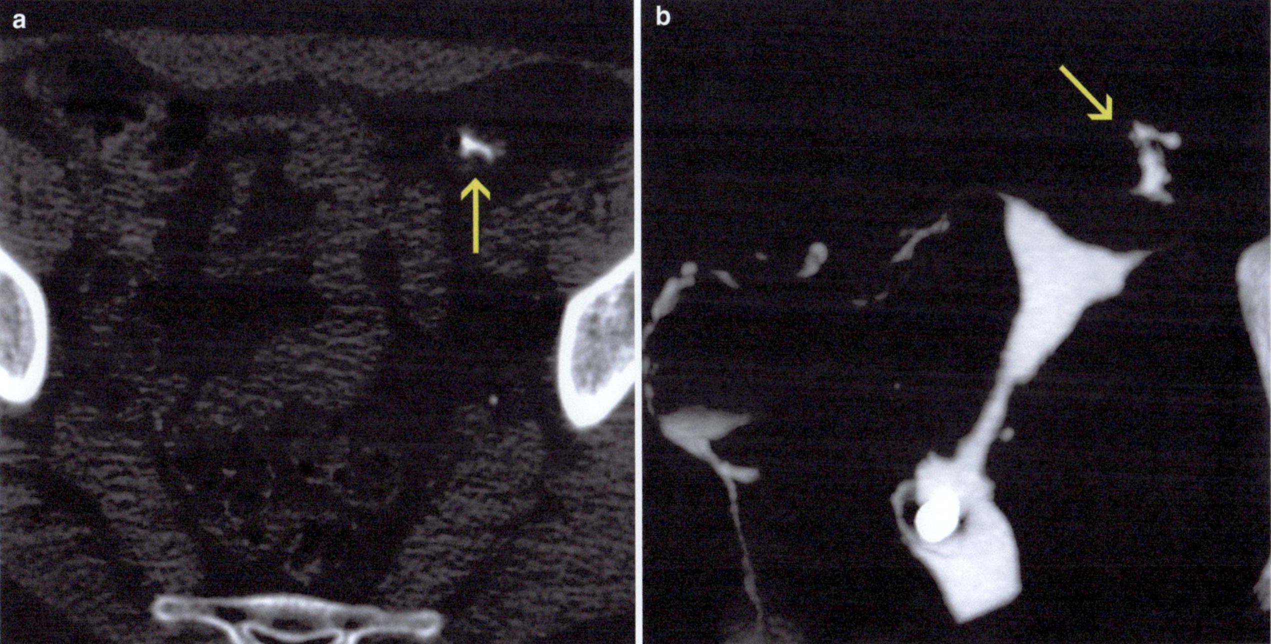

Fig. 11.10 Tubal-colonic fistula in a 38-year old patient with infertility and a history of pelvic inflammatory disease. (**a**) Axial VHSG image identifying contrast material in the sigmoid colon lumen (*arrow*). (**b**) With maximum intensity projection (MIP) image the normal right tube is observed, while the left tube is occluded in its medial portion is adjacent to the contrast material in the colon (*arrow*). (**c**, **d**) Sagittal MIP and 3D volume rendering images showing the continuity of the left uterine tube with the adjacent colon (*arrow*)

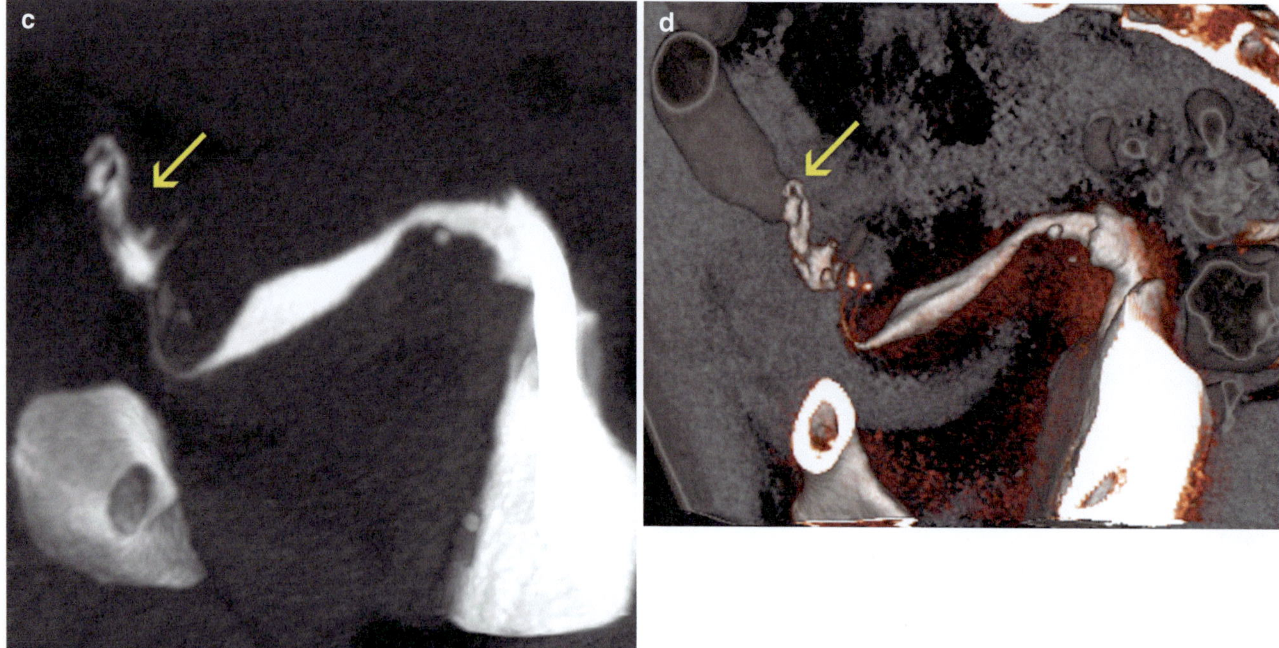

Fig. 11.10 (continued)

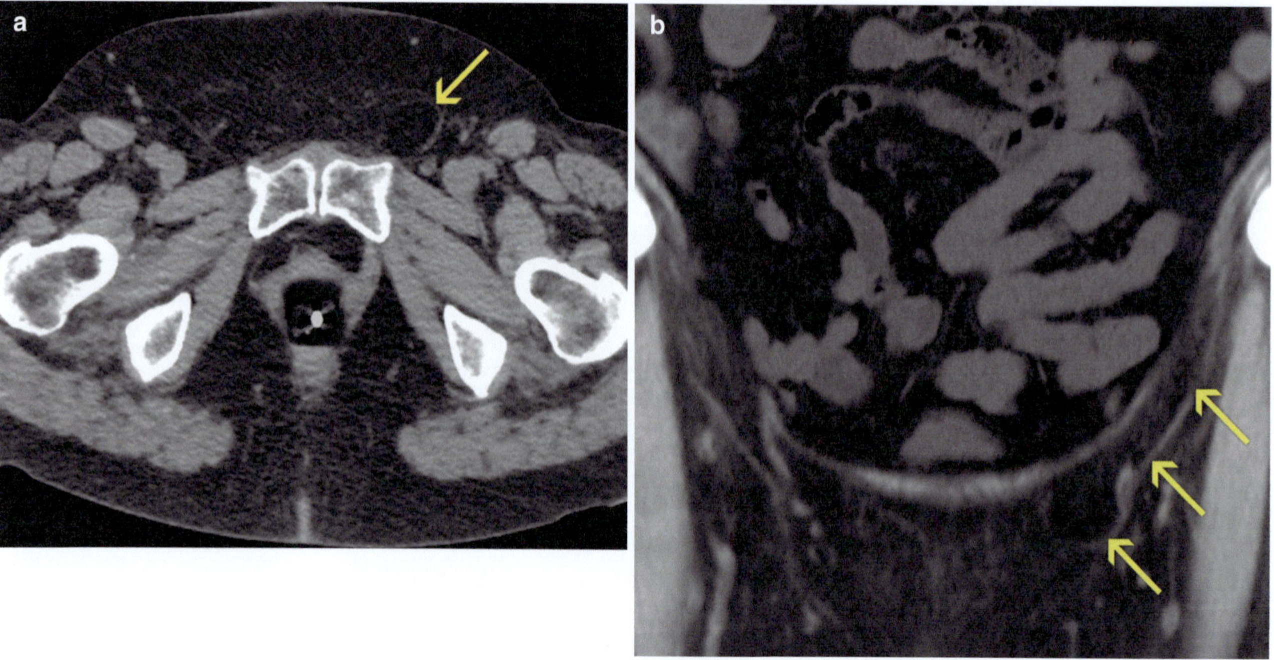

Fig. 11.11 Small inguinal hernia. (**a**, **b**) Axial and coronal VHSG images showing fat tissue pushing through the left inguinal canal (*arrows*)

Pelvic Lymph Nodes

There exist various lymphatic chains which are phases of lymphatic dissemination of regional pathologic processes, such as iliac, inguinal, presacral, and mesenteric chains. The detection and evaluation of the lymph nodes is based on their size and shape. When the lymph node diameter on the short axis is larger than 10 mm, it is considered adenomegaly. The morphological criteria of the lymph node pathology encompass irregular margins, a heterogeneous density and signs of central necrosis [14]. When these lymphadenopathies are detected in VHSG exams it should be reported and investigation is recommended (Fig. 11.12).

Pelvic Bone Evaluation

The VHSG has the advantage of being able to evaluate the bone structures with tomography quality. Therefore, the degenerative changes of the sacroiliac joints, of the pubic symphysis and of the hip are easily detected (Fig. 11.13). These findings are more frequent in patients over the age of 35. Other regular findings are bone islands which show up as regular focal images of high density (Fig. 11.14). When the lesions are undetermined, be them lytic or blastic (Fig. 11.15), the intrinsic characteristics are evaluated and, in general, require complementary studies in order to establish a diagnostic approximation.

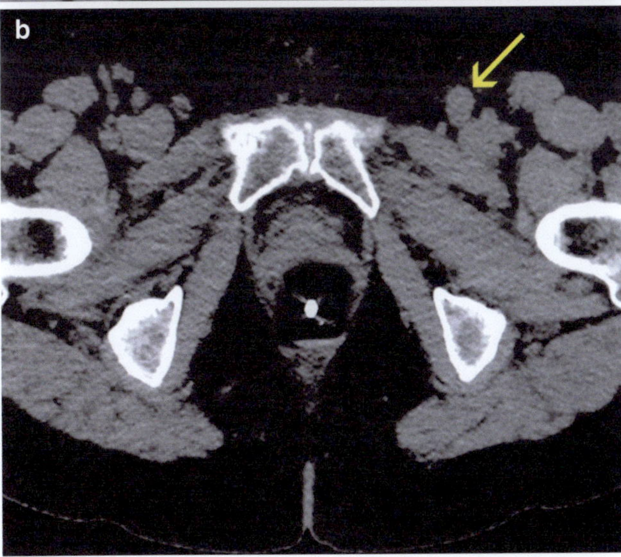

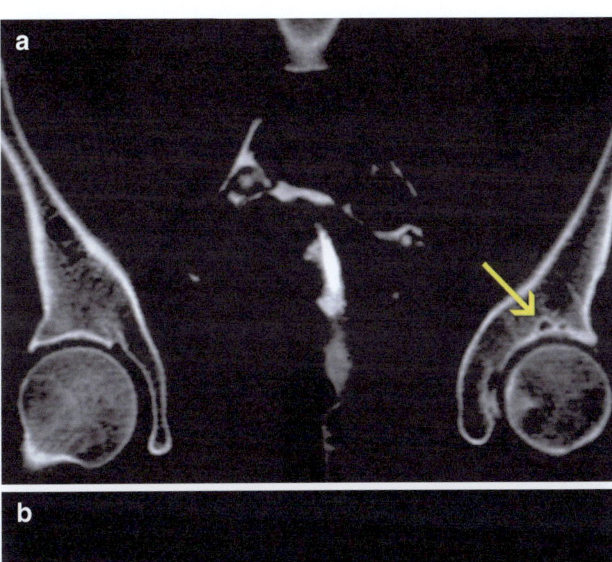

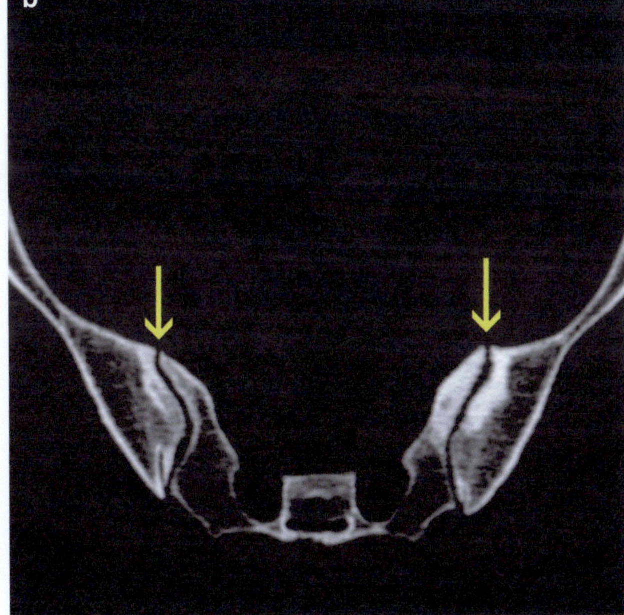

Fig. 11.12 Lymph nodes. (**a**) Coronal VHSG image showing bilateral lymph nodes (*arrows*). (**b**) Axial VHSG image showing a left inguinal adenopathy (*arrow*)

Fig. 11.13 Arthrosis. (**a**) Coronal multiplanar reconstruction image showing sclerosis on the articular surface of the left acetabulum, associated with subchondral geodes (*arrow*), as degenerative signs of arthrosis. (**b**) Axial CT image showing degenerative changes in both sacroiliac joints, manifested by sclerosis of the articular surfaces (*arrows*)

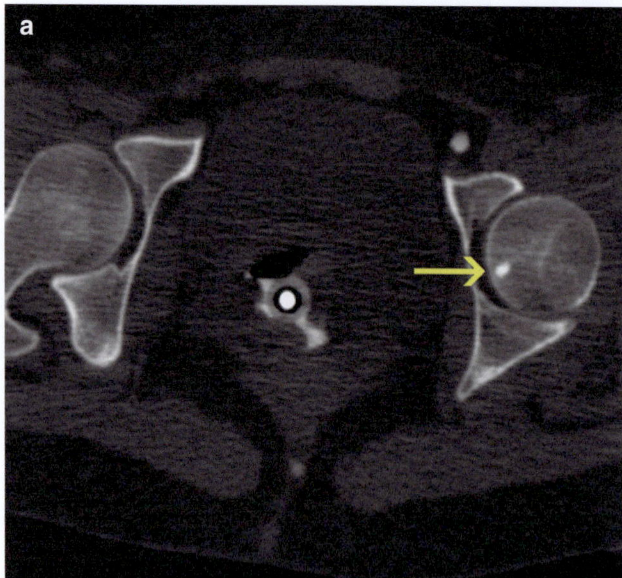

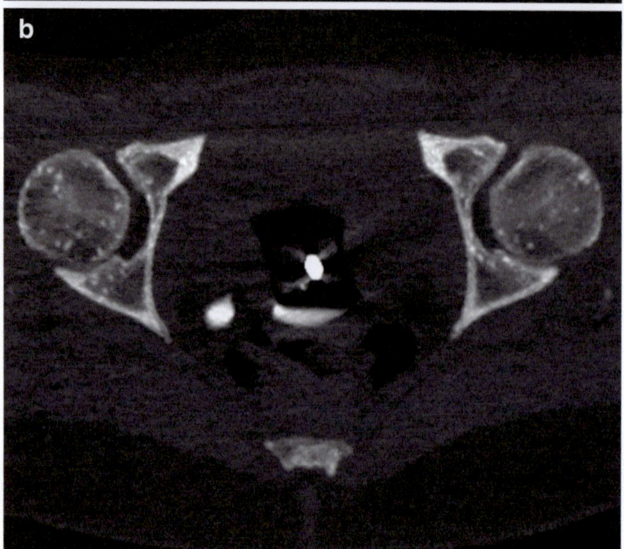

Fig. 11.14 (**a**) Axial CT image showing a focal sclerotic region of bone in the left femoral head (*arrow*), compatible with bone island. (**b**) Axial CT image showing multiple and small bone islands in the iliac bones and both femurs, in a patient with osteopoiquilia

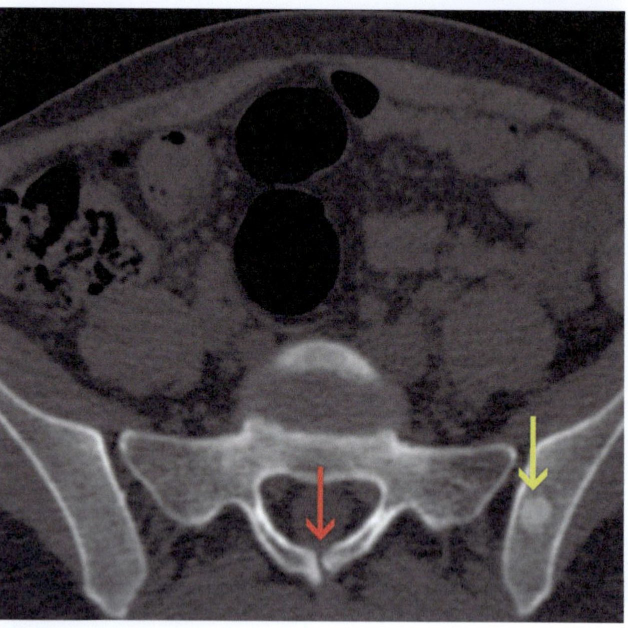

Fig. 11.15 Axial CT image showing a 10-mm focal blastic lesion with a small hypodense halo in the left iliac bone (*yellow arrow*), of unknown etiology. Note also the lack of fusion of the posterior arch of the sacrum vertebra (*red arrow*)

Conclusion

The capacity to evaluate the extra-uterine pelvic structures is an advantage of the VHSG in comparison to conventional studies. While the possibility of this analysis implies a longer time for the radiologist, it permits the detection of incidental findings, ranging from the ones that lack medical value to those with high clinical significance, hence a big benefit to the patient. This reflects the importance of the experience and training of the performing physician, and of his or hers responsibility in the global evaluation of the study.

References

1. Hellstrom M, Svensson MH, Lasson A. Extracolonic and incidental findings on CT colonography (virtual colonoscopy). AJR Am J Roentgenol. 2004;182:631–8.
2. Hara AK, Johnson CD, MacCarty RL, et al. Incidental extracolonic findings at CT colonography. Radiology. 2000;215:353–7.
3. Sosna J, Kruskal JB, Bar-Ziv J, et al. Extracolonic findings at CT colonography. Abdom Imaging. 2005;30:709–13.
4. Pickhardt PJ, Taylor AJ. Extracolonic findings identified in asymptomatic adults at screening CT colonography. AJR Am J Roentgenol. 2006;186:718–28.
5. Pickhardt PJ, Kim DH, Meiners RJ, et al. Colorectal and extracolonic cancers detected at screening CT colonography in 10,286 asymptomatic adults. Radiology. 2010;255(1):83–8.
6. Chin M, Mendelson R, Edwards J, et al. Computed tomographic colonography: prevalence, nature and clinical significance of extracolonic findings in a community screening programme. Am J Gastroenterol. 2005;100(12):2771–6.
7. Westbrook JI, Braithwaite J, McIntosh JH. The outcomes for patients with incidental lesions: serendipitous or iatrogenic? AJR Am J Roentgenol. 1998;171(5):1193–6.
8. Zalis ME, Barish MA, Choi JR, et al. CT colonography reporting and data system: a consensus proposal. Radiology. 2005;236:3–9.
9. Krysiewicz S. Infertility in women: diagnostic evaluation with hysterosalpingography and other imaging techniques. AJR Am J Roentgenol. 1992;159(2):253–61.
10. Mendelson EB, Friedman H, Neiman HL, et al. The role of imaging in infertility management. AJR Am J Roentgenol. 1985;144(2):415–20.
11. Steinkeler JA, Woodfield CA, Lazarus E, et al. Female infertility: a systematic approach to radiologic imaging and diagnosis. Radiographics. 2009;29(5):1353–70.
12. Tsili AC, Tsampoulas C, Charisiadi A, et al. Adnexal masses: accuracy of detection and differentiation with multidetector computed tomography. Gynecol Oncol. 2008;110(1):22–31.
13. Griffin N, Grant LA, Sala E. Adnexal masses: characterization and imaging strategies. Semin Ultrasound CT MR. 2010;31(5):330–46.
14. Walsh JW, Amendola MA, Konerding KF, et al. Computed tomographic detection of pelvic and inguinal lymph-node metastases from primary and recurrent pelvic malignant disease. Radiology. 1980;137(1):157–66.

In each virtual hysterosalpingography (VHSG) study there is a potential risk of carrying out an incorrect diagnosis. The VHSG has shown sensibility and specificity results similar to those of the conventional hysterosalpingography study [1, 2]. Nevertheless, a great number of false interpretations can affect the general validity of the method; the most efficient strategy to prevent the pitfalls is to appropriately solve the diagnostic errors which arise from false positives and negatives.

Anyhow, a considerable number of false diagnoses can be prevented, but not all of them. The perform of the diagnostic studies with an adequate preparation and an appropriate technical procedure is important for limiting the factors which entail errors [3]. It is also essential that the radiologist be familiarized with the spectrum of normal and pathological findings for a correct interpretation of the VHSG exams.

On occasions the false interpretations imply some clinical significance [4]. The false positive diagnosis is a perceptive error which occurs when a lesion is detected where in fact no such abnormality exists [5]. In the VHSG studies, in general, it occurs when elevated images of the uterine cavity exist which may suggest polipoid lesions or when, in the lack of opacification of the uterine tubes, they are interpreted as being obstructed. One false positive finding can lead to the execution of an unnecessary complementary study, with the added preoccupations, associated costs and risks that this entails. Even a wrong diagnosis can determine a change in the therapeutic conduct. Furthermore, false positives affect the specificity and positive predictive value when the validity of the method is evaluated [6].

A false negative diagnosis is an error that occurs when a lesion that in reality exists is not able to be identified. The experience of these false interpretations was acquired with research protocols along the years in our institution for the validation of the method. When one is aware of the existence of these potential errors, and applies the solutions to avoid them, they rarely occur [7]. A VHSG study in optimal technical conditions is considered an exam with few false negatives and, therefore, with a high negative predictive value. This way, the validity of the study also considerably depends on the occurrence of false negatives.

False Positives

Seudopolyps

In VHSG studies, elevated lesions can be characterized correctly in most of the cases. Even the detection of small lesions is possible thanks to the larger spacial resolution of studies performed with multislice tomography [8]. However, a variety of findings that can simulate polyps exist. To help minimize this situation, it is fundamental to implement a rigorous preparation and a standardized procedure. One of the frequent causes of errors is the persistence of endoluminal mucosa secretions (Fig. 12.1). They usually present themselves as free linear structures with one extremity leaning on the endometrial surface. In other occasions, they are well adhered to the wall and acquire a rounded aspect, simulating real sessile polyps (Fig. 12.2). To avoid the presence of residual secretions it is recommended to always perform the studies once finished the menstrual period. Also, in the event of diagnostic doubt, a second acquisition of images can be obtained, where the mucosa secretion usually modifies their position and morphology with respect to the first acquisition (Fig. 12.3), while, on the other hand, a polyp remains fixed and with the same shape it was before. The linear secretions can also be confused with synechiae when they are firmly adhered to the uterine wall on both extremes. In these cases, history of invasive procedures and gynecologic infectious processes, as well as the fibrous and irregular appearance of adhesions help perform the differential diagnosis.

Another case of misinterpretation is when the uterine folds are prominent and simulate elevated lesions in the endocervix as well as in the endometrium (Fig. 12.4). The prominent folds are of unknown etiology, and could be

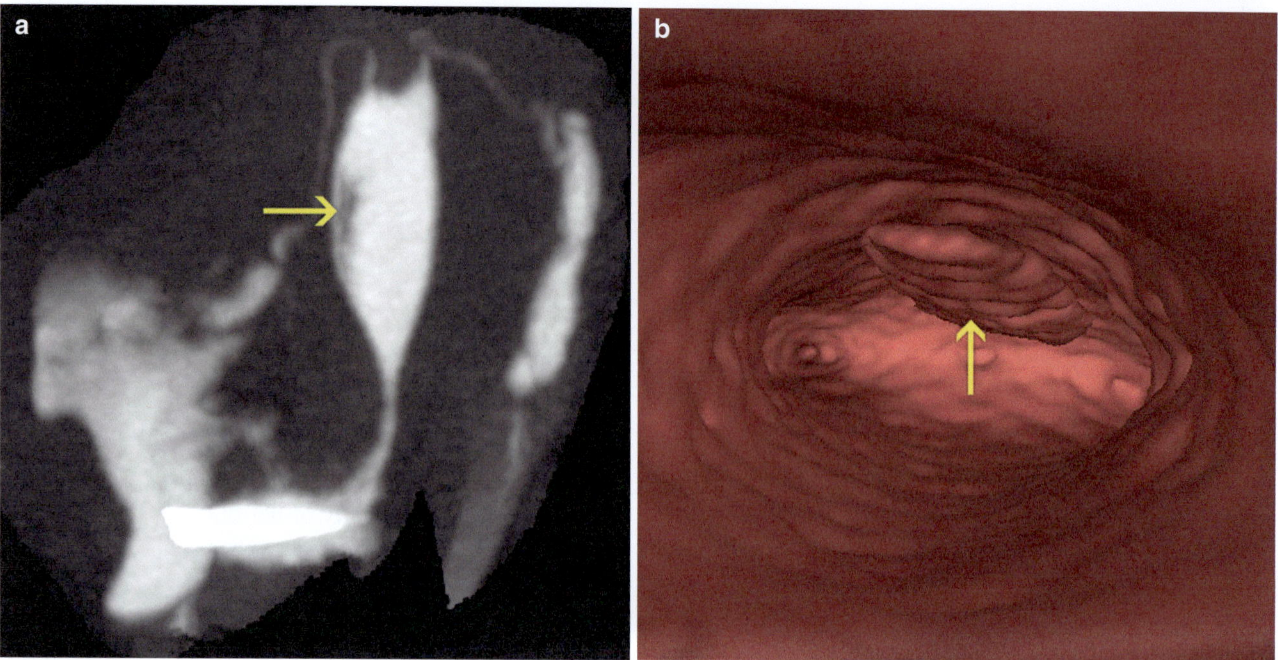

Fig. 12.1 Mucous secretions: (**a**) Maximum intensity projection image where a lineal filling defect is visualized adjacent to the anterior uterine wall (*arrow*), corresponding to secretions. (**b**) Virtual endoscopy image showing the mucous secretions (*arrow*)

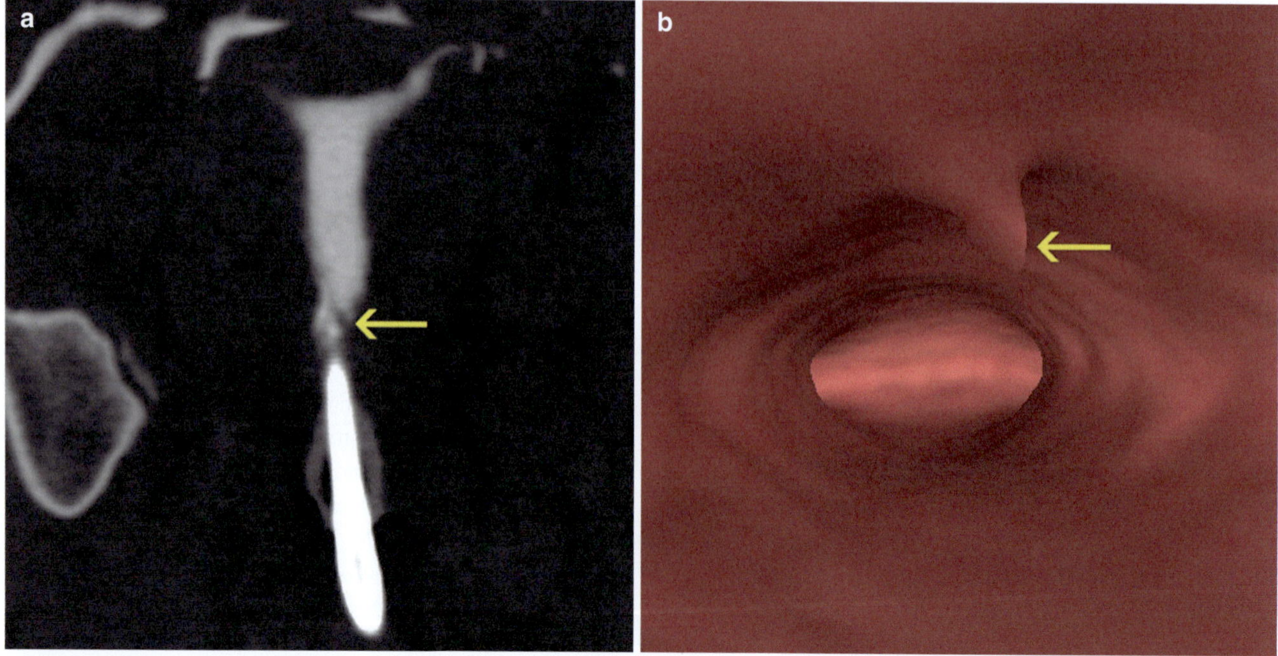

Fig. 12.2 Mucous secretions: (**a**) Coronal multiplanar reconstruction image showing a small lineal filling defect on the left anterolateral wall in the lower endometrial cavity (*arrow*). (**b**) Virtual endoscopy image showing the mucous secretion that acquires a polypoid appearance (*arrow*)

formed by the arrangement of longitudinal muscle bundle on the uterine wall. Likewise it has been reported that they correspond to remnants of the fusion of the Müllerian ducts [9]. In most cases they are easily distinguished due to the fact that they are elongated, parallel to the uterine longitudinal axis and their regular morphology (Fig. 12.5). A situation that favors their visualization is presented when an optimum distention of the cavity is not achieved. On occasions,

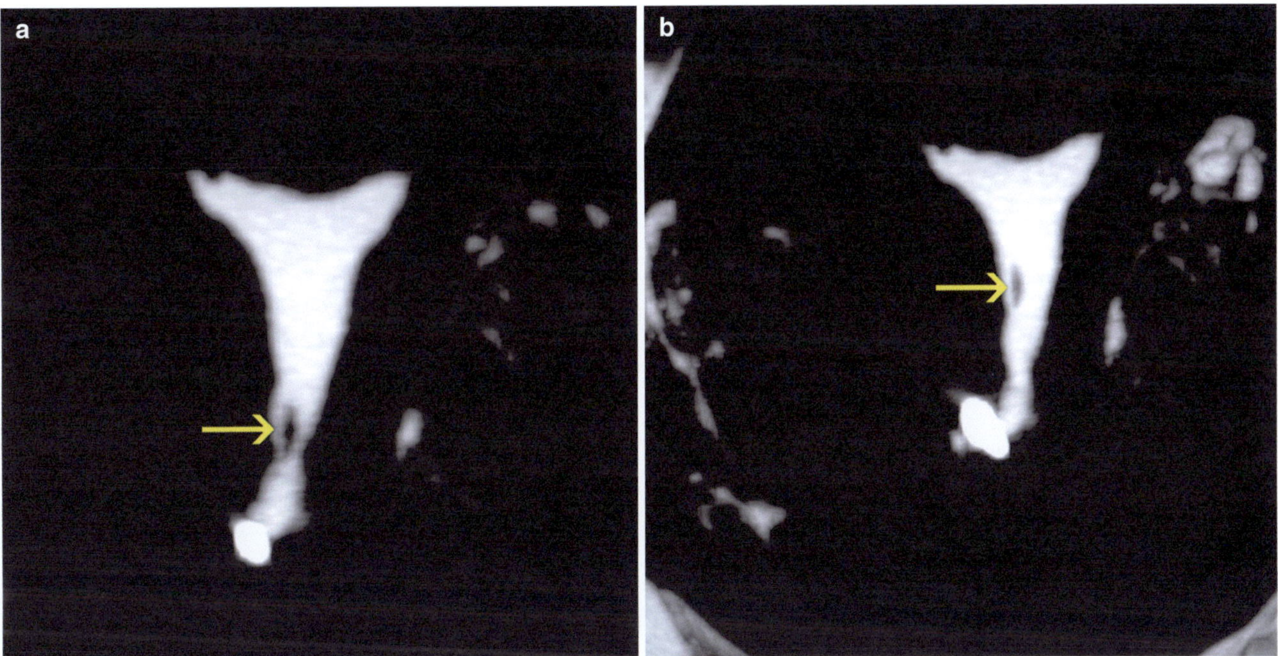

Fig. 12.3 Mucous secretions: (**a**) Coronal maximum intensity projection (MIP) image showing a lineal filling defect in the isthmic region of the endometrial cavity (*arrow*). (**b**) Delayed coronal MIP image demonstrating a change in the position of the filling defect, interpreted as a mobile mucous secretion (*arrow*)

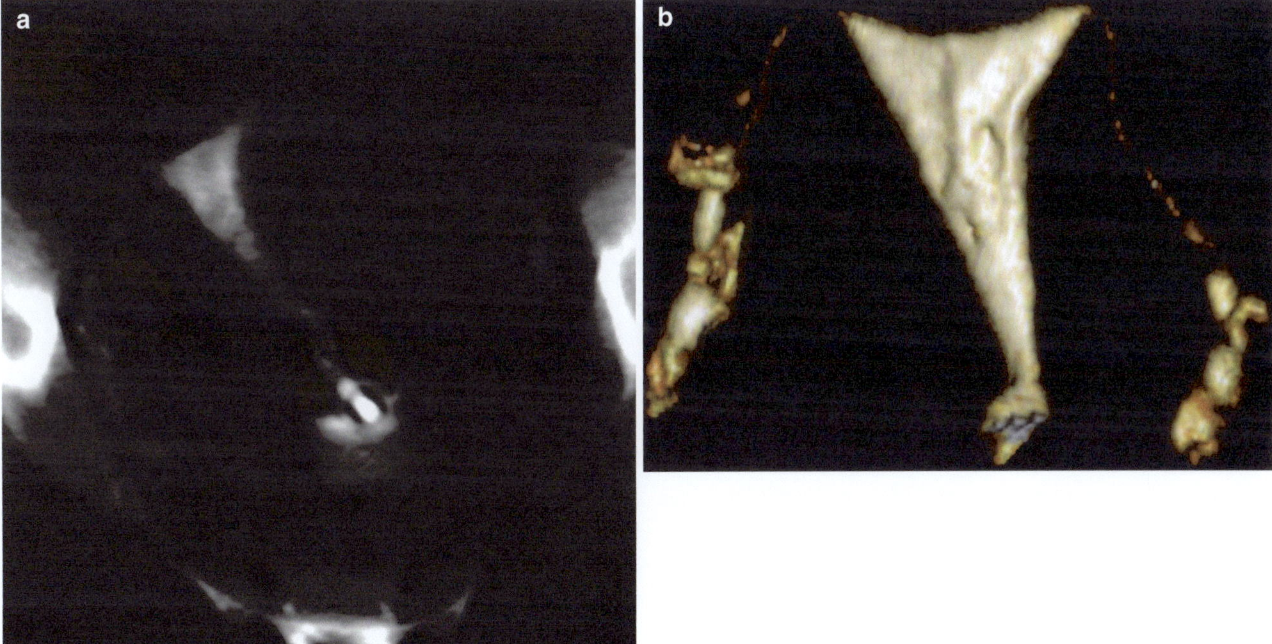

Fig. 12.4 Uterine folds. Lineal filling defects are visualized parallel to the uterus' axis, corresponding to prominent uterine myometrial folds. (**a**) Coronal multiplanar reconstruction image. (**b**) Coronal 3D volume rendering image

the prominent folds may generate confusion when the protrusion is more focused and bulbous than linear (Fig. 12.6).

A frequent cause of error in HSG studies occurs when air bubbles get into the uterine cavity through the cannula during the procedure. The bubbles can be mistaken for filling defects lesions on hysterosalpingograms (Fig. 12.7). This scenario does not repeat itself in VHSG due to the fact that air density is easily distinguished on bidimensional images

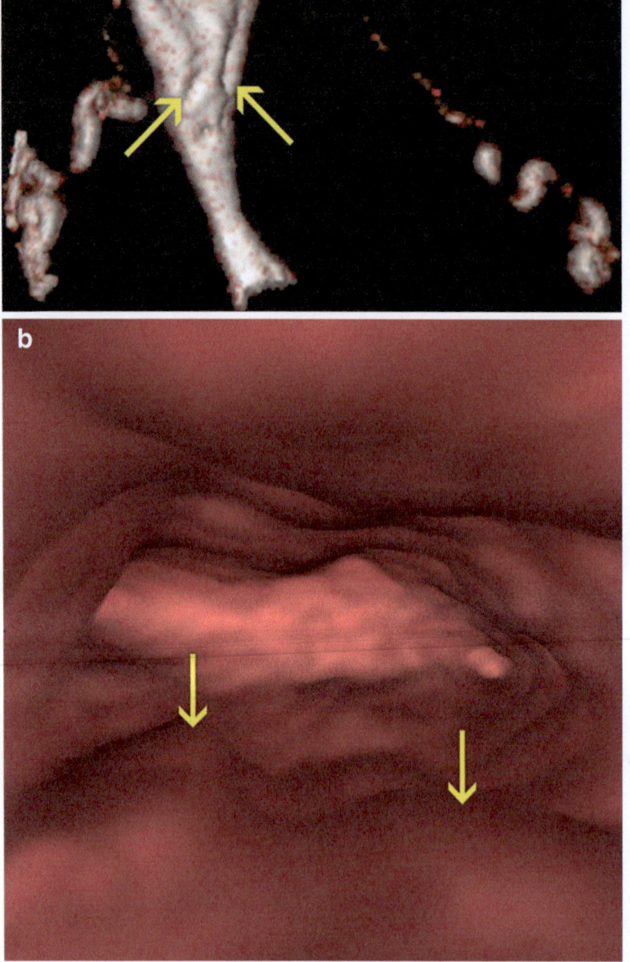

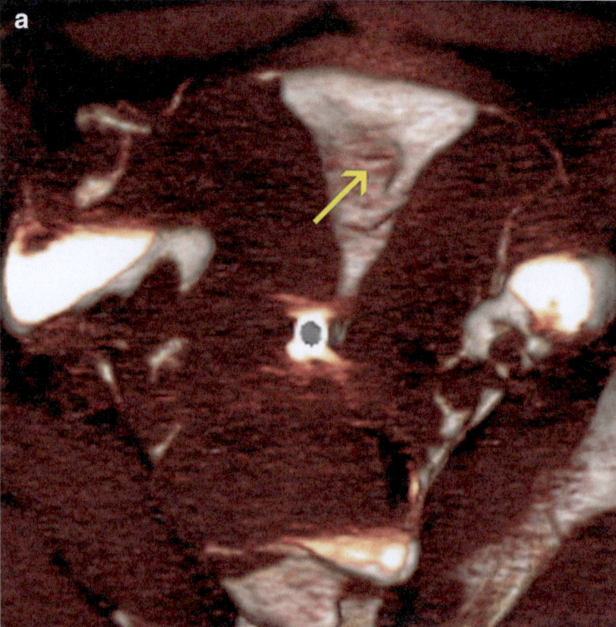

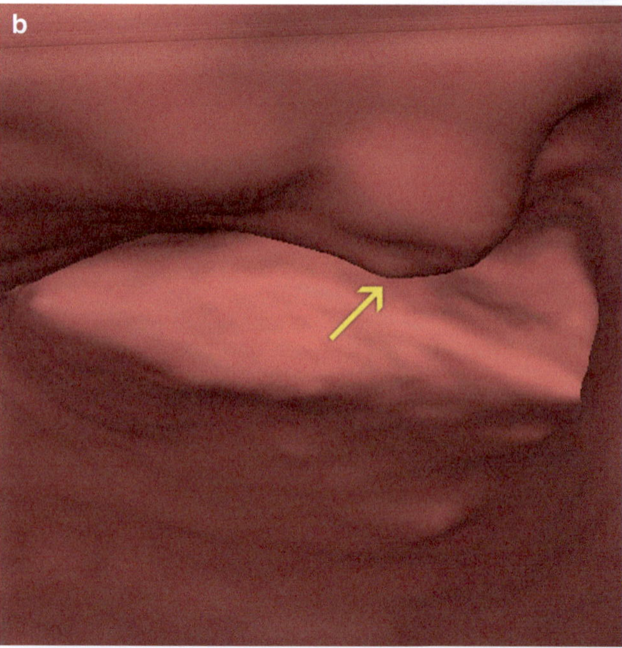

Fig. 12.5 Uterine folds. Linear filling defects are visualized parallel to the uterus' axis, corresponding to prominent uterine myometrial folds (*arrows*). (**a**) Oblique coronal 3D volume rendering image. (**b**) Virtual endoscopy image

(Fig. 12.8). They only can simulate a polyp on tridimensional and virtual navigation views (Fig. 12.9); hence the importance of use all analysis tools for an appropriate interpretation of the findings.

Fig. 12.6 Uterine fold. An indentation on the anterior surface of the uterine cavity is visualized (*arrows*) corresponding to an enlarged uterine fold simulating a polyp lesion. (**a**) Axial 3D volume rendering image. (**b**) Virtual endoscopy image

Tubal Seudo-obstructions

Conventional HSG is the adequate study to evaluate the tubal factor in infertile patients. However its performance is not high, with a sensibility of 65 % and a specificity of 83 % for tubal obstruction [10]. Moreover, when comparing the permeability results with the standard reference via laparoscopy and hysteroscopy, discrepancies exist in 10–17 % of cases [11]. Probable causes which explain the low yield are connected to technical factors such as an insufficient quantity of contrast, cornual spasms or mucus plugs [12]. On VHSG studies, tubal spasms can be avoided by the administration of oral antispasmodics 1 hour before the exam. In addition, an adequate preparation avoids intraluminal mucus plugs. The use of a power injector allows a controlled administration of the pressure and volume of the contrast medium. In cases where the instilled volume has been insufficient, another acquisition can be performed with a larger volume in order to achieve a complete tubal opacification (Fig. 12.10).

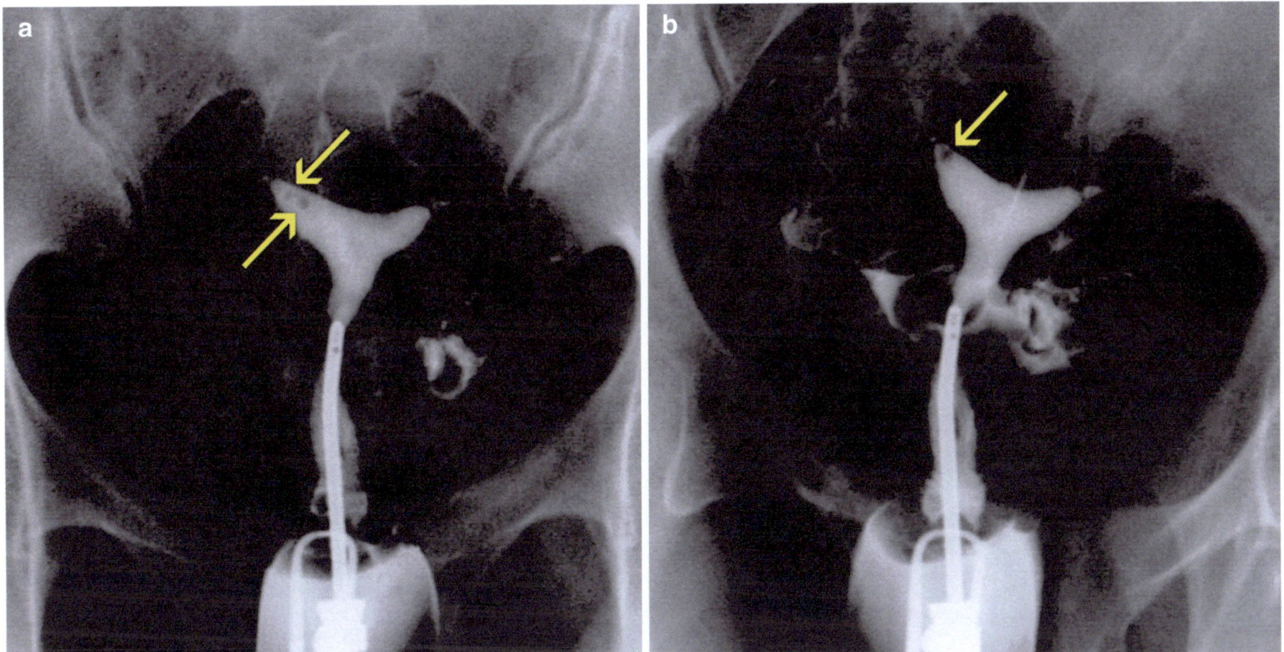

Fig. 12.7 Air bubbles. (**a**) HSG showing small filling defects in the right cornual region which simulate endometrial lesions (*arrows*). (**b**) Image demonstrating that the filling defects have change in position in a delayed acquisition (*arrow*), being compatible with air bubbles

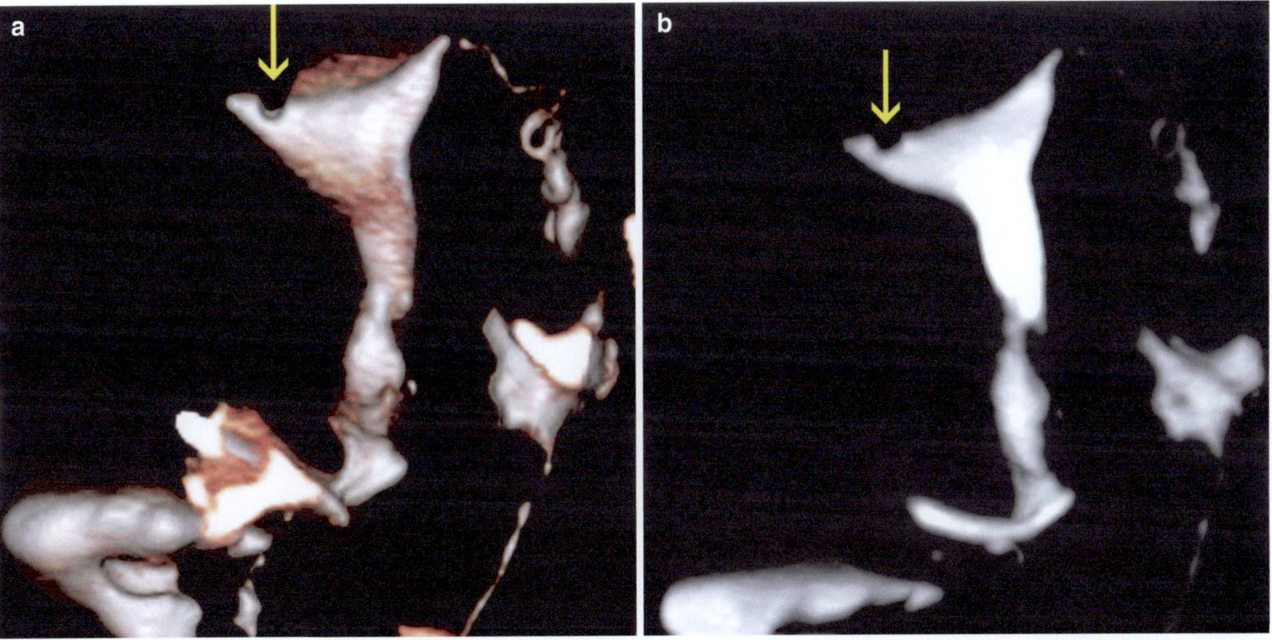

Fig. 12.8 Air bubble. A filling defect is visualized at the level of the right cornual region (*arrows*). (**a**) Coronal 3D volume rendering image. (**b**) Coronal maximum intensity projection image

Other Non-pathological Positive Findings

One normal finding that must not be considered as pathological is cornual lucencies, visible as small linear and regular filling defects, symmetrical in the proximity of the tubal ostium (Fig. 12.11). They correspond to the mark of a muscular ring in the intramural tubal portion [9]. In the cervix, it is not infrequent the observation of seudo-diverticular images that correspond to glandular structures which are filled with the contrast material (Fig. 12.12). The cesarean scars and myomectomies also simulate diverticula (Fig. 12.13); however, in most cases malinterpretations are not generated when the patient's surgical history is correlated.

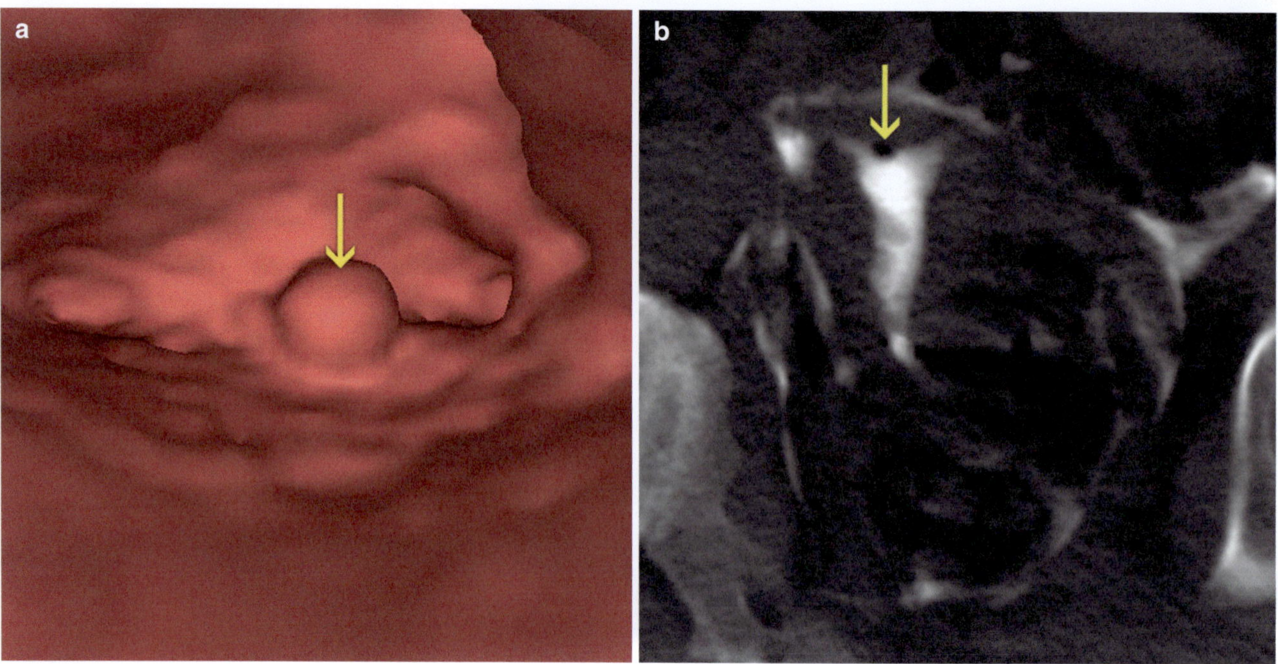

Fig. 12.9 Air bubble. (**a**) Virtual endoscopy image showing an elevated lesion in the uterine fundus, simulating a polyp lesion (*arrow*). (**b**) Axial CT image showing the presence of air density within the lesion (*arrow*), being compatible with an air bubble

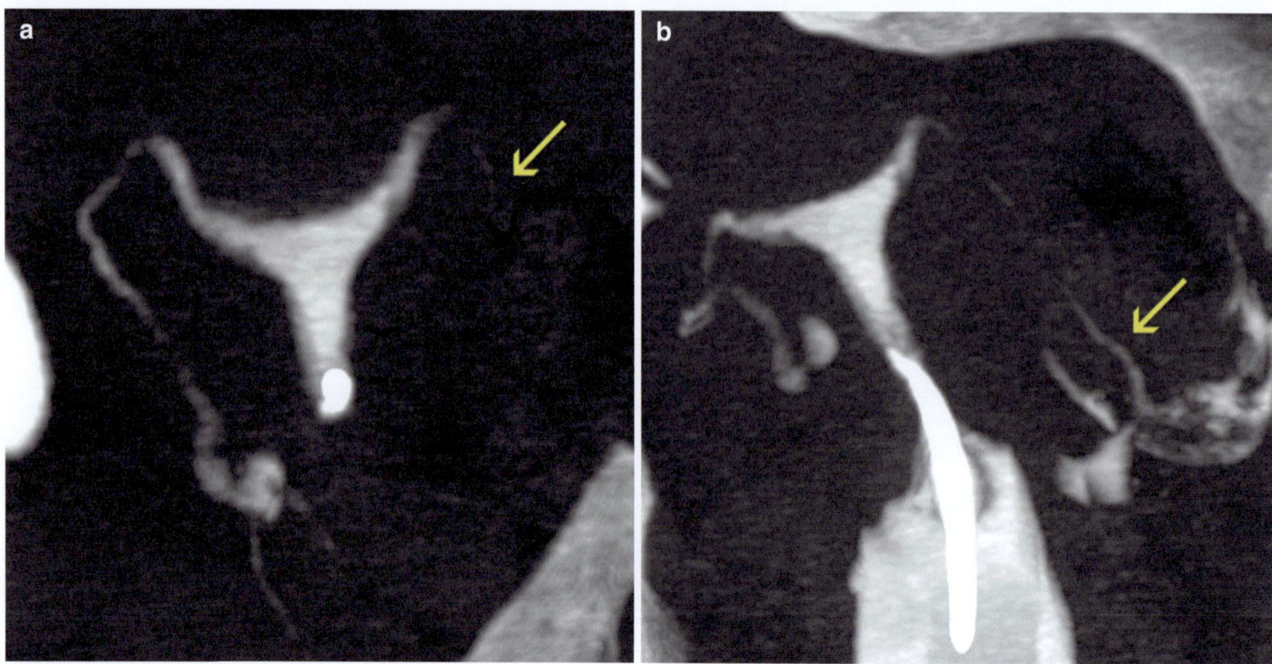

Fig. 12.10 Tubal pseudo-obstruction. (**a**) Coronal maximum intensity projection image showing partial and incomplete opacification of the left uterine tube (*arrow*), simulating a tubal obstruction. (**b**) Coronal maximum intensity projection image of a second scan where a complete filling of the left tube is observed, with passage of contrast to the peritoneal cavity (*arrow*)

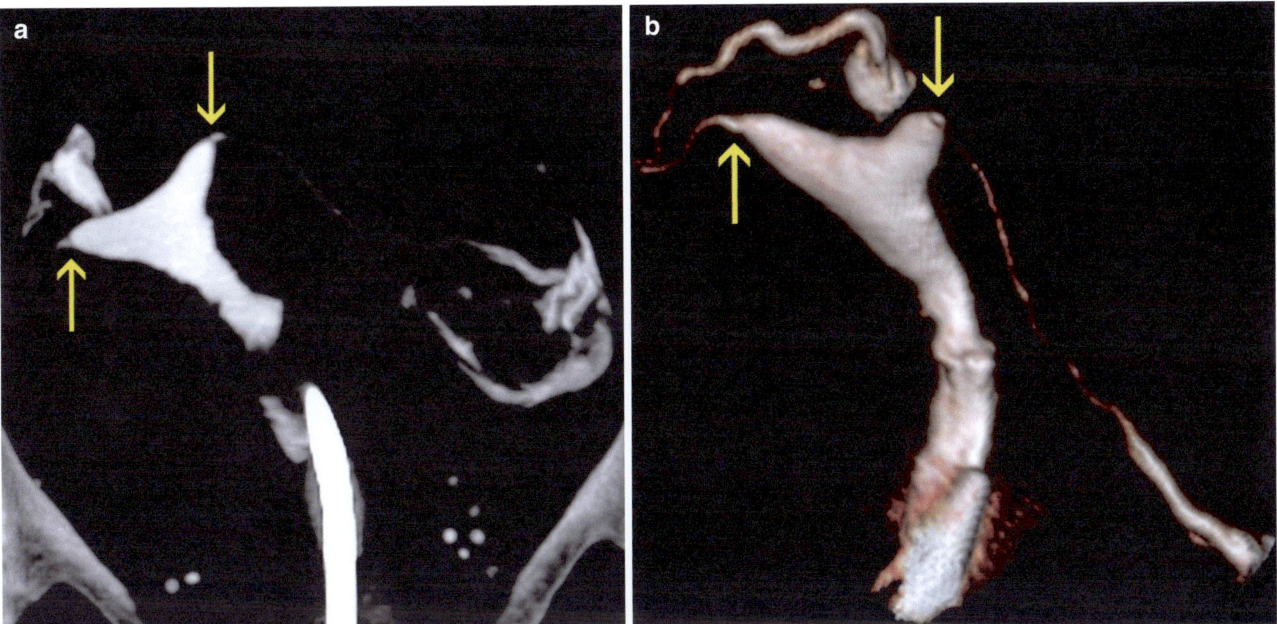

Fig. 12.11 Cornual lucencies. Small lineal filling defects in both cornual regions are visualized (*arrows*), without clinical value. (**a**) Coronal maximum intensity projection image. (**b**) Oblique coronal 3D volume rendering image

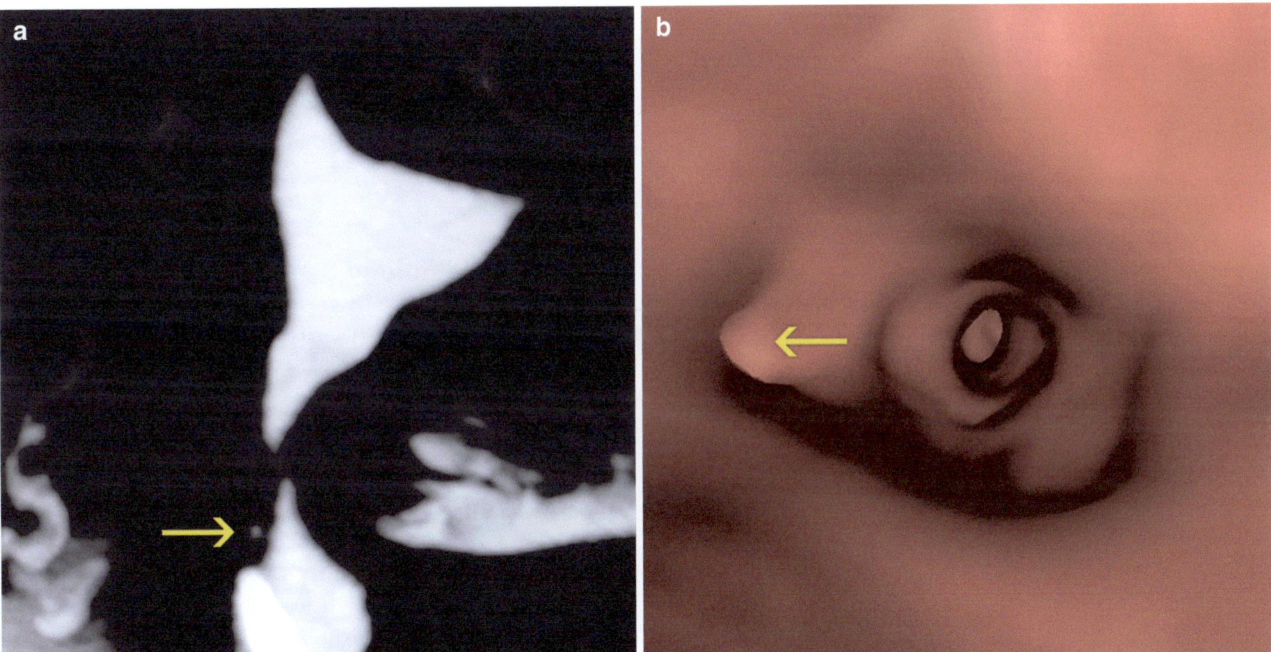

Fig. 12.12 Cervical glandular dilatation. (**a**) Coronal maximum intensity projection image showing a rounded pseudo-diverticular opacity adjacent to the right side of the cervical canal (*arrow*), corresponding to a cervical glandular dilatation. (**b**) Virtual endoscopy image where the orifice which communicates with the glandular dilatation is visualized (*arrow*)

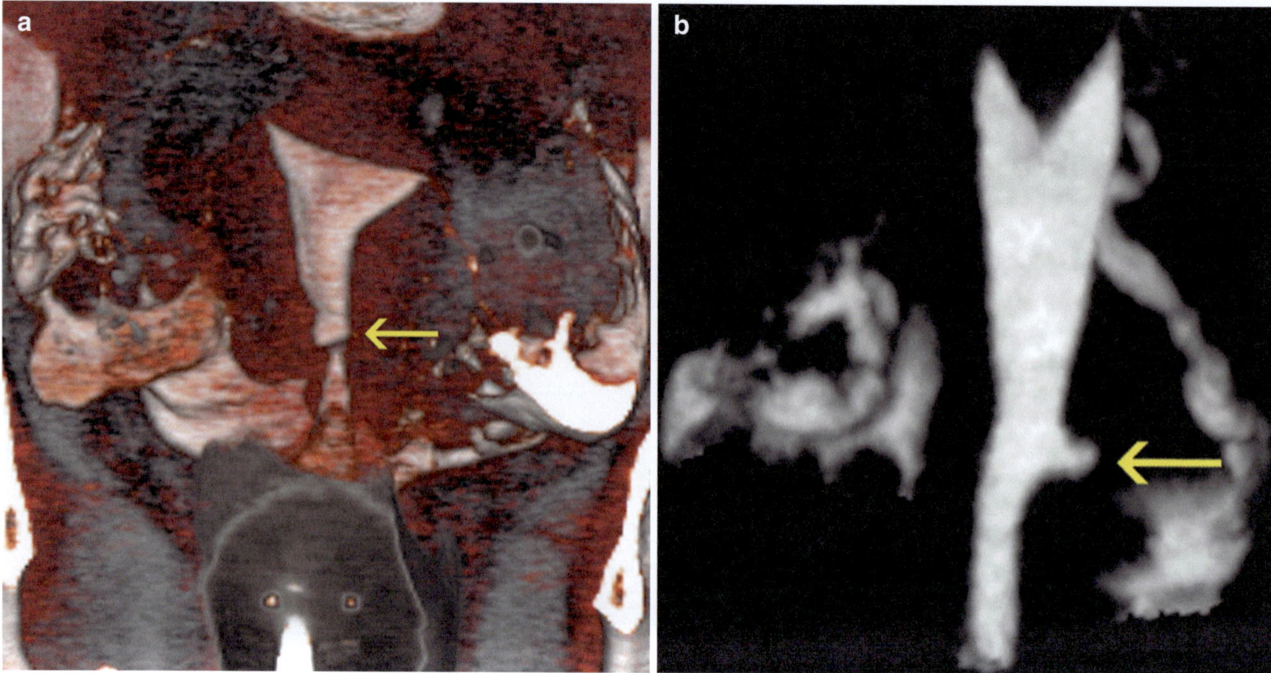

Fig. 12.13 Cesarean scar. (**a**) Coronal 3D volume rendering image showing a pseudo-diverticular dilatation at the level of the isthmic region (*arrow*) in a patient with a history of cesarean sections, compatible with the scar. (**b**) Oblique coronal maximum intensity projection image where another dilatation in the isthmus region is visualized corresponding to a cesarean scar (*arrow*)

False Negatives

Suboptimal Studies

When the preparation and procedure of the VHSG follow a protocol, an adequate visualization of the cervical canal, the endometrial cavity and tubes, along with the outlines of the uterine wall is achieved in most cases. In these optimal conditions, the occurrences of false diagnoses are infrequent. If, for some reason the exam cannot be carried out in the appropriate way, the probability of false negatives is increased. The causes of failure in the studies are due mainly to a wide cervical canal, which favors the reflux of contrast material. This occurs with higher frequency in multiparous patients and those with a history of cervical surgery. This problem can be countered with the use of plug devices which are placed on the end of the cannula, or resort directly to a balloon catheter that is introduced into the canal (Fig. 12.14) [13]. On the contrary, there exist occasions in which the external cervical orifice is too small for normal 12–16 F cannulas. In these cases, 16–22 G abbocath catheters which adapt to the end of the cannula and allow a normal instillation of contrast medium can be utilized. In any case, if the contrast volume which enters the cavity is insufficient, the lesions may remain hidden and the fallopian tubes will not fill. If this situation is irremediable, it is recommended to communicate to the patient and his/her doctor that the study was technically suboptimal.

Intramural Pathology

Unlike the HSG studies, the VHSG permits the visualization of the uterine wall. Nevertheless, the most frequent parietal pathologies, such as leiomyomas, usually have a similar density to the myometrium. It is for this reason that they can only be distinguished when generating an alteration on the surroundings. Hence, the submucosal and subserosal myomas can be easily observed because they protrude within the endometrial cavity or towards the peritoneum, respectively; instead the small intramural myomas, which do not generate deformities in the parietal surroundings, are imperceptible in the VHSG studies (Fig. 12.15) [14]. Accordingly, the adenomyosis nuclei that communicate with the superficial myometrial glands present themselves with the typical findings of multiple and small seudo-diverticula associated to a thickening in the width of the wall in the affected area. However, when the adenomyosis is deep, the VHSG cannot detect the abnormality (Fig. 12.16).

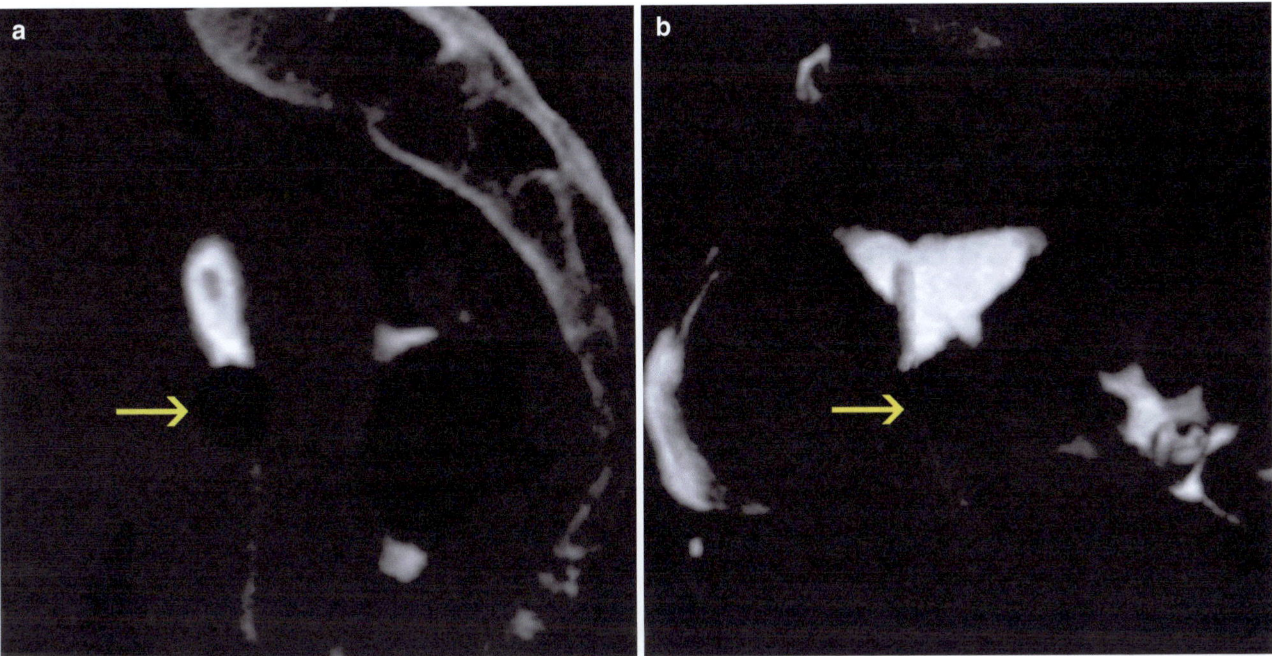

Fig. 12.14 Balloon catheter technique. Multiparous patient with abundant reflux of the contrast material during the VHSG procedure using conventional technique. A balloon catheter (*arrow*) was required for the administration of the contrast material. (**a**) Sagittal multiplanar reconstruction image. (**b**) Coronal maximum intensity projection image

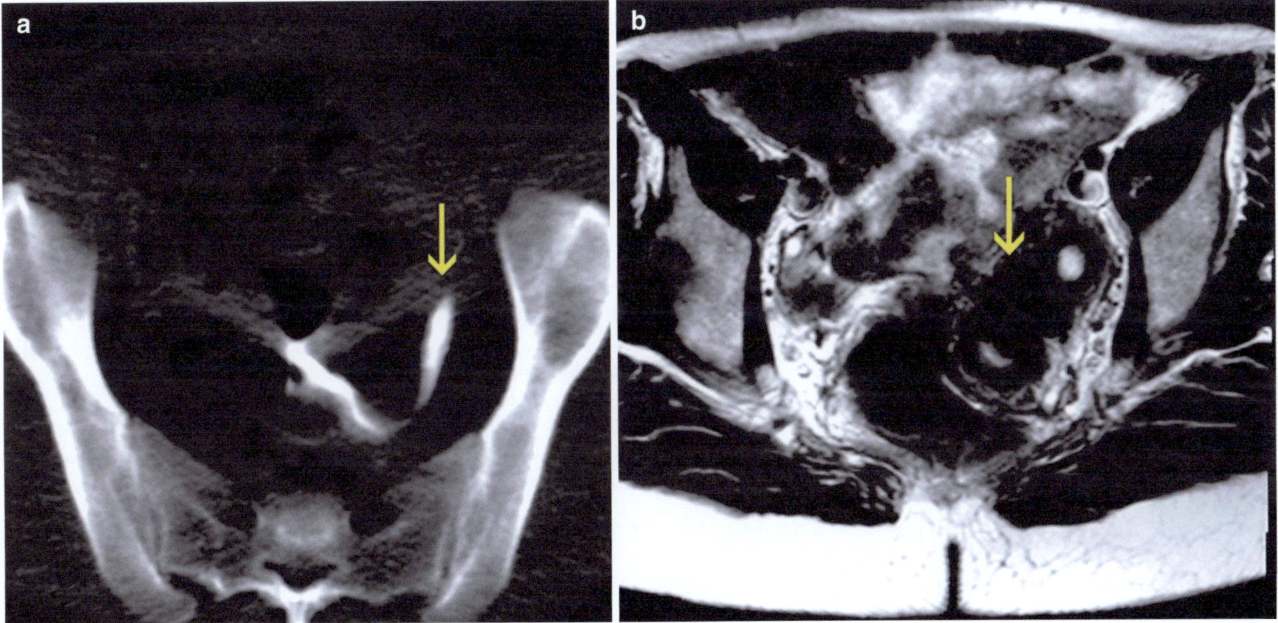

Fig. 12.15 Intramural myoma. (**a**) Axial CT image showing a left unicornuate uterus (*arrow*). (**b**) Axial T2 weighted MR image showing an intramural myoma on the right uterine wall (*arrow*), not visible in the VHSG exam

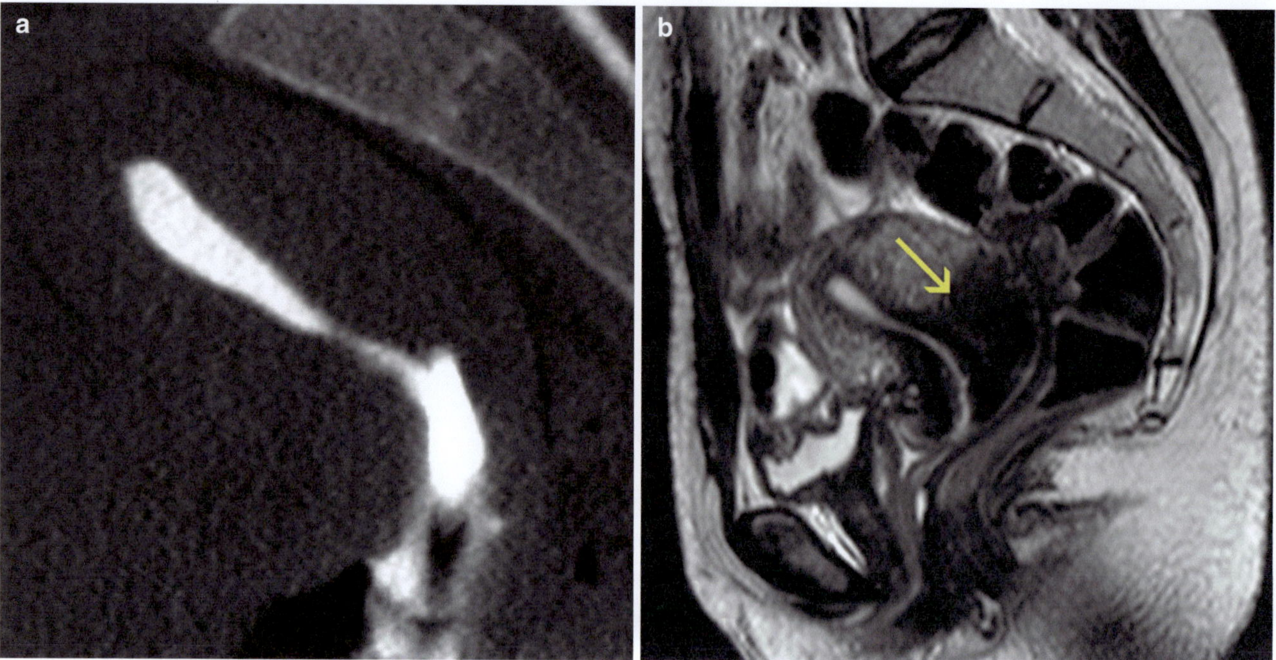

Fig. 12.16 Severe adenomyosis. (**a**) Sagittal multiplanar reconstruction image showing an anteverted uterus without evidence of pathology. (**b**) Sagittal T2 weighted MR image showing an ill-defined hypointense area in the posterior uterine wall (*arrow*), not visible in the VHSG study

Conclusion

The number of VHSG studies has increased over the last decade due to the advances in reproductive medicine. These studies fulfill a central role in the diagnosis of infertility. To ensure the success of the method and achieve good results, an emphasis on the rigorousness in the preparation and the technical procedures is required, as well as in the interpretation of the imaging findings. There exist different strategies to resolve the technical inconveniences. Thus, the occurrence of false diagnoses can be reduced to the minimum possible.

References

1. Carrascosa P, Baronio M, Capuñay C, et al. Multidetector computed tomography virtual hysterosalpingography in the investigation of the uterus and fallopian tubes. Eur J Radiol. 2008;67(3):531–5.
2. Carrascosa P, Baronio M, Capuñay C, et al. Clinical use of 64-row multislice computed tomography hysterosalpingography in the evaluation of female factor infertility. Fertil Steril. 2008;90(5):1953–8.
3. Mang T, Maier A, Plank C, et al. Pitfalls in multi-detector row CT colonography: a systematic approach. Radiographics. 2007;27:431–54.
4. Norman GR, Eva KW. Diagnostic error and clinical reasoning. Med Educ. 2010;44(1):94–100.
5. Mamede S, Schmidt HG, Rikers R. Diagnostic errors and reflective practice in medicine. J Eval Clin Pract. 2007;13(1):138–45.
6. Croskerry P. The importance of cognitive errors in diagnosis and strategies to minimize them. Acad Med. 2003;78(8):775–80.
7. Graber M, Gordon R, Franklin N. Reducing diagnostic errors in medicine: what's the goal? Acad Med. 2002;77(10):981–92.
8. Carrascosa PM, Capuñay C, Vallejos J, et al. Virtual hysterosalpingography: a new multidetector CT technique for evaluating the female reproductive system. Radiographics. 2010;30(3):643–61.
9. Ubeda B, Paraira M, Alert E, et al. Hysterosalpingography: spectrum of normal variants and nonpathologic findings. AJR Am J Roentgenol. 2001;177(1):131–5.
10. Practice Committee of American Society for Reproductive Medicine. Diagnostic evaluation of the infertile female: a committee opinion. Fertil Steril. 2012;98:302–7.
11. Steinkeler JA, Woodfield CA, Lazarus E, et al. Female infertility: a systematic approach to radiologic imaging and diagnosis. Radiographics. 2009;29(5):1353–70.
12. Ott DJ, Fayez JA. Tubal and adnexal abnormalities. In: Ott DJ, Fayez JA, Zagoria RJ, editors. Hysterosalpingography: a text and atlas. 2nd ed. Baltimore: Williams & Wilkins; 1998. p. 90–3.
13. Tur-Kaspa I. Hysterosalpingography with a balloon catheter versus a metal cannula: a prospective, randomized, blinded comparative study. Hum Reprod. 1998;13:75–7.
14. Carrascosa P, Capuñay C, Vallejos J, et al. Virtual hysterosalpingography: experience with over 1000 consecutive patients. Abdom Imaging. 2011;36(1):1–14.

In the daily practice of the imaging department, the virtual hysterosalpingography (VHSG) examination is performed with iodinated contrast; however, in patients with an allergic history, and in particular with radiographic dyes containing iodine, its usage is contraindicated [1–5].

There exist different iodinated contrast mediums which have been utilized throughout the years for the X-ray hysterosalpingographies. These contrast agents are classified in two categories, depending on if they are lipid-soluble or water-soluble. Within the lipid-soluble iodinated contrast agents, the iodized oil (Lipiodol; Guerbet, Roissy, France) is a mixture of ethyl esters of iodized fatty acids of poppy seed oil. Due to its possible effect on the production of pulmonary fat embolism, persistence of the contrast in the peritoneal cavity as a result of the lack of absorption and the necessity of doing a pelvic X-ray 24 h after its administration, the general utilization of this contrast medium was desisted in all X-ray hysterosalpingographies.

Within the group of water-soluble contrasts there are two according to their physical and chemical characteristics; ionic and non-ionic. The ionic iodinated contrast materials are hyperosmolal with respect to the plasma, up to five times superior. These contrasts were the ones initially utilized to perform the VHSG studies.

The non-ionic iodinated contrast agents, with the advantage of having less osmolality, present a diminished rate of moderate and severe adverse reactions, although no scientific evidence that they reduce deadly reactions exists. These are the contrasts currently utilized to perform routine VHSG.

The exact mechanism responsible for the secondary adverse reactions of the use of iodinated contrast media is unknown. The most clearly identified factor up to date is the osmolality. It is ideal that this be the lowest possible or similar with regards to the plasma.

At the time of deciding which contrast to utilize, the objective is to try to fully reduce the possibility of the patient presenting an adverse reaction. These can have different causes and severities. When deciding and choosing the contrast media it is of utmost importance to take into account and control, the risk of allergic reactions

Regarding the cause, the adverse reactions can be classified into two basic types:

Toxic reactions: Are produced by the action of the chemical structure of the compound on the blood vessel cells, circulating proteins and enzymatic systems, leading to hemodynamic changes in said organs and structures. Albeit they can occur in everyone, they result more frequent when associated diseases which predispose to renal or cardiac damage exist. Such reactions are related with the quantity of injected contrast and tend to be reversible, except for severe damage on the pre-existing disease. Dehydration is added as a clinical condition that predisposes renal damage. Therefore it is always recommended that the patients be well hydrated, as a simple measure to avoid renal or clinical damage.

Pseudoallergic (anaphylactoid) reactions: They are reactions which occur in some persons by direct action of the contrast materials on the cells of the organism that stores chemical mediators that, when released, can lead to allergic reactions like urticaria, edema, asthma, rhinitis and shock. In the true or anaphylactic allergic reactions, the antibody responsible of the liberation of the substances is the immunoglobulin E (IgE). Currently, a reaction to the contrast material in VHSG studies is unusual due to the fact that non-ionic iodinated contrast of low osmolality is utilized. Nevertheless there is the possibility of a systemic reaction such as venous or lymph intravasation, event which can be found in VHSG studies. The VHSG studies are performed with iodinated contrast diluted to the 70 % which means that most of the volume instilled endocavitary constitutes physiological solution and only scarce milliliters of hipoosmolal contrast (approximately 4 mL).

The contrast intravasation in VHSG produces a reticular pattern with multiple hyperdense lineal images which represents the opacification of the uterine wall vessels. The increases in the intrauterine pressure and uterine surgeries

P. Carrascosa et al., *CT Virtual Hysterosalpingography*,
DOI 10.1007/978-3-319-07560-0_13, © Springer International Publishing Switzerland 2014

are predisposing factors, but can occur in patients with no history of uterine abnormalities.

As far as severity, the adverse reactions can be divided in mild, moderate and serious:

Mild adverse reactions: Are the most frequent, occupying 99 % of all adverse reactions. They include symptoms such as nausea, generalized warmth, and facial blushing. They need no treatment and cease after a few minutes.

Moderate adverse reactions: Constitute 1 % of all adverse reactions. They exhibit themselves as diffuse hives, edema, mild bronchospasm and vomits. They require almost immediate treatment.

Serious adverse reactions: They are generalized hives, larynx edema, hypotension, bronchospasm or shock. They can appear in approximately 0.1 % of the total of reactions and require hospitalization. Eventually they can lead to death from cardiac failure, or irreversible neurologic damage from hypotension and hypoxia. These types of reactions are rare in patients undergoing this type of study. They are connected with more frequency to applications of intravenous contrast, than to endocavitary usage.

Hence in the case of patients with a history of iodine allergy, iodinated contrast media can be replaced with gadolinium.

The Research Team at Diagnóstico Maipú carried out a scientific investigation with the aim of testing gadolinium for the realization of these diagnostic studies.

Gadolinium, which is a paramagnetic substance utilized in magnetic resonance, has been used as a contrast medium in X-ray hysterosalpingographies to avoid possible complications caused by the iodinated contrast.

It must be taken into account that gadolinium is a safer contrast medium than iodine. An anaphylactic rate of 0.0003 % has been described in literature and a rate of adverse effects of 0.01 %, in intravenous injections. Hence the possible effect of endocavitary application is even lower.

Generally, the adverse reactions are mild, including nauseas, vomits, headaches and dizziness. The pruritus, maculopapular rash and other skin eruption of varying types are the most frequent and are rarely there is bronchospasm. Anaphylactic reactions are very infrequent (0.001–0.01 %).

Our research group evaluated the utility of gadolinium as a contrast agent to perform VHSG exams, and studied the intraluminal enhancement, the image quality and the discomfort of the patients compared to VHSG carried out with iodinated contrast, with the aim of determining if the gadolinium could be utilized as an alternative contrast in allergic patients. Fifty patients with a diagnosis of infertility were studied via VHSG performed in a 64-slice CT scanner (Brilliance 64; Philips Medical Systems, Cleveland, OH, USA). In 25 patients, the VHSG was performed with iodinated contrast and in the other 25 with gadolinium. The technical parameters used were the same for both acquisitions: 0.9 mm slice thickness; 0.45 mm reconstruction interval, pitch 0.64; gantry rotation time of 0.5 s; 120 kV and 100–150 mAs, with an average duration for each scan of 4 s.

The studies performed with iodinated contrast were done with a 15 % dilution in saline solution, and 40 % in the ones carried out with gadolinium. Twenty milliliters of dilution were used in each study. The endoluminal enhancement was evaluated in both studies hence a region of interest (ROI) was placed in the cervical canal and in the uterine cavity (Fig. 13.1). A quantitative analysis of the image quality was performed by an experimented radiologist with a scale of 0–10.

Complementarily, each patient participated in a query informing the discomfort produced in the study. It was classified in five levels:

- Level 0: no discomfort
- Level 1: slight discomfort
- Level 2: moderate discomfort
- Level 3: severe discomfort
- Level 4: intolerable

Description of the VHSG Procedure

The previous preparation of the patient was similar to the X-ray hysterosalpingography study. Nevertheless, due to the non invasiveness of the procedure, the prophylactic use of antibiotics was not required. The contraindications for the realization of the study were pregnancy and active pelvic infection. All the VHSG were performed between the 7th and 10th day of the menstrual cycle. All of the patients had to abstain from having sexual relations from the first day of the menstrual bleeding until 48 h after the realization of the exam.

Once the patient was in the room and located on the CT table in gynecologic position, the asepsis of the perineal region was performed prior to the placing of the speculum. When the uterine cervix was located, the asepsis was carried out. A scout view (localizer) was obtained with the purpose of planning the study before the instillation of the contrast solution (Fig. 13.2). A plastic catheter of a fine caliber was placed immediately after the external cervical orifice, through which the contrast dilution was instilled, using a power injector at a flow rate of 0.3 mL/s (Figs. 13.3 and 13.4). The acquisition of the study was performed with X-ray tube current modulation to reduce the radiation dose depending on the size of the patient on the z axis.

Once the images were acquired, they were sent to a workstation to reprocess them in bidimensional, tridimensional and endoscopic views.

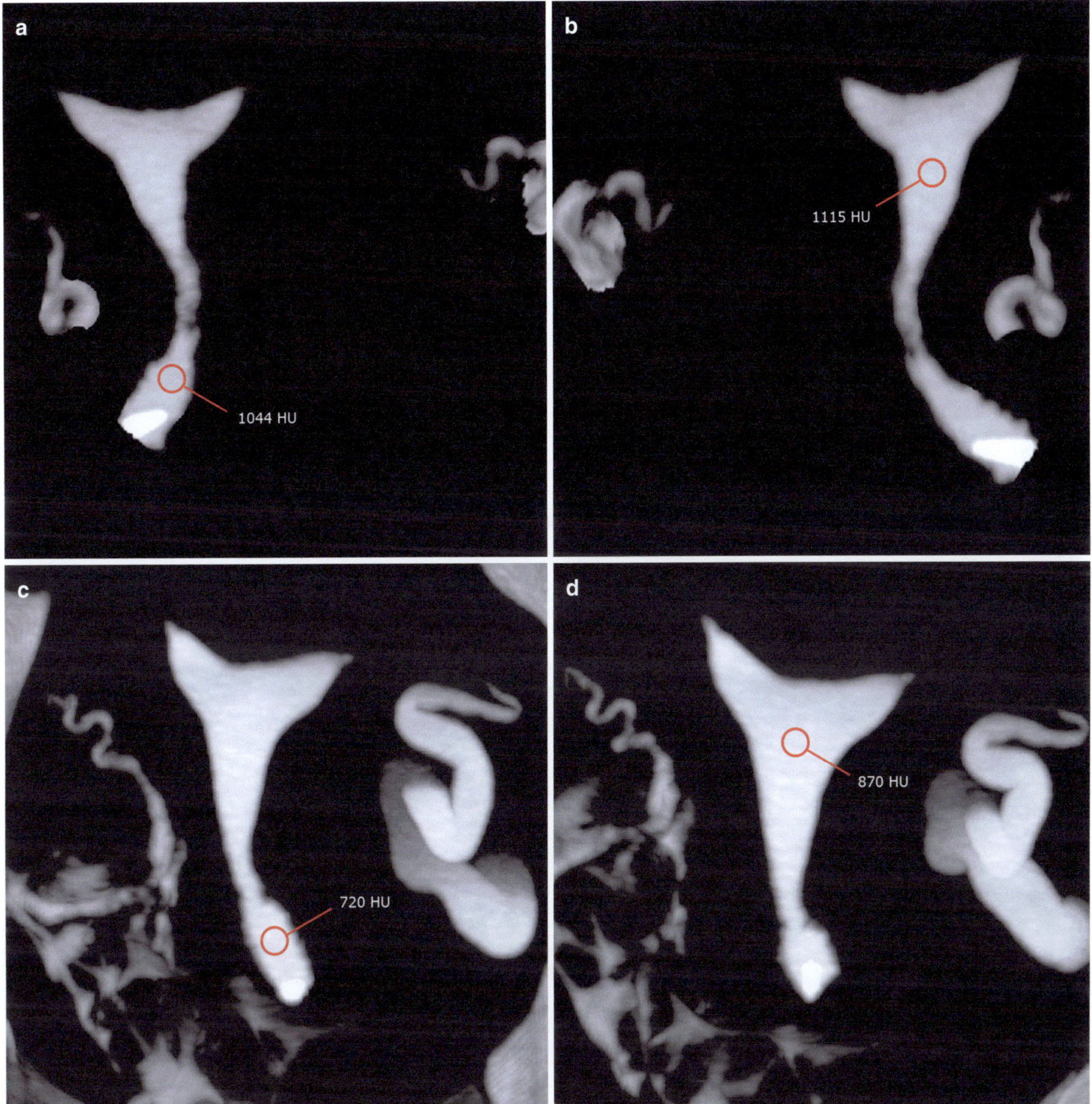

Fig. 13.1 CT density analysis in VHSG studies performed with iodine and gadolinium. (**a, b**) Measurements of the regions of interest (ROI) in the cervix and uterus in study with iodine. (**c, d**) ROI measurements in the cervix and uterus in study with gadolinium

A. Mulitplanar reformats: they were utilized in different planes: sagittal, coronal and curve. Images with soft tissue windows were analyzed with the aim of evaluating the neck, uterus, tubes and extrauterine structures.

   The curve reconstructions allowed the evaluation of the cervix, uterus and tubes in one same plane avoiding, in this way, the overlapping of anatomical structures.

B. Maximum intensity projections: this tridimensional reconstruction allowed the evaluation of the gynecologic structures with excellent anatomical detail especially of the uterine tubes.

C. Volume Rendering images: this tridimensional reconstruction allowed the evaluation of the totality of the reproductive system, displaying a wide spectrum of pathologies such as cervical stenosis, polyps, hydrosalpinx, etc.

D. Virtual Endoscopy: this post-processing algorithm complemented the gynecologic evaluation providing intraluminal images of the cervix, uterus and tubes similar to those obtained in a diagnostic hysteroscopy but non-invasively.

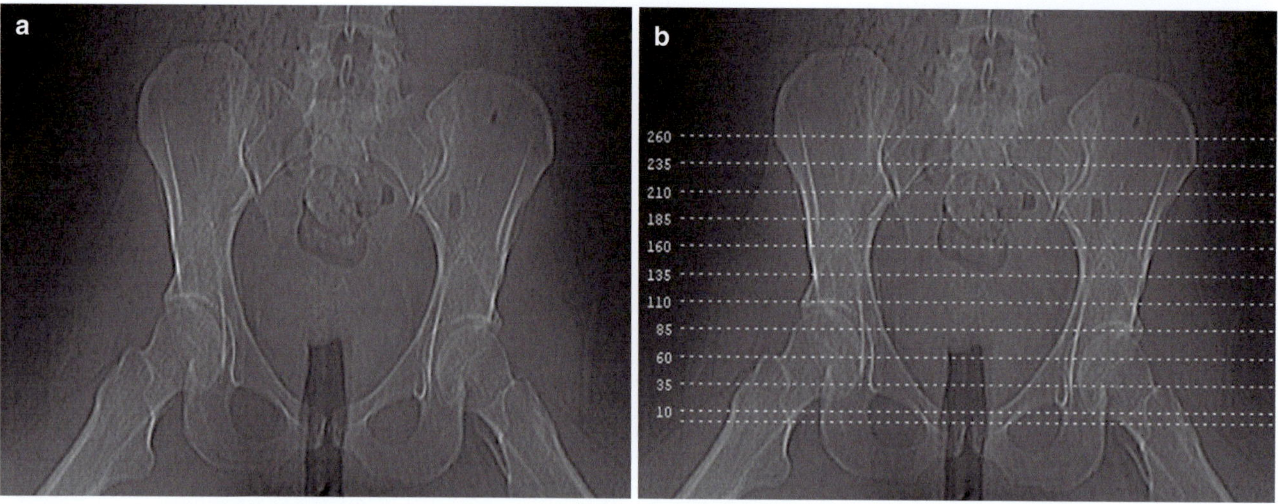

Fig. 13.2 (**a**) Scout view of the pelvis. (**b**) Scout view with the CT acquisition plan

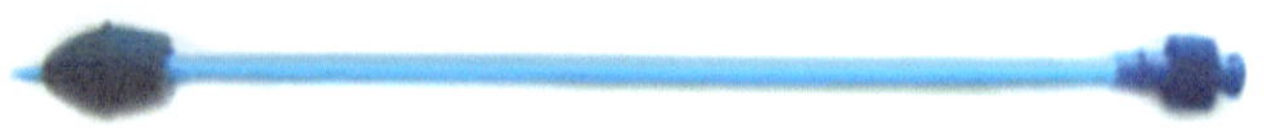

Fig. 13.3 Photo of plastic cannula utilized for the contrast media application

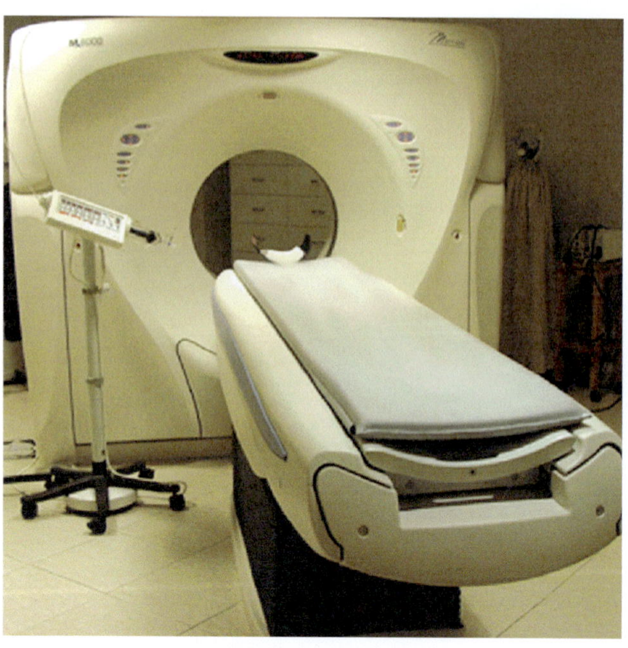

Fig. 13.4 Photo of the MSCT scanner and the injector pump. The pump permits an automatic contrast media application

The diverse reconstructions were performed on the acquisitions obtained with iodinated contrast and gadolinium alike (Figs. 13.5 and 13.6).

Regarding the results, there were no complications in the studies carried out with iodinated media or with gadolinium.

The radiation dose was 0.96 ± 0.08 mSv and 0.93 ± 0.10 mSv respectively.

The intraluminal enhancement in both studies did not find significant statistical differences in the cervical or uterine region (Table 13.1). Differences were also not identified in the image quality of both studies (Table 13.2).

Studies with similar diagnoses were compared with the aim of observing if differences existed regarding the evaluation of certain pathologies such as uterine synechiae (Figs. 13.7 and 13.8), endometrial polyps (Figs. 13.9 and 13.10), submucosal myomas (Figs. 13.11 and 13.12) and hydrosalpinx (Figs. 13.13 and 13.14).

The discomfort manifested by patients during the study using gadolinium showed a higher percentage of patients who did not suffer any type of discomfort during the procedure, 76 % versus 52 % in studies using iodinated contrasts. Nevertheless, in no case were severe or intolerable levels of discomfort observed. A more detailed explanation is displayed in Table 13.3.

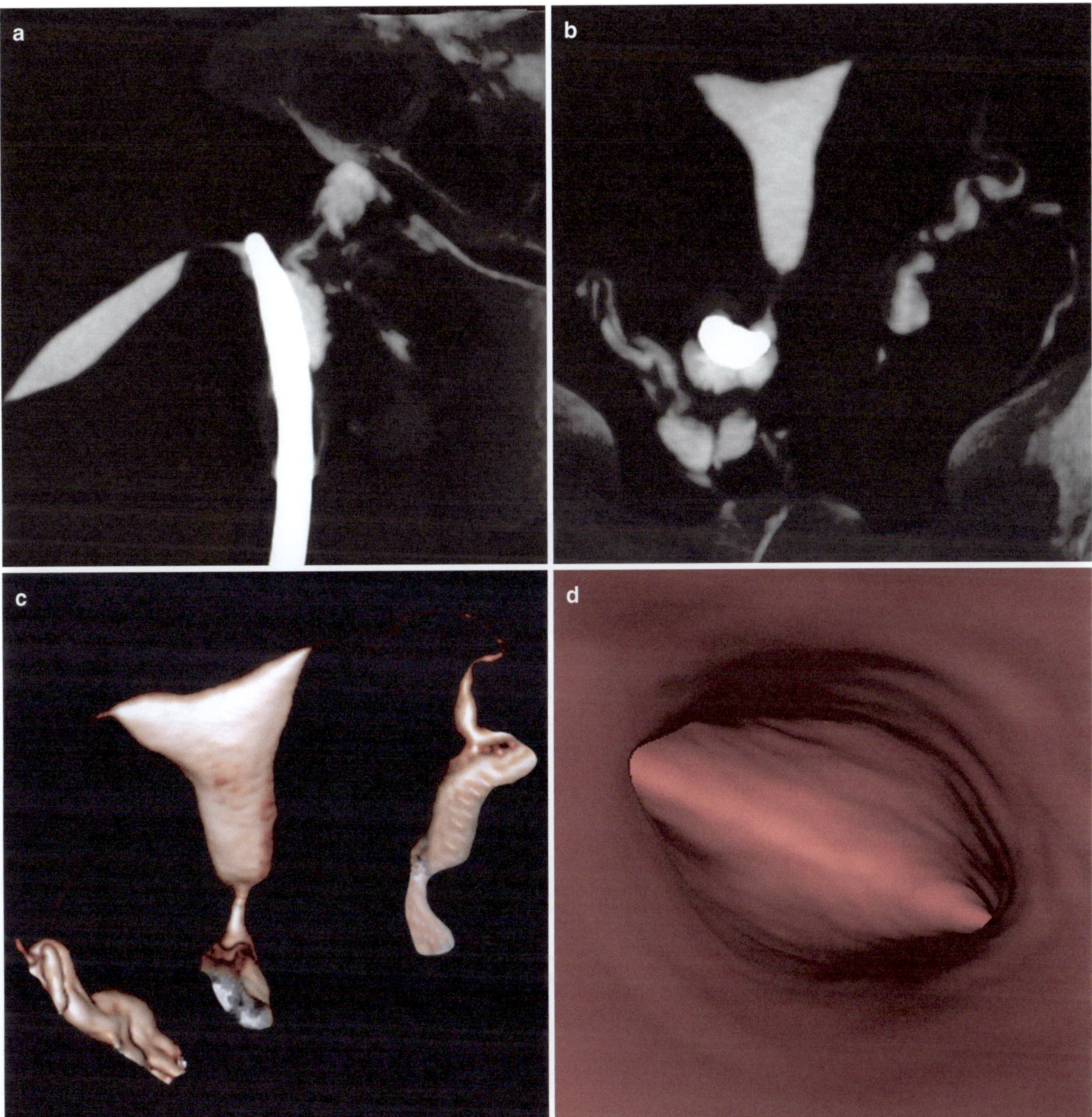

Fig. 13.5 Types of image reconstruction in iodine VHSG exams. (**a**) Sagittal multiplanar reconstruction image permits the visualization of the anteverted uterus position. (**b**) Maximum intensity projection image showing the gynecologic apparatus in its totality with clear evaluation of the Fallopian tubes. (**c**) 3D volume rendering image of the whole gynecologic apparatus. (**d**) Virtual endoscopy image of the interior of the uterine cavity

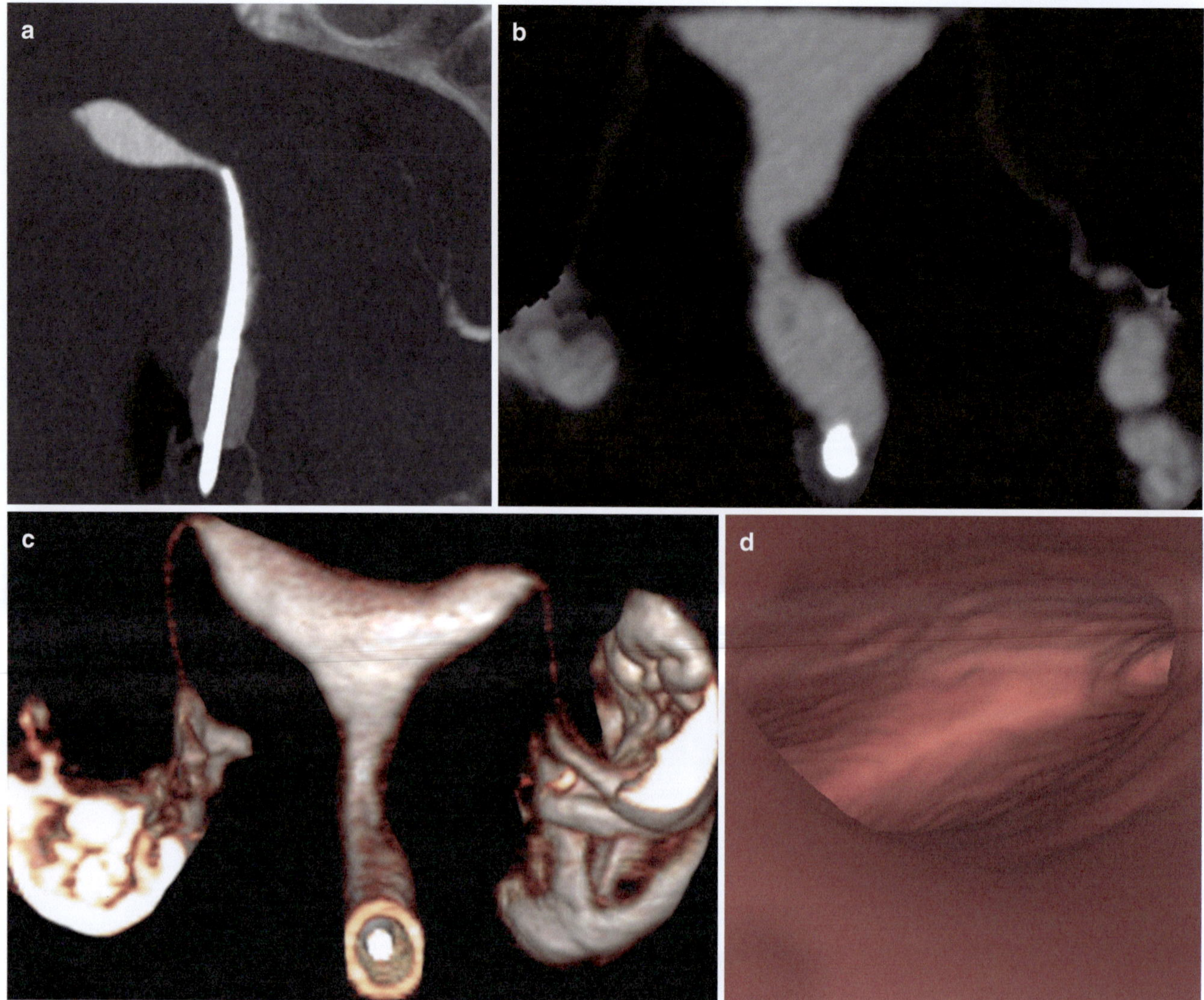

Fig. 13.6 Types of image reconstruction in gadolinium VHSG exams. (**a**) Sagittal multiplanar reconstruction image permits the visualization of the anteverted uterus position. (**b**) Maximum intensity projection image showing the gynecologic apparatus in its totality with clear evaluation of the Fallopian tubes. (**c**) 3D volume rendering image of the whole gynecologic apparatus. (**d**) Virtual endoscopy image of the interior of the uterine cavity

Table 13.1 Differences in intraluminal enhancement in iodine versus gadolinium studies

Enhancement	Iodine	Gadolinium	P
Cervix	1,090.15 HU	722	p<0.0001
Uterine cavity	1,127.20 HU	877.39	P<0.0001

Table 13.2 Image quality assessment between iodine and gadolinium (Scale 1–10)

Iodine	Gadolinium	P
9.29	8.83	P=0.07 (95 % CI 0.05–0.96)

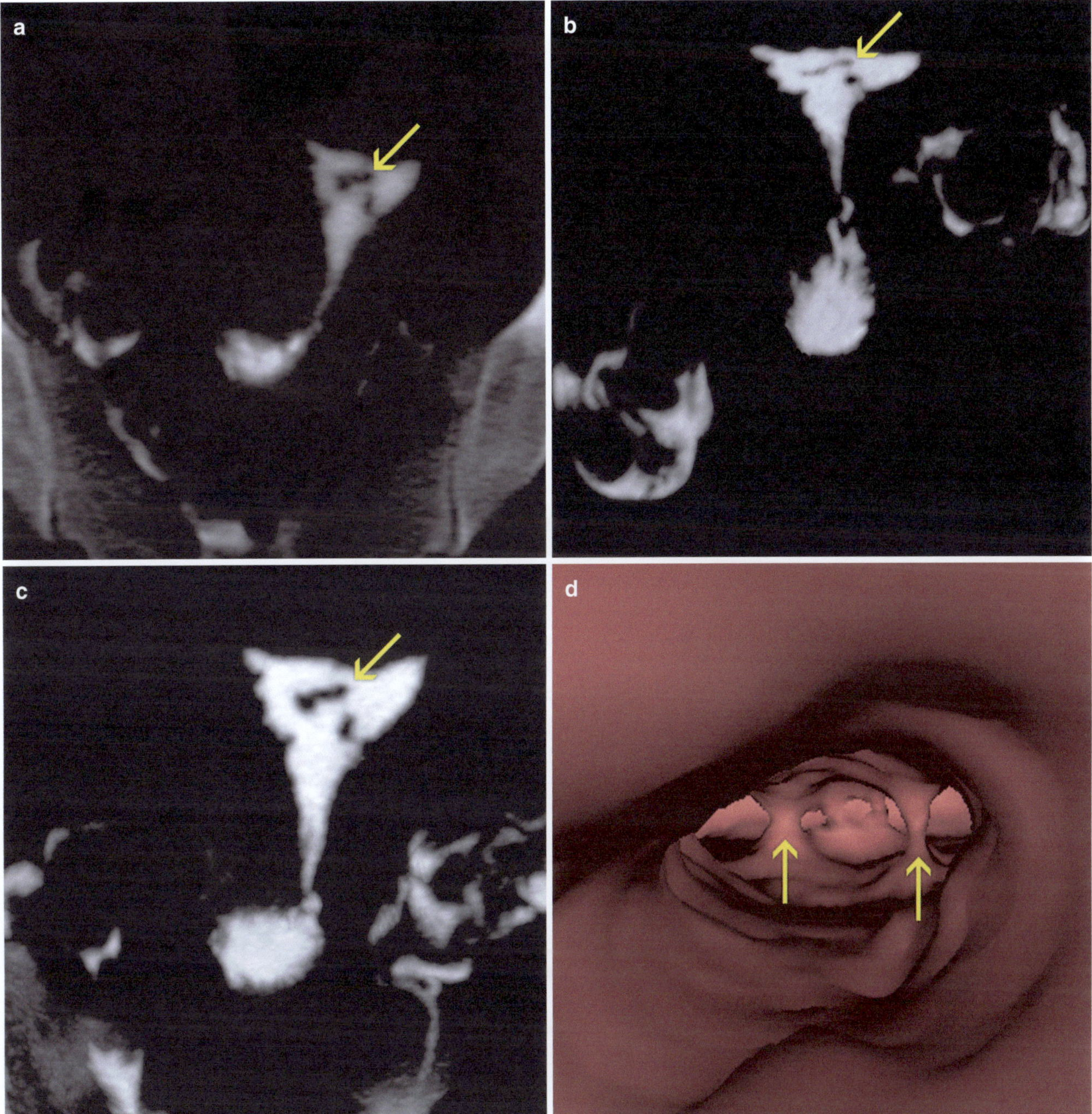

Fig. 13.7 Intrauterine synechiae in iodine VHSG exam. Central filling defects in the uterine cavity are observed (*arrows*).(**a**) Axial multiplanar reconstruction image. (**b**, **c**) Coronal maximum intensity projection images. (**d**) Virtual endoscopy image showing intraluminal lesions which reduce the lumen of the uterine cavity

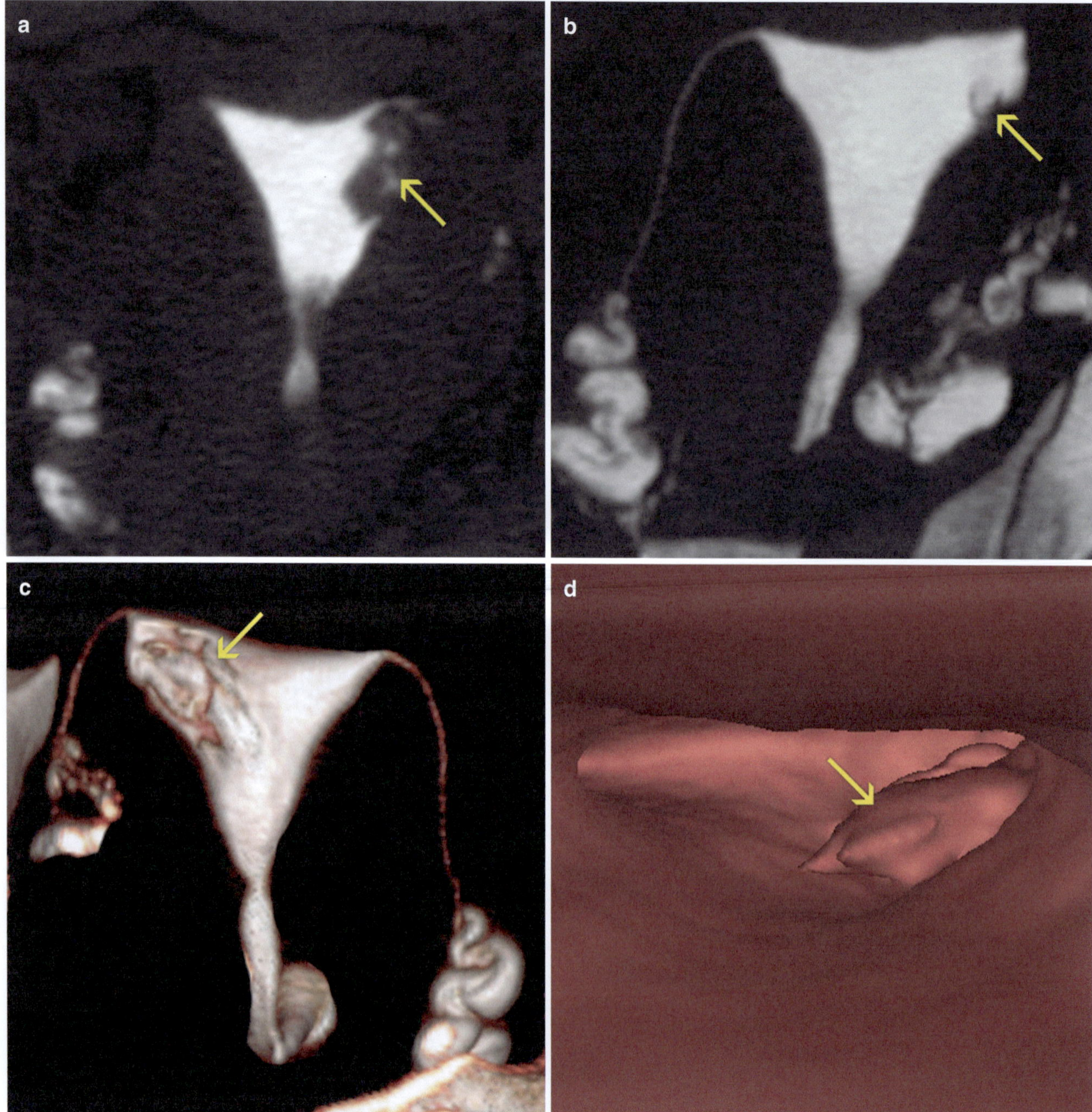

Fig. 13.8 Intrauterine synechiae in gadolinium VHSG exam. Filling defects adjacent to the left lateral wall of the uterine cavity are observed (*arrows*). (**a**) Coronal multiplanar reconstruction image. (**b**) Coronal maximum intensity projection image. (**c**) Coronal 3D volume rendering image, posterior view. (**d**) Virtual endoscopy image showing intraluminal lesions which reduce the lumen of the uterine cavity

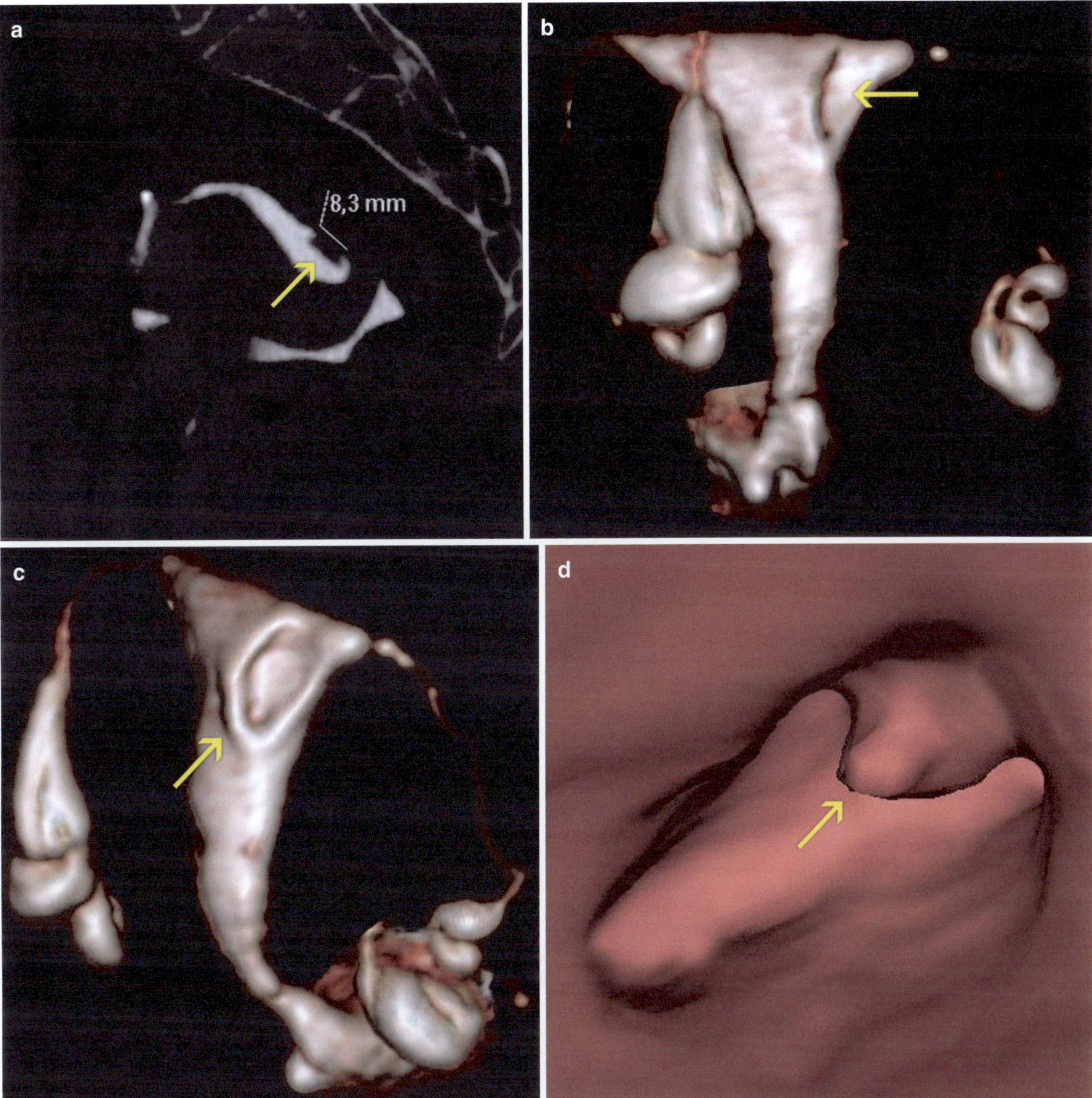

Fig. 13.9 Endometrial polyp (*arrows*) in iodine VHSG exam. (**a**) Sagittal multiplanar reconstruction image with soft tissue window showing an elevated lesion at the level of the uterine fundus. (**b, c**) 3D volume rendering images showing the filling defect in the uterine cavity. (**d**) Virtual endoscopy image showing an elevated lesion in the uterine cavity, compatible with a polyp

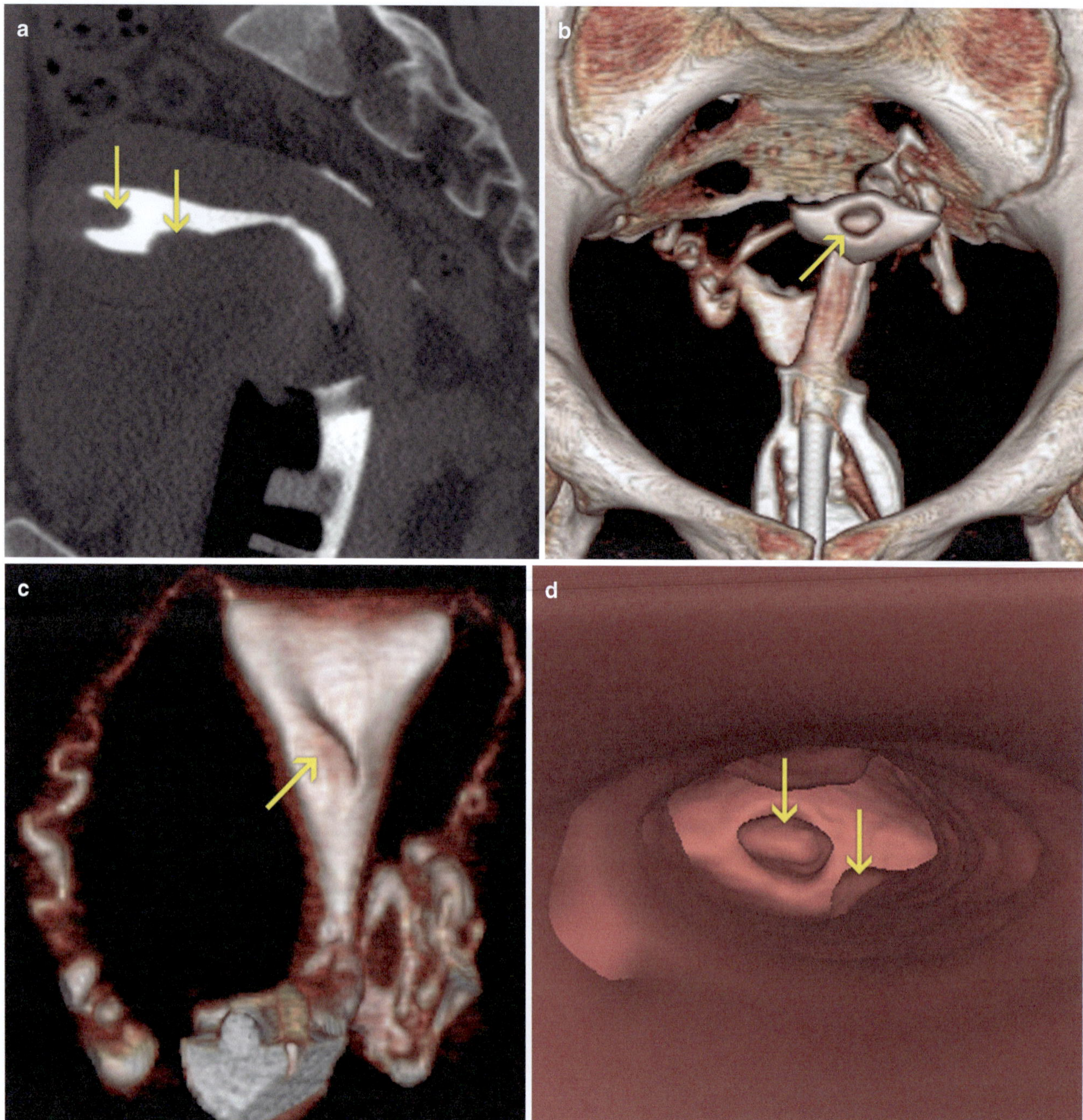

Fig. 13.10 Endometrial polyps (*arrows*) in gadolinium VHSG exam. (**a**) Sagittal multiplanar reconstruction image with soft tissue window. Two elevated lesions are visualized, one at the level of the anterior wall and the other in the uterine fundus. (**b**, **c**) Axial and coronal 3D volume rendering images. (**d**) Virtual endoscopy image

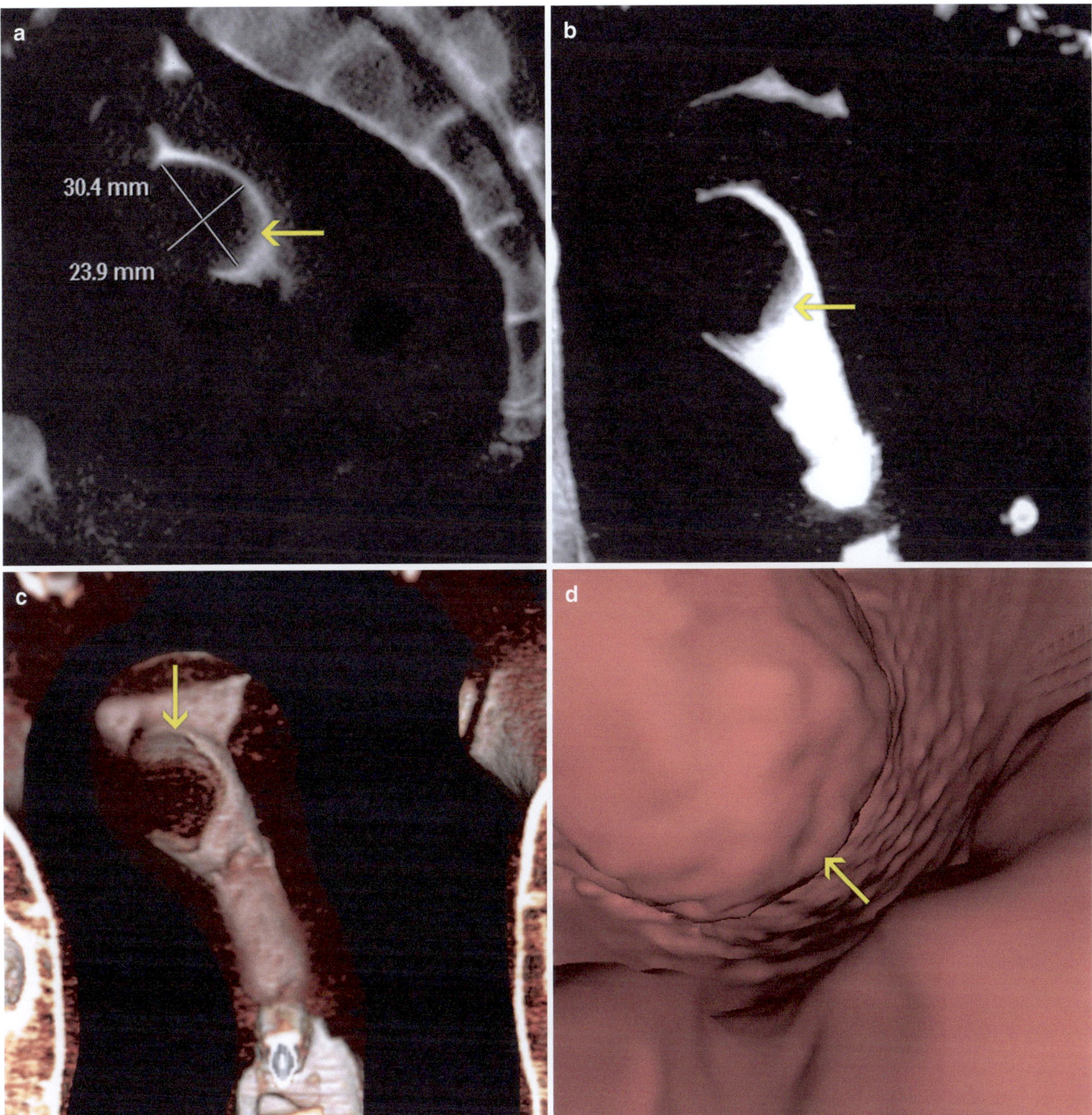

Fig. 13.11 Submucosal myoma (*arrows*) in iodine VHSG exam. (**a**) Sagittal multiplanar reconstruction image with soft tissue window showing an intramural myoma with submucosal projection in the anterior wall of the uterus. (**b**) Sagittal maximum intensity projection image. (**c**) Coronal 3D volume rendering image. (**d**) Virtual endoscopy image

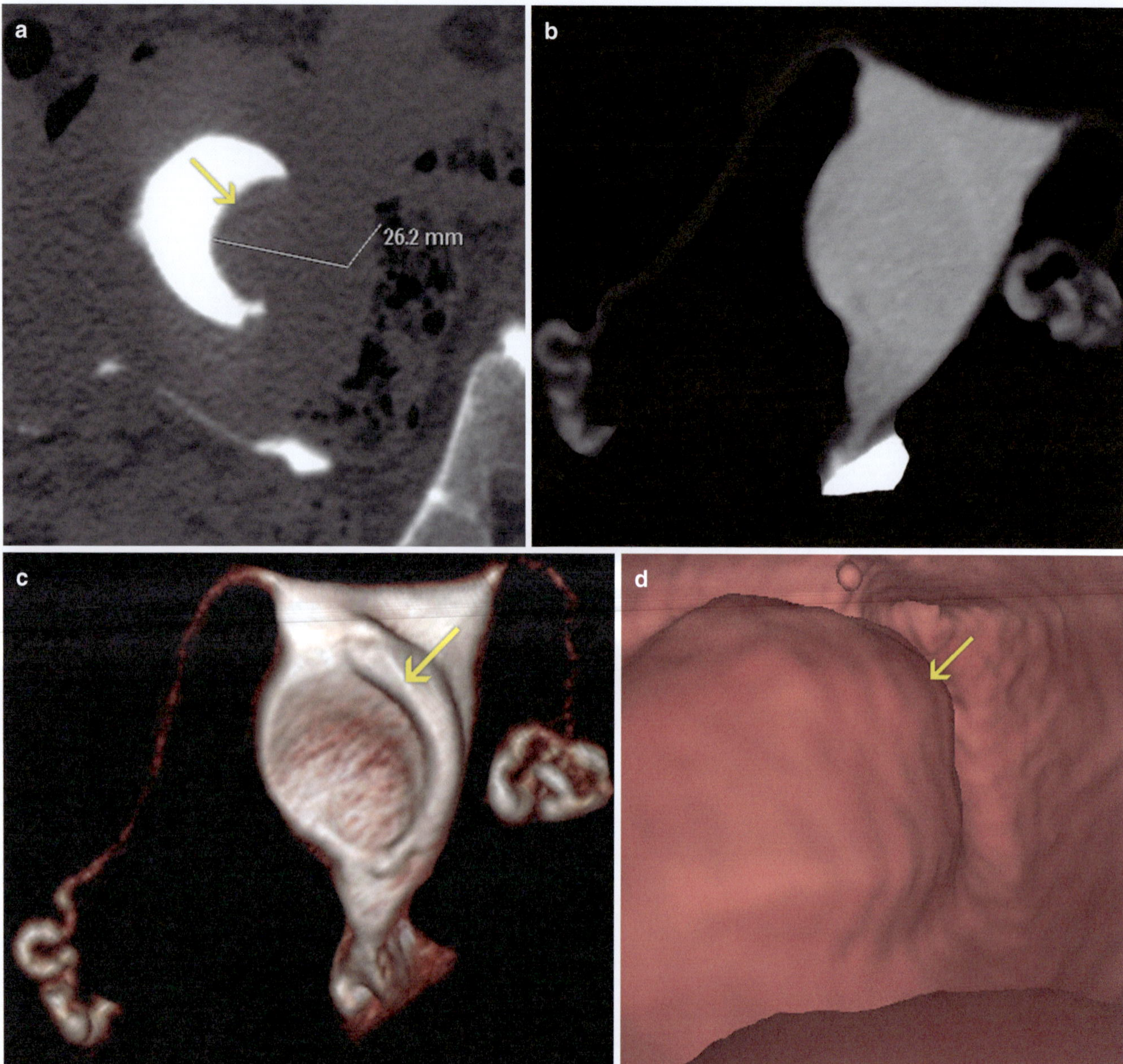

Fig. 13.12 Submucosal myoma (*arrows*) in gadolinium VHSG exam. (**a**) Coronal multiplanar reconstruction image with soft tissue window showing an intramural myoma with submucosal projection in the left lateral uterine wall. (**b**) Coronal maximum intensity projection image showing deformation of the uterine cavity. (**c**) Coronal 3D volume rendering image. (**d**) Virtual endoscopy image

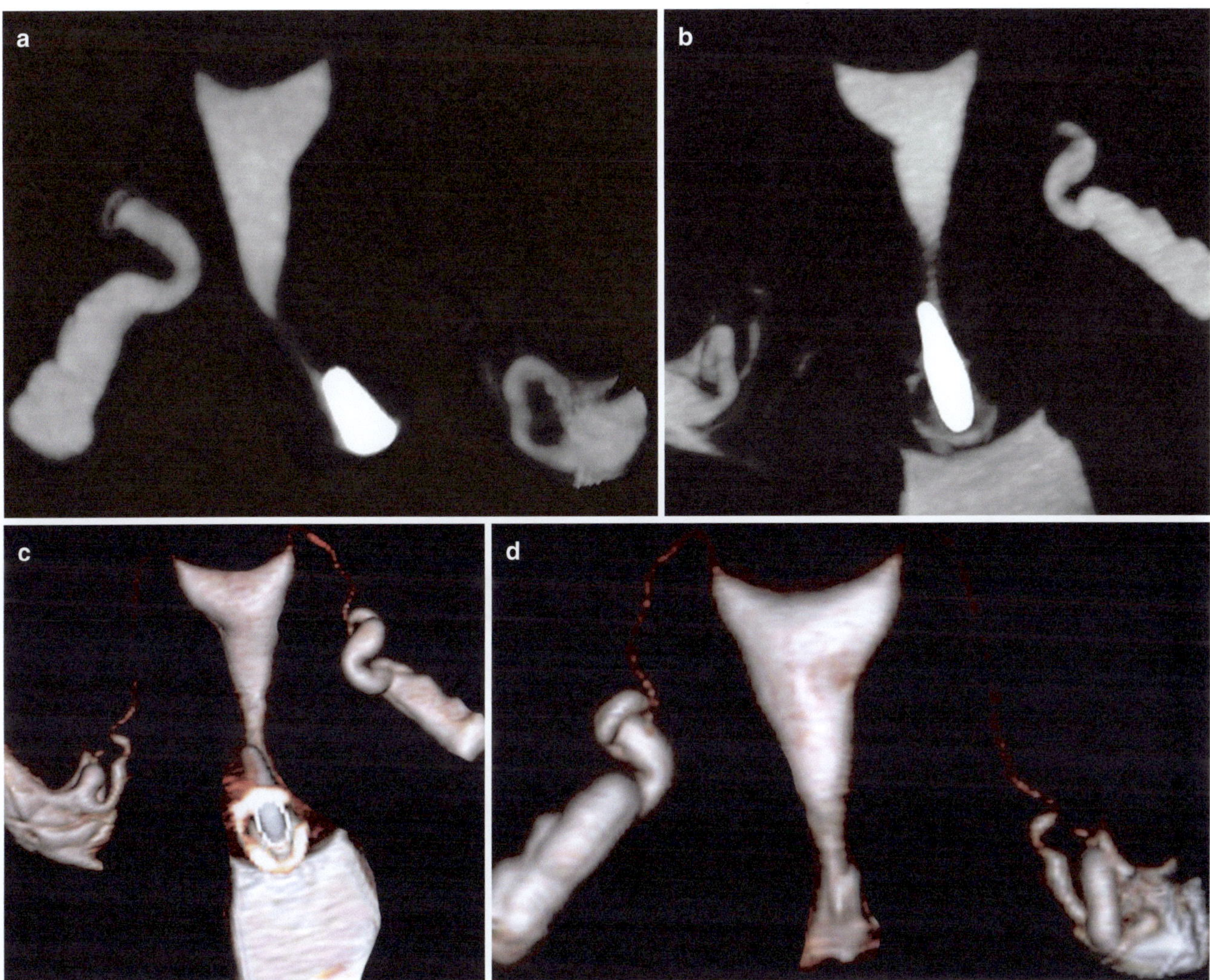

Fig. 13.13 Right hydrosalpinx in iodine VHSG exam. (**a**, **b**) Coronal maximum intensity projection images. (**c**, **d**) Coronal 3D volume rendering images

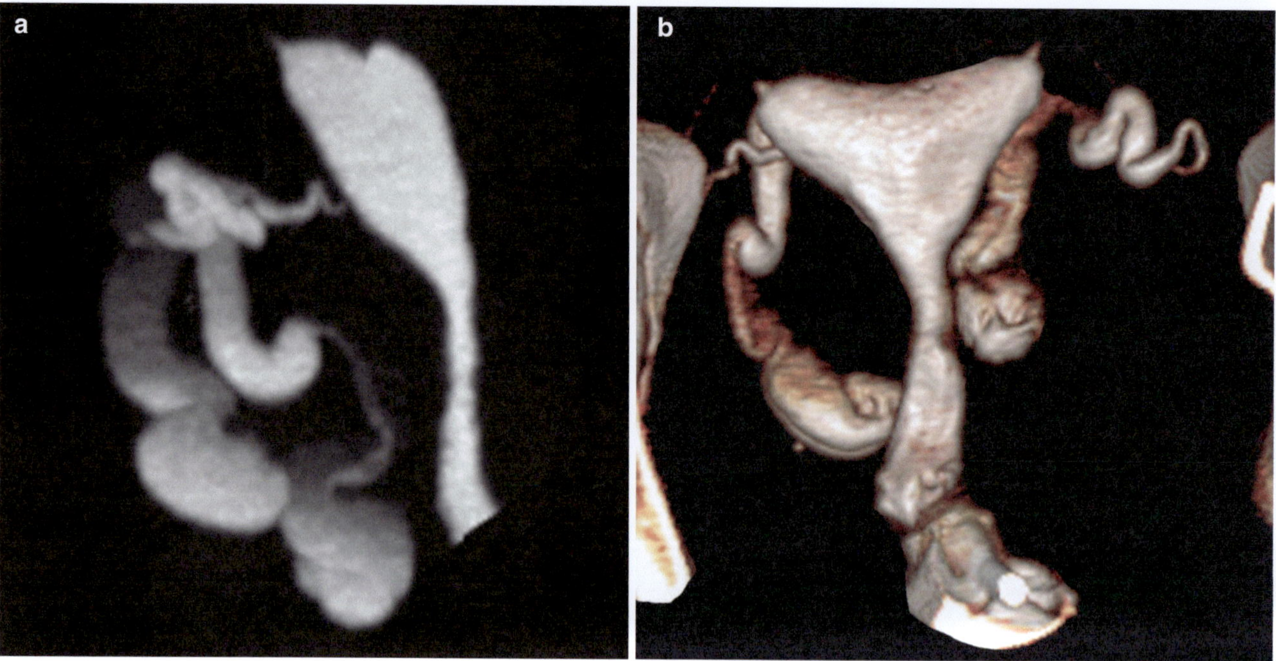

Fig. 13.14 Bilateral hydrosalpinx in gadolinium VHSG exam. (**a**) Oblique coronal maximum intensity projection image. (**b**) Coronal 3D volume rendering image

Table 13.3 Discomfort evaluation

Grade	Iodine	Gadolinium
0	13 (52 %)	19 (76 %)
1	6 (24 %)	2 (8 %)
2	6 (24 %)	4 (16 %)
3	0	0
4	0	0

Conclusion

The VHSG is a new noninvasive method useful in the evaluation of the entire woman's reproductive organs. It has shown via diverse researches excellent diagnostic results in the evaluation of the intracervical and intrauterine pathology in comparison with the gold standard method, the conventional hysteroscopy, as well as an excellent correlation in the evaluation of the tubarian pathology [3–5].

The diverse published works have been performed with an iodinated contrast dilution. It is for this reason that the demonstration of similar diagnostic quality and discomfort for the patient in studies using gadolinium would allow this alternative contrast agent to be utilized in patients allergic to iodinated ones.

A question which may present itself is why not utilizing gadolinium in 100 % of the patients and the answer lies in the costs of it, being three times higher than iodine in our country.

The VHSG performed with gadolinium has exhibited the same results as iodinated contrast with regard to diagnostic quality. In our experience the studies carried out with gadolinium have shown less intraluminal attenuation but no differences existed when it came to the image quality when compared to studies performed with iodinated contrast. In turn, the patients exhibited a very low percentage of studies with mild or moderate discomfort with a high percentage (76 %) of studies with no type of discomfort. That is why gadolinium could be considered as an alternative contrast to be utilized in VHSG studies in patients who are allergic to iodinated contrasts.

References

1. Carrascosa P, Baronio JM, Borghi M, et al. Histerosalpingoscopía virtual. Una técnica novedosa y no invasiva para diagnosticar patología intrauterina. Reproduccion. 2006;21:19–26.
2. Carrascosa P, Baronio M, Capuñay C, et al. Clinical use of 64-row multislice computed tomography hysterosalpingography in the

evaluation of female factor infertility. Fertil Steril. 2008; 90:1953–8.

3. Carrascosa P, Capuñay C, Mariano B, et al. Virtual hysteroscopy by multidetector computed tomography. Abdom Imaging. 2008; 33:381–7.

4. Carrascosa P, Baronio M, Capuñay C, et al. Multidetector computed tomography virtual hysterosalpingography in the investigation of the uterus and fallopian tubes. Eur J Radiol. 2008;67:531–5.

5. Carrascosa P, Capuñay C, Baronio M, et al. 64-Row multidetector CT virtual hysterosalpingography. Abdom Imaging. 2009;34:121–33.

The advantages of computed tomography (CT) are immense and have revolutionized the practice of medicine. Since its birth, the applications of CT have extended to different regions and areas of the body, allowing vast advances in the non invasive diagnosis of numerous diseases. Currently, most of the radiation applied for diagnostic purposes arises from the use of CT [1, 2], nuclear medicine and fluoroscopy. Furthermore, in the last decade with the oncoming of multislice CT (MSCT), there occurred a sustained increase in the utilization of this modality worldwide, with the consequent rise of the radiation dose in the population [3]. This fact has caught the attention of health authorities, the medical community in general and, specially, of radiologists, becoming a topic of high interest and importance around the globe.

The global concern over the possible consequences of the high radiation doses has led to a tendency of diminishing the radiation generated by CT studies [4, 5]. The largest existing evidence on the potential risks is based on publications which describe the relationship between the exposure to ionizing radiation of survivors of the atomic bombing of Japan and the development of cancer and cardiovascular diseases [6, 7]. Up until now the published works present no conclusive statistical evidence on the carcinogenic effect, and hence of any known risk, of doses below 100 mSv. Moreover, the carcinogenicity has been inferred via statistical calculations and extrapolations since enough time has not elapsed for the apparition of malignancies in individuals exposed to the radiation of CT [8, 9]. Despite information derived from survivors of the atomic bomb in Japan and other events which suggest that the expansion of the use of imaging techniques which utilize ionizing radiation will result in a higher occurrence of cancer in the exposed population, the problem can probably be minimized via the prevention of the inadequate use of diagnostic methods and the optimization of the studies performed to obtain the best image quality with the least radiation dose.

Due to the constant technological development and the numerous research works on CT which describe new and practical applications, the number of studies will continue rising as is often the case during the many years which are required for a new technique to reach its equilibrium. The radiologic community plays in this process an important role in the handling and control of the factors which influence the radiation dose received by the patient. Each of them must be analyzed taking into account the age, gender and state of health. The knowledge of the technical parameters and their adapted modification for each case subject to study, allows adjusting the necessary dose, avoiding excessive radiation [10]. Besides, in the last years new tools have been developed which are able to substantially reduce the radiation dose of the CT, without significantly diminishing the diagnostic quality of the study [11].

Radiation and Hysterosalpingography

The hysterosalpingography (HSG) is a radiologic procedure for the evaluation of the uterine cavity and the Fallopian tubes which has been utilized especially in the diagnostic algorithm of patients with primary or secondary infertility. The recent concern over the risks of the radiation related to diagnostic modalities, is even larger in HSG studies due to the fact that the examined anatomical region affects the gonads, and the patients which are subject to these studies compromise a young age group who which to become pregnant.

The HSG studies are performed via fluoroscopic control. During the gradual introduction of the contrast medium, various exposures and radiographic captures are effectuated to document the filling of the uterine cavity, the opacification of the tubes and the passage of the contrast to the peritoneum. The average time of exposure to the fluoroscopy which is employed during the exam is 2 min, while the number of radiographies obtained is an average of 6 in each HSG study. Both exposures, the fluoroscopic and radiographic, radiate primarily the gonads and determine the radiation dose employed [12].

P. Carrascosa et al., *CT Virtual Hysterosalpingography*,
DOI 10.1007/978-3-319-07560-0_14, © Springer International Publishing Switzerland 2014

The deleterious effects associated to the HSG refer to the radiogenic risk of the future embryo, as well as the risk of cancer induction of the exposed woman [13]. The scientific unit most utilized for the measurement of radiations is the millisievert (mSv). Each organ and tissue has a different sensibility to radiation; therefore, the radiogenic risk varies in each study according to the explored area and technique employed. The term "effective dose" refers to the radiation quantification taking into account the relative sensibilities of the different exposed tissues [14]. Little data exists on the literature which refers to the radiation dosimetry in HSG procedures. The effective dose in HSG was informed in only two publications [12, 13]. An estimation of the risks associated to HSG was reported in a recent study [15]. However, there exists a noticeable variation in the HSG technique utilized in different centers regarding the quantity of fluoroscopic exposure (0.3–8.5 min) and the number of radiographies obtained (0–14) [13]. Hence, the effective dose calculated for a HSG study which utilizes 2 min of radioscopy and six radiographic exposures is 5 mSv. Furthermore, the fact that different radioscopic control systems exist must be taken into account: conventional, remote and digital, consequently the data presented previously can be non applicable to patients subject to HSG procedures with the use of different units and technical parameters, and according to the case, a dosimetry must be carried out for each patient in particular [16, 17].

Evolution of the Radiation Dose in Virtual Hysterosalpingography

Since the development of the virtual hysterosalpingography over 10 years ago, the technology has evolved and the acquisition technical parameters modified in the search for better image quality, better results, and also, the lowest radiation dose possible. In its beginnings, the virtual hysterosalpingography studies were performed with the same technical parameters utilized in routine pelvic CT exams. For the study of an area of 15 cm of length, with a tube voltage of 120 kV and a current of 250 mA, the estimated effective dose is of 2.6 mSv [18]. In these studies, the acquisition parameters, among them the radiation dose, were adjusted to obtain an image which would allow the distinction of subtle density contrasts between the different soft tissues, and also to diminish the noise in the image. But when a specific distended organ is examined (uterus and tubes) with positive contrast material (hyper-dense), a great attenuation difference is created between the uterine cavity and the adjacent structures. In this way, the existing high contrast gave way to modifications in the scanning protocols and to significantly diminishing the radiation dose. The tube current was the corrected factor, utilizing between 100 and 150 mA, depending

on the habitus of patients. Furthermore, the scan length was reduced to 10 cm, adjusting the plane of study to the region of interest. The estimated radiation dose with these parameters varies between 0.9 and 1.3 mSv [19]. Recently, with the incorporation of new programs which perform reconstructions of raw data in order to diminish the noise and enhance the image resolution (iterative reconstruction), the tube voltage was able to be reduced with no damage to the quality of the study. Thus the current protocols employ 80 kV and 100–150 mA, with an estimated effective dose of 0.3–0.4 mSv (Fig. 14.1). In Table 14.1 the comparison of the radiation dose utilized in different radiographic and tomographic studies is shown.

Factors Which Influence the Radiation Dose in Virtual Hysterosalpingography Studies

Theoretically, there exist three principal reasons for incrementing the radiation dose in virtual hysterosalpingography studies. One of them is the use of multislice units, taking into account that these studies must be performed with scanner of 64 or more rows of detectors. Without a correct adjustment of the acquisition parameters, this implies a larger radiation dose in comparison with helical units due to a geometric defect, called penumbra effect [20]. Another of the reasons is the slice collimation necessary of 1 mm or less, in search of obtaining an increased spatial resolution, but with the inevitable cost of increasing the effective dose to try to achieve the diminishing of the noise in the image. The final factor is occasional and has to do with the procedure itself; it is the necessity of additional acquisitions in cases where the first image is incomplete or insufficient, which would lead to an increase in the radiation dose for the patient.

The use of adequate acquisition technical parameters, amid which we must highlight the collimation, pitch, voltage and x-ray tube current, has a direct effect on the radiation dose which each patient receives. Next, the managing of these variables, which determine the different strategies for diminishing the radiation as low as possible, without causing detriment on the quality of the images.

Choosing the Technical Parameters

The effective dose depends mainly on the quantity of radiation utilized during the exam, relating directly with the level of effective mAs (miliamper per second). The latter is determined by the tube current (in mA), the tube rotation time (in seconds) and the pitch. With the adequate use of these parameters an excessive exposure to radiation can be avoided. The easiest way to reduce the dose is to lessen the tube current, with a low rotation time, and a stable pitch close to 1. This is

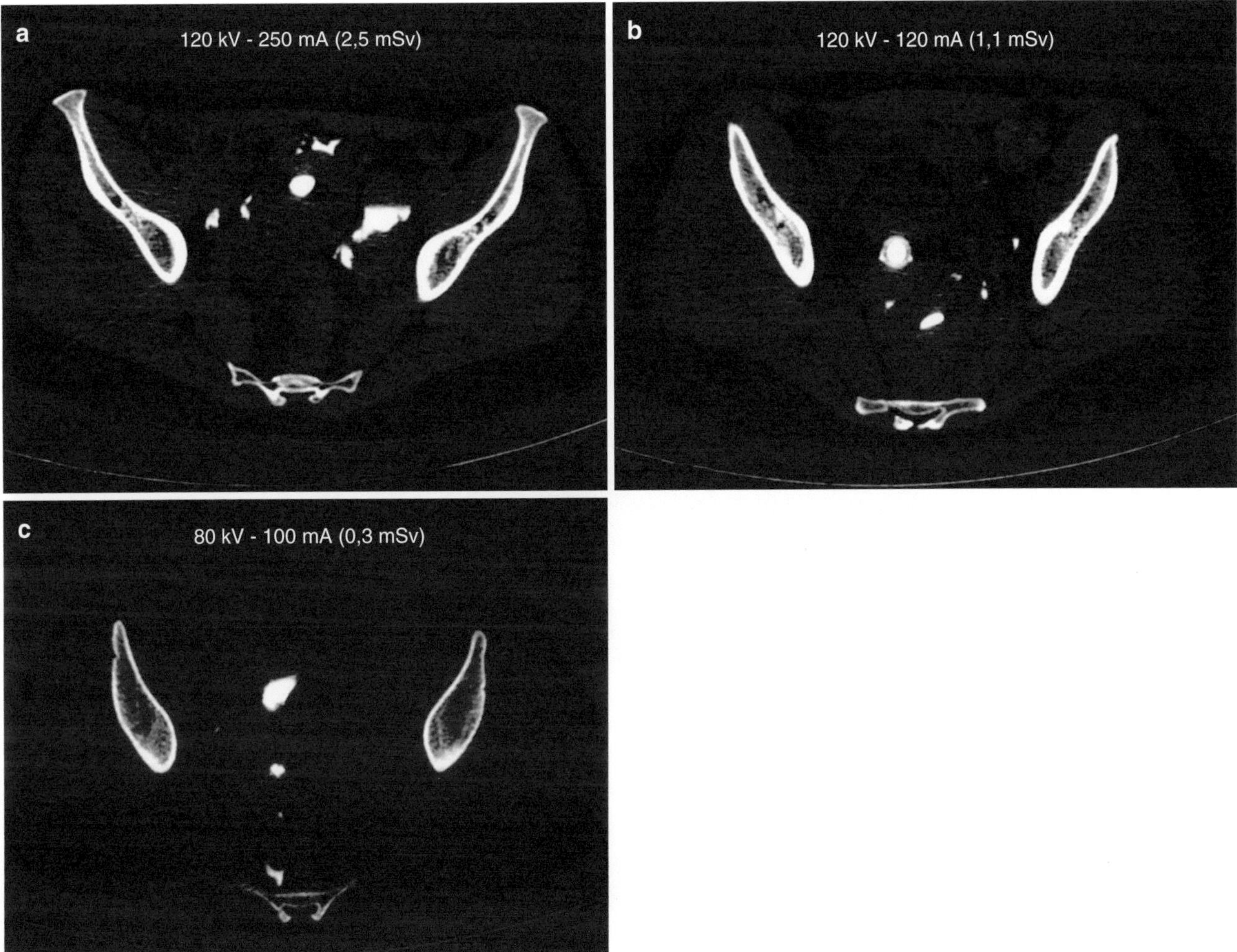

Fig. 14.1 Evolution of radiation exposure in VHSG studies. (**a**) Axial 64-slice image, with 120 kV and 250 mA (2.5 mSv), the same technical parameters used in a pelvic CT study. Adequate tissue discrimination between the soft tissues and a scarce image noise is appreciated. (**b**) Axial 64-slice image, with 120 kV and 120 mA (1.1 mSv). A high contrast between the opacified endometrial cavity and the adjacent structures is appreciated. The radiation dose was adjusted without detriment in image quality. (**c**) Axial 256-slice image, with 80 kV and 100 mA (0.3 mSv). With this technique, a significant reduction in the radiation dose is achieved, but an increase in the image noise exists; however, due to new raw data reconstruction algorithms, improvement in image quality is achieved, without altering the diagnostic outcome

Table 14.1 Radiation doses in x-ray and CT exams

Modality	Effective radiation dose (mSv)	Additional risk to fatal cancer due to exam
Chest x-ray	0.1	Minimum
Lumbar spine x-ray	1.5	Very low
Barium enema	8	Low
Intravenous Urogram	3	Very Low
Hysterosalpingography	5	Low
Mammography	0.4	Minimum
CT abdomen and pelvis	15	Low
CT colonography	10	Low
CT virtual hysterosalpingography	0.3	Minimum

determined taking into account the age, gender, habitus and the region to examine of each patient, among other factors [21, 22].

Another element which directly influences the effective dose is the tube voltage (Fig. 14.2). In most studies 120 kilovolts (kV) are utilized, although a higher (140 kV) or

Fig. 14.2 The voltage of the tube is a determining factor of the radiation dose and image quality. (**a**) Axial CT image with 80 kV–100 mA. (**b**) Axial CT image with 100 kV–100 mA. (**c**) Axial CT image with 120 kV–100 mA. At lower tube voltage an increase in noise can be appreciated, but the visualization of the endoluminal pathology is still possible with a low kV. However, only with iterative reconstruction, a reduction in the image noise and an improvement in image quality is achieved, allowing the use of low tube voltage

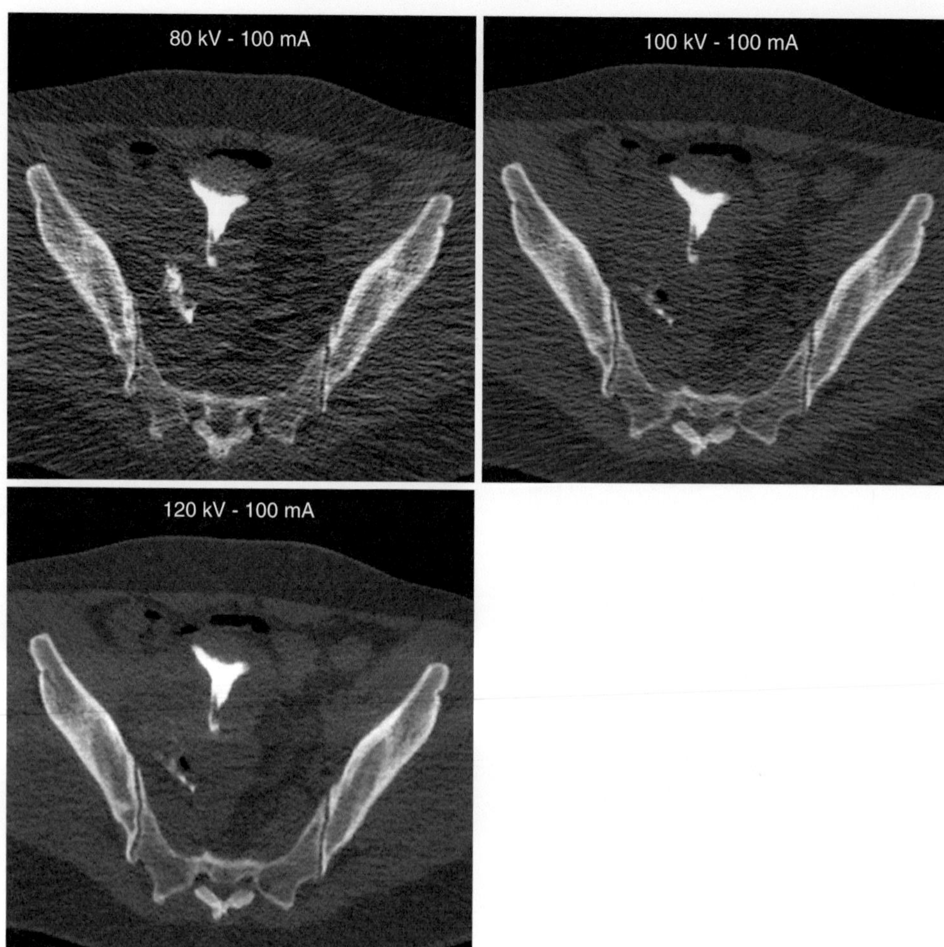

lower (80 or 100 kV) voltage can be useful in specific situations. However, the choice of the tube's voltage has a great impact on the effective dose: in comparison with the standard use of 120 kV, when 140 kV are utilized (for example, on obese patients) an increase of the effective dose by a factor of 1.3–1.6 exists. Furthermore, when choosing 100 kV (for example, on thin patients) a reduction by a factor of 1.5–1.7 is achieved; and when using 80 kV (for example, on pediatric patients) the achieved reduction reaches a factor of 3–4.

Effect of the Radiation on the Quality of the Study

The quality of the virtual hysterosalpingography studies is determined by the noise, the contrast and the definition of the images. The noise depends directly on the quantity of radiation, which in turn, according to the utilized effective mAs and voltage, determines the number of photons generated. Hence a reduction by a factor of 4 in the level of effective mAs doubles the noise in images. In the same way, when the voltage of the tube is reduced and less number of photons are generated which penetrate the tissues with less power due to their diminished energy, the noise increases. However, the negative effect of a noisy image is compensated by an increase of the contrast in the image. When positive contrasts are utilized, the contrast between a lesion and the tissues that surround it depend fundamentally on the utilized voltage. For low voltages, the contrast between structures with a low atomic number (endoluminal lesion) and high atomic number (iodine and barium) increases, balancing partially the increase of noise in the image. For this reason, for a same radiation dose, the reduction of the tube potential provides a better contrast-noise ratio (Fig. 14.3).

The primary objective of the search for an adequate contrast-noise balance is achieving a good image definition for an optimum visualization of the 2D and 3D reconstructions (Fig. 14.4). Besides, so as to obtain high quality images, the spatial resolution must be isotropic, this means that decrement of the image quality does not exist when switching the plane of visualization. With the MSCT units, very thin slices can be obtained, even sub-millimetric, allowing an increase in the spatial resolution. But while the width of the slice is less, the noise in the image increases. This effect is minimized by combination of the slices at the moment of carrying out the image reconstructions, diminishing the noise and increasing the definition.

Lastly, the fact that protocols with low doses may occasionally affect negatively the visualization quality of

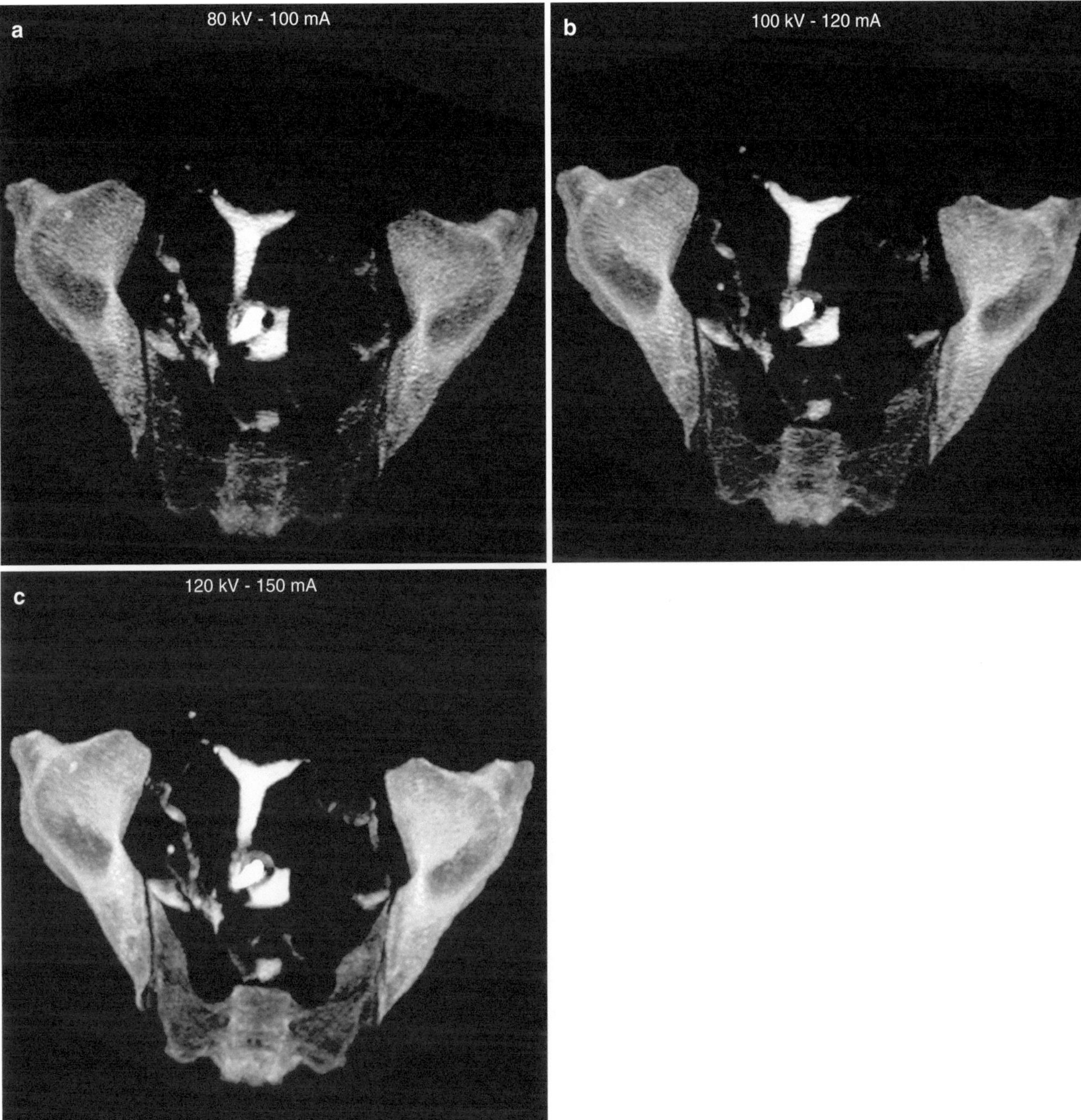

Fig. 14.3 Effect of the technical parameters on the quality of 2D CT images. Axial maximum intensity projection CT images with three different tube voltage and current combinations. (**a**) 80 kV–100 mA; (**b**) 100 kV–120 mA; (**c**) 120 kV–150 mA. The tubal permeability is measurable with the different techniques utilized

extra-gynecologic intra-pelvic organs must be taken into account. Nevertheless, the detection of the pelvic pathology with clinical relevance has not varied significantly when utilizing low doses. The International Commission on Radiological Protection (ICRP), via the ALARA principle (As Low As Reasonably Possible), recommends the establishment of adequate cut points and the modification of acquisition protocols so as to optimize the radiation dose, while maintaining an acceptable image quality in all CT studies [4].

New Strategies and Techniques to Optimize the Radiation Dose

Improvements in Scanner Designs

With the constant technological advance of CT, different applications to minimize the radiation exposition in each exam have been developed. When the multislice units were incorporated, the effective dose was larger in comparison with the scanner of only one row of detectors, due to the

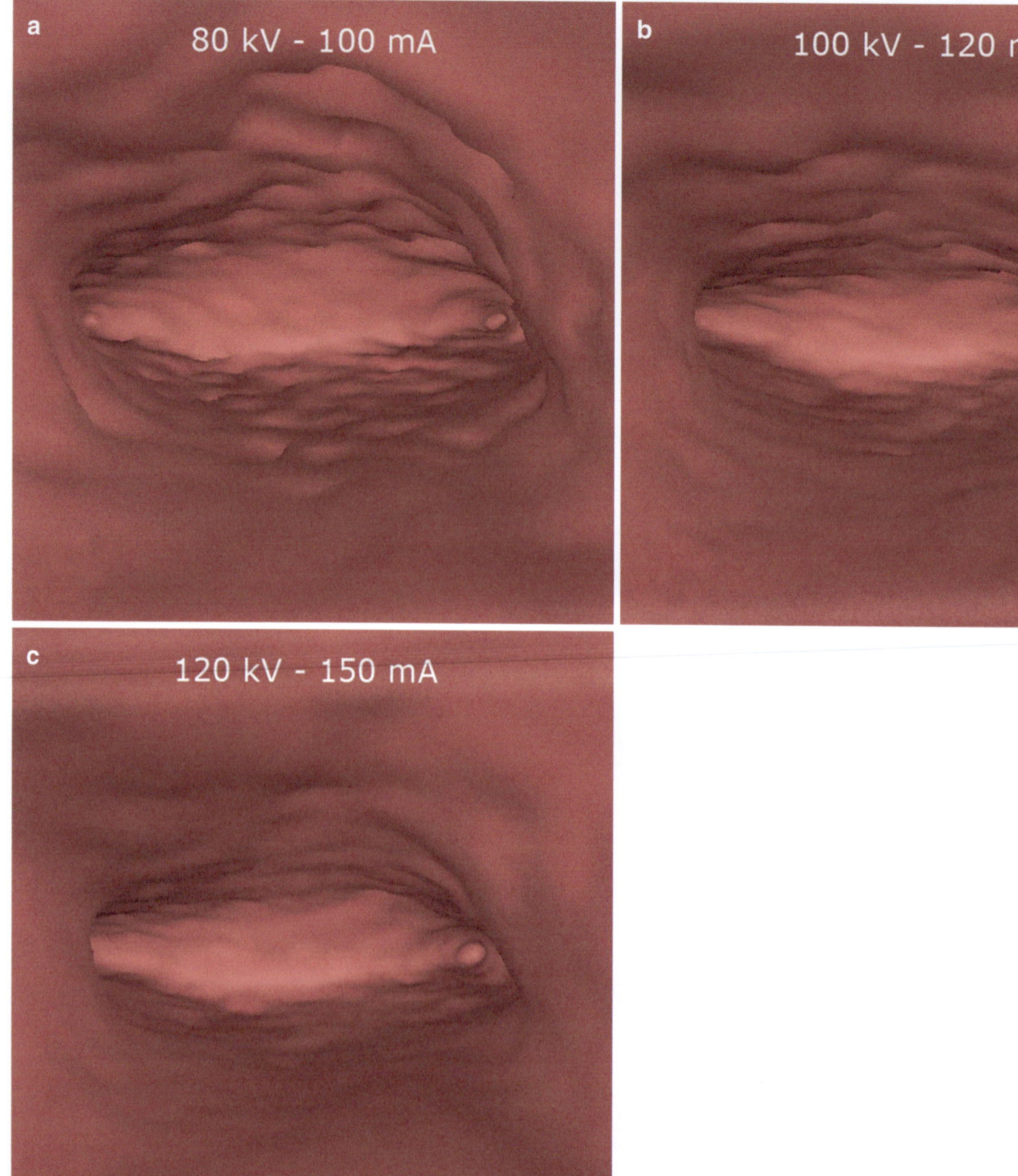

Fig. 14.4 Effect of the technical parameters on the quality of 3D CT images. Virtual endoscopy images of the uterine cavity with three different tube voltage and current combinations. (**a**) 80 kV–100 mA; (**b**) 100 kV–120 mA; (**c**) 120 kV–150 mA. Even thought the image quality is modified, the visibility of the cavity is maintained with the different techniques utilized

penumbra effect. This is generated by the inefficient geometric design of the tube which generates an X rays beam with a certain quantity of photons which fall outside of the active detector rows, mainly in equipment with four rows of detectors [23]. The latter designs of 16, 64 and 256 rows of detectors have minimized the penumbra effect, with the consequent diminishment of radiation (Fig. 14.5). This improvement was achieved with algorithms which allow a follow up of the focal point during the emission of the ray of photons. Furthermore, the increase in the longitudinal coverage by using a more rows of detectors limits the instances where the penumbra falls outside the active rows of detectors.

Another source of inefficiency of the radiation in helical scanner, including the multislice, is the necessity of scanning

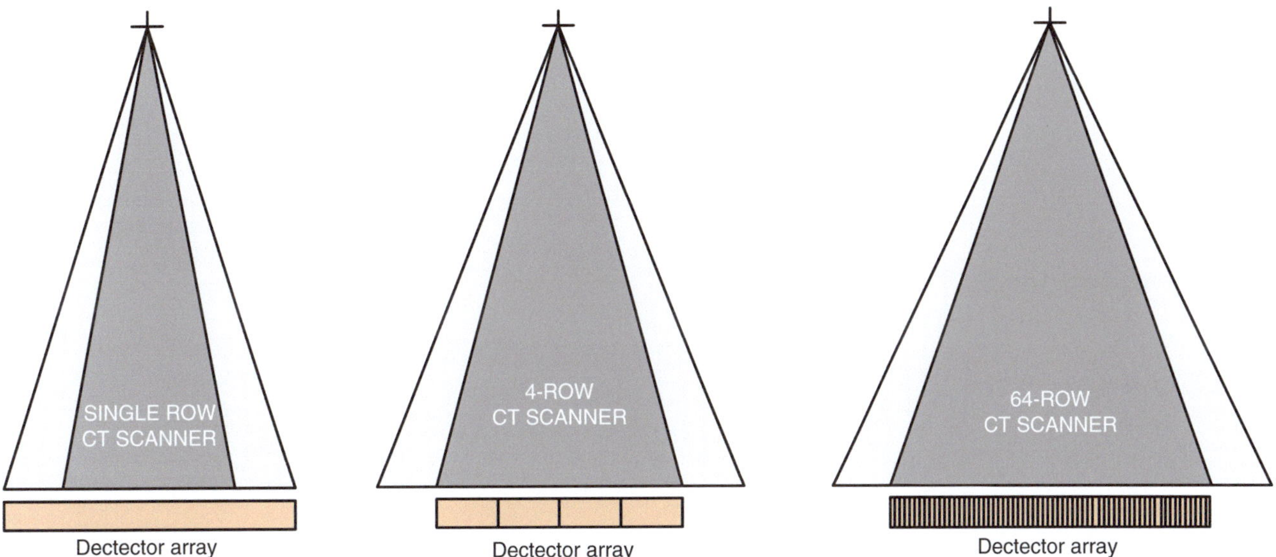

Fig. 14.5 Penumbra effect: in helical units of single detector row, the X-ray beam coincides with the detector coverage. In units with multiple detector rows, certain photons fall outside of the detector coverage (penumbra effect). As the number of detector rows increases, the longitudinal coverage increases and the penumbra effect decreases

the body tissue adjacent to the upper and lower limits of the volume in study, required for the reconstruction of the first and final slices. This effect of over-scanning on the z longitudinal axis increases as the total coverage expands, in other words, as the rows of detectors increase. The recently incorporated multislice units with 256 rows of detectors would produce an increase in the radiation dose via the over-scanning effect, when being utilized helically [24]. Hence, according to the area and type of study being carried out, these units must operate, for the study of small regions, axially which reaches coverage close to 10 cm with only one tube shot.

Tube Modulation

Many researchers have proven the existence of a relationship between the physique of the patient and the noise, and therefore, the quality of the image. As mentioned previously, the simplest strategy to avoid insufficient or excessive doses of radiation is to customize the study protocols and adapt them for each patient in particular. In turn, and so as to achieve a better optimization of the radiation, the unit manufacturers have developed automatic tools which permit the adjustment of the radiation dose in each patient, taking into account mainly the physique [25]. These tools receive the name of tube modulation and consist of two strategies. In one of them the unit calculates the width of the body during the initial scanogram, and with that measurement, estimates automatically the adequate tube current for the patient [11].

This way more exact adjustments are achieved and an average reduction of 25 % of the total radiation. The second modulation strategy takes into account the variations of the body width of the patient on the z longitudinal axis and the resistance to the X rays beam offered by tissues in different areas of the study [26]. This modulation is performed live and simultaneously during the tube rotation; thus, the current decreases in thin areas and relatively "transparent" to the X rays, and increases in areas of great width and where tissues with high resistance to photons exist, for example in the pelvis (Fig. 14.6).

Both modulation techniques carried out jointly manage to accurately adjust and synergistically reduce 40 % of the radiation dose applied on each patient.

Reduction of the Noise by Reprocessing the Raw Data

Regardless of the strategy utilized to decrease the radiation dose, its negative effect is manifested by an increase in the image noise. One way of minimizing a noisy image consists in a reprocessing technique of the raw data, applying an algorithm of raw data softening called iterative which substantially diminishes the noise and increases the quality of images, with the cost of slightly reducing their sharpness [27]. With this technique, study protocols with low radiation doses can be performed without decreasing the quality of the exam (Fig. 14.7).

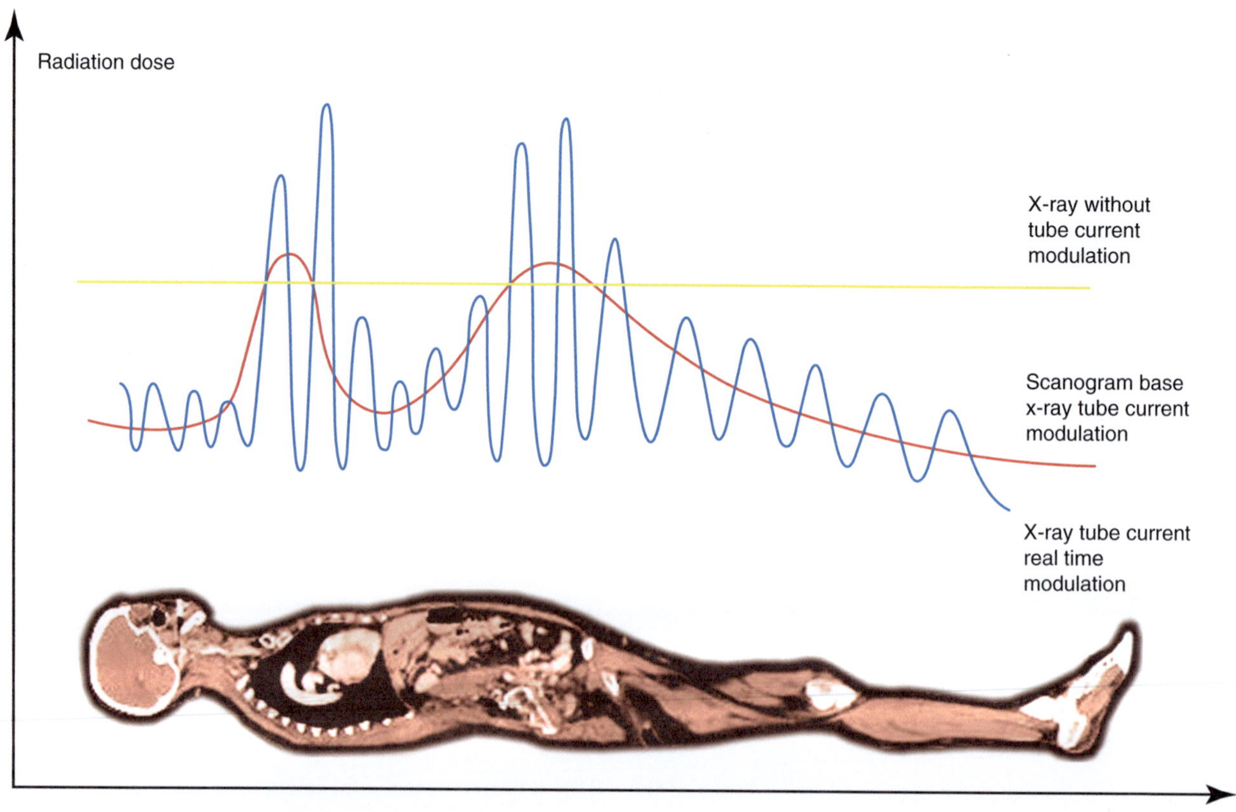

Fig. 14.6 X-ray tube current modulation. The *yellow line* represents a study without tube current modulation and indicates that the employed radiation dose does not modify during the study. The *red line* corresponds to the tube current modulation, automatically calculated by the CT scanner during the scan, determining an adequate dose for the region of study. The *blue line* represents the tube current modulation which is performed in real-time, slice by slice on the longitudinal z axis

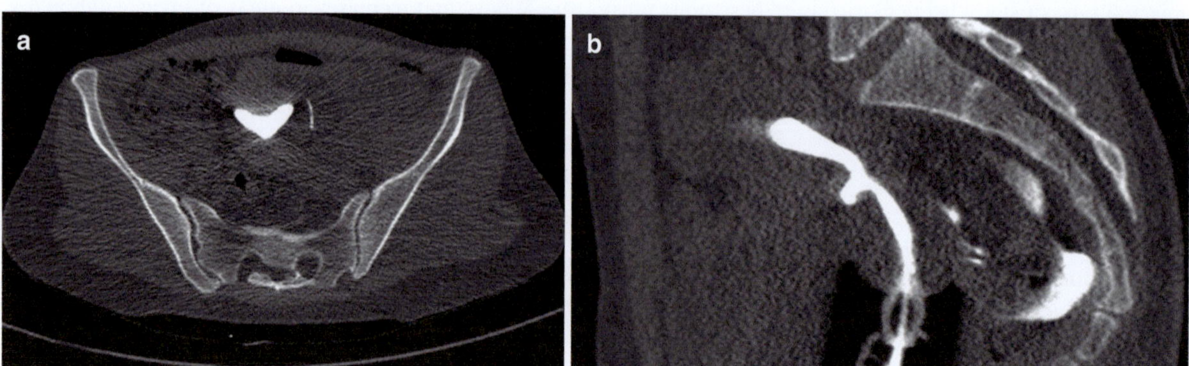

Fig. 14.7 CT raw data reconstruction. Axial CT images, sagittal multiplanar reconstruction images, axial maximum intensity projection images and virtual endoscopy images utilizing a low radiation exposure with 80 kV and 100 mA. On the left column, images are reconstructed with traditional raw data reconstruction algorithm (filtered back projection). Noisier images with less diagnostic quality are visualized. On the right column, images are reconstructed with iterative data reconstruction algorithm. Improvement in the image quality is achieved

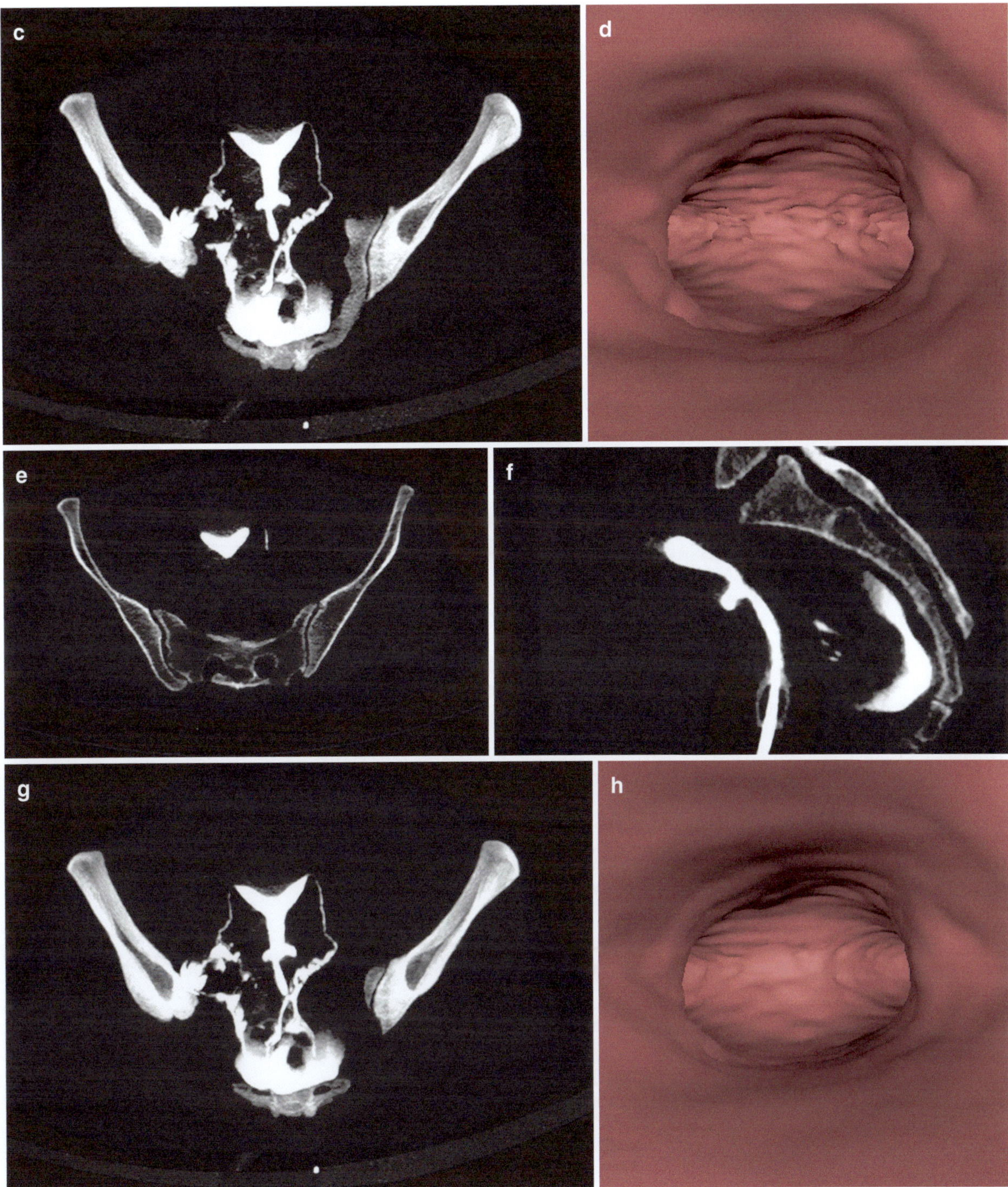

Fig. 14.7 (continued)

Conclusion

The need to reduce the radiation dose in CT studies is due to the possible harmful effects of the X rays on the human body. Even though controversies still exist on the magnitude of the risk associated with radiation, the need to decrease the dose is considered a priority, especially when utilized in screening studies.

When it comes to the decision of perform the virtual hysterosalpingographic study the risk-benefit balance for the patient must be estimated. For the vast majority of exams on infertile patients, the ratio in favor of carrying out the CT is 100:1 or more. A decrease of the radiation dose is also important for the acceptance of the study on behalf of the patient, in order to reduce the fear to radiation exposure.

With the novel tools and techniques which adequate the radiation dose in each study and for each patient and optimization of the effective dose is achieved without significantly affecting the quality of the images.

References

1. Wiest PW, Locken JA, Heintz PH, et al. CT scanning: a major source of radiation exposure. Semin Ultrasound CT MR. 2002;23:402–10.
2. Applegate KE, Amis Jr ES, Schauer DA, et al. Radiation exposure from medical imaging procedures. N Engl J Med. 2009;361:2289–90.
3. Brenner DJ, Hall EJ. Computed tomography: an increasing source of radiation exposure. N Engl J Med. 2007;357:2277–84.
4. National Council on Radiation Protection and Measurements, NCRP Report No. 160, Marzo de 2009.
5. De "White Paper: Initiative to reduce unnecessary radiation exposure from medical imaging". En sitio web: http://www.fda.gov.
6. Preston DL, Ron E, Tokuoka S, et al. Solid cancer incidence in atomic bomb survivors: 1958–1998. Radiat Res. 2007;168:1–64.
7. Shimizu Y, Kodama K, Nishi N, et al. Radiation exposure and circulatory disease risk: Hiroshima and Nagasaki atomic bomb survivor data, 1950–2003. BMJ. 2010;340:b5349.
8. Smith-Bindman R, Lipson J, Marcus R, et al. Radiation dose associated with common computed tomography examinations and the associated lifetime attributable risk of cancer. Arch Intern Med. 2009;169:2078–86.
9. Brenner DJ, Doll R, Goodhead DT, et al. Cancer risks attributable to low doses of ionizing radiation: assessing what we really know. Proc Natl Acad Sci U S A. 2003;100:13761–6.
10. McCollough CH, Bruesewitz MR, Kofler Jr JM. CT dose reduction and dose management tools: overview of available options. Radiographics. 2006;26:503–12.
11. Lee CH, Goo JM, Ye HJ, et al. Radiation dose modulation techniques in the multidetector CT era: from basics to practice1. Radiographics. 2008;28:1451–9.
12. Fernández JM, Vañó E, Guibelalde E. Patient doses in hysterosalpingography. Br J Radiol. 1996;69(824):751–4.
13. Perisinakis K, Damilakis J, Grammatikakis J, et al. Radiogenic risks from hysterosalpingography. Eur Radiol. 2003;13(7):1522–8.
14. Fife IA, Wilson DJ, Lewis CA. Entrance surface and ovarian doses in hysterosalpingography. Br J Radiol. 1994;67(801):860–3.
15. Papaioannou S, Afnan M, Coomarasamy A, et al. Long term safety of fluoroscopically guided selective salpingography and tubal catheterization. Hum Reprod. 2002;17:370–2.
16. Gregan AC, Peach D, McHugo JM. Patient dosimetry in hysterosalpingography: a comparative study. Br J Radiol. 1998;71(850):1058–61.
17. Karande VC, Levrant SG, Pratt DE, et al. What is the radiation exposure to patients during a gynaecoradiologic procedure? Fertil Steril. 1997;67:401–3.
18. Carrascosa P, Capuñay C, Baronio M, et al. 64-Row multidetector CT virtual hysterosalpingography. Abdom Imaging. 2009;34(1):121–33.
19. Carrascosa PM, Capuñay C, Vallejos J, et al. Virtual hysterosalpingography: a new multidetector CT technique for evaluating the female reproductive system. Radiographics. 2010;30(3):661–2; discussion 663.
20. McCollough CH, Zink FE. Performance evaluation of a multi-slice CT system. Med Phys. 1999;26:2223–30.
21. Kalra MK, Maher MM, Toth TL, et al. Strategies for CT radiation dose optimization. Radiology. 2004;230:619–28.
22. Wilting JE, Zwartkruis A, van Leeuwen MS, et al. A rational approach to dose reduction in CT: individualized scan protocols. Eur Radiol. 2001;11:2627–32.
23. Kulama E. Scanning protocols for multislice CT scanners. Br J Radiol. 2004;77:S2–9.
24. Mori S, Endo M, Obata T, et al. Properties of the prototype 256-row (cone beam) CT scanner. Eur Radiol. 2006;16:2100–8.
25. Kalra MK, Maher MM, Toth TL, et al. Techniques and applications of automatic tube current modulation for CT. Radiology. 2004;233:649–57.
26. Kalra MK, Maher MM, Toth TL, et al. Comparison of z-axis automatic tube current modulation technique with fixed tube current CT scanning of abdomen and pelvis. Radiology. 2004;232:347–53.
27. La Rivière PJ. Penalized-likelihood sinogram smoothing for low-dose CT. Med Phys. 2005;32:1676–83.

Virtual Hysterosalpingography (VHSG) is a new non-invasive technique that evolved from our group's prior experience with virtual colonoscopy studies [1]; as stated in prior publications [2], it allows us to evaluate the entire gynecologic tract in a single study, including the cervix, uterus [3] and fallopian tubes [4].

Infertile patients, unable to achieve conception after 12 months of unprotected intercourse, could benefit from VHSG, as many of the causes of infertility will be tested in great detail, as we will show in the present chapter. The causes of infertility are due to female causes in 40 % of the cases, male factor in 30 % and shared causes in 15 %; unexplained infertility is found in 15 %, and is encountered when a full evaluation of the infertile couple fails to identify abnormal studies. Table 15.1, shows the list of the most common factors involved in female infertility.

The diagnostic studies play an important role in the definition and diagnosis of the multiple causes of infertility, and as such, help us decide on the best therapeutic management, according to the type of pathology encountered [5, 6]. Focusing on the female factors, the diagnostic tests ought to determine whether the fallopian tubes are abnormal, as if they were, the transport of gametes and embryos will be compromised; also, the pathology of the uterus itself, inside the cavity as well as on the uterine wall, may be responsible for the patient's inability to get pregnant.

At present, the imaging studies that are most commonly performed in the infertile female patient, are the vaginal ultrasound and the conventional hysterosalpingography (HSG). Other studies, like MRI, are used to help or confirm

Table 15.1 Female causes of infertility

Tuboperitoneal factor	30 %
Ovulation problems	40 %
Cervical factor	10 %
Luteal phase disorders	5 %
Uterine factor	5 %
Idiopathic factors	10 %

the data initially obtained in patients with suspected endometriosis, adenomyosis, myomas or uterine malformations; also, performing a diagnostic in-office hysteroscopy may help in completing the evaluation.

Virtual hysterosalpingography (VHSG) gives similar information to the conventional HSG, but with far greater anatomic details and diagnostic precision, furthermore, it offers similar information to the MRI in cases of uterine malformations [7–10]. It is clear that this new diagnostic technique requires a learning curve for its interpretation, not only for the radiologist but also for the gynecologist, that is managing and referring the patient for the study.

That is why in our opinion, the study of the female reproductive tract ideally should have a high degree of spatial resolution, and also should be able to identify very small to large lesions, provide accurate information on their location, and to better help the gynecologist determine their clinical significance and best therapeutic approach; also, the study should be safe and free of major complications, as well as accessible to the majority of the infertile patients that need the study.

Which Diagnostic Procedures Are Best for the Infertile Female Patient?

The tubo-peritoneal factor is recognized as one of the main causes of infertility, existing in some cases with an associated uterine component. That is why the infertile female patient requires a complete evaluation of the reproductive tract, in search of accurate information about the cervix, uterus, fallopian tubes and ovaries, to detect the full spectrum of pathological processes that may be present. The conventional HSG does not provide information about the ovaries, while the VHSG gives only limited information. Both modalities offer valuable information on the cervix, uterine cavity and patency of the fallopian tubes; yet VHSG has the advantage of a better spatial resolution and the capability to accurately diagnose smaller size lesions. Also, while ultrasound and MRI evaluate

P. Carrascosa et al., *CT Virtual Hysterosalpingography*,
DOI 10.1007/978-3-319-07560-0_15, © Springer International Publishing Switzerland 2014

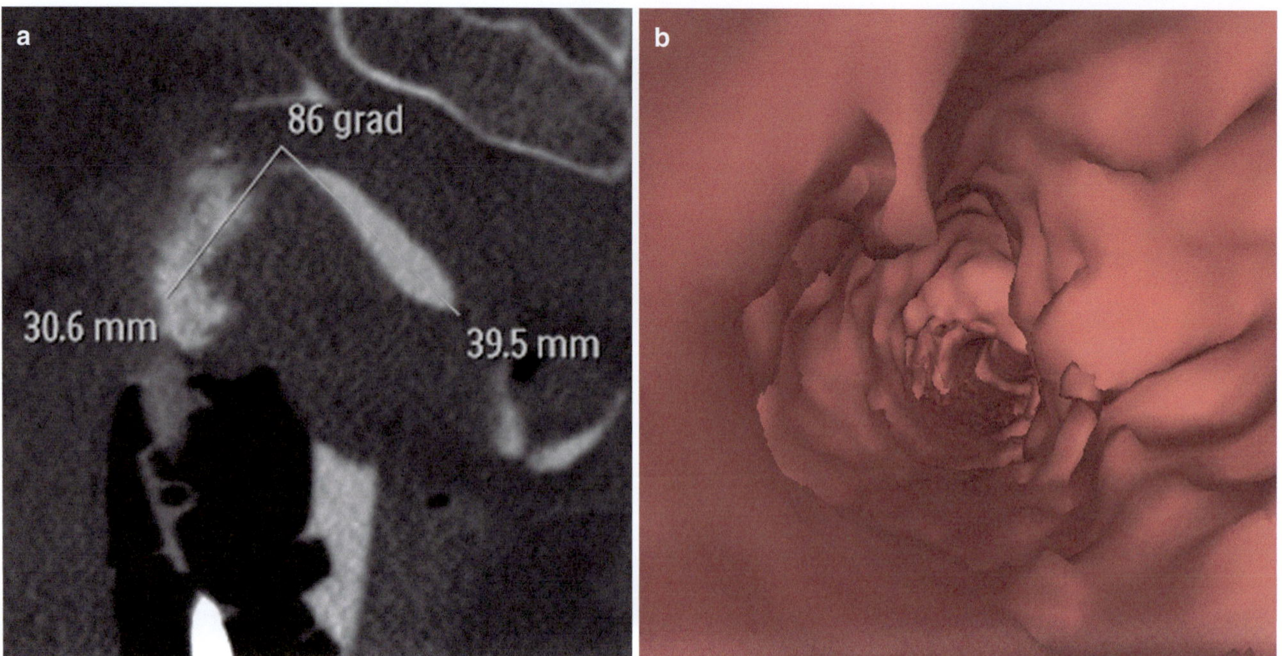

Fig. 15.1 VHSG study. Evaluation of the cervical canal. (**a**) Sagittal maximum intensity projection image whit measurement of the cervical angle. (**b**) Virtual endoscopy image with assessment of cervical folds

the uterus and ovaries with great diagnostic accuracy, they offer limited information on the fallopian tubes; so in summary, all these diagnostic modalities to a degree complement each other, in order to provide a full structural information on the female reproductive tract and the pathological processes that may be present, as well as to disclose their clinical significance, but is our opinion that VHSG stands out as one of the most comprehensive and cost effective techniques available today for the evaluation of the female reproductive tract.

Contributions (Advantages?) of Virtual Hysterosalpingography

VHSG is a new imaging diagnostic technique, performed through a volumetric acquisition by CT multi-slice of the pelvic region, after the instillation of contrast into the uterine cavity. The procedure is of short duration and very well tolerated by patients; as a matter of fact those patients that have gone through a conventional HSG before, provide input of having significantly less discomfort after having a VHSG.

This is probably due to the fact that there is no instrumentation of the cervix (traction of the cervix with a tenaculum), also, that the completion of the study takes only a few seconds, significantly shortening the patient-portion of the study and the possible discomfort that comes along with it. The reconstruction of the images post-study (raw data) is known

as advanced interactive reconstruction, obtaining images of excellent diagnostic quality, with the advantage of exposing the patient to a very low level of radiation in an average study (0.3–0.6 mSv).

Among the important contributions by this diagnostic method is worth mentioning the evaluation of the cervical canal, providing information of great value to the REI physician, in relation to the shape and trajectory of the canal (direction and angulation), and offering valuable information about the possible difficulties they may find at the time of performing an intrauterine insemination or an embryo transfer. VHSG, also has the capacity to provide endoscopic virtual images of the cervical canal and uterine cavity, similar to those obtained during a diagnostic hysteroscopy. Intracavitary myomas, uterine polyps, uterine congenital malformations are all well identified and characterized by VHSG as shown in Figs. 15.1, 15.2, 15.3, 15.4, 15.5 and 15.6. The type of uterine malformation present, the degree of intracavitary invasion by a submucous myoma, the size of a polyp, as well as its pedicle attachment, are all factors that allow the gynecologist to better prepare and determine the best surgical approach to use in each individual patient.

The evaluation of the fallopian tubes is also greatly benefited by performing a VHSG, since not only determines the morphology and patency of the tubes, but also the presence or absence of intraluminal pathology, like polyps or intratubal

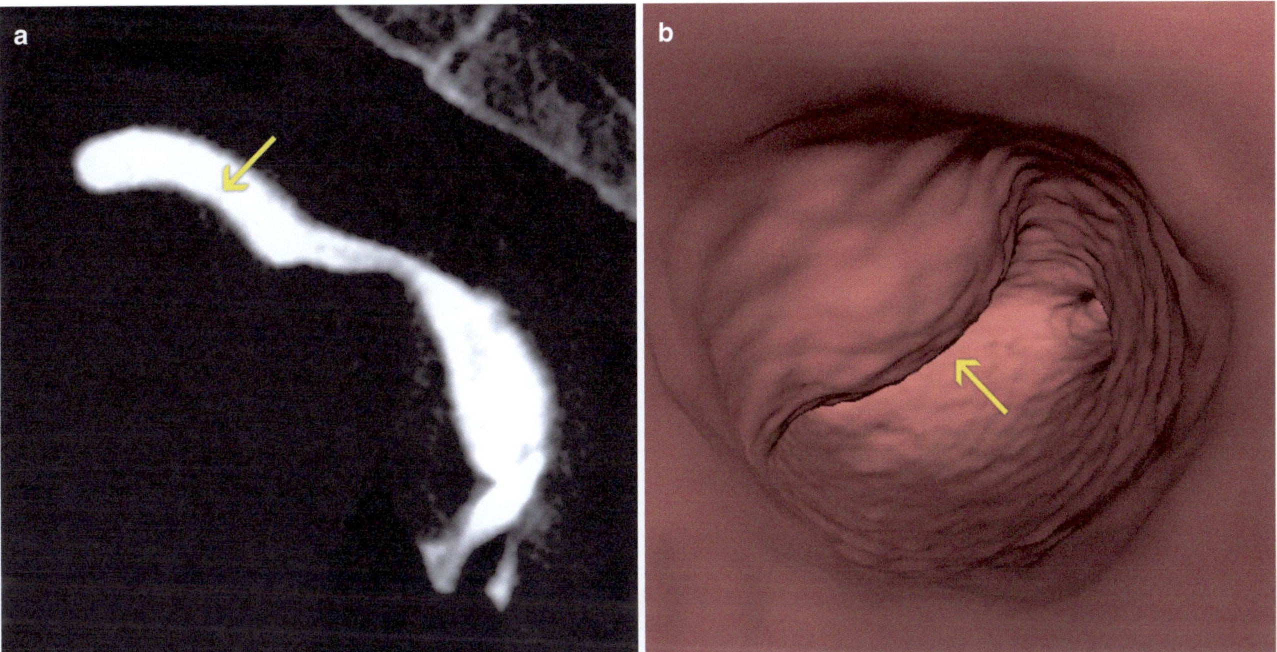

Fig. 15.2 VHSG study. Submucous myoma on the anterior uterine wall (*arrows*). (**a**) Sagittal maximum intensity projection image. (**b**) Virtual endoscopy image

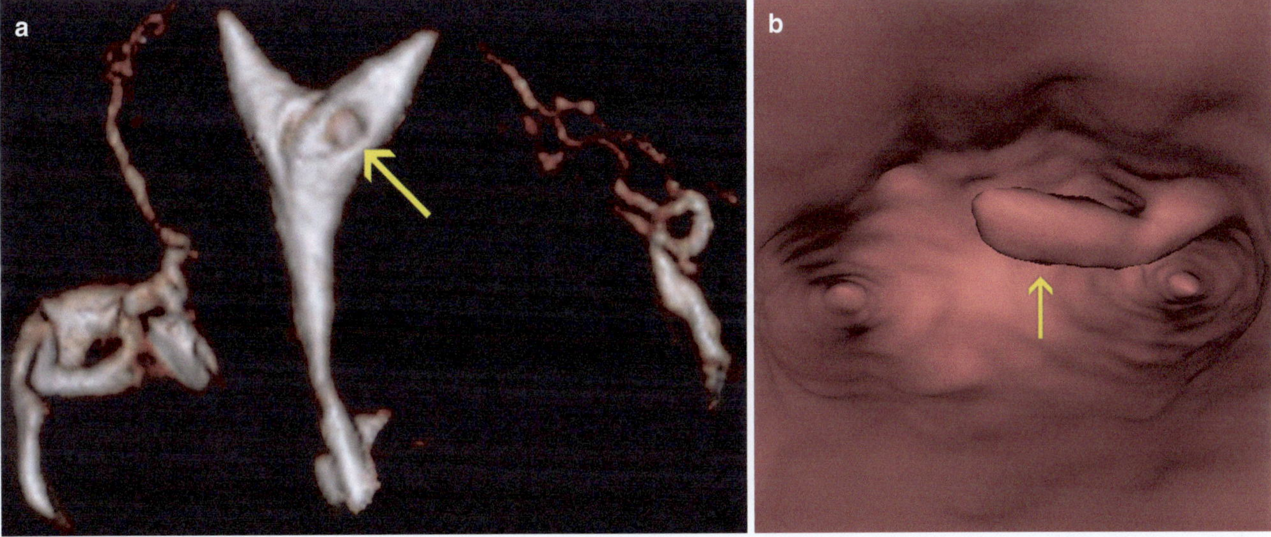

Fig. 15.3 VHSG study. Endometrial polyp on the posterior uterine wall (*arrows*). (**a**) 3D volume rendering image, left posterior-lateral view. (**b**) Virtual endoscopy image

adhesions. In cases of hydrosalpinges, one can obtain endoscopic views, impossible to produce with other non invasive diagnostic modalities.

Table 15.2 shows the main advantages of VHSG, in comparison to other conventional diagnostic imaging studies. Among the most significant advantages one can quote the lesser discomfort, less radiation and shorter time of the procedure; also, from a diagnostic viewpoint is worth mentioning the virtual endoscopic evaluation of the cervical canal, uterine cavity and fallopian tubes, as well as the assessment of the outer contour of the uterine wall.

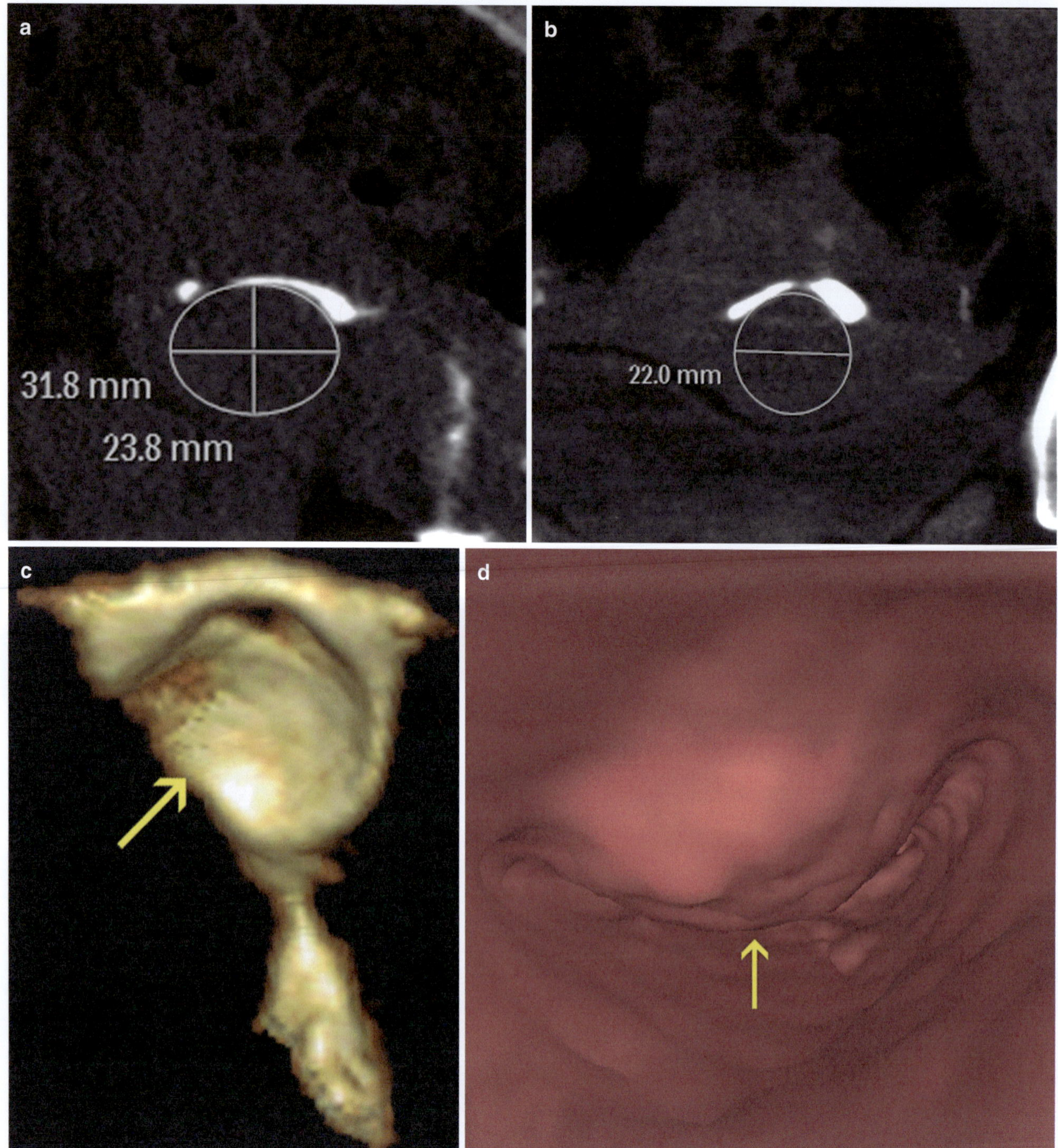

Fig. 15.4 VHSG study. Assessment of submucous myoma on the anterior uterine wall (*arrows*). (**a**) Sagittal maximum intensity projection (MIP) image. (**b**) Coronal MIP image. (**c**) Coronal 3D volume rendering image, anterior view. (**d**) Virtual endoscopy image

Fig. 15.5 VHSG study. Partial septate uterus. (**a**) 10-mm coronal multiplanar reconstruction image. (**b**) Coronal maximum intensity projection (MIP) image. (**c**) Coronal 3D volume rendering image. (**d**) Virtual endoscopy image. (**e**) Coronal MIP image after the removal of the uterine septum. (**f**) Post-treatment virtual endoscopy image

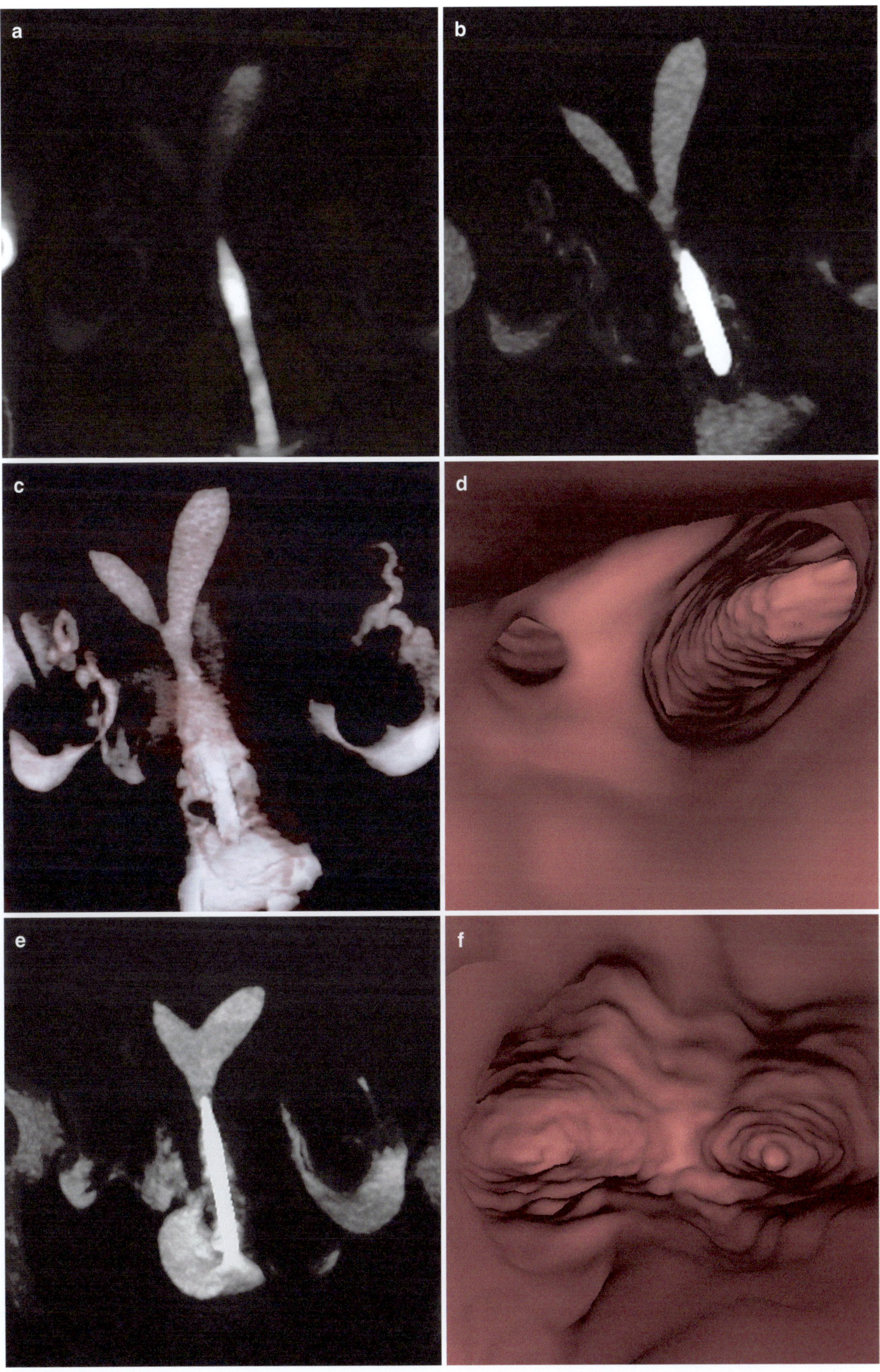

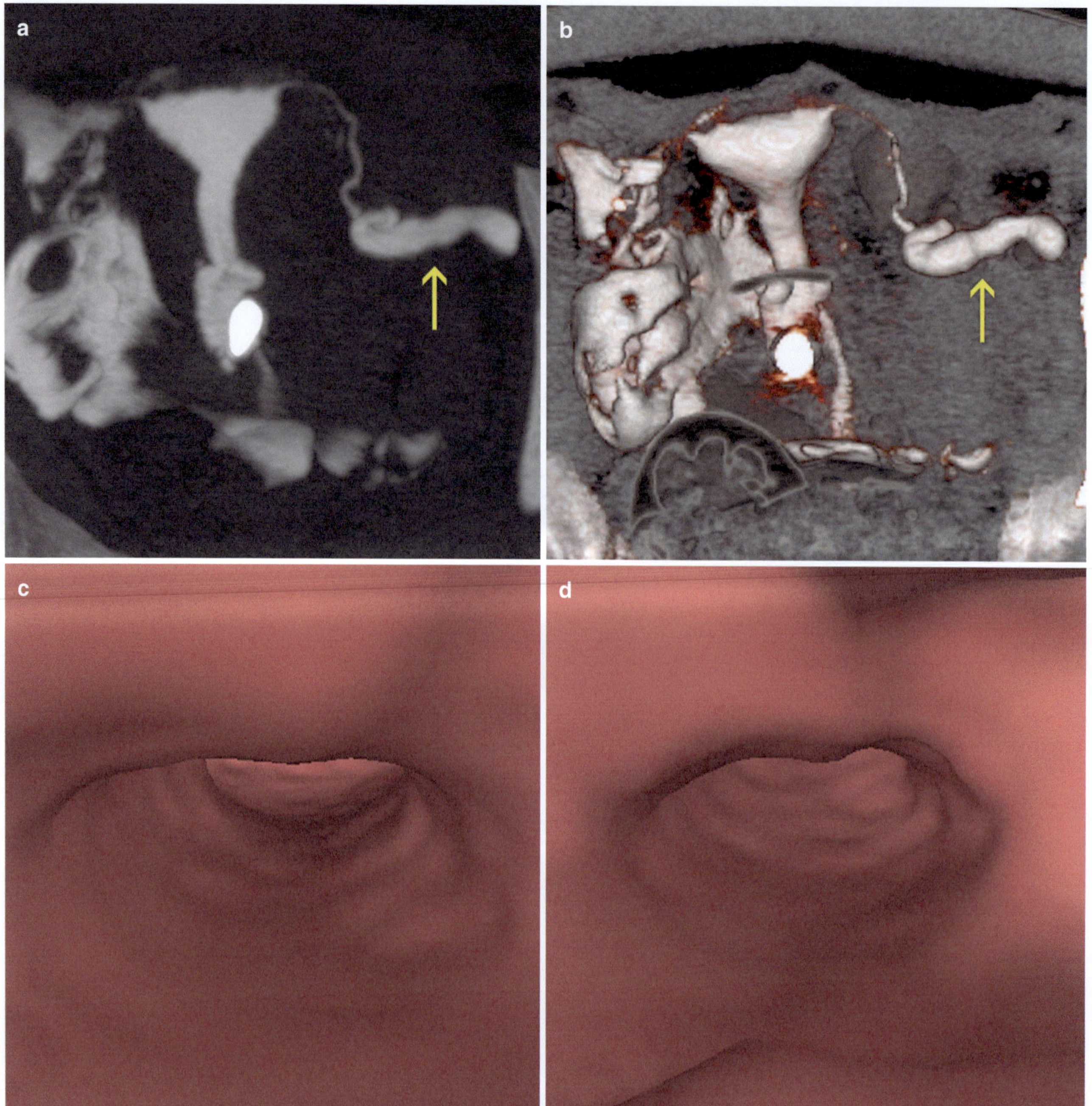

Fig. 15.6 VHSG study. Assessment of the uterine tubes. Dilatation of the left uterine tube (*arrows*). (**a**) Coronal maximum intensity projection image. (**b**) Coronal 3D volume rendering image. (**c, d**) Virtual endoscopy images

Table 15.2 Main advantages of virtual hysterosalpingography

Advantages for the patient
Less discomfort
Less complications
Less radiation dose
Less study duration
Advantages for the diagnosis
Cervical canal evaluation
Endoscopic evaluation of the uterine cavity and cervical canal
Endoluminal evaluation of the fallopian tubes
Uterine contour evaluation

Conclusions

The role of the imaging studies in the evaluation of the infertile female are significant, and contribute greatly to the diagnostic and therapeutic steps involved in the process; VHSG, as shown by our large experience with this procedure, has the ability to integrate most of the advantages of the diagnostic methods mentioned previously, becoming a valuable tool for the gynecologist in the evaluation and treatment of the infertile female. Whether it should completely replace the use of standard conventional HSG among infertile females, or be used as a back up to HSG, and indicated only when questionable or abnormal findings are encountered, is something that should be determined after clinicians gain significant experience with VHSG and consider all the pros and cons of each procedure.

The cost benefit ratio, which varies from country to country, is an important variable that should be determined on an individual basis; yet overall we are confident that VHSG has a bright future given its many diagnostic advantages.

References

1. Lobo RA. Infertility: etiology, diagnostic evaluation, management, prognosis. In: Katz VL, Lentz GM, Lobo RA, Gershenson DM, editors. Comprehensive gynecology. 5th ed. Philadelphia: Mosby Elsevier; 2007. cap.41.
2. Jose-Miller AB, Boyden JW, Frey KA. Infertility. Am Fam Physician. 2007;75(6):856–94.
3. Rebar RW, Erickson GF. Reproductive endocrinology and infertility. In: Goldman L, Ausiello D, editors. Cecil medicine. 24th ed. Philadelphia: Saunders Elsevier; 2011. cap.244.
4. Speroff L, Fitz M, editors. Clinical gynecologic endocrinology and infertility. 7th ed. Philadelphia: Lippincott Williams & Wilkins; 2005.
5. Trantham P. The infertile couple. Am Fam Physician. 1996;54(3): 1001–10.
6. De Sutter P. Rational diagnosis and treatment in infertility. Best Pract Res Clin Obstet Gynaecol. 2006;20(5):647–64.
7. Carrascosa P, Capuñay C, Baronio M, et al. 64-Row multidetector CT virtual hysterosalpingography. Abdom Imaging. 2009;34: 121–133.37.
8. Baronio M, Carrascosa P, Capuñay C, et al. Diagnostic performance of CT virtual hysteroscopy in 69 consecutive patients. Fertil Steril. 2010;94(Suppl):S77.
9. Carrascosa P, Capuñay C, Vallejos J, et al. Virtual hysterosalpingography: a new multidetector CT technique for evaluating the female reproductive system. Radiographics. 2010;30:643–61.
10. Carrascosa P, Capuñay C, Vallejos J, et al. Virtual hysterosalpingography: experience with over 1000 consecutive patients. Abdom Imaging. 2011;36(1):1–14.

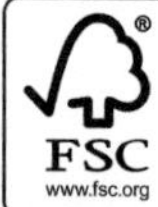